NUTRITION AND DIET RESEARCH PROGRESS

NUTRITIONAL INSIGHTS AND FOOD SAFETY

NUTRITION AND DIET RESEARCH PROGRESS

Additional books in this series can be found on Nova's website under the Series tab.

Additional E-books in this series can be found on Nova's website under the E-books tab.

PUBLIC HEALTH IN THE 21ST CENTURY

Additional books in this series can be found on Nova's website under the Series tab.

Additional E-books in this series can be found on Nova's website under the E-books tab.

NUTRITION AND DIET RESEARCH PROGRESS

NUTRITIONAL INSIGHTS AND FOOD SAFETY

JAROSLAVA ŠVARC-GAJIÆ
EDITOR

Nova Science Publishers, Inc.
New York

Library of Congress Cataloging-in-Publication Data

Nutritional insights and food safety / editor, Jaroslava
Svarc-Gajiæ
p. cm.
Includes bibliographical references and index.
ISBN 978-1-61122-130-5 (hardcover)
1. Food adulteration and inspection. 2. Food--Safety measures. I.
Svarc-Gajiæ, Jaroslava.
TX531.N88 2010
363.19'264--dc22
2010049153

Published by Nova Science Publishers, Inc. † New York

Contents

Preface

The nutritional value of the food is one of its most significant features. Even though the exact definition of this term is difficult to present, the term "nutritional value" usually denotes the content of building and functional elements in food necessary for human`s normal grow and development. This includes macroconstituents such as proteins, lipids and carbohydrates which provide both energy and constitutional (building) units. Vitamines and microelements from food support the function of bodily enzymes and enable complex biochemical processes to undergo in humans body. Many other substances naturally present in food fall into diverse chemical categories and exhibit different physiological effects in humans.

Balanced and healthy diet is prerequisite for a good health and wellbeing. To humans, balanced diet represents the source of energy, building and functional elements, as well as a pleasure. Dietary natural or introduced components can contribute in high extent to the development of certain diseases, such as in the case of carcinogenesis and cardiovascular illness, or may postpone or counteract their development in individuals' with high genetic susceptibility to certain disease. Nowdays, when environment has become severely contaminated with anthropogenic pollutants and when human awareness about physiological effects of natural food components has reached high level grace to science development, healthy nutrition has became a luxury. Several past decades are marked with intense promotion of organic food. Unfortunately due to its high price not everyone can afford its benefits and enjoy in safe and contaminants-free food.

The relationship food-health is so strongly stressed in scientific communities and in all media accessible to wider population, that many consumers put healthy food ahead of a foods palatability neglecting the hedonistic elements of nourishment. Some individuals, thus, choose to use the food predominantly as a mean of sustaining a good health and follow the principle defined by Socrates (469 BC–399 BC) " The pleasure of eating should not be the purpose of mans life; eating serves only to support the life". Seeking a food which would provide the most nutrients, fibers, minerals or vitamins, and at the same time avoiding the "unhealthy" food, these individuals are often exposed to health threats, because the potential risk is not anticipated, usually due to the lack of information's or knowledge. Uniform diet and diet predominantly relying on a particular food sources, usually of plant origin, may overexpose the consumer with the components which in balanced diet normally do not pose a risk, but in cases of monotonous diet may bring the concentration of potentially dangerous components to alerting level. Besides the risk of adverse health influence by food due to overconsumption of natural latent toxins and saturation of the organism by naturally-occurring latent threats, excessive specific food might compromise the health when it is contaminated.

Food essentiality and its beneficial effects on human health and life are unquestionable, however unpleasant food experience might arise when individual experiences food poisoning, most often resulting from microbial and other toxins, generated by food spoilage, inadequate food processing or storage. These factors can cause acute food poisoning, whereas chronic food poisoning arises when habitually consuming food containing some dangerous naturally occurring components (selenium in food from regions with seleniferous soil, lathyrogens in diet relying on leguminose, mycotoxins etc.), or when great portion of the prolonged diet is composed of food contaminated with anthropogenic pollutants. Anthropogenic pollutants, such as pesticides, polychlorinated biphenyl's, dioxins or heavy metals, are particularly dangerous since they are not efficiently biodegraded, and are also the subject of biomagnification in food chain, exposing humans to their high levels and residing in humans' body for a long time.

Besides organic food contaminants originating from industrial sources, dangerous organic compounds can also be formed during food processing in the course of cooking, frying or roasting. The products of Maillard reaction, heterocyclic amines, furans and polycyclic aromatic hydrocarbons are examples of such compounds. Other organic food contaminants result from microbiological processes normally undergoing during technological process or food storage. Yeast activity, for example, is responsible for increased levels of carbamates in alcoholic beverages and some fermented foods. Carbamates have attracted the attention of food specialists and analytical chemists due to their recognized genotoxicity. They are formed in reaction of microbially produced alcohol and urea which is produced by aminoacids metabolism. Histamine and other bioactive amines are produced by bacterial action in food and may cause very unpleasant experience mimicking food intolerance or severe allergic reactions.

Providing valuable nutrients to humans, plants also naturally produce components which play a certain protective role in them, but may act as toxins to humans exploiting different mechanisms. Some of these substances are natural defense mechanisms of plants created to protect them from pests and animals, thus, acting as natural pesticides or repellents. Majority of plant substances toxic to humans are plant secondary metabolites. Furthermore the plants are able to produce hormone-like substances acting as goitrogens (substances that suppress the function of the thyroid gland) and estrogens, or inhibiting some bodily enzymes (cholinesterase inhibitors e.g. physostigmin, solanine, chaconine). Many chemically diverse plant secondary metabolites cause severe symptoms by exhibiting very potent neurotoxicity by disturbing the transmittion of neural impulses.

Seafood may be an important source of naturally occurring toxins. Many marine organisms are able to produce venoms originally intendent to protect them from predators. These substances are normally very toxic to humans too. One of the most potent neurotoxins is tetrodotoxin produced by more than 90 species of pufferfish which are considered a delicacy in certain cuisines due to tingling sensation that they produce during their consumption. The fish are edible because the toxin is mostly concentrated in specific organs, such as ovaries, skin, liver, intestines and roe. Even after removal of fish organs containing the toxin, every meal of a puffer fish carries certain risk of poisoning. Ciguatoxin, a cholinesterase inhibitor, is produced by more than 300 fish species. The risk of poisoning by ciguatoxin can not completely be eliminated by avoiding toxin-producing species, since the toxin finds its way to many other marine species feeding on dinoflagellates which also produce the toxin. The fact that ciguatoxin can be found in numerous marine species makes the risk of ciguatoxin poisoning unpredictable. Similarly, saxitoxin poisoning arises due to accumulation of the toxin originally produced by dinoflagellates in clams, mussels and other shellfish.

Foodborne diseases caused by microorganisms can be related to either direct infection involving the pathogen itself, or may involve only the toxins or metabolites produced by pathogens. Direct food poisoning occurs when the food infected by microorganism is consumed. The symptoms of poisoning arise due to subsequently produced toxins. Indirect contamination occurs when toxic metabolites are passed to humans through animal-derived food. Typical example is the transmittion of aflatoxin metabolites by milk of livestock feeding on contaminated feed. Besides mycotoxin metabolites, milk may contain pesticide residues, veterinary drug residues and can concentrate certain heavy metals resembling calcium, e.g. lead. Since xenobiotics like veterinary drugs and pesticides are mostly metabolized in liver and are mostly excreted by kidneys, these edible animal organs, often considered a delicacy, are likely to contain the highest levels of these compounds.

The use of food additives has become a common practice in food industry and has enabled to preserve the food, to prolong the shelf-life and to improve its nutritional and sensory properties. Major classes of food additives include nutrients, preservatives, colorants, sweeteners, antioxidants and flavor ingredients. In order to be approved by FDA (Food and Drug Administration) all food additives follow very strict process of safety evaluation. Nevertheless many questions related to their impact on human health remain open. Some of concerns related to the presence of additives in food are due to food intolerance that has frequently been linked to consumption of specific food rich in additives, others are related to their safety in long-term consumption. When discussing safety concerns linked to food additives, consumers ought to be informed that food additives are not only synthetically produced substances, and that large group of food additives includes many natural compounds, such as vitamins, natural pigments and organic acids. In this respect it should be mentioned that not every "E" on food packaging should be considered as synthetic and dangerous.

Food and beverages can be chemically very aggressive and might interact with the materials they are in contact with. This includes the contact with food packaging materials, as well as food preparation surfaces and cooking utensils. In contact with food, packaging materials may release certain components which may compromise the food safety and quality. Migrating substances may impair the color and odor of the food and may negatively influence affectability in consumers. Most frequently used packaging materials include plastics, paper, glass and metal alloys. The release of metals from glass and metal packaging into food is highly influenced by the food acidity and composition. The food with high fat content which is packed in plastics, is likely to "extract" the plasticizers, used in plastic production, as well as transformation products formed during manufacturing of plastic, such as the compounds formed by decomposition and recombination of catalysts and initiators of polymerization. There is also a possibility of migration of oligomeric products that may be formed from reactive monomers during plastic production. Toxic printing inks and adhesives are not intended to come into contact with the food but can also contaminate it under certain circumstances.

In addition to listed potential dietary threats, the food safety also strongly depends on the possibility of food allergic reactions and food intolerance. Past century is marked with increasing incidence of food allergies. The response to specific food is difficult to predict in susceptible individuals, since there is a great number of different types of abnormal responses to specific food and offending ingredients can be present in distinct food products. Some of the types of food intolerance have an immunological background, while others arise by unelucidated mechanisms making them very difficult to predict. The use of genetically modified organisms in food production further spreads the occurrence of potential allergens increasing the health risk.

The given exhaustive overview of potential dietary health risks stresses the fact that the term "safe food" includes many different aspects, some of which are covered by this book. As much as the elaborated topics by this book seem broad, the material presents only limited aspects of food safety. More exhaustive approach would include some other nutritional, medical, biochemical and social aspects, often controversial. The main intention of this book is to demonstrate that the principle of golden mean is applicable in nutrition and that only balanced diet equilibrates dietary benefits and potential dietary risks. The book presents the scientific facts and evidences related to nutrition that will help the readership to create its own picture and attitude about the food safety, since the essence of the food safety can not be discussed excluding the philosophical approach. The book also demonstrates that food has changed in past millennium, it has adjusted itself to the needs and requirements of a modern man. By presenting traditional and modern concepts of food safety, this book helps the readership to make their own choices concerning nutritional and dietary habits.

Jaroslava Švarc-Gajiæ

In: Nutritional Insights and Food Safety
Editor: Jaroslava Švarc-Gajiæ

ISBN: 978-1-61122-130-5

Chapter I

Antinutrients in Food

Anamarija Mandić, Marijana Sakač and Aleksandra Mišan
Institute for Food Technology – FINS; Bulevar cara Lazara 1; 21 000 Novi Sad; Serbia

Abstract

Antinutrients in food, usually of plant origin, have long been recognized as undesirable chemicals which evolved as a part of their chemical defence against various insects, pests and humans. Regarding the vast literature on this topic, and the incoming information pointing out their beneficial effects to human health, the authors of this chapter have set themselves an ambitious task to discuss the information, sometimes even controversial, on their biological activity.

Antinutrients with beneficial effects include, among many other phytochemicals, polyphenols, tannins, phytic acid, saponins and phytosterols. Better understanding of the chemistry and biochemistry of phytochemicals, supported by new analytical tools may leed to a serious re-evaluation of their dietary importance. Thus, we found it challenging to make a critical review on analytical techniques most frequently used for their determination and to emphasize the major problems involved in their application.

Introduction

Antinutrients are natural or synthetic compounds that interfere with the absorption of nutrients, in the way to reduce their bioavailability and intake from food (Osagie, 1998). Antinutrients in food have long been recognized as undesirable chemicals, usually of plant origin, which evolved as a part of their chemical defence against various insects, pests and humans. The presence of antinutrients and toxins plays a great role in limiting the wider use of many plants. Apart from antinutient properties, same compounds exert beneficial effects, such as antioxidant activity (Ćetković et al., 2008, Čanadanović-Brunet et al., 2006), antimicrobial and (Čanadanović-Brunet et al., 2009) antiproliferative activities (Čanadanović-Brunet et al., 2008).

Due to the high diversity of compounds possessing anti-nutritional properties, it is difficult to make a classification which would encompass all the known groups of antinutrients. The classification of antinutrients is usually made on the basis of their chemical structure, function or their biosynthetic origin.

According to Soetan and Oyewole (2009), all antinutritional compounds may be divided into two major categories:

- Proteins (such as lectins and protease inhibitors) which are sensitive to normal processing temperatures, and
- Other substances which are stable or resistant to these temperatures. Examples of these natural compounds of plant origin are saponins, flavonoids, alkaloids, tannins, oxalates, non-protein amino acids and galactomannan gums.

Referring to Aletor (1993), the most significant antinutrients in plants used for human foods and animal feeds are: (i) Enzyme inhibitors (trypsin and chymotrypsin inhibitors, plasmin inhibitors, elastase inhibitors), (ii) Lectins (concanavalin A, ricin), (iii) Plant enzymes (urease, lipoxygenase), (iv) Cyanogenic glycosides (phaseolunatin, dhurrin, linamarin, lutaustralin), (v) Goitrogens (pro-goitrins and glucosinolates), (vi) Oestrogens (flavones and genistein), (vii) Saponins (soya sapogenin), (viii) Gossypol from Gossypium species e.g. cotton, (ix) Tannins (condensed and hydrolysable tannins), (x) Amino acid analogues (BOAA, DAP, mimosine, N-methyl-1-alanine), (xi) Alkaloids (solanine and chaconine), (xii) Anti-metals (phytates and oxalates), (xiii) Anti-vitamins (anti-vitamins A, D, E and B12) and (xiv) Favism factors.

Regarding the vast literature on the topic of antinutrients and their extreme diversity, only certain groups of antinutrients are described in this chapter.

1. Plant Lectins

Plant lectins, otherwise known as phytohemagglutinins or hemagglutinins, are a group of highly diverse proteins of non-immune origin that contain at least one non-catalytic domain which enables them to selectively recognize and reversibly bind to specific free sugars or glycans present on glycoproteins and glycolipids, or polysaccharides with high affinity, without altering the structure of the carbohydrate (Goldstein & Hayes, 1978; Peumans & Van Dammem, 1995). Based on their structure, sugar specificity and sequence homology, almost all plant lectins known today can be grouped into twelve different lectin families (Van Damme et al., 2008).

The search for the toxic principle in castor beans (*Ricinus communis*, Euphorbiaceae), conducted by Stillmark in 1888, revealed that extracts from castor beans and other Euphorbiaceae plants are able to agglutinate blood cells of different animals (Rüdiger & Gabius, 2001). On the basis of carbohydrate recognition, the reaction of red blood cells with blood-group-specific-lectins (the therminal-linked monosaccharides GalNAc (group A), Gal (group B) and Fuc (group O)), purified lectins are used to determine the blood type (ABO) (Rüdiger & Gabius, 2001).

Lectins have been identified in all kingdoms of life ranging from viruses, fungi and bacteria to animals and plants, including important food crops such as soybean, tomato, potato, bean and wheat (Lannooa & Van Damme, in press). Since they represent the largest family of these proteins, lectins of the legumes occupy a special position, and their biological properties have been extensively investigated (Nasi et al., 2009). According to Nasi et al. (2009), lectin content in investigated legume seeds varied from 0.09–0.16 g/kg raw seed in *Ulex europaeus* (gorse) to ~ 21 g/kg raw seed in *Canavalia ensiformis* (jack bean).

At the beggining, plant lectin research focussed on the purification and characterization of lectins that can be found in high amounts in seeds and vegetative storage tissues (Lannooa & Van Damme, in press). The majority of plant lectins that have been studied so far are secretory proteins, which means that they enter the secretory system and subsequently accumulate either in vacuoles or in the cell wall and intracellular spaces. For example, concanavalin A, soybean agglutinin, pea lectin, and favin can be found at relatively high levels and accumulate in vacuoles in the cotyledons (1% to 8% of total protein), and at lower levels in the embryonic axes of the seeds (Chrispeels & Raikhel, 1991). These lectins are synthesized during seed development together with the more abundant seed storage proteins. Similar to storage proteins, lectins are broken down to provide amino acids for the growing seedlings during germination and seedling grow. Lectins are also often quite abundant in vegetative plant organs such as roots, leaves, rhizomes, and stems. Some of these are vacuolar while others, such as the chitin-binding Datura seed lectin, are extracellular. Vacuolar lectins also occur in cereal seeds, but are much less abundant (1 μg/dry grain) and occur only in specific cell layers of the embryo (e.g. wheat germ agglutinin in the coleorhiza and rootcap of the wheat embryo) (Etzler, 1986). Although many roles have been proposed for plant lectins (Etzler, 1986), it is believed that the most likely function for the vacuolar lectins is in plant defense (Chrispeels & Raikhel, 1991).

During the last decade, evidence has been accumulating indicating that plants also synthesize small amounts of lectins in response to some specific stress factors and changing environmental conditions (Van Damme et al., 2008). Since lectin activity cannot be detected in normal tissues but is clearly upregulated after stress conditions, these lectins are referred to as 'inducible' lectins. It has been shown that many of these inducible lectins locate to the nuclear/cytosolic compartments where they probably fulfil a specific role (Van Damme et al., 2004).

1.1. Antinutritional Properties

It is known that lectins bind to sugar moieties in cell walls or membranes and thereby change the physiology of the membrane. One of the most nutritionally important features of plant lectins is their ability to survive digestion by the gastrointestinal tract of consumers, which means that they are resistant to stomach acid and digestive enzymes. This allows the lectins to bind to membrane glycosyl groups of the cells within the digestive tract and thereby change the physiology of the membranes to cause agglutination, mitosis, or other biochemical changes in the cell (agglutination-clumping; mitosis-multiplication or division of a cell forming two daughter cells) (Vasconcelos & Oliveira, 2004). Consequently, a series of harmful local and systemic reactions are triggered qualifying this class of molecules as antinutritive and/or toxic substances. In gastrointestinal tract, they can affect the turnover and loss of gut epithelial cells, damage the luminal membranes of the epithelium, interfere with nutrient digestion and absorption, stimulate shifts in the bacterial flora and modulate the immune state. Systemically, they can disrupt lipid, carbohydrate and protein metabolism, promote enlargement and/or atrophy of key internal organs and tissues, and alter the hormonal and immunological status. At high intakes, lectins can seriously threaten the growth and health of consuming animals (Vasconcelos & Oliveira, 2004). For example, lectins from the castor bean are highly toxic and can kill if ingested in even small amounts. They are also detrimental to numerous insect pests of crop plants although less is presently known about their insecticidal mechanisms of action (Vasconcelos & Oliveira, 2004).

1.2. Pharmacological Effects

During the last decade much attention has been given to the pharmacological effects of natural peptides and proteins, among them lectins. Plant lectins have received special attention for their potential as microbicide. These agents have been shown to interact with the glycans of the viral envelope (gp120) of HIV and block viral entry into its target cells. The plant lectins derived from *Hippeastrum* hybrid (HHA) and *Galanthus nivalis* (GNA) of the Amaryllidaceae family are 50 kDa mannose-specific tetramers which selectively inhibit a wide variety of HIV-1 and HIV-2 isolates (Balzarini et al., 2005).

Using an *in vitro* assay, Gaidamashvili and van Staden (2006) reported the cyclooxygenase inhibitory activity of lectins from South African medicinal plants used in traditional healing of inflammation, suggesting that some lectins have good potential as anti-inflammatory agents exhibiting cyclooxygenase inhibitory activity in high levels.

In the last two decades, plant lectins have been used as recognizing tools to differentiate malignant tumours from benign and the degree of glycosylation associated with metastasis (Gorelik et al., 2001). Meanwhile, several lectins such as mistletoe lectins have been adopted for alternative cancer therapy (Schumacher et al., 2003). Furthermore, they are indicated for the reduction of treatment-associated side-effects as adjuvant agents during chemotherapy and radiotherapy in Europe for several years (Valentiner et al., 2003). Recently, many studies have further presented the antitumour activities of plant lectins on a variety of malignant cells (Choi et al., 2004; De Mejía & Prisecaru, 2005). Several typical lectins such as MLs (Lyu et al., 2002), ricin (Mikkat et al., 2001; Plattner et al., 2008) and WGA (Battelli, 2004) have been reported to possess remarkable anti-tumour activities by inducing apoptosis in cancer cells.

1.3. Isolation of Lectins

Initially, the general methods used for proteins were employed for the purification of lectins, without exploiting their special characteristics (Rüdiger & Gabius, 2001). These methods included precipitation by salts, acids and organic solvents. As expected, the preparations obtained were far from pure and the results had to be interpreted with caution (Rüdiger & Gabius, 2001).

Introduction of preparative chromatographic methods with ion exchangers, gel filtration (size exclusion chromatography) media and, above all, affinity absorbents enabled the progress in this area. Originally developed for isolating enzymes by means of immobilized inhibitors, the principal strategy was transferred to lectinology, and cross-linked dextrans found versatile application in one-step purification schemes for Glc-binding plant lectins (Agrawal & Goldstein, 1967). Agarose, a commercially available natural polysaccharide containing Gal, was used as an affinity absorbent for Gal-binding lectins such as those from *Ricinus communis*, *Bauhinia purpurea*, *Glycine max* and *Wisteria floribunda*, and chitin, a polymer of *N*-acetylglucosamine (GlcNAc), for the purification from the lectin II from *Griffonia simplicifolia* (Lis & Sharon, 1981). By selecting suitable glycoproteins as ligands, it has even become feasible to devise an affinity matrix presenting a panel of carbohydrate epitopes as potential ligands. Such a matrix can prove its value when screening extracts with different lectins within one binding step followed by washing and differential elution. For this purpose, gastric mucin or ovomucoid were successfully tested as ligands (Freier et al., 1985). For eluting a lectin, the obvious method is to exploit the haptenic sugar as cometitive inhibitor following the principle of dissociating antibody-antigen complexes by the soluble hapten group (Landsteiner & van der Scheer, 1931). In the case of monosaccharides this is generally achievable. Certain lectins, however, bind to oligosaccharides which are not readily accessible or are expensive. In such cases lectin elution can be perfformed by lowering the pH of the buffer with immediate neutralization of the eluant. When run as a gradient, it has even been possible to fractionate isolectin mixtures (Rüdiger, 1977).

In recent years there has been considerable interest in designing new methods to capture target products directly from crude unclarified process liquors and thereby fuse the three classical steps—clarification, concentration, and initial purification—into one unit operation. At the present time the so-called "expanded bed adsorption" (EBA) is probably the benchmark technique in this field (Hjorth, 1997). Lectin extraction from aqueous solution by reverse micelles is another process that has been successfully applied to isolate plant lectins (Choe et al., 2000). It utilises basic techniques such as classical liquid–liquid extraction, and hence has also the potential for industrial application. This process can be used to separate proteins which have been solubilized in organic solvents using surfactants, without affecting their functional properties.

1.4. Analysis of Lectins

First method to detect lectins was based on their ability to agglutinate erythrocytes, while their carbohydrate-binding specificity was established most conveniently by semiquantitative assay, hapten inhibition of hemagglutination, using various sugars and sugar derivatives as inhibitors (Nachbar & Oppenheim, 1980). Although the hemagglutination assay is the most common method for the detection of lectin activity in different matrices, it has limitations: (i) it is applicable only for lectins with affinity to abundant glycans expressed at the cell surface, (ii) it is applicable only for multivalent lectins to cross-link glycans expressed at the surface of different cells, and (iii) relatively large amounts of lectins and saccharides are required, which are often not available (Wu et al., 2009).

Nowadays, a variety of approaches for the investigation of sugar-binding specificities of proteins exist. These include enzyme-linked immunosorbent assay (ELISA) (Blixt et al., 2003), equilibrium dialysis coupled with high performance liquid chromatography (Mega & Hase, 1991) and isothermal titration calorimetry (Dam & Brewer, 2004).

The enzyme-linked immunosorbent assay (ELISA) is based on the reaction between antibody and antigen in 96-well microtiter plates. Application of this method to lectins was initially based on binding the lectin to the antigen-coated surface of the well, followed by binding an anti-lectin antibody (Duk et al., 1992). ELISA is a very convenient and easy to perform test, but obtaining an antibody for each lectin is troublesome.

High performing technologies such as e.g. glycan array screening, surface plasmon resonance and frontal affinity chromatography are now available to study in much more detail the fine specificity of lectins and carbohydrate–protein interactions (Blixt et al., 2004; Paulson et al., 2006; Tatenov et al., 2007; Hirabayashi, 2008; Liang et al., 2008).

In recent years, the microtiter plate methods have lead to the development of micro-array techniques. Microarrays are solid surfaces which carry a great number of small spots-bound glycans. Lectin binding to immobilized glycans allows rapid analysis of their specificity and is useful for detecting even weak interactions due to multivalent display of ligands on the surface. Different ways of derivatization and immobilization of glycans and of determination of lectin binding are described in the literature.

To characterize the structure of lectin molecules, after isolation, mass spectrometric sequence confirmation or structural characterisation of lectins can be carried out according to the gel electrophoresis based or to electrophoresis-free proteomic strategies. In the case of glycosylated lectins, identification of glycosylation site(s) can be accomplished following the general scheme: 1. proteolytic digestion; 2. capture of the glycopeptides by choosing among several possible strategies including hydrophilic interaction chromatography (HILIC), affinity enrichment by lectins and hydrazide resin glycol-capture (Zhang et al., 2003); 3. chemical or enzymatic de-glycosylation (by peptide N-glycosidase F in the case of the N-glycosylation), preferably in $H_2{}^{18}O$; 4. LC-ESI MS/MS sequencing of deglycosylated peptides for identification of the linker amino acid (Nasi et al., 2009).

A number of methods have been developed for the detailed analysis of the profile of sugar moiety, on a species of glycoproteins. After cleavage from proteins and purification, two of the major techniques include high performance liquid chromatography (HPLC) and mass spectrometry (MS).

2. Phytic Acid

Phytic acid (myo-inositol hexaphosphate) (Figure 1) is presented in many cereals, legumes, oil seeds and nuts (1-5%) and represents the major phosphorous storage compound in plant seeds (Cheryan, 1980; Wu et al., 2009). It may account in the range of 60-90% of the total phosphorus content (Eeckhout & De Paepe, 1994; Lolas & Markakis, 1975; Zhou & Erdman, 1995). It exists in the form of mixed salts of Ca-Mg-K, i.e. phytate, and occurs in many locations within the kernel.

In cereals, approximately 1-2% of the weight of the seed is phytic acid, and it can even reach 3-6% (Febles et al., 2002). Phytic acid is mainly located in the bran fraction of whole-grain cereals, especially within the aleurone layer (Hídvégi & Lásztity, 2002).

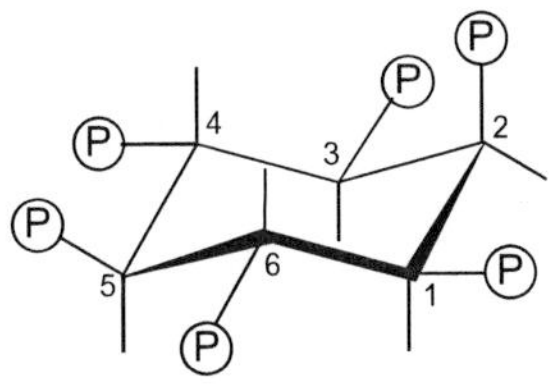

Figure 1. Phytic acid (myo-inositol hexaphosphate).

Rice. As rice is one of the most important cereal crops worldwide, the phytic acid content for 72 cultivars of rice was detected and it ranged from 0.685% to 1.03% (Liu et al., (2005). It is primarily accumulated in the outer layers of kernel while in an endeosperm there is no detectable phytic acid.

Barley. It is reported that more than 80% of phytic acid in barley grain (cca 1%) is localized in the aleurone layer, and the remainder in the germ (O'Dellet et al., 1972).

Maize. In maize the majority of the kernel phytic acid (90-95%) is found in the embryo, with the remainder in the aleurone layer (O'Dell et al., 1972; Lin et al., 2005).

Wheat. The content of phytic acid in wheat differs between soft wheat (1.13%) and hart wheat (2.43%) (Cheryan, 1980; Dost & Tokul, 2006).

The cereal flours showed values ranging between 3-4 mg/g for soft wheat, 9 mg/g for hard wheat and 22 mg/g for whole wheat. Febles et al. (2002) determined the phytic acid concentrations within the range 2-4 mg/g for refined wheat flours and 6-10 mg/g for the whole ones.

Corn, millet and sorghum flours reported a mean of 10 mg/g and oat, rice, rye and barley between 4 and 7 mg/g. Wheat brans had wide ranges (25±58 mg/g) of phytates. The phytic acid for oat brans was half that of wheat bran (20 mg/g) and higher value (58 mg/g) than that for rice bran. The breads made with single or mixture cereal fours exhibited ranges of phytic acid between 1.5 and 7.5 mg/g (García-Estapa et al., 1999).

2.1. Antinutritional Properties

Phytic acid has been considered as an antinutrient due to its strong ability to bind minerals and thus to change their solubility, functionality, absorption and digestibility (Fox & Tao, 1989; Rickard &Thompson, 1997; Zhou & Erdman, 1995). In fact, only myo-inositol hexaphosphate and myo-inositol pentaphosphate have a negative effect on a bioavailability of minerals. Other hydrolytic products which can be formed enzymatically of phytases or chemically during storage, fermentation, germination, and food processing, have a poor capacity to bind minerals, or the complexes formed are more soluble (Cheryan, 1980; Maga, 1982; Sandberg et al., 1989; Tao et al., 1986). Phytic acid is also reported to have the ability to react with some proteins to form complexes, which make the proteins less soluble, and affect enzymatic degradation and peptic digestion (Carnovale et al., 1988; Elsheikh et al., 2000).

Phytic acid-mineral complexes, especially those with zinc, calcium and iron, are insoluble at physiological pH and consequently they exhibit low bioavailability (Harland &

Harland, 1980; Weaver & Kannan, 2002). Therefore, humans and nonruminants excrete a large fraction of these complexes. This phenomenon can contribute to human mineral deficiency, particularly with respect to zinc (Karunaratne et al., 2008; Lönnerdal, 2000), iron (Hallberg et al., 1989; Minihane & Rimbach, 2002), calcium (Weaver et al., 1991), and manganese (Davidsson et al., 1995) in the populatios that live mainly on grains and legumes (Raboy, 2001).

Among the essential minerals, zinc is one of the most affected by phytic acid (Sandström & Lönnerdal, 1989). It was proposed that phytate depresses zinc bioavailability to monogastric animals and people because zinc coprecipitates as a Zn-Ca-phytate complex (Becker & Hoekstra, 1971). An inhibitory effect of phytate on zinc absorption has been demonstrated in numerous studies, including investigations with endogenous phytate (Oberleas & Harland, 1981; Saha et al., 1994; Sandström et al., 1987; Zhou et al., 1992) and with purifed sodium phytate (Turnland et al., 1984). Ma (2007) recently proposed that when phytate and zinc are present in a molar ratio of 16:1, the zinc is no longer bioavailable.

Several studies indicate a reduction of iron absorption at marginal dietary iron supply due to phytic acid in humans (Hallberg et al., 1989) and other monogastric animals (Thompson & Erdman, 1984). Phytate forms insoluble complex with iron and this complex may coprecipitate as Fe-Ca-phytate and become unavailable for absorption. The inhibiting effect of phytate on Fe absorption does not depend on the protein composition of the test meals (Reddy et al., 1996).

The effective mineral uptake in the digestive tract is affected not only by the presence of phytic acid, but the fibre, carbohydrate and phytase. Thus, inhibition of iron absorption as a result of dietary phytate can also be partially counteracted by activation of native or the addition of extrinsic phytase to phytate-rich diets (Sandberg et al., 1996; Pallauf et al., 1999).

Additionaly, some types of prosessing such as malting, fermentation and soaking result in the hydrolysis of phytate into intermediate myo-inositol phosphates. Soaking of millet, soya bean, maize, sorghum, and mung bean at 30 °C for 24 h decreased the contents of phytic acid by 4–51% (Lestienne et al., 2005), and soaking of sorghum flour (80% extraction) at room temperature for 24 h reduced phytic acid levels by 16-21% (Mahgoub & Elhag, 1998). The use of moist conditions to stimulate germination is another technique for reducing phytate levels. Germination of sorghum for 4 h reduced phytic acid by 68–87% (Mahgoub & Elhag, 1998).

There is some evidence that fermentation occurring during bread dough making can degrade phytic acid (Larsson & Sandberg, 1991; Natubu & Markakis, 1983). It can be broken down by phytases in a pre-fermentation step, such as that occurring in sourdough breads at pH 5-5.5 (Leenhardt et al., 2005), which significantly increases mineral bioavailability, especially that of iron and zinc (Lopez et al., 2003). As inositol penthaphosphate and hexaphosphate from bread were evidenced to exhibit an inhibitory effect on iron absorbtion more that lower-phosphorylated derivatives (Sandberg et al., 1996), it was concluded that bread dough fermentation reduces the loss in mineral absorption. Fermentation treatment was most effective in decreasing phytic acid (56–96% removal), followed by soaking at 10 °C after preheating (42–59%) in the case of rice (Liang et al., 2008). After 12 h of accelerated fermentation, 60% of phytic acid in sorghum was degraded (Mahgoub & Elhag, 1998).

Various thermal treatments can destroy phytic acid to the different destruction rates (Maga, 1982). Autoclaving for 30 min resulted in low phytate loss in the case of soy, while after 2 h approximately 70% of soy phytate was lost whereas rice, wheat and sesame had only 5-25% of lost (De Boland et al., 1975).

Phytic acid in rapeseed and mixture made of rapeseed and some crops (corn, barley, triticale, wheat and alfalfa) could be destroyed by dry extrusion in the range of 20-25% (Sakač et al., 2007). Lower levels of destruction in the case of rapeseed meal during toasting (approximately 9%) were registered by Mansour et al. (1993) and Park et al. (2000).

Antinutritive nature of phytic acid has directed the efforts made by scientists to reduce phytic acid content in grains throught fertilization (Elsheikh et al., 2000). Saastamoinen et al., (1992) reported that the phytic acid content in oat grains was increased by nitrogen and phosphorus fertilizer application as well as by high mean temperature during grain filling stage, and was decreased by high precipitation. Understanding of factors that affect phytic acid accumulation in barley grains is essential for breeders to develop low phytic acid barley cultivars (Dai et al., 2007).

2.2. Pharmacological Effects

Although phytic acid has been considered as an antinutrient for a long time, there are many data about its beneficial effects on human health through its significant influence on functional characteristics of foods (Harland et al., 1995; Rhou & Erdman, 1995; Thompon, 1993). Extensive studies show that phytic acid is a chemopreventive agent against cancers of the breast, colon, liver, leukemia, prostate, and skin (Fox & Eberl, 2002). Mechanisms of action have been proposed that include gene alteration, increase in immunity, antioxidant properties and metal-chelating ability as an anti-cancer activity (Fox & Eberl, 2002; Graf & Eaton, 1993).

Regarding its relatively high binding affinity towards minerals, especially to iron, phytic acid was recognized as a potent antioxidant (Graf & Eaton, 1990). It is a potent inhibitor of iron-catalyzed hydroxyl radical formation by chelating iron required for generation of hydroxyl radical via the Fenton-type reaction (Rimbach & Pallauf, 1998). Obata (2003) reported that phytic acid exhibited antioxidant effect by suppression iron (II)-enhanced hydroxyl radical formation induced by 1-methyl-4-phenylpyridinium ion (MPP^+) in rat striatum. That finding confirmed that iron-mediated oxidative damage involved in progression of Parkinson's disease could be inhibited by phytic acid (Dexter et al., 1989).

Phytic acid may reduce the incidence of colonic cancer by a similar mechanism, and protect against other inflammatory bowel diseases, especially in populations consuming a vegetarian-type diet (Graf & Eaton, 1990; Shamsuddin et al., 1997). Generally, xanthine oxidase, which generates superoxide anion during oxidation of xanthine, is distributed most abundantly in the intestine (Battelli et al., 1972). Dietary iron remains largely unabsorbed also in the intestine (Babbs, 1990), suggesting that the hydroxyl radical is generated through interaction of iron with superoxide anion produced by xanthine oxidase in the intestine. Hydroxyl radical generated by the action of xanthine oxidase or by colon bacteria causes DNA damage (Halliwell & Aruoma, 1991) and, consequently, could promote colonic cancer. Muraoka and Miura (2004) found out that phytic acid and myo-inositol demonstrated antioxidant activity not only by inhibition of xanthine oxidase-induced superoxide-dependent DNA damage, but also by preventing formation of ADP-iron-oxygen complexes.

The anticancer action of phytic acid is mostly attributed to its antioxidative action, i.e. iron chelating activity in inhibition of iron-catalyzed lipid peroxidation and DNA damage, due to the phosphorus moieties of the phytic acid molecule (Graf & Eaton, 1990; Graf et al., 1987; Miyamoto et al., 2000; Thompson & Zhang, 1991). However, phytate hydrolysis catalysed by microbial phytase as well as myoinositol had no effect of DMPO/•OH spin adducts. It is hypothesized that the 1,2,3 equatorial-axial-equatorial trisphosphate grouping in phytate has a conformation that provides a specific intramolecular interaction with iron to inhibit its ability to catalyse hydroxyl radical formation (Phillippy & Graf, 1997).

Some other experiments demonstrated anticancer effects of phytic acid in preventive and therapeutic actions (Midorikawa et al., 2001; Shamsuddin, 2002). Phytic acid inhibited the formation of 8-oxo-7,8-dihydro-2'-deoxyguanosine in cultured cells treated with an H_2O_2-generating system, although it did not scavenge H_2O_2.Site-specific DNA damage by H_2O_2 and Cu(II) at GG and GGG sequences was inhibited by phytic acid, but not by *myo*-inositol. Phytic acid alone did not cause DNA damage and thus, it should not act as a prooxidant (Midorikawa et al., 2001).

Furthermore, Hirose et al. (1991) showed that a supplement of 2% phytic acid inhibited development of neoplasmatic lesions in the liver and pancreas. *In vitro* studies clearly demonstrated that phytic acid also reduced cell proliferation rate in different cell lines, including erythroleukemia (Shamsuddin et al., 1992) and human mammary cancer (Shamsuddin et al., 1996). Furthermore, lower inositol phosphates, such as inositol tetraphosphate and inositol triphosphate, may play roles in mediating cellular responses and have been noted as having a function in second messenger transduction systems (Berridge & Irvine, 1989). Also, phytic acid exhibited benefits concerning a decrease in plasma cholesterol and triglycerides (Katayama, 1995).

The possibility of utilization of phytic acid as the antioxidant in processing and storage of foods was also documented. Graf et al. (1987) established that phytate prevented the peroxidation of arachidonic acid driven by ascorbic acid and iron. These authors proved that phytic acid caused a substantial shift in redox potential of iron, i.e. it accelerated $Fe^{2+} \rightarrow Fe^{3+}$ by molecular oxygen, which could explain the inhibition of lipid peroxidation. This occurs especially at high phytate:iron ratios.

When phytic acid was tested by measuring its ability to inhibit generation of peroxyl radical-N-*tert*-butyl-α-phenylnitrone spin adducts (PBN-OOL) during thermal and catalytic oxidation of hydroperoxyde-enriched soybean oil, it was established that it did not inhibit the thermal oxidation of the oil, but exhibited antioxidative effect on its catalytic oxidation by chelating Fe^{2+} ions (Sakač et al., 2008). This finding was in accordance with the statement of Ahn et al. (2004) who did not detect DPPH radical scavenging activity of phytic acid because it did not act as the chainbreaking antioxidant, capable of scavenging free radicals and thus preventing lipid oxidation.

Lee et al. (1998) found that phytic acid was effective for inhibition of the oxidative changes in a model beef system, i.e. it could act as food preservative. Positive effects of phytic acid on oxidative stability of raw and cooked meat was documented by Stodolak et al. (2007) who found out that effects of phytic acid were more pronounced in cooked meat than in raw because during cooking iron was liberated from myoglobin and interacted with phospholipids to catalyze lipid peroxidation (Graf & Eaton, 1990). Phytic acid and lower inositol phosphates were evidented to inhibit the marine oil oxidation with Fe^{2+} and they demonstrated strong synergistic effects with α-tocopherol (Uchida et al., 2001).

It seems reasonable to control phytic acid contents in edible parts of crops to a level in which the medical and health functions of the food may be maintained and bioavailability of minerals is not much altered (Febles et al., 2002). Nevertheless, in phytic acid-rich foods, trials for reducing phytic acid, including physical or chemical processing, genetic manipulation or enzymatic hydrolysis have been performed (Siddhuraju et al., 2002). Mutation breeding through γ-irradiation (Larson et al., 2000; Yuan et al., 2007) or chemically induced mutagenesis (Raboy et al., 2000; Dorsch et al., 2003) has been described for various cereals and legumes. Some cereals, including corn, barley, and rice mutants, have been developed that have significantly lower levels of phytic acid without reducing the total phosphorus (Larson et al., 2000). In addition, genetic engineering has been successfully applied to produce low phytic acid (*lpa*) crops (Kuwano et al., 2006; Shi et al., 2007). Low phytic acid mutants of various crops were shown to result in an enhanced utilization of phosphorus, calcium and zinc when fed to animals or consumed by humans (Raboy, 2007).

2.3. Analysis of Phytic Acid

There are many indirect methods for the determination of phytic acid based on a stoichiometric relationship between ferric ion and phytate. Harland and Oberleas (1977) extracted phytic acid directly with 1.2% HCl, followed with elution through an ion-exchange resin to separate inorganic phosphorus, then subsequently digesting it with concentrated H_2SO_4 and HNO_3 in order to measure the phosphorus content in foods, and converting it to the phytate equivalent. It formed the basis for developing an AOAC method (No. 986.11).

Haug and Lantzsch (1983) based their method on heating the sample with iron(III) solution and determining the decrease in iron content colorimetrically by adding thioglycolic acid (mercapto acetic acid) with 2,2'-bipyridine.

The rapid colorimetric method for determination of phytate based on the reaction between ferric ion and sulfosalicylic acid was described by Latta and Eskin (1980).

Mentioned methods based on precipitation, ion-exchange or colorimetric determination are useful for measuring phytic acid contents in unprocessed products, but in processed foods their application results in overestimating the phytic acid contents. Food processing is often accompanied by hydrolysis of phytate into intermediate myo-inositol phosphates which can not be separated using these methods.

HPLC methods can separate and determine myo-inositol hexaphosphate and lower myo-inositolphospates, and, therefore, are suitable to quantify them, especially in processed foods. Tangendjaja et al. (1980) first applied HPLC for determination of phytic acid. Lehrfeld (1989) also developed a procedure for the analysis of phytic acid by HPLC.

Dost and Tokul (2006) proposed a rapid and simple analytical procedure to determine the phytic acid content in food stuffs by reverse phase high performance liquid chromatography in parallel with a spectrophotometric detection method. The method was based on phytic acid replacing the metal from a coloured complex, iron(III)-thiocyanate.

Chen et al. (2008) described a novel synchronous fluorescence method for determining phytic acid in food samples, based on the formation of a ternary complex among phytate, 1,10-phenanthroline, and Fe^{3+}.

3. Saponins

Saponinsare generally known as non-volatile, surface-active compounds that are widely distributed in nature, occurring primarily in the plant kingdom (Hostettmann & Marston, 2005; Lasztity et al., 1998; Oleszek, 2002). Their surface-active properties are what distinguish these compounds from other glycosides. They dissolve in water to form colloidal solutions that foam upon shaking (Tyler et al., 1981).

Saponins are found in a wide variety of foods including legume seeds, such as peas, soybeans, lentils and lupin (Lasztity et al., 1998), asparagus, beans (navy beans, haricot beans, kidney beans), blackberries, lucerne, peas, potatoes, sugar beet and tea (Dini et al., 2001; Fenwick & Oakenfull, 1981). They occur in nearly 100 plant families – Alliaceae (Corea et al., 2003; Zou et al., 2001), Amaranthaceae (Michl et al., 2000), Dracaenaceae (Yokosuka et al., 2000; 2002), Leguminosae (Bialy et al., 1999), Solanaceae (Fujiwara et al., 2003) and many others.

Saponins consist of nonpolar aglycones coupled with one or more monosaccharide moieties (Oleszek, 2002) and can be classified into two groups based on the nature of their aglycone skeleton (Abe et al., 1993). The first group consists of the steroidal saponins, which are almost exclusively present in the monocotyledonous angiosperms. The second group consists of the triterpenoid saponins, which are the most common and occur mainly in the dicotyledonous angiosperms (Bruneton, 1995).

Steroidal saponins consist of a steroidal aglycone, a C27 spirostane skeleton, generally comprising of a six-ring structure (Figure 2A). In some cases, in fresh plant material, the hydroxyl group in the 26-position is engaged in a glycosidic linkage, and so the aglycone structure remains pentacyclic. This is referred to as a furostane skeleton (Figure 2B). Triterpenoid saponins consist of a triterpenoid aglycone, which consists of a C30 skeleton, comprising of a pentacyclic structure (Figure 2C).

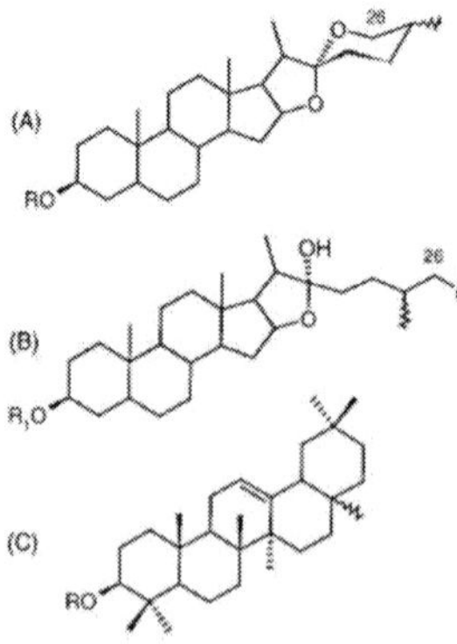

Figure 2. Aglycone skeletons of (A) steroidal spirostane, (B) steroidal furostane, and (C) triterpenoid saponins. R = sugar moiety

Saponins have a diverse range of properties, which include sweetness and bitterness (Grenby, 1991; Heng et al., 2006; Koziol, 1991; Price et al., 1985), foaming and emulsifying properties (Price et al., 1987), pharmacological and medicinal properties (Attele et al., 1999), hemolytic properties (Oda et al., 2000; Sparg, Light & van Staden, 2004), as well as antimicrobial, insecticidal, and molluscicidal activities (Sparg et al., 2004). Saponins have found wide applications in cosmetics (Petit et al., 1995; Price et al., 1987; Uematsu et al., 2000) and pharmaceutical products (Estrada et al., 2000; Sparg et al., 2004).

3.1. Antinutritional Properties

One of the major biological and pharmacological properties of saponins is their hemolytic activity, which implies their ability to rupture erythrocytes. The haemolytic properties are generally attributed to the interaction between the saponins and the sterols of the erythrocyte membrane. As a result, the membrane bursts, causing an increase in permeability and a loss of hemoglobin. Baumann et al. (2000) investigated the effects of saponins on the membrane structure through hemolysis of human erythrocytes. The findings showed that saponin-lysed erythrocytes do not reseal, and therefore indicate that saponin damage to the lipid bilayer is irreversible.

The level of haemolytic activity is attributed to the type of aglycone and the presence of sugar side chains. Therefore, structure-activity relationships are of the major significance for establishing the structural feature for hemolytic activity of saponins (Sparg et al., 2004). Although toxic to cold-blooded species, if taken orally by warm-blooded species, saponins have only a weak toxicity (Bruneton, 1995), which is probably attributed to low absorption rates.

There are different data about the influence of processing on saponin content. Domestic processing and cooking methods including soaking, ordinary and pressure cooking of soaked and unsoaked seeds and sprouting significantly lowered saponin content of mungbean (*Vigna radiata* L.) seeds. Loss of the saponins was greater when soaked instead of unsoaked seeds were cooked (Kataria et al., 1989). On the contrary, Fenwick and Oakenfull (1981) found that saponins were not destroyed by processing or cooking.

3.2. Pharmacological Effects

Many saponins isolated from plant sources produce an inhibition of inflammation. Just et al. (1998) reported that a bidesmosidic saponin isolated from *Bupleurum fruticescens* L. (Apiaceae) exhibited the highest anti-inflammatory activity of all saponins tested in the mouse edema assays. These authors suggested that the anti-inflammatory activity of saponins isolated from *Bupleurum fruticescens* was related to their chemical structure. Triterpenoid saponins from the stem bark of *Kalopanax pictus* Nakai (Araliaceae) also showed significant anti-inflammatory activity (Li et al., 2002).

Many saponins were tested for both antiyeast and antifungal activity (Escalante et al., 2002), as well as antimicrobial activity (Killeen et al., 1998). Steroidal saponins from *Yucca schidigera* Roezl. ex Ortgies (Agavaceae) (Mohave yucca) were shown to exhibit effective growth-inhibitory activities aginst food-deteriorating yeasts, film-forming yeasts, and dermatophytic yeasts and fungi (Miyakoshi et al., 2000). Also, triterpenoid saponins from the seeds of *Chenopodium quinoa* Willd. (Chenopodiaceae) have been reported to demonstrate antifungal activity (Woldemichael & Wink, 2001).

There are numerous scientific results indicating cytotoxic properties of many saponins. Many isolated steroidal saponins have been shown to be either cytostatic or cytotoxic to HL-60 human leukemia cell lines (Mimaki et al., 2001; Yokosuka et al., 2002). Triterpenoid saponins have also shown cytotoxicity against human cell lines. Xiao et al. (1999) isolated a novel triterpene saponin from the root bark of *Aralia dasyphylla* Miq. (Araliaceae) which showed significant cytotoxic activity against KB and HeLa-S3 cells. Some cytotoxic saponins also possess antitumor properties (Sparg et al., 2004). Lee et al. (1999) isolated a novel saponin metabolite (IH-901) from *Panax ginseng* C.A.Meyer (Araliaceae) which showed *in vitro* antitumor activity. Yun (2003) investigated the anticancer properties of *Panax ginseng* C.A. Meyer (Araliaceae) and concluded that the activity of ginseng saponins were non-organ specific and that the anticarcinogenicity or human cancer preventative effect of *Panax ginseng* was due to the ginsenoside saponins Rg3, Rg5 and Rh2.

Saponins have also been reported to have antiviral activities. A mixture of tea-seed saponins from *Camellia sinensis* L. var *sinensis* (Ternstroemiaceae) were reported to inactivate human type A and B influenza viruses. Triterpenoid saponins from the Fabaceae family have been reported to have anti-herpes virus activity (Kinjo et al., 2000). Anti-herpes simplex virus activity was found to be structure related. Saponins with glucosyl unit in the central sugar moiety seemed to show greater anti-herpes virus activity.

Antioxidant nature of some saponins was also investigated. Huong et al. (1998) investigated the antioxidant activity of Vietnamese ginseng (*Panax vietnamensis* Ha and Grushv., Araliaceae) saponins. The results of the study showed that Vietnamese ginseng saponins exerted protective action against free radical-induced tissue injury.

Saponins from *Argania spinosa* at a non-hemolytic concentration diminished erythrocyte hemolysis induced by free radicals. Also, a combination of *A. spinosa* saponins and vitamin E protected against free radical-induced erythrocyte hemolysis, indicating that *A. spinosa* saponins enhanced the antioxidant effect of vitamin E (Amzal et al., 2008).

The results obtained by Li et al. (1998) suggested that *Panax quinquefolium* saponins demonstrated antioxidant properties and that reduction of LDL oxidation by these saponins may provide a protective effect against the detrimental actions of oxidized low-density lipoproteins.

The protective effects of the saponins isolated from the roots of *Platycodon grandiflorum* A. DC (Campanulaceae) and Changkil saponins (CKS), on the *tert*-butyl hydroperoxide (*t*-BHP)-induced oxidative injury (hepatotoxicity) in cultured rat primary hepatocytes and in rat livers were investigated (Lee et al., 2004). The authors concluded that CKS provided good protection from the *t*-BHP-induced production of intracellular reactive oxygen species and DNA damage. In addition, CKS was able to quench 1,1-diphenyl-2-picrylhydrazyl (DPPH) free radicals and the superoxide radicals and, consequently, they protected cells from oxidative stress.

Two triterpenoid saponins have been isolated from the seed kernels of *Entada rheedii* and were tested for their antiproliferative activity against T98G, A431, PC3 and B16-F1 cell lines, and for their antioxidant properties (Nzowa et al., 2010). Moderate cytotoxic potency and antioxidant properties were found.

The list of other biological activities of saponins is wide. Saponins extracted from *Acorus calamus* L. (Araceae) were tested for hyperlipidemic activity. Treatments of hyperlipidemic rats with saponins significantly decreased the serum cholesterol and triglyceride levels (Milgate & Roberts, 1995; Parab & Mengi, 2002). Saponin fractions from *Allium* species have been shown to decrease the plasma total cholesterol levels (Matsuura, 2001). The active fractions contained steroid saponins which are thought to be responsible for the cholesterol lowering effects of garlic. Oakenfull and Sidhu (1990) also confirmed the beneficial effects of saponins for hypercholesterolemia.

3.3. Analysis of Saponins

Some saponins show hemolytic activity which have been used for semiquantitative tests for saponin determination. In the simplest hemolytic method, saponin-containing material or its water extract is mixed with blood or with washed erythrocytes in isotonic-buffered solution (0.9% NaCl). After 20–24 h samples are centrifuged and hemolysis is indicated by the presence of haemoglobin in the supernatant. For the evaluation of hemolytic activity, European Pharmacopoeia uses a unit the haemolytic index (HI), which is defined as the number of milliliters of ox blood (2%, v/v) that can be hemolyzed by 1 g of crude saponins or plant material. The saponin mixture of *Gypsophila paniculata* L. (HI = 30 000) or Saponin white (Merck, HI = 15 000) are usually used as reference. Another modification of the hemolytic method is the hemolytic micromethod in which cow's blood stabilised with sodium citrate (3.65%, w/v) is mixed with gelatine solution (Jurzysta, 1979). Using these methods it has been documented that saponins differ in their hemolytic activities depending on their structures and that hemolytic methods are approximate and they do not distinguish between different saponins.

The biological methods including growth of sensitive fungus colony (Shany et al., 1970), and spectrofotometric methods, for example for determination of total steroidal sapogenin (Baccou et al., 1979) still being used, provide results on saponin concentrations, but they are not appropriate for the detection and quantification of individual saponins.

Thin-layer chromatography on normal and reversed-phases (TLC, HPTLC, 2D-TLC) provides excellent qualitative information and in combination with on-line coupling of a computer with dual-wavelength flying-spot scanner and two-dimensional analytical software can be used for routine determination of saponins in plant material (Oleszek, 2002). Determination of some saponins by TLC-densitometry was used to estimate the saponin content of 20 common food plants and also of foods prepared from some of them (Fenwick & Oakenfull, 1981).

Gas-liquid chromatography has limited application for determination since saponins are quite big molecules and are not volatile compounds. Therefore, there are only few applications of GC for determination of intact saponins. The saponins of roots, leaves and flowers in *Panax ginseng* were determined by gas-liquid chromatography after trimethylsilylation (Bombardelli et al., 1980). The GC method has been used for determination of TMS, such as mentioned, or acetyl or methyl derivatives of aglycones released during saponin hydrolysis. However, structurally different saponins show different rates of hydrolysis and precise optimisation of hydrolysis conditions is essential. Besides, during hydrolysis a number of compounds can be formed which can influence the final results (Oleszek, 2002).

High-performance liquid chromatography is the most powerful and the most frequently used technique for saponin determination due to the fact that it can deal effectively with non-volatile, highly polar compounds. It has been used extensively for determination of both aglycones and intact saponins. The separations are performed usually on normal (silica gel) and reversed-phase (C_8, C_{18}) columns, of which C_{18} has been preferred. The main problem in HPLC analysis of saponins is detection due to the absence of chromophores necessary for UV detection for majority of saponins. Therefore, the separation of intact glycosides or their aglycones has to be traced at lower UV wavelengths ranging from 200 to 210 nm. There are numerous papers dealing with HPLC determination of saponuns using low wavelength UV (Besson et al., 1989; Domon et al., 1984; Petersen & Palmqvist, 1990) or RI (refractive index) detection (Kaizuka & Takahashi, 1983). Also, pre-column derivatisation of saponins to introduce chromophores has been conducted (Besso et al., 1979; Oleszek et al., 1999).

4. Polyphenols

Polyphenolic compounds, ubiquitous in plant kingdom, are an integral part of the human diet. Ranging from simple molecules such as phenolic acid, to highly polycondensed compounds like tannins, the occurence and amount of polyphenols in food may vary extrimely. Traditionally, polyphenols have been considered and clasified as antinutrients. However, interest in plant phenolics has been steadily increasing owing to their antioxidant activities and possible beneficial effects on human health. Polyphenols are the most abundant antioxidants in a diet. Their total dietary intake could be much higher than that of other classes of phytochemicals and other dietary antioxidants.

Fruit juices, tee, coffee, red wine are considered main dietary sources, while vegetables, cereals, chocolate and legumes also contribute to the total polyphenol intake (Scalbert et al., 2005).

More than 8,000 different substances which differ according to their structure have been clasified as polyphenolics, the plants secondary metabolites. They possess aromatic ring with one or more hydroxyl groups in their structure (Croft, 1999). In plants, these compounds mainly occure as conjugates, with one or two sugar moieties. The most common sugar compound is glucose, but it could be other monosaccharide, disacharide, or even an oligosaccharide. Association with other compounds, such as amines, lipids, organic and carboxylic acids are also common. Some of the compunds belong to this class due to their metabolic pathway, although they do not possess niether phenolic gorups or the aromatic ring. The examples are cinnamic, elenoic, shikimic and hinic acid (Robards et al, 1999). During 60's, criteria for the clasification of polyphenolics included their occurence in plant (widely spread or not), their role and significance in plant, humans and animals (Milić et al., 2000). Up to date, there is no unique classification of polyphenolics although it is based on chemical structure (Ribereau-Gayon, 1972; Harborne, 1989). Flavonoids represent the most common and widely distributed group of plant phenolics. Their basic structure is diphenylpropane (C6-C3-C6) and consists of two aromatic rings linked through three carbons that usually form an oxygenated heterocycle (Figure 3). Flavonoids are further divided into several subclasses, including chalcones, dihydrochalcones, aurones, flavones, flavonols, dihydroflavonols, flavanones, flavanols, flavandiols, anthocyanidins, isoflavonoids, biflavonoids and proanthocyanidins (Bravo, 1998).

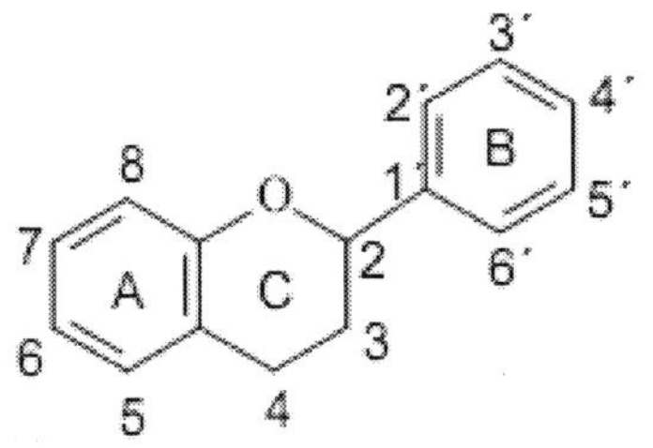

Figure 3. Basic structure of flavonoids.

4.1. Antinutritional Properties

Polyphenols react with digestive enzymes and/or dietary proteins reducing their digestibility and/or increasing endogenous protein elimination (de Mira et al., 2009). Presence of tannins in food has been considered as an antinutritional aspect due to their well known capacity to bind and precipitate proteins. Tannin-protein complexes are usually formed via hydrogen bonds and hydrophobic interactions. Also, insoluble complexes of tannins could be formed with starch and other carbohydrates, reducing the digestibility of these nutrients as well (Carbonaro et al., 1996).

Polyphenols form complexes with metal cations through their hydroxyphenyl and carboxyl groups, and thus, interfere with the intestinal absorption of minerals, especially with iron(III) (de Mira et al., 2009). The chelating ability of polyphenolics increases a risk of iron depletion in people with marginal iron status (Mennen et al., 2005). Catechins, chlorogenic acid, polymers in black tea and cocoa, and wine polyphenols showed significant reduction on nonheme iron absorption. Negative effects of some polyphenols on reduced absorption of zink, sodium and aluminium, but not on manganese, calcium and magnesium is observed. On the other hand, chelation of metals is a way in which polyphenols exert their antioxidant activity. Bravo (1998) gives the overview of the main nutritional effects of polyphenolic compounds as well as a description of the chemistry, dietary sources and metabolism of flavonoids.

4.2. Pharmacological Effects

Research on plant polyphenolics has been intensified after the discovery of the French paradox, the observation that the incidence of coronary heart disease is lower in French, despite having a diet relatively rich in saturated fats. There is a lack of medicinal consensus about the moderate consumption of wine and the longevity.

Flavonoids and other polyphenolic compounds have been studied as a potential protective agents against the risk of chronical deseases, but the real contributions of such compounds to health and the mechanisms of their action still remains unclear (Halliwell et al., 2005). Proposed antioxidant effects of flavonoids are not supported by strong evidence *in vivo*.

It is believed that oxidative stress is involved in the pathology of many diseases such as cancer, arteriosclerosis, malaria, rheumatoid arthritis and ageing processes (Štajner et al., 1998). Plant-derived antioxidants, first of all polyphenols, may function as free-radical scavengers, reducing agents, metal ion chelators, quenchers of singlet and triplet oxygen, and inhibitors of lipid peroxidation (Sakač et al., 2009). Evaluation of antioxidant activity of plants and food products enriched with natural antioxidants has been in focus for decades (Štajner et al., 2004; Mišan et al., 2006; Mišan et al., 2009b). Among all antioxidants, plant polyphenolics are considered to be the most investigated ones.

The capacity to act as antioxidants *in vitro* is the best described property of polyphenolic compounds. Comprehensive review of methods for determining antioxidant activity is given by Moure et al., 2001. In food related systems, polyphenolics exert their antioxidant activity as primary chain-breaking antioxidants and/or secondary, the ones which reduce the rate of chain initiation. Another clasification divides polyphenolics on free radical scavengers, and metal chelators. Therefore, the antioxidant activity should be evaluated using different tests for different mechanisms.

Reported results of antioxidant capacity in research papers usually include the application of few tests which do not reflect the overall antiradical activity. The most often used test for that purpose is DPPH assay. The antiradical activity that implies ability to quench hydroxyl radical ($OH^{\cdot}$) and superoxide radical ($O_2^{\cdot -}$), the biologically important most reactive oxygen species (ROS), responsible for the oxidative stress as the trigger leading to many chronic diseases is not often tested, especially by ESR. ESR is considered to be a reliable direct method for measurement of the radical scavenging properties of antioxidants (Figure 4). Phenolic compounds, which are known as powerful chainbreaking antioxidants inhibit lipid peroxidation by decreasing concentration of peroxyl radicals via hydrogen atom transfer from the antioxidant to the lipid peroxyl radical, deactivating lipid peroxyl radicals by single electron transfer and chelating transition metals to suppress the initiation of radical formation during metal-catalyzed lipid peroxidation. Therefore, AOA, reducing activity and chelating activity on Fe^{2+} of the investigated extracts should be performed. Reported values of antioxidant activity are usually given as a percent of radical scavenging activity, or obtained antioxidant activity for the tested concentration of the plant extract. For the easier and better comparison of the activities among extracts the results should be expressed as IC_{50} values, defined as the concentration of an antioxidant extract which was required to quench 50% of the initial amount of free radical under the given experimental conditions. Up to now, results obtained using *in vitro* methods for the measurement of the antioxidant capacity were dependent on applied extraction procedure. New "quencher" approach for the direct measurement of total antioxidant capacity of foods has been proposed by Gökmen et al. (2009). Apart from used *in vitro* assays for assessing the antioxidant activity of food, data on *in vivo* studies are of great importance.

Conclusions of the review of the intervention studies on bioavailability and bioefficacy of polyphenols in humans showed that bioavailability varies widely among polyphenols and, for some of compounds, among dietary sources. The polyphenols that are most well absorbed in humans are isoflavones and gallic acid, followed by catechins, flavanones, and quercetin glucosides, with different kinetics. The least well-absorbed polyphenols are the proanthocyanidins, the galloylated tea catechins, and the anthocyanins.

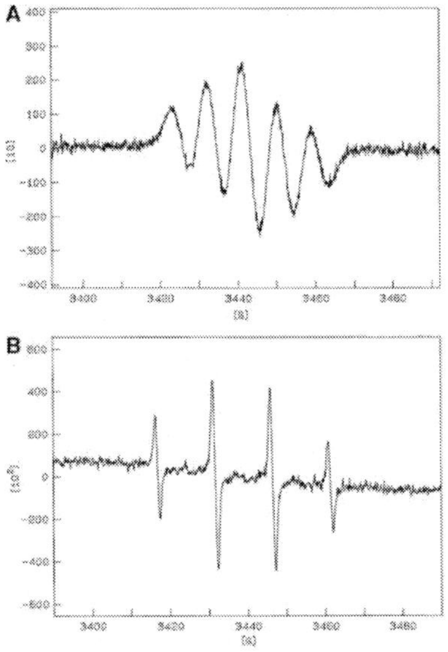

Figure 4. ESR spectra of (A) DPPH radicals and (B) DMPO-OH spin adducts (Ćetković et al., 2008).

The plasma kinetics also differ among polyphenol classes (Manach et al., 2005). According to Williamson and Manach (2005), many human intervention studies show biological effects, but the exact effects depend on the class of polyphenol used. Most of the studies were short term, and there is a necessity for longer-term studies. Furthermore, very few studies demonstrated a dose response relationship, which is also needed for convincing evidence. Finally, metabolism by microflora needs to be understood, because the gut microflora probably plays a major role in the biological activity of many polyphenols (Williamson & Manach, 2005).

The major effect of polyphenolics may be the result of their radical scavenging, and the another possible mechanism by which they act is through interaction with various enzyme systems, and furthermore, some effects may be a result of a combination of radical scavenging and an interaction with the enzyme functions (Nijveldt et al., 2001).

According to the overview of the potential hazards of polyphenol consumptions given by Mennen et al. (2005), the risk of consuming high doses of polyphenols from food naturally rich in polyphenol is considered to be low. Dietary reference intake (DRI) values do not exist for polyphenols, but bioavialability and dose-effects, including toxic levels, need to be established before the DRI. Recently, polyphenols have been discussed as „lifespan essentials“ because they are needed to achieve the full lifespan by reducing a risk of a range of chronic diseases (Williamson & Holst, 2008).

Review of the literature which support the argument that food rather than supplements should be considered when addressing the nutritional requirements, bioavalability of nutrients and health effects, is given by Jacobs et al. (2009).

4.3. Analysis of Polyphenols

Extraction of polyphenols from the sample matrix is commonly applied prior their identification and quantification using an appropriate method. The choice of an extraction method is affected by structural diversity of plant polyphenolics and the nature of the sample. Isolation of the polyphenolics from the food matrices involves 3 principal techniques that may be used:

1. Extraction using solvents
2. Solid-phase extraction
3. Supercritical extraction

The application of recently developed techniques, including microwave-assisted extraction, membrane extraction, solid-phase micro extraction and pressurized liquid or fluid extraction, broaden the possibility to obtain the representative extract for the further analysis (Escribano-Bailon & Santos-Buelga, 2003).

Hydrolysis step is often included aiming to obtain more simple chromatographic data and/or to elucidate the structure of present glycosides and esters. Hydrolysis could be acidic, alkaline or enzymatic, sometimes resulting in destruction and rearrangement of some polyphenolics. In addition, the acidic hydrolysis is sometimes applied to reflect the fate and the metabolism of polyphenolics in humans, although this approach has many disadvantages. Alkaline hydrolysis could be employed to reveal the fate of polyphenolics after the used alkali treatment in food processing. Hydrolysis conditions used in sample preparation for the chromatographic determination have been reviewed by Robards (2003).

Clean-up of the crude extracts is used to avoid potential interferences of the present carbohydrates and/or lipids on the determination of polyphenolics. It is also used to isolate targeted polyphenolic compounds, i.e. separation of oligomeric and polymeric proanthocyanidins. These methods include gel permeation and affinity chromatography, solid phase extraction, liquid/liquid extraction and precipitation.

Determination of the polyphenolics content by introducing spectrophotometric assays is often used, although these methods lack specificity. The most widely used assay for the determination of total polyphenolics in an extract is the one using Folin-Ciocalateu reagent (Singleton & Rossi, 1965). It is based on the reducing power of the phenolic hydroxyl groups and therefore all polyphenolics could be determined, but with variable sensitivity. The result is expressed as the molar equivalent of a certain polyphenolic compound which has been used for the calibration and which occures in the extract in high amount. Very often used is gallic acid equivalent (GAE). Simple, sensitive and specific spectrophotometric assays have been developed, like vanillin assay for the determination of narrow range of flavanols (monomers and olygomers) and dihydrohalcones that have a single bond at the 2,3 – position and free meta oriented hydroxyl groups on the B-ring (Sun et al., 1998, Nakamura et al., 2003).

Identification and determination of individual polyphenolic compounds is performed using liquid chromatography (HPLC). Merken and Beecher (2000) have presented a detailed tabulated review on the chromatographic conditions for the HPLC determination and the sample preparation methods of food flavanoids. In general, reversed-phase HPLC columns have been used for the separation of the compounds. As a mobile phase, acetonitrile and/or methanol in combination with water containing acid has been employed. The most frequently used acids are formic and acetic acid. Gradient elution starting with 0-20% of organic solvent, and ending with 50-100% of organic solvent is applied for a run which is usually an hour long.

New generation of reversed phase chromatography columns, with smaller particles, packed in shorter columns increase the speed of analysis and provide enough efficiency to maintain resolution equivalent to longer columns packed with larger particles. In Figure 5 is presented the separation of 17 compounds belonging to different polyphenolic classes on a short reversed phase analytical column packed with 1.8 μm silica-based particles.

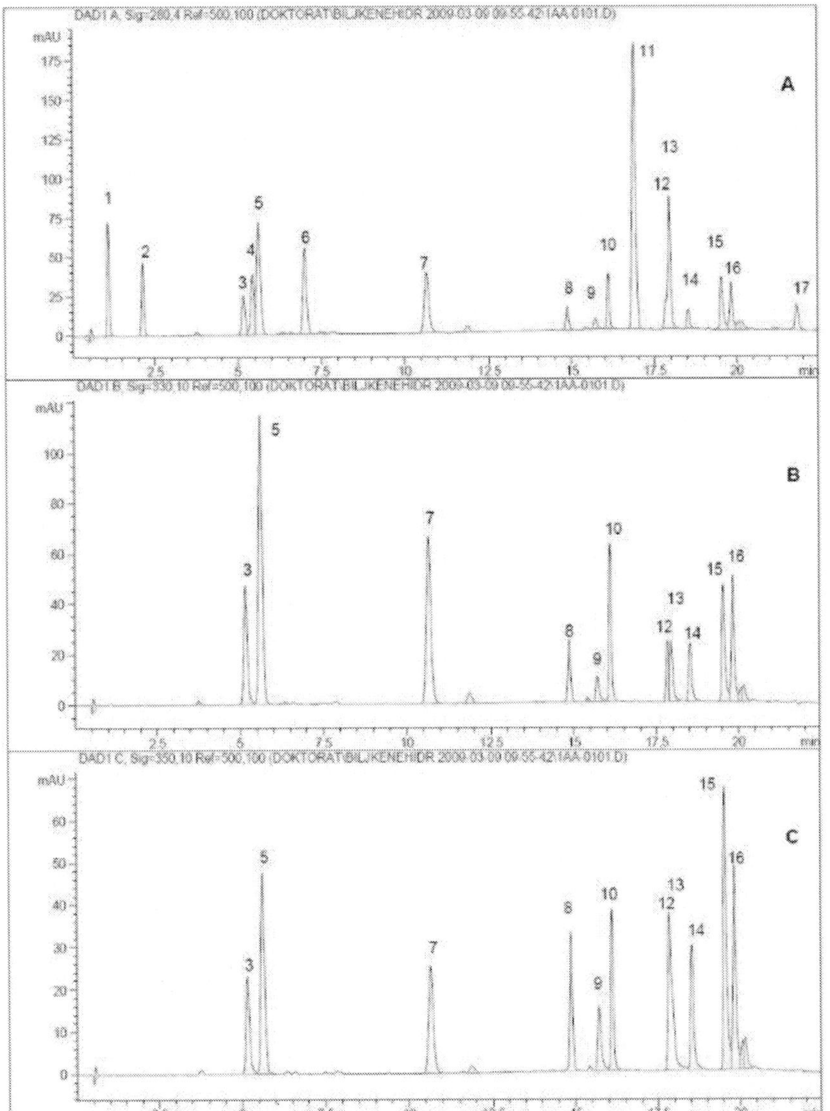

Figure 5. Chromatogram of external standard mixture, absorbance at A-280 nm, B-330 nm and C-350 nm: 1-gallic acid, 2-protocatechuic acid, 3-caffeic acid, 4-vanillic acid, 5-chlorogenic acid, 6-syringic acid, 7-ferulic acid, 8-rutin, 9-myricetin, 10-rosmarinic acid, 11- *trans*-cinnamic acid, 12-quercetin, 13-naringenin, 14-luteolin, 15-kaempferol, 16-apigenin and 17-aloe-emodin. Using Agilent 1200 series rapid resolution HPLC with Eclipse XDB-C18, 1.8 μm, 4.6 x 50 mm column, at a flow-rate of 1 mL min^{-1} and DAD detector (Mišan et al., 2009a).

Phenols absorb in UV region, and therefore the UV-VIS or diode-array (DAD) are the most often used detectors (Figure 6.). Overview of the wavelenghts used for the polyphenols (simple polyphenols, flavonoids, catechins and theaflavins, chalcones, anthocyanins and anthraquinones) detection is presented by Sakakibara et al. (2003). For the structural characterization of aglycones and substituents (sugars, acyl groups, etc.) mass spectrometry (MS) could be used as a detector. A triple-quadropole MS with an electrospray ionisation source is a powerfull tool for the characterization of the polyphenolic compounds, confirmation and identification of novel flavonoids MALDI-TOF-MS (Matrix-Assisted Laser Desorption/Ionization Time-of-Flight MS) could be used. 1D and 2D NMR spectroscopy have been used for the characterization and quality control of food. The detailed overview of spectrophotometric techniques used for flavonoid determination is given by Fossen and Andersen (2006).

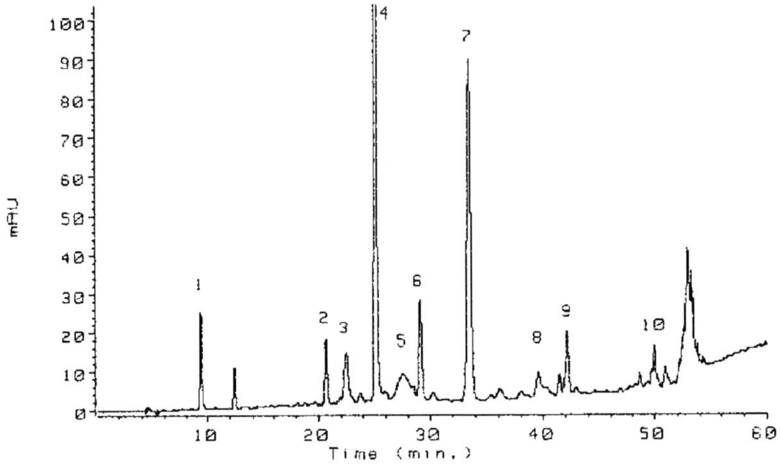

Figure 6. HPLC chromatogram of a grape seed extract, recorded at 277 nm. Peak assignment (t_R, min): 1. gallic acid (9.3); 2. procyanidin-B_3 (20.6); 3. procyanidin-B_1 (22.4); 4. (+)-catechin (25.0); 5. procyanidin-B_4 (27.5); 6. procyanidin-B_2 (29.1); 7. (-)-epicatechin (33.4); 8. procyanidin-C_1 (39.5); 9. dimer gallate (42.1); 10. procyanidin-B_5 (49.9). (Mandić et al., 2008).

Expected position of polyphenol subclasses on reversed-phase column is shown in Figure7. In one run, up to now developed HPLC methods can detect flavonoids across one, two, or three subclasses (Ćetković et al., 2007). Since food may contain several subclasses, an ideal method is needed for the simultaneous measurement of present polyphenols in a single run.

Conclusion

Although many different and potentially dangerous compounds have been isolated from many of the potentially useful plants, little emphasis is placed on their beneficial effects in comparison to their toxic and antinutritive effects. Antinutrients with beneficial effects include, among many other phytochemicals, polyphenols, tannins, phytic acid, saponins and phytosterols.

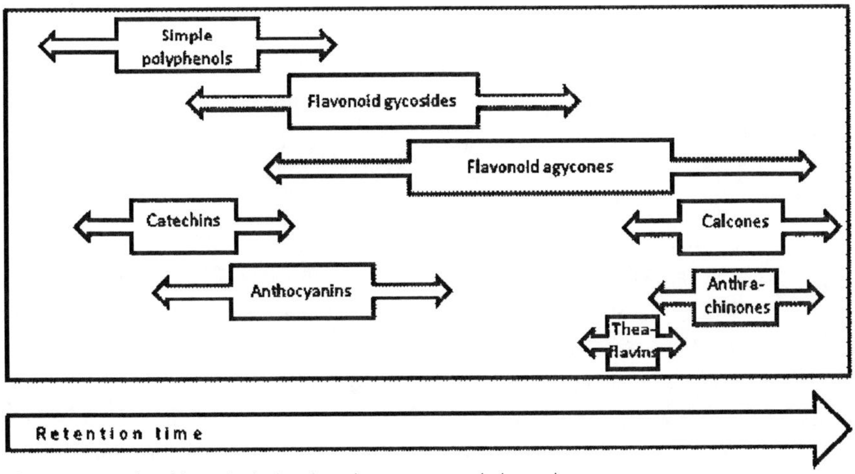

Figure 7. Expected positions of polyphenol subclasses on reversed-phase column.

The concept of food sinergy is based on a proposition that the interrelations between constituents in foods are singnificant. The food sinergy concept supports the intake of nutrient rich foods and dietary variety, rather than food suplements. The viability of the food sinergy concept is reinforced by the lack of effects for manny isolated compounds shown in clinical trials (Jacobs et al., 2009). Major focus in research of the chronic diseases prevention is placed on dietary antioxidants. Holst and Williamson (2008), propose that *in vitro* work should be driven by *in vivo* results, and not vice versa.

Modern plant biotechnology techniques including tissue culture, genetic manipulation and other plant breeding methods will play a vital role in optimising the pharmacological and other beneficial effects of the antinutrients in plants. Better understanding of the chemistry and biochemistry of phytochemicals, supported by new analytical tools may leed to a serious re-evaluation of their dietary importance.

References

Abe, I., Rohmer, M., and Prestwich, G. C. (1993). Enzymatic cyclization of squalene and oxidosqualene to sterols and triterpenes. *Chemical Reviews*, *93*, 2189-2206.

Agrawal, B.B.L. and Goldstein, I.J. (1967). Protein carbohydrate interaction. VI. Isolation of concanavalin A by specific adsorption on cross-linked dextran gels. *Biochim. Biophys. Acta*, *147*, 262-271.

Ahn, H-J., Kim, J-H., Jo, C., Kim, M-J., and Byun, M-W. (2004). Comparison of irradiated phytic acid and other antioxidants for antioxidant activity. *Food Chemistry*, *88*, 173-178.

Aletor, V.A. (1993). Allelochemicals in plant foods and feeding stuffs. Part I. Nutritional, Biochemical and Physiopathological aspects in animal production. *Vet. Human Toxicol.*, *35(1)*, 57-67.

Amzal, H., Alaoui, K., Tok, S., Errachidi, A., Charof, R., Cherrah, Y., and Benjouad, A. (2008). Protective effect of saponins from *Argania spinosa* against free radical-induced oxidative haemolysis. *Fitoterapia*, *79,* 337-344.

Attele, A. S., Wu, J. A., and Yuan, C. S. (1999). Ginseng pharmacology. Multiple constituents and multiple actions. *Biochemical Pharmacology*, *58*, 1685-1693.

Babbs, C. F. (1990). Free radicals and the etiology of colon cancer. *Free Radical Biology and Medicine*, *8*, 191–200.

Baccou, J. C., Lambert, F., and Sauvaire, Y. (1979). Spectrophotometric method for the determination of total steroidal sapogenin. *Analyst*, *102*, 458-465.

Balzarini, J.; Van Laethem, K.; Hatse, S.; Froeyen, M.; Peumans W. & Van Damme, E. *et al.*, (2005). Carbohydrate-binding agents cause deletions of highly conserved glycosylation sites in HIV gp120: a new therapeutic concept to hit the Achilles heel of HIV. *Journal of Biological Chemistry*, *280*, 41005–41014.

Battelli, M. G., Corte, E. D., and Stirpe, F. (1972). Xanthine oxidase type D (dehydrogenase) in the intestine and other organs of the rat. *Biochemical Journal*, *126*, 747-749.

Battelli, M.G. (2004). Cytotoxicity and toxicity to animals and humans of ribosome 431 inactivating proteins. *Mini Rev. Med. Chem.*, *4*, 513–521.

Baumann, E., Stoya, G., Völkner, A., Richter, W., Lemke, C., and Linss, W. (2000). Hemolysis of human erythrocytes with saponin affects the membrane structure. *Acta Histochemica*, *102*, 21-35.

Becker, W. M., and Hoekstra, W. G. (1971). The intestinal absorption of zinc. In: Skoryna, S.C. and Waldron-Edward, D. (Eds.), *Intestinal Absorption of Metal Ions, Trace Elements and Radionuclides*. Pergamon Press, New York, pp. 229-256.

Berridge, M. J., and Irvine, R. F. (1989). Inositol phosphates and cell signaling. *Nature*, *341*, 197–205.

Besso, H., Saruwatari, Y., Futamura, K., Kunihiro, K., Fuwa, T., and Tanaka, O. (1979). High performance liquid chromatographie determination of ginseng saponin by ultraviolet derivatisation. *Planta Medica*, 37, 226-333.

Besson, V., Lavaud, C., Massiot, G., Le Men-Olivier, L., Bianchi, S., Flament, P., and Datee, Y. (1989). Medicagenic acid and saponins in callus and suspension cultures of alfalfa. *Phytochemistry*, *28*, 1379-1380.

Bialy, Z., Jurzysta, M., Oleszek, W., Piacente, S., and Pizza, C. (1999). Saponins in alfalfa (*Medicago sativa* L.) root and their structural elucidation. *Journal of Agricultural and Food Chemistry*, *47*, 3185-3192.

Birgit, H., and Williamson G. (2008). Nutrients and phytochemicals: from bioavailability to bioefficacy beyond antioxidants. *Current Opinion in Biotechnology*, *19*, 73-82.

Blixt, O.; Collins, B.E.; Van Den Nieuwenhof, I.M.; Crocker, P.R. and Paulson, J.C. (2003). Sialoside specificity of the siglec family assessed using novel multivalent probes: Identification of potent inhibitors of myelin-associated glycoprotein. *J. Biol. Chem, 278(33)*, 31007–31019.

Blixt, O.; Head S. and Mondala, T. et al., (2004). Printed covalent glycan array for ligand profiling of diverse glycan binding proteins. *Proc. Natl. Acad. Sci. U. S. A, 101*, 17033–17038.

Bombardelli, E., Bonati, A., Gabetta, B., and Martinelli, E. M. (1980). Gas-liquid chromatographic method for determination of ginsenosides in *Panax ginseng*. *Journal of Chromatography A*, *196*, 121-132.

Bravo, L. (1998). Polyphenols: Chemistry, dietary sources, metabolism, and nutritional significance. *Nutrition Reviews*, *56*, 317-333.

Bruneton, J. (1995). *Pharmacognosy, Phytochemistry, Medicinal Plants*. Lavoisier Publishing, Paris, pp. 538-544.

Čanadanović-Brunet, J., Ćetković, G., Djilas, S., Tumbas, V., Bogdanović, G., Mandić A., Markov S., Cvetković D., and Čanadanović V. (2008). Radical scavenging, antibacterial and antiproliferative activities of *Melissa officinalis* L. extracts. *J. Med. Food, 11(1)*, 133-143.

Čanadanović-Brunet, J., Ćetković, G., Djilas, S., Tumbas, V., Savatović S., Mandić A., Markov S., and Cvetković D. (2009). Radical scavenging and antimicrobial activity of horsetail (*Equisetum arvense* L.) extracts. *Int. J. Food Sci. Technol.*, *44*, 269-278.

Čanadanović-Brunet, J.M., Djilas, S.M., Ćetković, G.S., Tumbas, V.T., Mandić, A.I., and Čanadanović, V.M. (2006). Antioxidant activities of different *Teucrium montanum* L. extracts. *International Journal of Food Science and Technology*, 41(6), 667-673.

Carbonaro, M., Cappelloni, M., Nicoli, S., Lucarini, M., and Carnovale, E. (1997). Solubility-digestibility relationship of legume proteins. *Journal of Agricultural and Food Chemistry*, *45*, 3387–3394.

Carnovale, E., Lugaro, E., and Lombardi-Boccia, G. (1988). Phytic acid in faba bean and pea: Effect on protein availability. *Cereal Chemistry*, *65*, 114–117.

Ćetković, G., Čanadanović-Brunet, J., Djilas, S., Savatović S., Mandić A., and Tumbas, V., (2008). Assessment of polyphenolic content and *in vitro* antiradical characteristics of apple pomace. *Food Chem.*, *109*, 340-347.

Ćetković, G., Mandić, A., Čanadanović-Brunet, J., Djilas, S., and Tumbas, V. (2007). HPLC Screening of phenolic compounds in winter savory (*Satureja montana* L.) extracts. *Journal of Liquid Chromatography and Related Technologies*, *30(2)*, 293-306.

Chen, Y., Chen, J., Luo, Z., Ma, K. ,and Chen, X. (2008). Synchronous fluorescence analysis of phytate in food. *Microchim. Acta*, *2*, 1-5.

Cheryan M. (1980). Phytic acid interactions in food systems. *CRC Critical Reviews in Food Science and Nutrition*, *13*, 297-335.

Choe, J.; Zhang, F.; Wolff, M.W.; Murhammer, D.W.; Linhardt, R.J. and Dordick, J.S. (2000). Separation of alpha-acid glycoprotein glycoforms using affinity-based reversed micellar extraction and separation, *Biotechnol. Bioeng*, *70*, 484–490.

Choi, S.H.; Lyu S.Y. & Park, W.B. (2004). Mistletoe lectin induces apoptosis and telomerase inhibition in human A253 cancer cells through dephosphorylation of Akt. *Arch. Pharm. Res., 27*, 68–76.

Chrispeels, M.J. and Raikhel, N.V. (1991). Lectins, lectin genes, and their role in plant defense. *Plant Cell.*, *3(1)*, 1-9.

Corea, G., Fattorusso, E., and Lanzotti, V. (2003). Saponins and flavonoids of *Allium triquetrum*. *Journal of Natural Products*, *66*, 1405-1411.

Croft, K.D. (1999). Antioxidant effects of plant phenolic compounds. In: T.K. Basu, N.J. Temple, and M.L. Garg, (Eds.), *Antioxidants in Human Health*, United Kingdom: CAB International.

Dai, F., Wang, J., Zhang, S., Xu, Z., and Zhang, G. (2007). Genotypic and environmental variation in phytic acid content and its relation to protein content and malt quality in barley. *Food Chemistry*, *105*, 606-611.

Dam, T.K. and Brewer, C.F. (2004). Multivalent protein–carbohydrate interactions: Isothermal titration microcalorimetry studies. *Methods Enzymol, 379*, 107–128.

Davidsson, L., Almgren, A., Jullerat, M. A., and Hurrell, R. F. (1995). Manganese absorption in humans: the effect of phytic acid and ascorbic acid in soy formula. *American Journal of Clinical Nutrition*, *62*, 984–987.

De Boland, A. R., Garner, G. B., and O'Dell, B. L. (1975). Identification and properties of phytate in cereal grains and oilseed products. *Journal of Agricultural and Food Chemistry*, *23*, 1186-1189.

De Mejía, E.G. and Prisecaru, V.I. (2005). Lectins as bioactive plant proteins: a potential in cancer treatment. *Crit. Rev. Food Sci. Nutr.*, *45*, 425–445.

De Mussi, M.N.V., Louro, M.I., de Iglesias, S.C.P.C., and Lanfer, M.U.M. (2009). Comparative study of phenolic compounds in different Brazilian rice (*Oryza sativa* L.) genotypes. *Journal of Food Composition and Analysis*, *22(5)*, 405-409.

Dexter, D. T., Carter, C. J., Wells, F. R., Javoy-Agid, F., Agid, Y., Lees, A., Jenner, P., and Marsden, C. D. (1989). Basal lipid peroxidation in substantia nigra is increased in Parkinson's disease. *Journal of Neurochemistry*, *52*, 381-389.

Dini, I., Schettino, O., Simioli, T., and Dini, A. (2001). Studies on the constituents of *Chenopodium quinoa* seeds: isolation and characterization of new triterpene saponins. *Journal of Agricultural and Food Chemistry*, *49*, 741-746.

Domon, B., Dorsaz, A. C., and Hostettmann, K. (1984). High-performance liquid chromatography of oleanane saponins. *Journal of Chromatography A*, *315*, 441-446.

Dorsch, J. A., Cook, A., Young, K. A., Anderson, J. M., Bauman, A. T., Volkmann, C. J., Murthy, P. P. N., and Raboy, V. (2003). Seed phosphorus and inositol phosphate phenotype of barley low phytic acid genotypes. *Phytochemistry*, *62*, 691–706.

Dost, K., and Tokul, O. (2006). Determination of phytic acid in wheat and wheat products by reverse phase high performance liquid chromatography. *Analytica Chimica Acta*, *558*, 22-27.

Duk, M.; Mitra, D.; Lisowska, E.; Kabat, E.A.; Sharon, N. and Lis, H. (1992). Immunochemical studies on the combining site of the A + N blood type specific Moluccella laevis lectin. *Carbohydr. Res.*, *236*, 245–258.

Eeckhout, W., and De Paepe, M. (1994). Total phosphorus, phytate-phosphorus and phytase activity in plant feedstuffs. *Animal Feed Science and Technology*, *47*, 19-29.

Elsheikh, E. A. E., Fadul, I. A., and El Tinay, A. H. (2000). Effect of cooking on anti-nutritional factors and in vitro protein digestibility (IVPD) of faba bean grown with different nutritional regimes. *Food Chemistry*, *68*, 211–212.

Escalante, A. M., Santecchia, C. B., López, S. N., Gattuso, M. A., Ravelo, A. G., Monache, F. D., Sierra, M. G., and Zacchino, S. A. (2002). Isolation of antifungal saponins from *Phytolacca tetramera*, an Argentinean species in critic risk. *Journal of Ethnopharmacology*, *82*, 29-34.

Escribano-Bailon, M., and Santos-Buelga, C. (2003). Polyphenol extraction from foods. In: C. Santos-Buelga, and G. Williamson (Eds.), *Methods in Polyphenol Analysis* (pp. 1-16), Cambridge, United Kingdom: RSC Publishing.

Estrada, A., Katselis, G. S., Laarveld, B., and Barl, B. (2000). Isolation and evaluation of immunological adjuvant activities of saponins from *Polygala senega* L. Comparative Immunology. *Microbiology and Infectious Diseases*, *23*, 27-43.

Etzler, M.E. (1986). Distribution and function of plant lectins. In I.E. Liener; N. Sharon, and I.J. Goldstein (Eds.), *The Lectins.*, pp. 371-435, San Dieg, Academic Press.

Febles, C. I., Arias, A., Hardisson, A., Rodriguez-Alvarez, C., and Sierra, A. (2002). Phytic acid level in wheat flours. *Journal of Cereal Science*, *36*, 19-23.

Fenwick, D. E., and Oakenfull, D. (1981). Saponin content of food plants and some prepared foods. *Journal of the Science of Food and Agriculture*, *34*, 186-191.

Fossen, T, and Andersen O.M. (2006). Spectroscopic techniques applied to flavonoids. In: O.M. Andersen, and K.R. Markhan (Eds.), *Flavonoids: Chemistry, Biochemistry and Application* (pp. 37-142). Boca Raton, USA: CRC Press Taylor and Francis Group.

Fox, C. H., and Eberl, M. (2002). Phytic acid (IP6), novel broad spectrum anti-neoplastic agent: a systematic review. *Complementary Therapies in Medicine*, *10*, 229–234.

Fox, M. R. S., and Tao, S. H. (1989). Antinutritive effects of phytate and other phosphorilated derivatives. *Nutrition Toxicology*, *3*, 59-62..

Freier, T.; Fleischmann, G.; Rüdiger, H. (1985). Affinity chromatography on immobilizes hog gastric mucin and ovomucoid. A general method for the isolation of lectins. *Biol. Chem. Hoppe-Seyler*, 366, 1023-1028.

Fujiwara, Y., Yahara, S., Ikeda, T., Ono, M., and Nohara, T. (2003). Cytotoxic major saponin from tomato fruits. *Chemical and Pharmaceutical Bulletin*, *51*, 234-235.

Gaidamashvili, M. and van Staden, J. (2006). Prostaglandin inhibitory activity by lectin-like proteins from South African medicinal plants. *South African Journal of Botany, 72(4)*, 661-663.

García-Estapa, R. M., Guerra-Hernández, E., and García-Villanova, B. (1999). Phytic acid content in milled cereal products and breads. *Food Research International*, *32*, 217-221.

Goldstein, J. and Hayes C.E. (1978). The lectins: carbohydrate-binding proteins of plants and animals. *Adv. Carbohydr. Chem. Biochem.*, *35*, 127–340.

Gorelik, E.; Galili U. and Raz, A. (2001) On the role of cell surface carbohydrates and their binding proteins (lectins) in tumor metastasis. *Cancer Metast. Rev.*, *20*, 245–277.

Graf, E. and Eaton, J. W. (1990). Antioxidant functions of phytic acid. *Free Radical Biology and Medicine*, *8*, 61-69.

Graf, E., and Eaton, J. W. (1993). Suppression of colonic cancer by dietary phytic acid. *Nutrition and Cancer*, *19*, 11–19.

Graf, E., Empson, K. L., and Eaton, J. W. (1987). Phytic acid. A natural antioxidant. *Journal of Biological Chemistry*, *262*, 11647-11650.

Grenby, T. H. (1991). Intense sweeteners for the food industry: an overview. *Trends in Food Science and Technology*, *2*, 2-6.

Hallberg, L., Brune, M., and Rossander, L. (1989). Iron absorption in man: ascorbic acid and dose-dependent inhibition by phytate. *American Journal of Clinical Nutrition*, *49*, 140–144.

Halliwell, B., and Aruoma, O. I. (1991). DNA damage by oxygen-derived species. Its mechanism and measurement in mammalian systems. *FEBS Letters*, *281*, 9-19.

Harborne, J.B. (1989). *Methods in Plant biochemistry, I: Plant Phenolics*. London, United Kingdom: Academic Press.

Harland, B. F. and Oberleas, D. (1977). A modified method for phytate analysis using an ion-exchange procedure: application to textured vegetable proteins. *Cereal Chemistry*, *54*, 827-832.

Harland, B. F., and Harland, J. (1980). Fermentative reduction of phytate in rye, white and whole wheat breads. *Cereal Chemistry*, *57*, 226-229.

Harland, B. F., Morris, E. R., and Eugene, R. (1995). Phytate: A good or a bad food component? *Nutrition Research*, *15*, 733–754.

Haug, W., and Lantzsch, H.-J. (1983). Sensitive method for the rapid determination of phytate in cereals and cereal products. *Journal of the Science of Food and Agriculture*, *34*, 1423-1426.

Heng, L., Vincken, J.-P., van Koningsveld, G. A., Legger, L., Gruppen, H., van Boekel, M. A. J. S., Roozen, J. P., and Voragen, A. G. J. (2006). Bitterness of saponins and their content in dry peas. *Journal of the Science of Food and Agriculture*, *86*, 1225-1231.

Hídvégi, M., and Lásztity, R. (2002). Phyitic acid content of cereals and legumes and interaction with proteins. *Periodica Polytechnic Chemical Engineering*, *46*, 59-64.

Hirabayashi, J. (2008). Concept, strategy and realization of lectin-based glycan profiling. *J. Biochem.*, *144*, 139–147.

Hirose, M., Ozaki, K., Tabaka, K., Fukushima, S., Shirai, T., and Ito, N. (1991). Modifying effects of the naturally occurring antioxidants g-oryzanol, phytic acid, tannic acid and *n*-tririacontane-16,18-dione in a rat wide-spectrum organ carcinogenesis model. *Carcinogenesis*, *12*, 1917–1921.

Hjorth, R. (1997). Expanded-bed adsorption in industrial bioprocessing: recent developments. *Trends Biotechnol*, *15*, 230–235.

Hostettmann, K., and Marston, A. (2005). *Saponins. Chemistry and Pharmacology of Natural Products*. Cambridge University Press, Cambridge.

Huong, N. T. T., Matsumoto, K., Kasai, R., Yamasaki, K., and Watanabe, H. (1998). *In vitro* antioxidant activity of Vietnamese ginseng saponin and its components. *Biological and Pharmaceutical Bulletin*, *21*, 978-981.

Jacobs, D.R., Jr, Gross M.D, and Tapsell, L.C. (2009). Food synergy: an operational concept for understanding nutrition. *Am. J. Clinical Nutrition*, *89*, 1543S - 1548S.

Jurzysta, M. (1979). Hemolytic micromethod for rapid estimation of toxic alfalfa saponins. *Acta Agrobotanica*, *32*, 5-11.

Just, M. J., Recio, M. C., Giner, R. M., Cuéllar, M. J., Māñez, S., Bilia, A. R., and Ríos, J.-L. (1998). Anti-inflammatory activity of unusual lupine saponins from *Bupleurum fruticescens*. *Planta Medica*, *64*, 404-407.

Kaizuka, H., and Takahashi, K. (1983). High-performance liquid chromatographic system for a wide range of naturally occurring glycosides. *Journal of Chromatography A*, *258*, 135-146.

Karunaratne, A. M., Amerasinghe, P. H., Sadagopa Ramanujam, V. M., Sandstead, H. H., and Perera, P. A. J. (2008). Zinc, iron and phytic acid levels of some popular foods consumed by rural children in Sri Lanka. *Journal of Food Composition and Analysis*, *21*, 481– 488.

Kataria, A., Chauhan, B. M., and Punia, D. (1989). Antinutrients and protein digestibility (*in vitro*) of mungbean as affected by domestic processing and cooking. *Food Chemistry*, *32*, 9-17.

Katayama, T. (1995). Effect of dietary sodium phytate on the hepatic and serum levels of lipids and on the hepatic activities of NADPH-generating enzymes in rats fed on sucrose. *Bioscience and Biotechnological Biochemistry*, *59*, 1159–1160.

Killeen, G. F., Madigan, C. A., Connolly, C. R., Walsh, G. A., Clark, C., Hynes, M. J., Timmins, B. F., James, P., Headon, D. R., and Power, R. F. (1998). Antimicrobial saponins of *Yucca schidigera* and the implications of their in vitro properties for their in vivo impact. *Journal of Agricultural and Food Chemistry*, *46*, 3178-3186.

Kinjo, J., Yokomizo, K., Hirakawa, T., Shii, Y., Nohara, T., and Uyeda, M. (2000). Anti-herpes virus activity of fabaceous triterpenoidal saponins. *Biological and Pharmaceutical Bulletin*, *23*, 887-889.

Koziol, M. J. (1991). Afrosimetric estimation of threshold saponin concentration for bitterness in quinoa (*Chenopodium quinoa* Willd). *Journal of the Science of Food and Agriculture*, *54*, 211-219.

Kuwano, M., Ohyama, A., Tanaka, Y., Mimura, T., Takaiwa, F., and Yoshida, K. T. (2006). Molecular breeding for transgenic rice with low-phytic-acid phenotype through manipulating myo-inositol 3-phosphate synthase gene. *Molecular Breeding*, *18*, 263–272.

Landsteiner, K.; van der Scheer, J. (1931). On the specifity of serological reactions with simple chemical compounds (inhibition reactions). *J. Exp. Med*, *54*, 295-305.

Lannooa, N.E. & Van Damme, J.M. Rewiev, Nucleocytoplasmic plant lectins, *Biochimica et Biophysica Acta (BBA)* - General Subjects, Article in Press, Corrected Proof.

Larson, S. R., Rutger, J. N., Young, K. A., and Raboy, V. (2000). Isolation and genetic mapping of a non-lethal rice (*Oryzae sativa* L.) low phytic acid mutation. *Crop Science*, *40*, 1397–1405.

Larsson, M., and Sandberg, A.-S. (1991). Phytate reduction in bread containing oat flour, oat bran and rye bran. *Journal of Cereal Science*, *14*, 141-149.

Lasztity, R., Hidvegi, M., and Bata, A. (1998). Saponins in food. *Food Reviews International*, *14*, 371-390.

Latta, M., and Eskin, M. (1980). A simple and rapid colorimetric method for phytate determination. *Journal of Agricultural and Food Chemistry*, *28*, 1313-1315.

Lee, B. J., Hendricks, D. G., and Cornforth, D. P. (1998). Antioxidant effects of carnosine and phytic acid in model beef system. *Journal of Food Science*, *63*, 394-398.

Lee, K. J., Choi, C. Y., Chung, Y. C., Kim, Y. S., Ryu, S. Y., Roh, S. H., and Jeong, H. G. (2004). Protective effect of saponins derived from roots of *Platycodon grandiflorum* on *tert*-butyl hydroperoxide-induced oxidative hepatotoxicity. *Toxicology Letters*, *147*, 271-282.

Lee, S.-J., Sung, J.-H., Lee, S.-J., Moon, C.-K., and Lee, B.-H. (1999). Antitumor activity of a novel ginseng saponin metabolite in human pulmonary adenocarcinoma cells resistant to cisplatin. *Cancer Letters*, *144*, 39-43.

Leenhardt, F., Levrat-Verny, M. A., Chanliaud, E., and Remesy, C. (2005). Moderate decrease of pH by sourdough fermentation is sufficient to reduce phytate content of whole wheat flour through endogenous phytase activity. *Journal of Agricultural and Food Chemistry*, *53*, 98-102.

Lehrfeld, J. (1989). High-performance liquid chromatography analysis of phytic acid on a pH-stable, macroporous polymer column. *Cereal Chemistry*, *66*, 510-515.

Lestienne, I., Icard-Vernière, C., Mouquet, C., Picq, C., and Trèche, S. (2005). Effects of soaking whole cereal and legume seeds on iron, zinc and phytate contents. *Food Chemistry*, *89*, 421–425.

Li, D. W., Lee, E. B., Kang, S. S., Hyun, J. E., and Whang, W. K. (2002). Activity-guided isolation of saponins from *Kalopanax pictus* with anti-inflammatory activity. *Chemical and Pharmaceutical Bulletin*, *50*, 900-903.

Li, J., Huang, M., Teoh, H., and Man, R. Y. K. (1998). Panax quinquefolium saponins protects low density lipoproteins from oxidation. *Life Sciences*, *64*, 53-62.

Liang, J., Han, B.-Z., Nout, M. J. R., and Hamer, R. J. (2008). Effects of soaking, germination and fermentation on phytic acid, total and *in vitro* soluble zinc in brown rice. *Food Chemistry*, *110*, 821-828.

Liang, P.H.; Wu, C.Y.; Greenberg W.A. and Wong, C.H. (2008). Glycan arrays: biological and medical applications. *Curr. Opin. Chem. Biol.*, *12*, 86–92.

Lin, L., Ockenden, I., and Lott, J. N. A. (2005). The concentrations and distribution of phytic acid-phosphorus and other mineral nutrients in wild-type and low phytic acid1-1 (*lpa1-1*) corn (*Zea mays* L.) grains and grain parts. *Canadian Journal of Botany*, *83*, 131-141.

Lis, H. and Sharon, N. (1981). Affinity chromatography for the purification of lectins. *J. Chromatogr,* 215, 361-372.

Liu, Z., Cheng, F., and Zhang, G. (2005). Grain phytic acid content in japonica rice as affected by cultivar and environment and its relation to protein content. *Food Chemistry*, *89*, 49-52.

Lolas, G. M., and Markakis, P. (1975). Phytic acid and other phosphorus compounds in beans. *Journal of Agriculture Food Chemistry*, *23*, 13-15.

Lönnerdal, B. (2000). Dietary factors influencing zinc absorption. *Journal of Nutrition*, *30*(5S Suppl.), 1378s–1383s.

Lopez, H. W., Duclos, V., Coudray, C., Krespine, V., Feillet-Coudray, C., Messager, A., Demigne, C., and Remesy, C. (2003). Making bread with sourdough improves mineral bioavailability from reconstituted whole wheat flour in rats. *Nutrition*, *19*, 524-530.

Lyu, S.Y.; Choi, S.H. & Park, W.B. (2002). Korean mistletoe lectin-induced apoptosis in hepatocarcinoma cells is associated with inhibition of telomerase via mitochondrial controlled pathway independent of p53. *Arch. Pharm. Res., 25*, 93–101.

Ma, G. (2007). Iron and zinc deficiencies in China: Existing problems and possible solutions. Ph.D. Thesis. Wageningen University, Wageningen.

Maga, J. (1982). Phytate: its chemistry, occurrence, food interactions, nutritional significance, and methods of analysis. *Journal of Agricultural and Food Chemistry*, *30*, 1-9.

Mahgoub, S. E. O., and Elhag, S. A. (1998). Effect of milling, soaking, malting, heat-treatment and fermentation on phytate level of four Sudanese sorghum cultivars. *Food Chemistry*, *61*, 77–80.

Manach, C., Williamson, G., Morand, C., Scalbert, A., and Rémésy, C. (2005). Bioavailability and bioefficacy of polyphenols in humans. I. Review of 97 bioavailability studies. *Am. J. Clin. Nutr., 81(suppl)*, 230S– 242S.

Mandic, A.I., Đilas, S.M., Ćetković, G.S., Čanadanović-Brunet, J.M., and Tumbas, V.T. (2008). Polyphenolic composition and antioxidant activities of grape seed extract. *International Journal of Food Properties*, *11*, 713-726.

Mansour, E. H., Dworschák, E., Lugasi, A., Gaál, Ö., Barna, É., and Gergely, A. (1993). Effect of processing on the antinutritive factors and nutritive value of rapeseed products. *Food Chemistry*, *47*, 247-252.

Matsuura, H. (2001). Saponins in garlic as modifiers of the risk of cardiovascular disease. *The Journal of Nutrition*, *131*, 1000S–1005S.

Mega, T. & Hase, S. (1991). Determination of lectin-sugar binding constants by microequilibrium dialysis coupled with high performance liquid chromatography. *J. Biochem., 109(4)*, 600–603.

Mennen, L.I, Walker, R., Bennetau-Pelissero, C., and Scalbert, A. (2005). Risks and safety of polyphenol consumption. *Am. J. Clinical Nutrition*, *81*, 326S - 329S.

Michl, G., Abebe, D., Bucar, F., Debella, A., Kunert, O., Schmid, M. G., Mulatau, E., and Haslinger, E. (2000). New triterpenoid saponins from *Achyranthes aspera* Linn. *Helvetica Chimica Acta*, *83*, 359-363.

Midorikawa, K., Murata, M., Oikawa, S., Hiraku, Y., and Kawanishi, S. (2001). Protective effect of phytic acid on oxidative DNA damage with reference to cancer chemoprevention. *Biochemical and Biophysical Research Communications*, *288*, 552-557.

Mikkat, U.; Damm, I.; Kirchhoff, F.; Albrecht, E.; Nebe B. and Jonas, L. (2001). Effects of lectins on CCK-8-stimulated enzyme secretion and differentiation of the rat pancreatic cell line AR42J. *Pancreas, 23,* 368–374.

Milgate, J., and Roberts, D. C. K. (1995). The nutritional and biological significance of saponins. *Nutrition Research*, *15*, 1223-1249.

Milić, B.Lj., Đilas, S.M., Čanadanović-Brunet, J.M. and Sakač, M.B. (2000). *Biljni polifenoli.* Novi Sad, Serbia: Univerzitet u Novom Sadu, Tehnološki fakultet.

Mimaki, Y., Yokosuka, A., Kuroda, M., and Sashida, Y. (2001). Cytotoxic activities and structure-cytotoxic relationships of steroidal saponins. *Biological and Pharmaceutical Bulletin*, *24*, 1286-1289.

Minihane, A. M., and Rimbach, G. (2002). Iron absorption and the iron binding and anti-oxidant properties of phytic acid. *International Journal of Food Science and Technology*, *37*, 741-742.

Mišan, A., Mandić, A., Mimica-Dukić, N., Sakač, M., Sedej, I., and Milovanović, I. (2009a). HPLC determination of medicinal plant phenolics in crude extracts. *4th International Symposium on Recent Advances in Food Analysis*, Prague, Czech Republic: 4-6 November, Book of Abstracts, pp. 556.

Mišan, A., Šimurina, O., Psodorov, Đ., Sakač, M., Sedej, I., Mandić, A., and Kevrešan, Ž. (2009b). Evaluation of antioxidant activity of medical plant extracts and their application in biscuits. In D. Mihailović, and M. Vojinović-Miloradov (Eds.) *Environmental, Health and Humanity Issues in the Down Danubian Region, Multidisciplinary Approaches* (pp. 165-171) Singapore: World Scientific Publishing Co. Pte. Ltd.

Mišan, A., Štajner, D., Kraljević-Balalić, M., Kakaš, M., and Kapor A. (2006). Antioxidative enzyme activities in wheat genotypes. *Cereal Research Communications*, *34*, 997-1004.

Miyakoshi, M., Tamura, Y., Masuda, H., Mizutani, K., Tanaka, O., Ikeda, T., Ohtani, K., Kasai, R., and Yamasaki, K. (2000). Antiyeast steroidal saponins from *Yucca schidigera* (Mohave yucca), a new anti-food-deteriorating agent. *Journal of Natural Products*, *63*, 332-338.

Miyamoto, S., Kuwata, G., Imai, M., Nagao, A., and Terao, J. (2000). Protective effect of phytic acid hydrolysis products on ironinduced lipid peroxidation of liposomal membranes. *Lipids*, *35*, 1411–1413.

Moure, A., Cruz, J.M., Franco, D., Domínguez, J.M., Sineiro, J., Domínguez, H., Núñez M.J., and Parajó, J.C. (2001). Natural antioxidants from residual sources. *Food Chemistry*, *72* 145-171.

Muraoka, S., and Miura, T. (2004). Inhibition of xanthine oxidase by phytic acid and its antioxidative action. *Life Sciences*, 74, 1691-1700.

Nachbar, M.S. & Oppenheim, J.D. (1980). Lectins in the United States diet: a survey of lectins in commonly consumed foods and a review of the literature. *The American Journal of Clinical Nutrition, 33*, 513-521.

Nakamura, Y., Tsuji, S., and Tonogai, Y. (2003). Analysis of proanthocyanidins in grape seed extracts. Health foods and grape seed oils. *Journal of Health Science*, *49*, 45-54.

Nasi, A.; Picariello, G. & Ferranti, P. (2009). Proteomic approaches to study structure, functions and toxicity of legume seeds lectins. Perspectives for the assessment of food quality and safety. *Journal of Proteomics, 72(3),* 527-538.

Natubu, N. R., and Markakis, P. (1983). Effect of fermentation time on the inositol phosphates of bread. *Journal of Food Science*, *48*, 262-263.

Nijveldt, R.J., van Nood, E., van Hoorn, D.E.C., Boelens, P.G., van Norren, K. and van Leeuwen., P.A.M. (2001). Flavonoids: a review of probable mechanisms of action and potential applications. *Am. J. Clin. Nutr.*, *74*, 418-425.

Nzowa, L. K., Barboni, L., Teponno, R. B., Ricciutelli, M., Lupidi, G., Quassinti, L., Bramucci, M., and Tapondjou, L. A. (2010). Rheediinosides A and B, two antiproliferative and antioxidant triterpene saponins from *Entada rheedii*. *Phytochemistry*, *71*, 254-261.

O'Dell, B. L., de Boland, A. R., and Koirtyohann, S. T. (1972). Distribution of phytate and nutritionally important elements among the morphological components of cereal grains. *Journal of Agricultural and Food Chemistry*, *20*, 718–721.

Oakenfull, D., and Sidhu, G. S. (1990). Could saponins be a useful treatment for hypercholesterolaemia? *European Journal of Clinical Nutrition*, *44*, 79-88.

Obata, T. (2003). Phytic acid suppresses 1-methyl-4-phenylpyridinium ion-induced hydroxyl radical generation in rat striatum. *Brain Research*, *978*, 241-244.

Oberleas, D., and Harland, B. F. (1981). Phytate content of foods: Effect on dietary Zn bioavailability. *Journal of American Dietetic Association*, *79*, 433-436.

Oda, K., Matsuda, H., Murakami, T., Katayama, S., Ohgitani, T., and Yoshikawa, M. (2000). Adjuvant and haemolytic activities of 47 saponins derived from medicinal and food plants. *Biological Chemistry*, *381*, 67-74.

Oleszek, W. A. (2002). Chromatographic determination of plant saponins. *Journal of Chromatography A*, *967*, 147-162.

Oleszek, W., Junkuszew, M., and Stochmal, A. (1999). Determination and toxicity of saponins from *Amaranthus cruentus* seeds. *Journal of Agriculture and Food Chemistry*, *47*, 3685-3687.

Osagie, A.U. (1998). Antinutritional factors. In A.U. Osagie, & O.U. Eka (Eds.), *Nutrition Quality of Plant Foods. Benin City*, pp. 229–230, Post Harvest Research Unit Publication.

Pallauf, J., Pippig, S., Most, E., and Rimbach, G. (1999). Supplemental sodium phytate and microbial phytase influence iron availability in growing rats. *Journal of Trace Elements in Medicine and Biology*, *13*, 134–140.

Parab, R. S., and Mengi, S. A. (2002). Hypolipidemic activity of *Acorus calamus* L. in rats. *Fitoterapia*, *73*, 451-455.

Park, W.-Z., Matsui, T., Yano, F., and Yano, H. (2000). Heat treatment of rapeseed meal increases phytate flow into the duodenum of sheep. *Animal Feed Science and Technology*, *88*, 31-37.

Paulson, J.C.; Blixt, O. and Collins, B.E., (2006). Sweet spots in functional glycomics. *Nat. Chem. Biol., 2,* 238–248.

Petersen, T. G., and Palmqvist, B. (1990). Utilizing column selectivity in developing a high-performance liquid chromatographic method for ginsenoside assay. *Journal of Chromatography A, 504,* 139-149.

Petit, P. R., Sauvaire, Y. D., Hillaire-Buys, D. M., Leconte, O. M., Baissac, Y. G., Posin, G. R., and Ribes, G. R. (1995). Steroid saponins from fenugreek seeds: extraction, purification, and pharmacological investigation on feeding behaviour and plasma cholesterol. *Steroids, 60,* 674-680.

Peumans, W.J. & Van Damme, E.J.M. (1995). Lectins as plant defense proteins. *Plant Physiol., 109,* 347–352.

Phillippy, B.Q., and Graf, E. (1997). Antioxidant functions of inositol 1,2,3-trisphosphate and inositol 1,2,3,6-tetrakisphosphate, *Free Radical Biology and Medicine, 22,* 939–946.

Plattner, V.E.; Wagner, M.; Ratzinger, G.; Gabor, F. and Wirth, M. (2008). Targeted drug delivery: binding and uptake of plant lectins using human 5637 bladder cancer cells. *Eur. J. Pharm. Biopharm., 70,* 572–576.

Price, K. R., Griffiths, N. M., Curl, C. L., and Fenwick, G. R. (1985). Undesirable sensory properties of the dried pea (*Pisum sativum*). The role of saponins.. *Food Chemistry, 17,* 105-115.

Price, K. R., Johnson, I. T., and Fenwick, G. R. (1987). The chemistry and biological significance of saponins in foods and feedstuffs. *Critical Reviews in Food Science and Nutrition, 26,* 27-135.

Raboy, V. (2001). Seeds for a better future: 'Low phytate' grains help to overcome malnutrition and reduce pollution. *Trends in Plant Science, 6,* 458–462.

Raboy, V. (2007). Seed phosphorus and the development of low-phytate crops. In: Turner, B.L., Richardson, A.E., and Mullaney, E.J. (Eds.), *Inositol Phosphates. Linking Agriculture and the Environment.* CAB International, Wallingford, Oxfordshire, UK, pp. 111–132.

Raboy, V., Gerbasi, P. F., Young, K. A., Stoneberg, S. D., Pickett, S. G., Bauman, A. T., Murthy, P. P. N., Sheridan, W. F., and Ertl, D. S. (2000). Origin and seed phenotype of maize low phytic acid 1-1 and low phytic acid 2-1. *Plant Physiology, 124,* 355-368.

Reddy, M. B., Hurrell, R. F., Juillerat, M. A., Cook, J. D. (1996). The influence of different protein sources on phytate inhibition of nonheme-iron absorption in humans. *American Journal of Clinical Nutrition, 63,* 203-207.

Rhou, J. R., and Erdman, J. V. (1995). Phytic acid in health and disease. *CRC Critical Reviews in Food Science and Nutrition, 35,* 495-502.

Ribereau-Gayon, P. (1972). *Plan Phenolics,* Edinburgh, United Kingdom: Oliver and Boydd.

Rickard, E. S., and Thompson, L. U. (1997). Interactions and effects of phytic acid. In F. Shahidi (Ed.), *Antinutrients and Phytochemicals in Foods.* Washington, DC: American Chemical Society.

Rimbach, G., and Pallauf, J. (1998). Phytic acid inhibits free radical formation in vitro but does not affect liver oxidant or antioxidant status in growing rats. *Journal of Nutrition, 128,* 950-955.

Robards, K. (2003). Strategies for the determination of bioactive phenols in plants, fruit and vegetables. *Journal of Chromatography A., 1000,* 657-691.

Robards, K., Prenzler, P., Tucker, G., Swatsitang, P., and Glover, W. (1999). Phenolic compounds and their role in oxidative processes in fruits. *Food Chemistry*, *66*, 401-436.

Rüdiger H. & Gabius, H-J. (2001). Rewiev Plant lectins: Occurrence, biochemistry, functions and applications. *Glycoconjugate Journal*, *18*, 589-613.

Rüdiger, H. (1977). Purification and properties of blood group specific lectins from *Vicia cracca*. *Eur. J. Biochem.*, *72*, 317-322.

Saastamoinen, M., Plaami, S., and Kumpulainen, J. (1992). Beta-Glucan and phytic acid content of oats cultivated in Finland. *Acta Agriculturae Scandinavica. Section B: Soil and Plant Science*, *42*, 6–11.

Saha, P. R., Weaver, C. M., and Mason, A. C. (1994). Mineral bioavailability in rats from intrinsically labeled whole wheat flour of various phytate levels. *Journal of Agriculture and Food Chemistry*, *42*, 2531-2535.

Sakač, B.M., Gyura, F.J., Mišan, Č.A., and Šereš, I.Z. (2009). Antioxidant properties of sugarbeet fibers. *Sugar Industry, 134*, 418-425.

Sakač, M., Filipović, S., Ristić, M., and Kormanjoš, Š. (2007). Thermal treatment and antinutritients in rapeseed, I International congress "Food Technology, Quality and Safety", XII Symposium "Feed Technology", Proceedings, 240-250, Novi Sad, Serbia.

Sakač, M., Mišan, A., Tumbas, V., Mandić, A., Kevrešan, Ž., and Sedej, I. (2008). Antioxidative effect of phytic acid on peroxyl radical formation, *International Scientific Conference on Cereals – their products and processing, Proceedings*, 207-213, Debrecen, Hungary.

Sakakibara, H., Honda, Y., Nakagawa, S., Ashida, H., and Kanazawa K. (2003). Simultaneous determination of all polyphenols in vegetables, fruits, and teas. *Journal of Agricultural and Food Chemistry*, *51*, 571-581.

Sandberg, A. S., Carlsson, N. G., and Svanberg, U. (1989). E€ects of inositol tri-, tetra-, penta-, hexaphosphates on *in vitro* estimation of iron availability. *Journal of Food Science*, *54*, 159-186.

Sandberg, A. S., Hulthen, L. R., and Turk, M. (1996). Dietary *Aspergillus niger* phytase increases iron absorption in humans. *Journal of Nutrition*, *126*, 476–480.

Sandström, B., and Lönnerdal, B. (1989). Promoters and antagonists of zinc absorption. In: Mills CF (ed.), *Zinc in Human Biology*. New York: Springer Verlag, pp. 59–68.

Sandström, B., Almgren, A., Kivistö, B., Cederblad, Å. (1987). Zinc absorption in humans from meals based on rye, barley, oatmeal, triticale and whole wheat. *Journal of Nutrition*, *117*, 1898-1902.

Schumacher, K.; Schneider, B.; Reich, G.; Stiefel, T.; Stoll G. and Bock, P.R.et al., (2003). Influence of postoperative complementary treatment with lectin-standardized mistletoe extract on breast cancer patients: a controlled epidemiological multicentric retrospective cohort study. *Anticancer Res.*, *23*, 5081–5087.

Shamsuddin, A. M. (2002). Anti-cancer function of phytic acid. *International Journal of Food Science and Technology*, *37*, 769-782.

Shamsuddin, A. M., Baten, A., and Lahwani, N. D. (1992) Effect of inositol hexaphosphate on growth and differentiation in K-562 erythroleukemia cell line. *Cancer Letters*, *64*, 195–202.

Shamsuddin, A. M., Vucenik, I., and Cole, K. E. (1997). IP6: A novel anti-cancer agent. *Life Science*, *61*, 343-354.

Shamsuddin, A. M., Yang, G. Y., and Vucenik, I. (1996) Novel anti-cancer functions of IP6: growth inhibition and differentiation of human mammary cancer cell lines in vitro. *Anticancer Research*, *16*, 3287–3292.

Shany, S., Gestetner, B., Birk, Y., and Bondi, A. (1970). Lucerne saponins III. – Effect of lucerne saponins on larval growth and their detoxification by various sterols. *Journal of the Science of Food and Agriculture*, *21*, 508-510.

Shi, J., Wang, H., Schellin, K., Li, B., Faller, M., Stoop, J. M., Meeley, R. B., Ertl, D. S., Ranch, J. P., and Glassman, K. (2007). Embryo-specific silencing of a transporter reduces phytic acid content of maize and soybean seeds. *Nature Biotechnology*, *25*, 930–937.

Siddhuraju, P., Makkar, H. P. S., and Becker, K. (2002). The effect of ionizing radiation on antinutritional factors and the nutritional value of plant materials with reference to human and animal food. *Food Chemistry*, *78*, 187–205.

Singleton, V.L. and Rossi, Jr. J.A. (1965). Colorimetry of total phenolics with phosphomolybdic-phosphotungstic acid reagent. *American Journal of Enology and Viticulture.*, *16*, 144-158.

Soetan, K. O. and Oyewole, O. E. (2009). The need for adequate processing to reduce the anti-nutritional factors in plants used as human foods and animal feeds: A review. *African Journal of Food Science, 3(9)*, 223-232.

Sparg, S. G., Light, M. E., and van Staden, J. (2004). Biological activities and distribution of plant saponins. *Journal of Ethnopharmacology*, *94*, 219-243.

Štajner, D., Čanadanović-Brunet, J., and Pavlović, A. (2004). *Allium schoenoprasum* L., as natural antioxidant, *Phytotherapy Research*, *18*, 522-524.

Štajner, D., Ćirin-Novta, V., and Pavlović, A. (1998). Scavenger properties of synthetic naphthenic methyl esters. *Z. Naturforsch C*, *63*, 871- 875.

Stodolak, B., Starzyńska, A., Czyszczoń, M., and Żyła, K. (2007). The effect of phytic acid on oxidative stability of raw and cooked meat. *Food Chemistry*, *101*, 1041-1045.

Sun, B.S., Ricardo-da-Silva J.M. and Spranger, I. (1998b). Critical factors of vanillin assay for catechins and proanthocyanidins. *Journal of Agricultural and Food Chemistry*, *46*, 4267-4274.

Tangendjaja, B., Buckle, K. A., and Wootton, M. (1980). Analysis of phytic acid by high-performance liquid chromatography. *Journal of Chromatography A*, *197*, 274-277.

Tao, S. H., Fox, M. R. S., Phillipy, B. Q., Fry, B. E. Jr., and Johnson, M. R. (1986). Effect of inositol phosphates on mineral utilization. *Federation Proceedings*, *45*, 819-823.

Tateno, H.; Nakamura-Tsuruta, S. & Hirabayashi, J. (2007). Frontal affinity chromatography: sugar–protein interactions. *Nat. Protoc.*, *2*, 2529–2537.

Thompon, L. U. (1993). Potential health benefits and problems associated with antinutrients in foods. *Food Research International*, *26*, 131–149.

Thompson, D. B., and Erdman, J. W. Jr (1984). The effect of soy protein isolate in the diet on retention by the rat of iron from radiolabeled test meals. *Journal of Nutrition*, *114*, 307-311.

Thompson, L. U., and Zhang, L. (1991). Phyitic acid and minerals: effect on early markers of risk for mammary and colon carcinogenesis. *Carcinogenesis*, *12*, 2041-2045.

Turnland, J. R., King, J. C., Keyes, W. R., Gong, B., and Michael, M. (1984). A stable isotope study of zinc absorption in young men: Effect of phytate and alpha-cellulose. *American Journal of Clinical Nutrition*, *40*, 1071-1077.

Tyler, V. E., Brady, L. R., and Robbers, J. E. (1981). *Pharmacognosy* (8th ed.) Lea and Ferbiger (eds.), Philadelphia, p. 67.

Uchida, T., Imai, M., Kuwata, G., Terao, J., Yoshida, N., Gotoh, N., and Wada, S. (2001). Antioxidant activity of phytic acid and its hydrolysis products for marine lipid. *Journal of the Japanese Society of Food Science and Technology*, *48*, 726–732.

Uematsu, Y., Hirata, K., and Saito, K. (2000). Spectrophotometric determination of saponin in Yucca extract used as food additive. *Journal of AOAC International*, *83*, 1451-1454.

Valentiner, U.; Fabian, S.; Schumacher U. & Leathem, A.J. (2003). The influence of dietary lectins on the cell proliferation of human breast cancer cell lines *in vitro*. *Anticancer Res.*, *23*, 1197–1206.

Van Damme, E.J.M.; Barre, A.; Rougé P. & Peumans, W.J. (2004). Cytoplasmic/nuclear plant lectins: a new story. *Trends Plant Sci.*, *9*, 484–489.

Van Damme, E.J.M.; Lannoo, N. and Peumans, W.J. (2008). Plant lectins. *Adv. Bot. Res.*, *48*, 107–209.

Vasconcelos, I.M. and Oliveira, J.T. (2004). Antinutritional properties of plant lectins. *Toxicon*, *44*, 385-403.

Vural, G., Arda, S., Vincenzo F. (2009). Direct measurement of the total antioxidant capacity of foods: the 'QUENCHER' approach. *Trends in Food Science and Technology*, *20*, 278-288.

Weaver, C. M., and Kannan, S. (2002). Phytate and mineral bioavailability. In: Reddy, N. R. and Sathe, S. K. (Eds.), *Food Phytates*. CRC Press LLC, Boca Raton, pp. 211–223.

Weaver, C. M., Heaney, R. P., Martin, B. R., and Fitzsimmons, M. L. (1991). Human calcium absorption from whole-wheat products. *Journal of Nutrition*, *121*, 1769–1775.

Williamson, G. and Holst B. (2008). Dietary reference intake (DRI) value for dietary polyphenols: are we heading in the right direction? *British Journal of Nutrition*, *99*, *Supplement S3*, S55-S58.

Williamson, G. and Manach C. (2005). Bioavailability and bioefficacy of polyphenols in humans. II. Review of 93 intervention studies. *Am J Clin Nutr*, *81(suppl)*, 243S–255S

Woldemichael, G. M., and Wink, M. (2001). Identification and biological activities of triterpenoid saponins from *Chenopodium quinoa*. *Journal of Agricultural and Food Chemistry*, *49*, 2327-2332.

Wu, A.M.; Lisowska, E.; Duk, M. and Yang, Z. (2009). Lectins as tools in glycoconjugate research. *Glycoconj. J.*, *26*, 899-913.

Wu, P., Tian, J.-C., Walker, C. E., and Wang, F.-C. (2009). Determination of phytic acid in cereals – a brief review. *International Journal of Food Science and Technology*, *44*, 1671-1676.

Xiao, K., Yi, Y.-H., Wang, Z.-Z., Tang, H.-F., Li, Y.-Q., and Lin, H.-W. (1999). A cytotoxic triterpene saponin from the root bark of *Aralia dasyphylla*. *Journal of Natural Products*, *62*, 1030-1032.

Yokosuka, A., Mimaki, Y., and Sashida, Y. (2000). Steroidal saponins from *Dracaena surculosa*. *Journal of Natural Products*, *63*, 1239-1243.

Yokosuka, A., Mimaki, Y., and Sashida, Y. (2002). Four new 3,5-cyclosteroidal saponins from *Dracaena surculosa*. *Chemical and Pharmaceutical Bulletin*, *50*, 992-995.

Yokosuka, A., Mimaki, Y., and Sashida, Y. (2002). Spirostanol saponins from the rhizomes of *Tacca chantrieri* and their cytotoxic activity. *Phytochemistry*, *61*, 73-78.

Yuan, F.-J., Zhao, H.-J., Ren, X.-L., Zhu, S.-L., Fu, X.-J., and Shu, Q.-Y. (2007). Generation and characterization of two novel low phytate mutations in soybean (*Glycine max* L. Merr.). *Theoretical and Applied Genetics*, *115*, 945–957.

Yun, T.-K. (2003). Experimental and epidemiological evidence on non-organ specific cancer preventive effect of Korean ginseng and identification of active compounds. *Mutation Research/Fundamental and Molecular Mechanisms of Mutagenesis*, *523/524*, 63-74.

Zhang, H.; Li, X.J.; Martin, D.B. & Aebersold, R. (2003). Identification and quantification of N-linked glycoproteins using hydrazide chemistry, stable isotope labeling and mass spectrometry. *Nat. Biotechnol, 21*, 660–666.

Zhou, J. R., and Erdman, J. W. (1995). Phytic acid in health and disease. *Critical Reviews in Food Science and Nutrition*, *35*, 495-508.

Zhou, J. R., Fordyce, E.J., Raboy, V., Dickinson, D. B., Wong, M. S., Burns, R. A., and Erdman Jr., J. W. (1992). Reduction of phytic acid in soybean products improves zinc bioavailability in rats. *Journal of Nutrition*, *122*, 2466-2473.

Zou, Z.-M., Yu, D.-Q., and Cong, P.-Z. (2001). A steroidal saponin from the seeds of *Allium tuberosum*. *Phytochemistry*, *57*, 1219-1222.

In: Nutritional Insights and Food Safety
Editor: Jaroslava Švarc-Gajiæ

ISBN: 978-1-61122-130-5

Chapter II

Naturally Occurring Food Toxicants

Jaroslava Švarc-Gajiæ
Faculty of Technology, University of Novi Sad, Bulevar cara Lazara 1,
21 000 Novi Sad, Serbia

Abstract

Naturally produced toxic food components can be found in food of animal and plant origin, as well as in higher fungi used as a food source. Dangerous food components fall into different chemical classes, including simple amines and aminoacids, fatty acids, organic acids, phenolic compounds, and encompass also more complex alkaloids, cyanogenic glycosides and very complex proteins. Being diverse in their chemical structure, the mode of toxic action varies considerably among naturally occurring food toxicants. The toxins may impair specific organs and systems, such as the skin or cardiovascular system, or may have systematic effects by binding to hormone receptors or affecting the nervous system. This chapter presents to the reader the dietary risks linked to different substances naturally found in food, encompassing the food of fungal, plant and animal origin, and also including the toxins in spice plants, as well as taking into consideration unusual, indigenous food specific for certain regions of the World. The occurrence and chemistry of food toxins and the mode of their action is presented for common food like potatoes, beans and carrots, but also for many specific and interesting food sources used in some world cuisines. The presented overview of numerous food toxins of different origin underlines that not only the food for which the toxic character and high acute toxicity are unambiguous and well established is dangerous, but that also common and everyday food carries the potential health risk in specific circumstances such as the uniform diet. The chapter covers major food toxicants including seafood toxins, alkaloids, mushroom toxins, biogenic amines, phenolics and many other chemical classes.

Introduction

Balanced diet comprises the food originating from many different sources and encompasses food products of animal and plant origin, as well as higher fungi. Where animal-derived food pose a risk to human health most often indirectly as a result of distribution and excretion of anthropogenic (Švarc-Gajić et.al., 2006, Švarc-Gajić et.al., 2009a) or microbial toxins in animals, numerous plants and mushrooms are able to produce by themselves many chemically different compounds toxic to humans. More than 2000 plants are cultivated as food plants and most of them include several cultivars. Naturally occurring toxins found in plant food encompass very broad, diverse chemical groups (Table 1) acting in human body by different mechanisms. Some of the dangerous toxins exhibit high acute toxicity, whereas others are toxic due to pronounced carcinogenic, procarcinogenic or teratogenic effects. Others can have negative effects in humans due to disruption of endocrine function. Hormone-like substances have been identified in grains like soybeans, wheat and rice, some vegetables (carrots, potatoes) and fruits (date, cherries, apples, pomegranate), as well as in spices like garlic, parsley and anis. These substances competively bind to hormone receptors acting as agonists or antagonists. Hemmaglutinins synthetized by leguminous plants such as castor bean, jack bean, soybean and other, act acutely very toxic by provoking clumping of blood cells. Acute toxicity of cyanogenic glycosides can be explained by instantaneous action of released cyanide in the course of food digestion. Numerous plant and mushroom toxins exhibit very potent neurotoxicity disturbing the signal transduction in synapses or at neuro-muscular junctions, by different mechanisms one of which includes the disturbances of acetylcholine esterase function. Some plants normally do not contain significant levels of toxins, but their synthesis is intensified when the plant is damaged and the plants defense mechanism is activated. Increased levels of solanum glycoalkaloids, such as solanine, chaconine and tomatine, can be found in damaged potatoes, eggplant, tomatoes and other vegetables and fruit, and have been shown to exhibit high acute toxicity and teratogenic potency. Similarly, mustard seed, horseradish and cauliflower generate and release their toxins only when plant tissue is damaged as a part of plants tendency to protect itself from invaders. Alkaloids are naturally produced by some plants, mushrooms and fungi as secondary metabolites. Many of them act neurotoxic and cause hallucinogenic effects. Different analogs of amino acids synthetized by diverse plant species represent the `hidden` and canning mean of plants defense system against predators, shown to be very effective even against much larger organism such as humans. Photosensitizing agents, such as those found in celery and parsley, provoke phototoxic dermal reaction after they have been distributed to the skin. Some of plant toxins are not biosynthesized within the plants, but are acquired from other plant species by parasitism. This includes relatively low levels of pyrrolizidine alkaloids found in the family Scrophulariaceae. Alkaloid levels in these plants are likely to be low, but unpredictable nature of plant parasitism and the cumulative nature of pyrrolizidine alkaloid toxicity raises the level of concern regarding the use of these plants.

Microbially produced food toxins are important class of compounds which include different chemical classes of mycotoxins, alkaloids, amines and other. Mycotoxins form a very large group of food toxins and encompass diverse chemical classes. As much as they represent the direct risk to humans due to their carcinogenic, goitrigenic or estrogenic effects, they might also indirectly reach the men through dairy products, or may cause damage to livestock. This large category of food toxicants will not be elaborated by this chapter, since detailed overview about the occurrence and effects of fungal toxins is given in Chapter XI. Some food toxins are produced in food under certain conditions by naturally undergoing microbial processes as a result of improper food storage. Increased levels of histamine and other biogenic amines in food result from microbial action and in some food can indicate hygienic food quality. Increased levels of histamine in food can be a cause of allergy-like manifestations and food intolerance. In addition to listed organic toxins that can be found in food, many inorganic compounds (Švarc-Gajić et al., 2005), such as nitrates and minerals which can be present in some food at high levels, may compromise the healthy diet if their source is consumed in excess.

This chapter covers many different classes of naturally occurring food toxicants. Even though the given overview of potential risks is quite broad, not all dangerous food is possible to encompass, predominantly due to enormous number of food varieties that are consumed worldwide. Some of them are very specific and indigenious to certain world regions, threatening mostly the local communities. On the other hand, the intention of this chapter was to present to the readership that even common, every day food might represent the health risk under certain circumstances (Kravić et al., 2009). Some compounds which are normally present in food at low levels pose a risk only in an uniform diet, chronically exposing a consumer (Kravić et al., 2010) and demonstrating their effects after prolonged period. In this respect the principle of `golden mean` best describes that the key to healthy diet lies in abstemious, versatile and balanced dietary habits.

When judging the "harmfulness" of specific food components many different aspects should be considered. Health effects of certain food must be judged only after evaluating overall effects that all food components demonstrate. Often besides containing offending components, other food constituents might have beneficial effects on human health or may counteract the negative impact of the compound in question. It is virtually impossible to define all coactivities of food components; it is even difficult mathematically to calculate the number of possible combinational experiments.

Table 1. Some naturally produced food toxicants

Alfalfa sprouts	Canavanine
Basil	Estragole
Beans	Hemagglutinins, Cyanogenic glycosides
Beer	Ethyl carbamate
Black pepper	Piperine; Safrole
Bracken fern	Tannins
Bread	Ethyl carbamate, Formaldehyde
Broccoli	Benzpyrene, Goitrin, Allyl isothiocyanate
Cabbage	Allyl isothiocyanate
Carrots	Carotatoxin
Cauliflower	Allyl isothiocyanate
Celery	Psoralens
Cinnamon	Safrole
Coffee	Caffeine, Hydrogen peroxide, Methyl glyoxal, Tannins
Fennel	Estragole
Fiddlehead greens	Ptaquiloside

Table 1. (Continued)

Horseradish	Allyl isothiocyanate
Mace	Safrole
Morel, false	Metyl hydrazine, Myromitrin, N-methyl-N-formylhydrazine
Mushroom, common	Hydrazines, Parahydrazinobenzoic acid
Mustard	Allyl isothiocyanate
Nutmeg	Myristicin; Safrole
Okra	Sterculic acid
Parsnips	Psoralens
Peanuts	Aflatoxin
Potatoes	Chaconine, Solanine
Red wines	Tannins
Rocket (arugula)	Allyl isothiocyanate
Sake	Carbamate
Shrimp	Formaldehyde
Soy sauce	Ethyl carbamate, Genistin, Daidzin, Coumesterol, Vasoactive amines
Spinach	Phytanic acid
Star anise	Safrole
Tarragon	Estragole
Tea	Tannins
Tomato	Tomatine, Quercetin glycosides, Methylglyoxal
Wine	Ethyl carbamate
Yogurt	Ethyl carbamate
Wheat germ	Phytoestrogens

Estimation whether the benefits gained by the consumption of certain food overweigh the negative effects should be a guideline to diet design. Consequently, often exaggerated alerts concerning specific food components should be judged reasonably, taking into account the health benefits provided by certain food, as well as the ingested food portion.

1. Alkaloids

Plants have the ability to synthesize numerous substances of different chemical classes such as amines, polyphenolics, acids, terpens, alkaloids etc. Alkaloids are nitrogen-containing class of compounds which are secondary metabolites and can be produced by a large variety of organisms, including bacteria, fungi, plants and animals. These compounds are indented to repel predators and to protect the organism from insects and fungus. Majority of natural alkaloids posses' very potent pharmacologic activity. These secondary metabolites are formed from proteins and are considered to be of the highest toxicity to predators and man, among all other naturally synthetized compounds.

Chemically, majority of natural alkaloids are heterocyclic, with the exception of some substances like mescaline, ephedrine and hordenine. Alkaloids encompass very broad spectrum of chemically diverse compounds and the classification of alkaloids is very complex. Usually alkaloids are classified on the basis of their chemical structure (Table 2) or on the basis of the producing species.

Table 2. Major structural classes of alkaloids

Alkaloid group	Representatives
Indole	tryptamines (serotonin, dimethyltryptamine, 5-methoxy-dimethyltryptamine, bufotenine, psilocybin) ergot alkaloids (ergine, ergotamine, lysergic acid derivatives) beta-carbolines (harmine, harmaline, tetrahydroharmine) yohimbans (reserpine, yohimbine) vinca alkaloids (vinblastine, vincristine) kratom alkaloids (mitragynine, 7-hydroxymitragynine) *Tabernanthe iboga* alkaloids (ibogaine, voacangine, coronaridine) *Strychnos nux-vomica* alkaloids (strychnine, brucine)
Indolizidine	senecionine, swainsonine
Isoquinoline	opium alkaloids (papaverine, narcotine, narceine), pancratistatin, sanguinarine, hydrastine, berberine, emetine, berbamine, oxyacanthine
Miscellaneous	capsaicin, cynarin, phytolaccine, phytolaccotoxin
Phenanthrene	opium alkaloids (morphine, codeine, thebaine, oripavine)
Phenethylamine	mescaline, ephedrine, dopamine
Purine	xanthines (caffeine, theobromine, theophylline)
Pyridine	piperine, coniine, trigonelline, arecoline, arecaidine, guvacine, cytisine, lobeline, nicotine, anabasine, sparteine, pelletierine
Pyrrolidine	phygrine, cuscohygrine, nicotine
Quaternary ammonium compounds	muscarine, choline, neurine
Quinoline	quinine, quinidine, dihydroquinine, dihydroquinidine, strychnine, brucine, veratrine, cevadine
Terpenoid	*Aconitum* alkaloids (aconitine) steroid alkaloids *Solanum* alkaloids (solanidine, solanine, chaconine) *Veratrum* alkaloids (veratramine, cyclopamine, ycloposine, jervine, muldamine) others (samandarin, conessine)
Tropane	atropine, cocaine, ecgonine, scopolamine, catuabine

1.1. Ergot Alkaloids

Claviceps purpurea (Hypocreacea family) is an alkaloid-producing fungus that grows on the rye and other cereals. Alkaloids produced by this fungus are denoted as ergot alkaloids and have been associated with numerous series of intoxications in Europe thought the history. Ergot alkaloids fall in the large group of indole alkaloids. Other indole alkaloids can be found in plants of the Apocynaceae, Rubiaceae, and Loganiaceae families and also include mushroom hallucinogens psilocin and psilocybin, very potent strychnine, reserpine and yohimbine, as well as many other extremely toxic substances. Humans are exposed to ergot alkaloids primarily by consuming contaminated flour.

Claviceps species produce two distinct types of substances, namely clavinet type alkaloids and lysergic acid amides. Diethyl-amide derivative of lysergic acid (LSD) is semisynthetic derivative (Figure 1) of ergot alkaloids that was first synthetized in 1938 by Albert Hofmann and is known for its hallucinogenic properties. Natural amides of lysergic acid contain peptide chain and can further be divided into water soluble and water insoluble groups. Water non-soluble derivatives of lysergic acid contain at least three amino acids in a peptide moiety and encompass numerous medicinally important compounds.

The clavine type of alkaloids, such as agroclavine and elymoclavine, are considered to be the precursors in biosynthesis of other ergot alkaloids. Nevertheless they also demonstrate powerful uterine stimulation and inhibition of prolactin release. These alkaloids have been also isolated from the higher plants of the Convolvulaceae family.

Ergonovine and methysergide are water-soluble amide derivatives of lysergic acid. Ergonovine provokes strong uterine contractions and has been used through history as a mean of abortion, while methysergide is pharmacologically used to treat severe migraines due to its specific vasodilatating properties in cranial brain regions.

Ergotamine, another ergot alkaloid, has also shown to be beneficial in relieving migraine headache due to ability to constrict peripheral blood vessels. The compound is a representative of water insoluble amides of lysergic acid. In its peptide chain hydroxyalanine, proline and phenylalanine constitute the peptide moiety. Peptide derivatives of isolysergic acid (dextrorotary, *d* isomers), ergotaminine and ergometrinine, are physiologically less active.

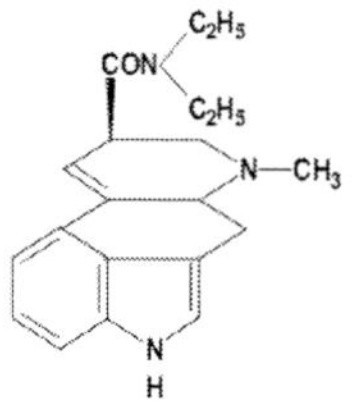

Figure 1. Semisynthetic lysergic acid diethylamide (LSD).

Upon ingestion of food contaminated with ergot alkaloids, two forms of ergotism can be recognized, gangrenous and convulsive, depending on the dominant type of the present alkaloids (Švarc-Gajić, 2009). Symptoms in intoxicated individuals depend on the alkaloid class which is predominantly produced by the growing fungus. Gangrenous ergotism first starts with tingling effects in fingers and toes, followed by the gangrene progression in limbs and in some cases complete loss of the limbs. In convulsive ergotism hallucinations, delirium and epileptic-type seizures are observed.

1.2. Nux-Vomica Alkaloids

The nux vomica tree (*Strychnos Nux-vomica*), is a small tree widely distributed in India, Sri Lanka, Thailand and northern Australia. The fruit of the plant resembles an orange and the seeds usually contain around 2-3 percents of powerful poisonous alkaloids strychnine and brucine (Figure 2) as well as hemitoxiferine, a degradation product of strychnine. The fruit pulp surrounding the seed contains high levels of the iridoid glycoside loganin, a biosynthetic precursor of strychnine. Other parts of the plant also contain toxins but in lesser extent. Strychnine can also be found in the leaves of the plant. Strychnine and brucine are similar in their structure, but brucine, a dimethoxy derivative of strychnine, exhibits several times lower toxicity in comparison to strychnine.

Due to very potent pharmacological activity, pure strychnine is nowadays intensively produced from the nux vomica tree with India being one of the most active exporters. Seeds of the plant are mostly used for isolating this medicinally important compound.

As a general stimulant, strychnine improves reflexes, quickens the pulse and rate of respiration and raises arterial pressure. Sharpness of the sight, hearing, and smell are notably improved by this alkaloid. Being a very potent stimulant, in low doses strychnine may be administrated as an aid in constipation activating the peristalsis by acting on a neuro-muscular junction in bowel. The substance has also shown to be effective in treating impotency and improving the sexual desire. The pain from menstrual colics, as well as from colics caused by lead poisoning, may be relieved by small doses of strychnine.

Poisoning with strychnine or nux vomica seeds are among the most violent and unpleasant poisonings. In fatal intoxications the death may occur after two hours, but in some cases the outcome can be delayed for six hours. Death usually occurs after several violent seizures which are triggered by minor stimuli, such as weak light beam, a sound stimuli or an air flow (Osweiler, 1983). Strychnine stimulates the spinal cord causing general tremor and provoking the contraction of all body muscles. Lethal outcome usually results from respiratory failure due to overstimulation of muscles of respiratory tract. In intoxicated individuals inhalation of chloroform and very strong vasodilatator amyl nitrite may be useful. Sedative chloral hydrate or an anticonvulsant potassium bromide may also be administrated to relieve the symptoms.

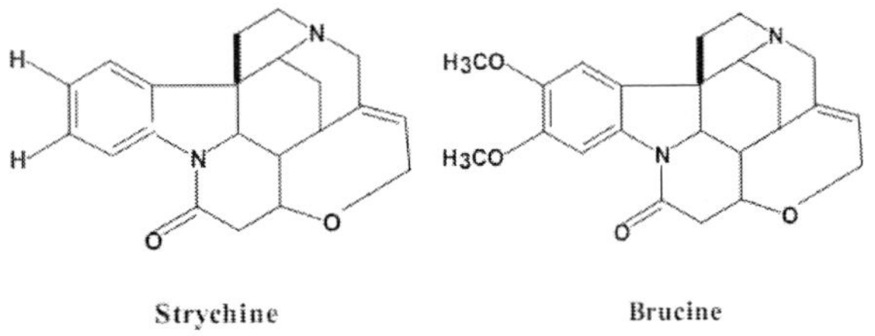

Figure 2. Alkaloids of *Strychnose Nux vomica*.

1.3. Physostigma Alkaloids

The seeds of leguminous plant, *Physostigma venenosum* (Calabar beans), native to Africa, have been traditionally used in rituals and witchcraft. Physiological potency of the seeds arises mostly from alkaloids physostigmin and calabarine which affect the cholinergic receptors by inhibiting choline-esterase (Zhao et al, 2004). Atropine acts antagonistically to physostigmin and is used as a part of the poisoning treatment. Upon ingestion physostigmin first increases salivary secretion, but later on the salivation can be completely arrested due to constriction of blood vessels supplying the glands. Also, accompanying strong feeling of pharynx constriction is due to physostigmin action on muscular fibers. Pharynx constriction may provoke vomiting. In first moments upon physostigmin absorption respiration is accelerated, but later on complete respiratory and heart arrest cause the death. On oppose to physostigmin, calabarine stimulates the motor and reflex functions of the spinal cord.

Due to strong pharmacological potency physostigmin is nowadays considered pharmaceutically highly appreciated chemical. It is widely used in ophthalmology and for the treatment of some serious medical conditions, for which other chemotherapeutics are not sufficiently effective, such as in the case of myasthenia gravis, Alzheimer's disease and paralysis.

1.4. Purine Alkaloids

Xanthines or purine alkaloids are commonly found in coffee, tea, and cocoa, with caffeine, theophylline and theobromine being major representatives. Three alkaloids differ only in a position of the methyl group. Caffeine (1,3,7-trimethylxanthin) is a naturally occurring water-soluble xantine alkaloid found in leaves, seeds and fruits of different plants such as tea, coffee, yerba mate and guarana berries (*Paullinia cupana*) where it plays a role of a natural insecticide. Theophylline is specific for tea plant and theobromine is mainly found in cacao beans.

Caffeine is a component of many common beverages, such as coffee, tea, energy drinks and cola. Certain precaution must be taken when consuming these products since caffeine exhibits influence on respiratory and vasomotor centers in the brain. In moderate doses caffeine is not toxic to humans, however in animals such as dogs and horse's even moderate doses might provoke intoxication. In humans caffeine in small doses induces fatty acid metabolism, increases the blood circulation and causes peripheral vasodilatation, as well as CNS stimulation via induction of adrenaline and noradrenalin release. It is also considered that caffeine in small doses is beneficial for the heart function since glycolysis and ATP production in heart mussel cells enhance after binding of caffeine to the receptors on the surface of heart muscle cells.

Average doses of caffeine (1-3 cups of coffee) may result in decreased fatigue, feelings of alertness and eased flow of thoughts, however chronic ingestion of high caffeine doses may be responsible for anxiety, insomnia and psychomotor agitation (Bolton & Null, 1981). Acute overdoses with caffeine may provoke panic attacks, seizures, tremors, phobia and instability of heart rate, while chronic overdosis with caffeine can induce bone porosity and miscarriage.

Theophylline (1,3-dimethylxanthin) provokes the release of adrenalin and noradrenalin by stimulating both adrenergic β_1 and β_2 receptors and can be used as an aid in the treatment of asthma and other pulmonary diseases. The alkaloid is commonly found in cocoa, green coffee, black and green tea, and mate (*Ilex paraguariensis*). The principal mechanism of theophylline toxicity arises from the excess of endogenous catecholamines (adrenalin and noradrenalin) which are abundantly produced after theophylline absorption.

Theobromine (3,7-dimethylxanthine) is a predominant xantine alkaloid of coca, acai berries, cola nuts (1.0-2.5%) and tea plant. The alkaloid exhibits stimulating properties similar to caffeine, but about ten times weaker, as well as diuretic and relaxing effects. The substance is not very toxic in humans, but in animals like dogs, horses, cats and parrots, it can induce seizures, heart attack and internal bleeding.

1.5. Pyrrolizidine Alkaloids

Many plants from the Boraginaceae, Compositae and Leguminosae families are able to synthetise pyrrolizidine alkaloids. Cereal crops may be contaminated with the weeds that produce these alkaloids and the substances can further reach humans provoking their poisoning. Also bees foraging on toxic plants can transfer the toxins in honey. Poisoning can also occur by consuming milk of animals feeding with pyrrolizidine-containing plants or by consuming specific teas and herbal preparations. The consumption of the popular Mexican herbal tea, *Gordolobo yerba*, obtained from *Gnaphalium*, has often been a cause of human poisoning with pyrrolizidine alkaloids, as well as typical Chinese herbal preparations, such as *zicao, kuandonghua, qianliguang, peilan*, and Indian herb *Heliotropium eichwaldii.*

Acute intoxication with pyrrolizidine alkaloids is usually characterized with gastrointestinal disturbance, accompanied with symptoms such as nausea, vomiting and stomach pain. Chronic ingestion of pyrrolizidine alkaloids over prolonged period, such as in the case of routine tea drinking, causes permanent liver damage in the form of liver cirrhosis which is indistinguishable from the cirrhosis of other etiology.

1.6. Solanum Alkaloids

Numerous plants belonging to Solanaceae family (potato, tomato, eggplant, chili pepper) produce very toxic alkaloids. Besides food plants, the family also comprises the plants like tobacco, petunia, deadly nightshade (*Atropa belladonna*) and Datura species, which predominantly produce tropane alkaloids like atropine, hyosciamine, cocaine and scopolamine, but are also able to produce other chemical groups of alkaloids. The alkaloids are present in all parts of the plants, including leaves, roots, flowers, stems, and fruits, being a part of plant defense mechanism against insects and predators.

Steroidal-like glycoalkaloids such as solanine (Figure 3), chaconine and tomatine, are produced by food plants like potato, eggplant and tomato at elevated levels under certain circumstances and can be responsible for poisoning with these plants. In small quantities solanine may also be produced by apples, bell peppers, cherries and sugar beet. The content of alkaloids is the highest in the peel. Tomatine is a glycoalkaloid found in tomatoes. Its aglycone is tomatidine. Solanine and chaconine have the same aglycone, solanidine, but the structure of their carbohydrate side chains is different. Chaconine exhibits similar toxicity and toxicological profile as solanine. The acute toxicity as well as teteratogenic potency of chaconine is estimated to be higher in comparison to solanine. Other glycoalkaloids or their aglycones including solamargine, demissidine, tomatidenol and 5β-solanidan-3α-ol, as well as α- and β- solamarine, deriving from tomatidenol, have been identified in potatoes (Sharma & Salunkhe, 1989). Commersonine and demissine, both deriving from demissidine, have been introduced in cultivated red potatoes by variety breeding.

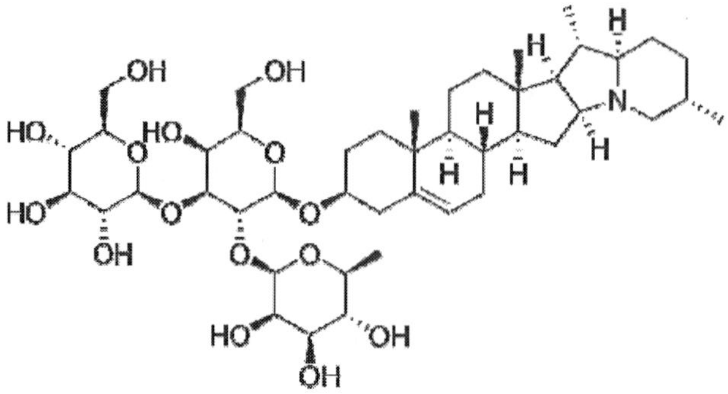

Figure 3. Solanine.

Potatoes do not generally contain more than 0.25 mg/g of solanine, however the production can be favored when the plant is damaged or exposed to a light, reaching the contents up to 1 mg/g and more. The content of solanine in unripe tomato is also elevated. A bitter taste and a green color of potatoes, which originates from chlorophyll and results from plants biochemical battle, can indicate the processes undergoing in the plant and can alert elevated solanine content.

Food processing influences differently the content of solanum glycoalkaloids which tend to be thermally relatively stable. Frying reduces the content of glycoalkaloids in food due to extraction by fats, while other processing procedures, like boiling, microwave heating or freezing do not significantly change the alkaloids content.

Solanine is known for its fungicidal properties and solanine-based insecticides have been produced, however the procedure for its isolation is quite expensive to be applied on an industrial scale.

The symptoms of solanine poisoning start demonstrating 8-12 hours upon ingestion, but the cases of symptoms development after as quickly as 30 minutes have been reported. The symptoms of poisoning appear after consuming potatoes containing approximately 2-5 mg/g of solanine and usually include gastrointestinal disturbances like vomiting, diarrhea, as well as dizziness, headache and sensation of throat burning. Solanine-induced neurological disturbances provoke hypothermia with fever, hallucinations, loss of sensation and paralysis. Recent studies have shown that many food plants in the Solanaceae family besides being a source of solanum alkaloids, also contain significant levels of calystegines, polyhydroxytropane alkaloids that are potent inhibitors of glucosidases (Asano et al., 1997). These alkaloids may also be involved in digestive disturbances through inhibition of gut enzymes.

Even though very toxic, some medicinal properties of solanine and other solanum alkaloids have been reported. Historically, solanine was used in the treatment of epilepsy and asthma, as well as for cough relieve. The sedative and anticonvulsant properties of solanine have also been reported, but were exploited only on a research level. Chaconine has been used as a nematicide, while anticarcinogenic properties of solamargine are speculated on the basis of animal studies. The studies also indicate that solamargine exhibits a potent cytotoxicity to human hepatocytes and skin fibroblasts.

1.7. Tropane Alkaloids

Tropane alkaloids are known for their occurrence in more then 3000 plant species of the family Solanaceae. Particularly high concentrations of these alkaloids have been found in *Datura stramonium* and *Datura ferox*, as well as in *Datura innoxia*. The most important natural tropane alkaloids produced by these plants are scopolamine and hyosciamine. Atropine represents racemic mixture of l- and d-hyosciamine. Datura plants pose a health risk primarily to livestock because they can contaminate feed materials, particularly those prepared from soybean and linseed.

Even though all parts of plants contain active substances, the highest concentration of tropane alkaloids is found in roots and seeds of Datura species. The composition of alkaloids and their content varies depending on the time of a year, soil at which the plant is grown and plant species.

Symptoms of poisoning with tropane alkaloids manifest 30 – 60 minutes upon ingestion and can last up to 48 hours. These alkaloids occupy muscarinic receptors in both central and peripheral nervous systems.

Initial signs of poisoning with tropane alkaloids include dry mucous membranes, photophobia, blurred vision and increased heart rate. First signs and symptoms of poisoning may be followed by confusion, agitation and hyperthermia, which end up with seizures, coma, and death. Intoxicated individuals have difficulties in performing urination and after recovery hardly recall the events due to amnesia.

1.8. Quinolizidine and Isoquinoline Alkaloids

Table 3. Isoquinoline alkaloids

Class	Producing plant species
Benzylisoquinolines	
reticuline	*Anonianthus dulcis*
turcomanidine	*Berberis turcomanica*
juziphine	*Fumaria bastardii*
reticuline	*Orophea hexandra*
thalprzewalskiinone	*Thalictrum przewalskii*
heterocarpine	*Ceratocapnos heterocarpa*
papaverine, noscapine, morphin	*Papaver somniferum*
codein	*Papaver bracteatum*
berberin	*Coptis chinensis, Hydrastis canadensis*
protopine	*Argemone mexicana*
tubocurarine	*Chondrodendron tomentosum,*
Bisbenzylisoquinolines	
aromoline, baluchistanamine, berbamine, isotetrandrine, obaberine, obamegine, oxyacanthine, tejedine	*Berberis vulgaris*
fenfangjine A, fenfangjine B, fenfangjine C	*Stephania tetrandra*
Ipecac alkaloids	
emetine, cephaeline, psychotrine protoemetine	*Psychotria ipecacuanha*
tubulosine, psychotrine	*Pogonopus speciosus*
isocephaeline	*Psychotria klugii*

Table 3 (Continued)

neocephaeline, emetine, cephaeline, psychotrine, protoemetine, 9-demethylprotoemetinol, isocephaeline	*Cephaelis acuminate*
Isoquinolines	
mescaline	*Lophophora williamsii, Echinopsis pachanoi, Echinopsis peruviana, Acacia berlandieri*
lophophorine, anhalonine, anhalonidine, anhalamine	*Echinocactus Williamsi, Echinocactus Lewenii*
pellotine	*Lophophora williamsi*
doryphornine, thalifoline	*Annona cherimola*
turcomanine	*Berberis turcomanica*
thalifoline	*Berberis vulgaris*
corydaldine, oxohydrastinine	*Fumaria bastardii*
oxohydrastinine	*Hypecoum leptocarpum*
N-methylcorydaldine	*Thalictrum przewalskii*
Naphthylisoquinolines	
korundamine A	*Ancistrocladus korupensis*
ancistrobrevine B, ancistrocladine, ancistrorobertsonine A, hamatine	*Ancistrocladus robertsonorium*
dioncophylline D, 8-*O*-methyldioncophylline D, 5A-*O*-demethyldioncophylline A, dioncophyllinol	*Triphyophyllum peltatum*
Phthalide-isoquinolines	
adlumiceine and adlumidiceine	*Fumaria agrarian*
bucuculline, corlumine and b-hydrastine	*Fumaria bastardii*
adlumiceine and adlumidiceine	*Fumaria capreolata*
adlumiceine and adlumidiceine	*Fumaria densiflora*
adlumiceine and adlumidiceine	*Fumaria muralis*
adlumiceine and adlumidiceine	*Fumaria officinalis*
adlumiceine, adlumidiceine, corledine, corlumidine, ahydrastine	*Fumaria parviflora*
adlumiceine, adlumidiceine	*Fumaria vaillantii*
hydrastine	*Hydrastis Canadensis*
severtzine	*Cordyalis severtzovii*
bicuculline	*Dicentra cucullaria, Adlumia fungosa, Fumariaceae, Corydalis*
narcotine (noscapine)	*Papaveraceae*
Protopines	
cryptopine, protopine	*Fumaria agraria, Fumaria capreolate, Fumaria parviflora, Fumaria vaillantii*
protopine	*Fumaria bastardii, Fumaria officinalis, Fumaria muralis, Hypercoum leptocarpum*
cryptopine	*Fumaria densiflora*
allocryptopine and protopine	*Thalictrum triternatum*
argemexicaines A and B	*Argemone mexicana* L.
Spirobenzylisoquinolines	
isohyperectine	*Hypecoum leptocarpum*
fumaricine, fumarophycine, *O*-methylfumarophycine, parfumine	*Fumaria vaillantii*
fumariline, fumaritine, *O*-methylfumarophycine, parfumine	*Fumaria parviflora, Fumaria bastardi*
fumaricine, fumariline, fumaritine, fumarophycine, *O*-methylfumarophycine, parfumine	*Fumaria officinalis, Fumaria densiflora, Fumaria capreolate, Fumaria agraria*
fumaricine, fumaritine, fumariline, parfumine	*Fumaria murali*

Isoquinoline alkaloids are produced by many different plant species and they encompass different subclasses (Table 3). Humans can be poisoned by isoquinoline alkaloids directly or indirectly. Indirect intoxication arises by consuming food contaminated with alkaloid-producing plants, or by consuming milk of the animals grazing at such plants, because many metabolites of isoquinoline alkaloids are excreted in milk. All isoquinoline alkaloids act neurotoxic provoking different neurological effects ranging from relaxation and euphoria to seizures (Bentley, 2000). The substances also act as gastrointestinal irritants (Howard & Michael, 1986).

Benzylisoquinoline class of isoquinolines includes narcotic alkaloids of the poppy plant (*Papaver somniferum*), among which morphine is the major compound. The alkaloids are produced in latex juice of ripened seed capsule of the plant, which in contact with air hardens. Morphin, isolated from the latex juice can further be chemically transformed to diacetyl derivative producing a heroin. Poppy seed used in human diet does not contain significant levels of morphin (opium) alkaloids and therefore do not pose a risk for humans. Opium or morphin alkaloids have also been isolated from the plants belonging to Argemone (prickly poppy) and Dicentra (family Fumariaceae) genera.

Another powerful isoquinoline alkaloid, belonging to benzylisoquinoline subclass, has been isolated from the lianas of South American *Chondodendron tomentosum* (Menispermaceae family). Active principle of the plant, an alkaloid D-tubocurarine, was widely used in traditional Brazilian remedies for healing the bruises, fever and edema (Takahata & Momose, 1993). In small doses the compound is beneficial for accelerating the removal of the kidney stones and for the treatment of psychosis. Historically, concentrated alkaloid was used together with frog venoms to tip the arrows in order to produce more fatal weapon. The toxicity of D-tubocurarine arises from blocking the neuromuscular junction and provoking the paralysis. Impaired conduction of nerve impulses appear first in ears, eyes and legs, finally attacking the muscles involved in respiration and provoking a respiratory arrest.

Several species from the genus Lupinus, the leguminous plants close to soybeans and belonging to the family Fabaceae, have a great agronomic significance. White lupin (*Lupinus albus*), blue lupin (*Lupinus angustifolius*) and Andean lupin (*Lupinus mutabilis*) are mostly used as livestock and poultry feed, while yellow lupin (*Lupinus luteus*) is the lupin which is predominantly used in human nutrition, even though humans consume other lupines as well. Lupin seeds are used for preparing typical Mediterranean dishes. The dishes are normally prepared from the seeds that were soaked for few days in salted water in order to reduce their toxicity. Lupin plants have high nutritional value, however they also contain great variety of antinutrients, such as tannins, saponins and numerous alkaloids of quinolizidine, piperidine and indole groups. Most abundant alkaloids in *Lupinus* species include sparteine, a tetracyclic quinolizidine alkaloid, and lupinine, a bicyclic quinolizidine alkaloid. According to alkaloid content *Lupinus* species are devided into two groups, bitter lupines which contain higher levels of alkaloids, and sweet lupines which are intended for human consumption and normally have lower alkaloid contents.

Lupin proteins are more and more used to replace animal proteins in many foodstuffs, such as meat products, imitation dairy products, bakery products and some beverages, introducing the risk of alkaloids poisoning. Both sparteine and lupinine act neurotoxic, however the modes of their action are different. Sparteine has been reported to block transmission of impulses in sympathetic and parasympathetic ganglia and to affects heart muscle. The substance also induces the contraction of uterus. Lupinine acts by blocking acetylcholine esterase in neural synapses.

Quinolizidine and isoquinoline alkaloids are also very widely distributed in numerous flowering plants, such as *Baptisia*, *Laburnum*, *Cytisus*, *Sophora*, *Argemone*, *Chelidonium* and *Corydalis* species. Cytisine, a tricyclic quinolizidine alkaloid found in these plant species, acts on muscarinic receptors influencing the function of gastrointestinal and central nervous systems (Michael, 2001). Throughout the history these plants have been dried and conserved for their stimulant effects and mild hallucinogenic properties. In India several cases of poisoning were reported and aroused due to addition of argemone oil as an adulterant to mustard oil or when using the oil for the massage. Argemone oil contains an isoquinoline alkaloid sanguinarine whose principal mode of toxic action includes the inhibition of liver (glutathione reductase, glutathione-S-transferase) and erythrocytes (glucose-6-phosphate) enzymes. It is speculated that regular consumption of argemone oil is responsible for increased incidence of gallbladder cancer in India. It was also established that consumption of grains containing Argemone seeds induces dropsy and glaucoma in humans (Cheeke, 1998).

2. Amines in Food

Many processed and fermented food products might contain significant levels of different amines adversely affecting human health. The effects of physiologically active amines from dietary sources are unlikely to be significant, however sensitive individuals and persons receiving antidepressant therapies (MAO inhibitors) might develop severe reactions after consuming food rich in amines.

Besides being a products of food processing and aging, amines are also produced naturally by some plants. Bananas, pineapple and avocado, for example, naturally contain high levels of serotonin, whereas a tryptamine was identified in tomatoes, plums and oranges, and noradrenalin in potatoes and bananas. Many other amines, such as phenylethylamine, adrenaline, dopamine, agmatine, histamine, cadaverin, octapamine, synephrine, as well as some aliphatic amines have also been identified in different food. In addition, numerous volatile aliphatic amines like dimethylamine, ethylamine, propylamine, isopropylamine and butylamine are synthetized by numerous food plants, such as bananas, potatoes, apples, cocoa, coffee, soybean, oat and tea plant.

Most foods that are high in biogenic amines are usually highly processed or fermented, such as cheese (Švarc-Gajić & Stojanović, 2011), beer, wine, sauerkraut, canned meats, pickled vegetables, fish and chocolate, or implies fermented sauces like soy, teriyaki and miso. The amines are produced by microbial processes responsible for decarboxilation of corresponding aminoacids (Švarc-Gajić & Stojanović, 2010), namely tyrosine and histidine for most abundant tryptamine and histamine, respectively. Free aminoacids in protein-rich food results from proteolytic processes normally undergoing in food.

Biogenic amines, such as adrenaline, noradrenalin, histamine, serotonin, tryptamine, are also frequently called vasoactive amines, due to their effects on blood vessels. Their role in human body is very complex. Human body has the ability to inactivate excess of these amines primarily via activity of two enzymes, diamine oxidase and histamine-N-methyltransferase. Persons receiving the therapy of monoamine oxidase inhibitors are particularly susceptible to consumption of amine-rich food and are prone to the development of dietary-linked adverse reactions.

The most common symptoms of the intolerance to dietary high amine content include headaches, flushing, hives, and arrhythmia, however in more severe cases asthma attacks, and anaphylactic shock might be expected. Severe migraine headaches arising after the consumption of amine-rich food can be explained by selective cerebral vasoconstriction followed by dilatation of the cranial vessels under the influence of amine excess.

Vasoactive amines are unable to cross the blood/brain barrier, however ingestion of vasoactive amines through food provokes the release of other, stored endogenous amines such as adrenaline, noradrenalin and dopamine which, in return, cause the hypertensive crisis, manifested as vasoconstriction, increased blood pressure and heart rate. In repeated dietary exposures to amines an apparent tolerance may develop due to reduced levels of consequently released endogenous amines. In tyramine exposure, for example, tyramine metabolite octopamine is stored in synaptic vesicles together with noradrenalin. After repeated tyramine exposure, vesicules will contain higher levels of octopamine and reduced amount of noradrenaline. Subsequent exposure to tyramine will result in less amount of the released noradrenaline, and consequently in less severe symptoms.

Toxic diamines cadaverin and putrecine are formed in the course of protein hydrolysis during spoilage of different protein-rich food. Cadaverin is formed by decarboxilation of the amino acid lysine, while putrescine is formed by decarboxilation of L-ornithine. Polyamines like spermine and spermidine usually accompany above mentioned diamines and are produced from precursor amino acids arginine and methionine.

Whereas the content of thyramine indicates the aging of food products and the level of histamine is firmly linked to the content of the parent aminoacid histidine, the content of cadaverine and putrescine might be considered as a good indicator of food spoilage. These diamines are also normally formed during putrefaction of the animal tissue and are produced in microalgae. Diamines cadaverin and putrecine are also ubiquitously found in plants where they bind to pectin, delaying fruit softening. In humans the polyamines, spermidine, spermine and the diamine precursor, putrescine, have shown to be essential for the normal cell growth and differentiation. The compounds are responsible for distinctive odor of urine and semen. In humans under physiological pH they occur in protonated form and electrostatically interact with negatively charged body macromolecules like proteins, DNA, RNA, phospholipids etc. The polyamines interact more strongly with essential molecules in comparison to inorganic cations. Furthermore the amines have exact distance in-between their positive charges, which is crucial for the specificity of interactions. Spermidine, spermine and putrescine have demonstrated the possibility to activate and block numerous cation channels and receptors. Upon their depletion from cells, the cells loose the ability to differentiate, but usually do not die.

Polyamines like cadaverin, putrescine, spermine and spermidine have demonstrated moderate acute toxicity in animal studies (Table 4) (Il et al., 1997). In quantities normally found in food they are not probable to cause the poisoning, however elevated levels of these amines can negatively impact sensory properties of the specific food.

Table 4. Acute toxicity of some food amines

Amine	Precursor aminoacid	Chemical structure of the amine	Acute toxicity
Tyramine	Tyrosine	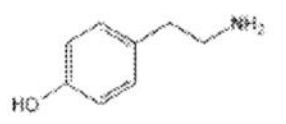	710 mg/kg (mouse, intraperitoneal)
Histamine*	Histidine	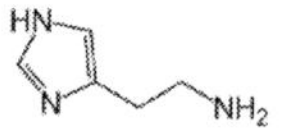	807 mg/kg (mouse, oral)
Cadaverine	Lysine		>2000 mg/kg (rat, oral)
Putrescine	L-ornithine	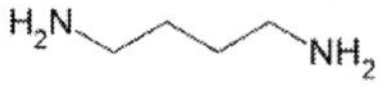	2000 mg/kg (rat/oral)
Spermidine	Methionine Arginine	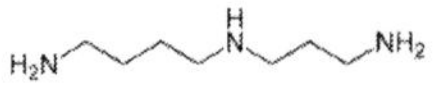	600 mg/kg (rat/oral)
Spermine	Methionine Arginine	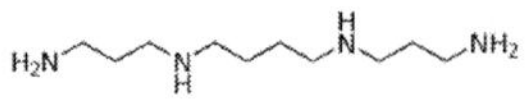	600 mg/kg (rat/oral)

*for histamine dihydrochloride.

3. Amino Acid Analogs

The analogs of protein amino acids are very numerous in nature and are produced by many different plant species (Table 5). Some of them, such as δ-aminolevulinic acid, are primary plant metabolites, while others are secondary plant metabolites, naturally tailored to protect the plant from microorganisms, insects or herbivores (Rosenthal, 1982). Compounds, structurally similar to protein amino acids, can also be produced in human body *in vivo* by the oxidation of the aminoacid side chain.

All amino acid analogs exhibit negative health effects in humans acting as antinutrients. The modes of action of aminoacid analogs may be different. Some of them, like β-N-methylamino-l-alanine, are dangerous due to direct neurotoxicity, while others incorporate into proteins instead of essential aminoacids producing aberrant and non-functional molecules.

Table 5. Plant derived structural analogues of protein amino acids

Protein amino acids	Structurally related plant amino acids
Arginine	Canavanine
Glutamic acid	β-N-methylaminoalanine (BMAA)
Leucine	Leucine hydroxides (e.g. 5-hydroxyleucine)
Phenylalanine	m-Tyrosine, o-tyrosine
Proline	Azetidine, proline hydroxides (e.g. *trans*-3-hydroxyproline, *trans*-4-hydroxyproline)
Tyrosine	3,4-Dihydroxyphenylalanine (DOPA)
Valine	Valine hydroxides (e.g. 4-hydroxyvaline)

3.1. Azetidine

Azetidine-2-carboxylic acid is a nonprotein, heterocyclic aminoacid, a homologue of proline, and is found in rhizomes and leaves of certain plants from Liliaceae (*Convallaria majalis*), Ruscaceae (*Polygonatum officinale*) and Fabaceae family (Rubenstein et al., 2008). The compound has also been detected in sugar and table beet.

The toxicity of azetidine-2-carboxylic acid stems from its misincorporation into proteins in place of proline. This process mostly effects and disturbs the synthesis of collagen, hemoglobin and keratin, where normally the content of proline is high. Besides producing aberrant proteins, the studies conducted in different animal species suggest very strong teratogenic potency of this amino acid analog.

3.2. Canavanine

Canavanine (2-amino-4-(guanidinooxy) butanoic acid) is the substance, structurally analogous to L-arginine and is produced by plants as a defense mechanism from herbivores and as a nitrogen source. It occurs in over 350 species of the Papilionoideae, a subfamily of the Leguminosae, and some plants have the ability to produce quite high amounts of canavanine. The highest content of canavanine, about 13% of dry weight, has been reported in *Dioclea megacarpa*, the highest concentration being in the seed of the plant. The seed of *Canavalia ensiformis* contains approximately 5% of canavanine. The leafs of Sutherlandia plant contain L-canavanine at levels of approximately 0.2%.

The toxicity of canavanine stems from the fact that it replaces arginine in many important enzymes and it also incorporates in cell nucleus disturbing the normal cellular division. Other negative impacts of L-canavanine reflect the thickness of the blood and provoke autoimmune reaction in which humoral immune cells attract the host's organs.

It is indubitable that canavanine posse's strong physiological activity but besides its toxicity some conducted animal studies have demonstrated several beneficial effects of the compound (Iskit et al, 1999; Liaudet et al, 1996). Administration of canavanine has shown beneficial effects in the treatment of pancreatic cancer, arthritis as well as in some brain disorders.

Legumes that produce canavanine often contain another toxic non-protein amino acid, called canaline (2-amino-4-(aminooxy)butyric acid) which has O-alkyl hydroxylamine functionality and very potent insecticidal properties. In plants canavaline is produced from canavanine by the activity of arginase (Rosenthal, 1990). The most common source of this amino acid is the jack bean, *Canavalia ensiformis*. The toxicity of canaline arises from the fact that after ingestion, the substance easily forms very reactive and dangerous oxymes in the body, especially with pyridoxal phosphate cofactors.

3.3. Djenkol

The large brown beans of *Archidendron pauciflorum* (*Pithecellobium jiringa*, *Pithecellobium lobatum* or *Archidendron jiringa*) are consumed in the countries of Southeast Asia, notably Malasya, Indonesia and Thailand, by preparing very popular meals such as curry or satay. Consumption of djenkol beans pose a health risk to humans due to presence of sulfur-containing non-protein amino acid called djenkolic acid (Figure 4). While djenkol beans contain up to 10-20 mg/kg per dry weight of djenkolic acid, other leguminous plants such as *Leucaena esculenta* and *Pithecolobium ondulatum* may contain 10 fold lesser amount of this aminoacid.

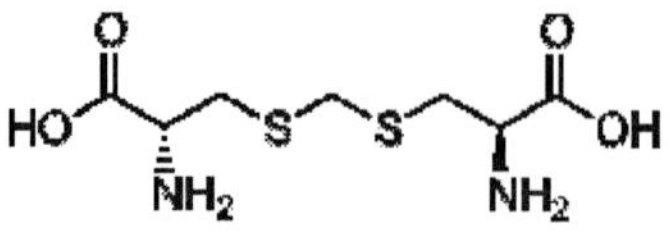

Figure 4. Djenkolic acid.

The most pronounced toxic effects of djenkolic acid are expressed in urinary tract where ingested djenkolic acid crystallizes and mechanically damages renal tubules. In the cases of poisoning with djenkol, the presence of needle-like crystals of djenkolic acid in urine can easily be confirmed by urine analysis. Mechanical obstruction in urinary tract provokes severe colics, hematuria, nausea, vomiting and general abdominal discomfort, which appear several hours upon ingestion (Vachvanichsanong & Lebel, 1997). In intoxicated individuals administration of alkali, such as sodium bicarbonate, and increased urine excretion by elevated water uptake, is recommended in order to dissolve and remove the acid crystals.

3.4. Hypoglycine

Hypoglycine is an aminoacid structurally similar to lysine and is found in typical Jamaican fruit, called ackee or akee (*Blighia sapida*). Even though ackee is considered typical Jamaican fruit and is most widely cultivated there, the fruit originates from West Africa and was brought to Jamaica in the 18th century. The fruit contains two types of hypoglycine, A and B. Hypoglycine A is found in both the seeds and the arils of the plant, while hypoglycine B is found only in the seeds. Unripened or inedible parts of the fruit are particularly dangerous, since they contain the highest amount of toxins. Today, the harvesting techniques of ackee are improved and optimized in Jamaica so cases of poisoning are rare and the fruit is not consumed until the fruit has not been opened fully, indicating decrease in hypoglycine content. Levels of hypoglycine A in the ackee arils peak at maturity but rapidly diminish to non-detectable levels in the opened fruit making it safe for consumption. Many tourists are not familiar with the toxicity of ackee fruit and the cases of random poisoning are quite frequent (Jamaican vomiting sickness).

The toxicity of hypoglycines arises from the fact that they competitively bind to several important enzymes involved in fatty acid metabolism, such as carnitine acyltransferases (I and II) and acyl-CoA dehydrogenase. They also bind irreversibly to coenzyme A and carnitine I, reducing their bioavailability and consequently inhibiting beta oxidation of fatty acids (Orane et al., 2006). Beta oxidation is closely linked to glycolysis, because it provides the body with ATP, NADH, and acetyl CoA, supplementing the energy from glycolysis. In the body hypoglycines are converted to methylenecyclopropyl acetic acid (MCPA) which acts in a similar manner as hypoglycine and is also very toxic (Feng & Patrick, 1958)

In individuals intoxicated with hypoglycines nausea and vomiting are first alerting symptoms which appear 2-3 hours upon ingestion. Inability to switch glucose metabolism to beta oxidation further leads to severe hypoglycemia. Occurring lethargy might further develop to unconsciousness and coma. As a result of altered fatty acid metabolism, increased urinary excretion of dicarboxylic acid, due to omega oxidation that occurs in the endoplasmatic reticulum, can be a reliable indicator of poisoning with ackee fruit.

3.5. Lathyrogens

Lathyrogens are naturally occurring derivatives of amino acids found in legumes (*Lathyrus sativus*) such as chick peas and vetch that have been demonstrated to cause very serious adverse health reactions in both the grazing animals and humans when the vegetables are consumed row. The poisoning with lathyrogens is especially frequent in the periods of drought, when the population is relying on diet rich in vetch, sweet pea (*Lathyrus odoratus*), or grass pea. Poisoning with lathyrogens is denoted as a lathyrism and is particularly frequent in India, China and some parts of Mediterranean (Spain).

Two types of lathyrism are recognized, neurolathyrism and osteolathyrism, in which nervous system, or bones and connective tissue are attacked, respectively. It is believed that males of age between 20 – 29 years old are particularly susceptible to neurolathyrism. Principal mechanism of neurolathyrism includes the antagonism with glutamic acid which is an important neurotransmitter. Very potent neurolathyrogen β-oxalyl-L-α,β-diaminopropionic acid (Figure 5) was isolated from *Lathyrus* grains and is considered responsible for neurological symptoms accompanying poisoning, such as loss of the strength in the lower limbs and irreversible paralysis. Isolated and, later on, well investigated neurotoxin, has shown to act by damaging mitochondria in motor neurons and provoking cell death.

The causative agent of osteolathyrism has been linked to another active principle, beta-aminopropionitrile (Figure 5), which inhibts copper-containing enzyme lysil oxidase, responsible for cross-linking of procollagen and proelastin in connective tissue (Wilmarth & Froines, 1992). The compound is produced in the course of biochemical transformation of the precursor substance present in lentils, grasspea and pea (Dawson et al., 2002). Other physiologically active amino-compounds like ureides, semicarbazides and thiosemicarbazides, can provoke similar effects as aminopropionitrile by chelating the copper-containing prosthetic group of lysil oxidase. Inhibited lysil-oxidase allows aminoacid lysine to be oxidized. Formed aldehyde undergoes several reactions with neighboring aldehydes or amines to create strong covalent cross-links between collagen tertiary structures in bones. For these reasons poisoning with osteolathyrogens is accompanied with the loosening of connective tissue and tinning of bones, coupled to bone deformities. These symptoms are likely to be irreversible. Osteolathyrogens can also offend the heart muscle by provoking damage to aorta.

a) b)

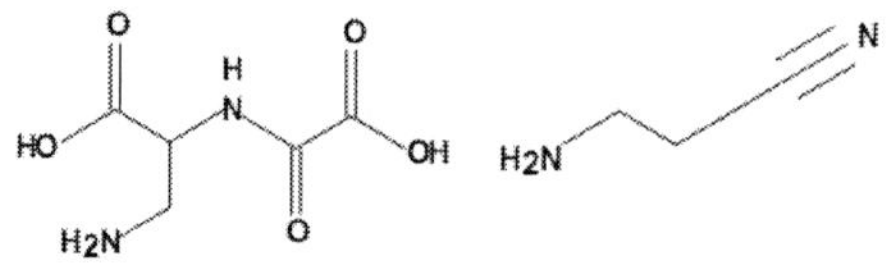

Figure 5. Lathyrogens of *Lathyrus* species (a) β-oxalyl-L-α,β-diaminopropionic acid; (b) beta-aminopropionitrile.

3.6. L-DOPA (L-3,4-Dihydroxyphenylalanine)

L-DOPA is physiologically active substance which is able to cross blood/brain barrier and is used for the treatment of Parkinsonism. Some species of beans contain significant amounts of this alanine analog. The seeds of various *Mucuna* species contain up to 6 % of L-DOPA, while the pods of *Vicia faba* may contain up to 0.25 % of the substance (Su et al., 1992). Other plants like *Phanera*, *Pileostigma*, *Cassia*, *Canavalia*, *Dalbergia* are also able to synthetise L-DOPA, but in significantly lower concentrations than the velvet bean (*Mucuna pruriens*).

Consumption of improperly boiled seeds of velvet bean (*Mucuna pruriens*) containing high levels of L-DOPA is known to cause increase in body temperature and skin damage. When large amounts are ingested vomiting and diarrhea are first poisoning symptoms to occur. Consumption of plants containing L-DOPA is particularly dangerous in individuals deficient in glucose-6-phosphate dehydrogenase in their erythrocytes. These individuals rapidly develop the symptoms of classical fauvism, in which the most common poisoning signs include severe headache, confusion, agitation and paranoid delusions, and in more severe cases can be accompanied with hemolysis (destruction of red blood cells).

The presence of L-DOPA in some food may also negatively affect the quality of prepared dishes. The aminoacid is very prone to oxidation, forming the conjugates with SH (cysteine) functionalities of proteins. Formed 5-S-cysteinyldopa cross links lead to polymerization of proteins. Also, oxidized L-DOPA forms an O-quinone, a highly unstable and highly reactive molecule, which subsequently reacts with other O-quinones, amino acids or proteins, leading to the formation of undesirable brown and red heterogeneous polymers which may compromise the sensory properties of the food.

3.7. Mimosine

Mimosine (β-(3-hydroxy-4-pyridone-1-yl)-L-alanine), the toxic, non-protein amino acid, contributes as much as 15% to the total nitrogen content of *Leucaena leucocephala*. The plant is fast growing evergreen leguminose and is used as animal feed. In Central America, Indonesia, and Thailand the leaves and seeds of the plant are used as human food and as an oil source.

The concentration of mimosine depends on the stage of the plant growth and is highest in the seeds. Mimosine content varies widely among various cultivars of white leadtree

(*Leucaena leucocephala*) and ranges from 2.2% to 10%. The content of mimosine in seed may be as high as 60% of the total free amino acids.

According to its chemical composition *Leucaena* plants are high quality feed, with nutritional values approaching soy of fish meal, however ingestion of mimosine may provoke undesirable health effect. It was first noticed that livestock fed with *Leucaena* looses the hair. Similarly to effects in livestock, alopecia was observed in humans. Other adverse health effects include growth retardation, cataract, goiter and decreased fertility. Several toxicity mechanisms have been proposed for mimosine. It is considered that mimosine interferes with the metabolic pathways of aromatic amino acids, tryptophan and glycine (Makkar et al., 2007). The substance also antagonizes the action of vitamin B6, and disturbs collagen biosynthesis. In ruminants mimosine is reduced to 3-hydroxy-4(1H)-pyridone, a goitrogen that inhibits the binding of iodine (Colegate & Dorling, 1994) It is assumed that hyperactivity in livestock, following consumption of mimosine-containing plants might be attributed to mimosine metabolite pyridone which interferes with enzyme systems responsible for the inactivation of adrenalin and noradrenalin. Mimosine also reduces weight gain and possibly provokes reproductive defects and cataracts (Cheeke, 1995).

3.8. Selenoaminoacids

Selenium is an essential element incorporated in many important bodily enzymes involved in iodine metabolism, immune response and protection from harmful peroxides, however selenium excess may produce many adverse effects. The form in which the selenium in incorporated in proteins includes different selenoaminoacids, the analogs of sulphur-containing aminoacids. The biochemical paths of functional sulphur-containing aminoacids and selenoaminoacids are very similar and selenium excess may cause the production of different non-functional proteins. Other mechanisms of selenium toxicity are also known (Švarc-Gajić, 2009). The content of selenium in plant depends on its content in soils on which the plant is grown (Suturović et al. 2005; Švarc-Gajić et al., 2009b) and the plants biochemistry. Many regions of the World, such as United States, China, Ireland, Australia and Israel, are known to contain high amounts of selenium in soils. The content of selenium in plant tissue also depends on the plant type. Selenium accumulators (*Oonopsis*, *Xylorrhiza,* some *Astragalus* spp.) can grow only on selenium-rich soils and may accumulate up to 15, 000 ppm of the element in their tissue. In selenium accumulators majority of selenium excess is not incorporated in proteins, but is present in the form of free selenium compound, such as Se-methyl-selenocystein. It is assumed that the synthesis of free selenium compounds represents a plants detoxification mechanism by which the plant protects itself from the incorporation of aminoacid analogs selenomethionine and selenocystein and production of nonfunctional proteins. Secondary selenium absorbers, such as *Aster* and *Atriplex* spp., accumulate the element in the amounts of several hundreds of ppm only if they grow on seleniferous soil, but they can equally well grow on a soil containing average selenium contents, so these plants pose a risk to animals and humans only if the soil on which they are grown is selenium rich. *Neptunia amplexicaulis*, for example, is Australian plant in the legume family Mimosaceae that selectively absorbs selenium and has frequently been a cause of selenium poisoning.

Due to high selenium content, the consumption of monkeys' coconut or *Lecythis ollaria* which grow in Venezuela and Brazil has been a cause of serious selenium intoxications and some of them had the lethal outcome. The plant belongs to Lecythidaceae family together with related Brazil nut (*Bertholletia excelsa*). Both trees produce woody, thick-walled seed capsules about the size of a large grapefruit. The toxic component of this selenium-accumulating plant is seleno-cystathionine (Figure 6) (Aronow & Kerdel-Vegas, 1965). Ingestion of the nut causes nausea, vomiting and loss of hair. In some cases the hair from whole scalp area is lost. Death cases were reported in children after consuming several nuts.

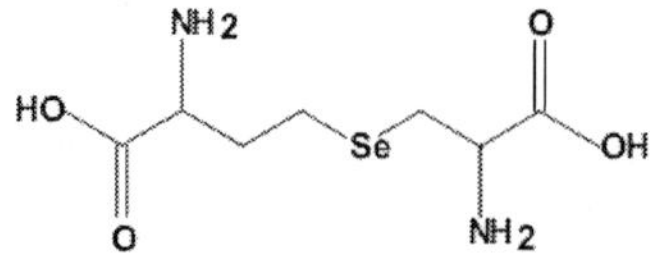

Figure 6. Seleno-cystathionine, a toxic factor in the seeds of *Lecythis ollaria*.

Chronic poisoning of animals which graze the selenium rich plants is called alkali disease and is hallmarked with stiff gait, loss of hair and sloughing of the hooves. Humans chronically exposed to moderate selenium doses via dietary sources have high incidence of skin discoloration, gastrointestinal disturbances and dental caries. Acute poisoning in humans is accompanied with dizziness, fatigue, dermatitis and loss of hair and nails.

3.9. 5-Hydroxytryptophan (5-HTP)

Griffonia simplicifolia is a plant growing in western African countries such as Ghana, Ivory Coast and Togo, which contains significant levels of 5-hydroxytryptophan. The content of free 5-hydroxytryptophan in the plant varies from 6-10%. 5-Hydroxytryptophan is physiologically active compound which is converted into serotonin in humans' brain after crossing the blood/brain barrier. Serotonin, as a known mood enhancer, exhibits beneficial effects in sleep disorders, depression and anxiety, and for these reasons the leafs and juice of *Griffonia simplicifolia* have a long history of use in some traditional medicines. Today various synthetic supplements containing 5-hydroxytryptophan are used as a sleep aid, to regulate mood, and control appetite.

Due to high content of 5-HTP in *Griffonia simplicifolia* occasional intoxications have been described by West Africans people. In intoxicated individuals tremors and hypersalivation were followed by the loss of light reflex and apparent blindness. The disturbances of cardiac rhythm were also reported and were accompanied with the necessity for deep breathing (Deshpande, 2002).

3.10. β-Cyanoalanine

β-cyanoalanine and its γ-L-glutamyl peptide are potent neurotoxins isolated from fava beans (*Vicia sativa*), extensively used in Latin American and Arab cuisines. The plant also contains other nitrogenous antinutrients, such as the cyanogenic glycosides vicianine and prunasin, as well as toxins isouramil, vicine and convicine, responsible for favism. Favism occurs as a result of glucose-6-phosphate dehydrogenase deficiency. Following ingestion of fava beans, or even inhalation of plants pollen, consequent severe hemolytic anemia and coma manifests after the period of tiredness. In addition, vicin and convicine significantly enhance the toxicity of β-cyanoalanine (Farran et al., 2002). Intoxication with β-cyanoalanine provokes characteristic neurological disturbances which start with stiffness and convulsions. Pyridoxal (one of the forms of vitamin B6) can delay and moderate the symptoms of β-cyanoalanine neurotoxicity. Besides being neurotoxic and acutely very threatening, it is also important to note that chronic ingestion of low β-cyanoalanine doses can provoke sulphur depletion in the body under specific circumstances. Animal studies have demonstrated that in sulphur deficient diets sulphur depletion occurs due to enhanced urinary excretion of thiocyanate and cystathionine induced by β-cyanoalanine.

3.11. β-N-Methylaminoalanine (BMAA)

The palm-like plants from Cycadaceae family include a single genus *Cycas* and are native to tropical Asia, Australia, and Polynesia, where the seeds of the plant are used as a dietary source. The seeds of the plants from *Cycas* genus contain β-N-methylaminoalanine (BMAA), an analog to glutamic acid, which is responsible for their toxicity. The compound was also recently found in a wide range of free-living cyanobacteria. Amino acid analog replaces glutamic acid in polypeptide chain and produces non-functional proteins. It is assumed that β-N-methylaminoalanine in fact is released from its precursor form in the body in the course of the digestion processes by acid hydrolysis.

Consumption of flour produced from the seeds of *Cycas circinalis* (*Cycas micronesica*) has been linked to high incidence of nerve degeneration disorder in Guam inhabitants. Guam is an island in the western Pacific Ocean and is the largest island of the Mariana group of islands in Micronesia. The syndrome of *Cycas* induced nerve degeneration involves progressive dementia and Parkinsonism. In Australia numerous cases of animal poisonings as a result of consumption of leaves and seeds of *Cycas* have also been reported. Consumption of as little as 0.6 kg of the seeds led to progressive weakness and death in livestock.

Neurodegenerative character of BMAA poisoning stems from the damage of motor neurons, important for controlling voluntary muscle movements. (Nunn & Ponnusamy, 2009) The poisoning with β-N-methylaminoalanine is commonly denoted as amyotrophic lateral sclerosis-Parkinsonism-dementia complex, because it is accompanied with progressive dementia and Parkinsonism-like symptoms, as well as general muscle weakness and atrophy throughout the body. Intoxicated persons may ultimately lose the ability to initiate and control all voluntary movements, as well as bladder and bowel sphincters. In most of the cases eye muscles activity remains undamaged. Besides neurotoxicity, in conducted animal studies other toxicological aspects of *Cycas* seeds were identified, revealing carcinogenic effects as well as hepato- and nephrotoxicity.

In attempt to explain the mode of β-N-methylaminoalanine toxicity, it has been demonstrated that the substance binds to ionotropic glutamate receptors in cell cultures, acting as a neuroexcitant. Conducted experiments on cell cultures revealed that BMAA can also occupy metabotropic receptors (Copani et al., 1990). This action was noticed only in the presence of bicarbonates, and it is assumed that neurotoxicity is mediated by the formation of carbamates. Carbamate formation may explain the convulsive activity of the amino acid in experimental animals.

Besides the major antinutrient β-N-methylaminoalanine, the seeds of plants from *Cycas* genus have been shown to contain a number of toxic azoglycosides, including cycasin and neocycasins (Kisby et al., 1992). The compounds share highly toxic common aglycone methylazoxymethanol. In animal studies it has been demonstrated that methylazoxymethanol acts as a potent methylating agent, speculating mutagenic character. Aglycone methylazoxymethanol has also been identified in the wild pineapple which belongs to *Macrozamia* genus of Zamiaceae family. Azoglycoside macrozamin produces similar neurological effects in man and animals as *Cycas* species.

3.12. Other Aminoacid Analogs

In addition to listed substances many other aminoacid analogs are synthetized by plants but they are usually present in low concentrations. Some of the toxic aminoacid analogs include proline hydroxides, valine hydroxides, leucine hydroxides, *m*-tyrosine, *o*-tyrosine and DOPA. Some of these compounds exhibit very potent phytotoxic activity by disturbing the root development in plants. *m*-Tyrosine is significantly more phytotoxic than its structural isomers *o*- and *p*-tyrosine. Assumed mode of action of *m*-tyrosine is similar to that of other nonprotein amino acids by substituting phenylalanine during translation in protein synthesis and resulting in dysfunctional proteins. Some researchers postulate that in plants *m*-tyrosine is converted to L-DOPA, a known phytotoxin. β-(3-isoxazolin-5-on-2yl)-alanine which is found in roots of pea (*Pisum sativa*) also demonstrates phytotoxic effects but less potent in comparison to *m*-tyrosine.

Data concerning human toxicity of *m*-tyrosine and other aminoacid analogs are very limited, however available data and experiments conducted in cell cultures demonstrate their cytotoxic character. Recognized cytotoxic character of these substances imposes a necessity for a precaution when ingesting significant amounts of plants containing these compounds or in prolonged, chronic exposures.

4. Carbamates

The occurrence of carbamates, mostly in the form of ethyl esters of carbamic acid, is widespread in alcoholic beverages and fermented foods, such as soy sauce, cheese, bred, olives, sauerkraut etc. Ethyl carbamate or urethane is formed by the reaction of ethanol and urea, where urea results from the yeast metabolism of aminoacids like arginine or citrulline. The reaction of esterification and carbamate formation is favored at higher temperatures, so higher content of carbamates are expected in distilled alcoholic beverages like whisky and brandy, up to levels of several ppm. Beverages like sake, beer and wine contain carbamates to lower extent.

Due to recognized genotoxicity of carbamates the content of ethyl carbamate in wines, alcoholic beverages and fermented food is in most countries regulated by low. Even though animal studies suggest carcinogenic character of carbamates, the carcinogenicity of the compound has not yet been proven in humans and the substance is classified by the World Health Organization's International Agency for Research on Cancer (IARC) as a "probably carcinogenic in humans".

5. Cyanogenic Glycosides

Cyanogenic glycosides are produced by many food plants as secondary metabolites and as a part of protective mechanism against herbivores. In digestion process cyanogenic glycosides release hydrogen cyanide, one of the most potent neurotoxins, contributing to the toxicity of the plant parts having high glycosides content. Cyanogenic glycosides are composed of alpha-hydroxynitrile type aglycone and of a sugar, usually D-glucose. The amount of the produced glycoside depends on the plants age, the variety of the plant, and the environmental factors. The number of plants which produce cyanogenic glycosides is very large, including families Fabaceae, Rosaceae, Linaceae, Compositae and others. Produced glycosides are concentrated in kernels and seeds of many fruits like cherries, plums, almonds, peaches, apricots and apples. Cassava, an important feed and a source of carbohydrates in human diet, contains significant amounts of cyanogenic glycosides among which linamarin and lotaustralin (Figure 7) are the most abundant. The content of these glycosides may reach 1 g/kg in the plants root. Prior consumption cassava is detoxified by soaking, cooking or fermentation, allowing the glycosides to break down. 100 g of cassava root produces approximately 53 mg of HCN, while the same amount of bitter almonds produces approximately 250 mg of HCN. Close amount of the cyanide is also released from the pasture grass (*Sorghum*) in which the principal cyanogenic component is dhurrin. In almonds the principal cyanogenic glycoside is amygdaline. Other related cyanogenic glycosides in plants include cyanohydrins such as mandelonitrile (Harborne, 1972).

Ingestion of large quantities of plant parts containing cyanogenic glycosides may induce severe poisoning. The enzyme activity in body rapidly detoxifies ingested cyanides, however the capacity of biotransformational enzymes is limited. Released cyanide rapidly inhibits the oxidative processes of cells provoking their death. Enzymatic capacities of a healthy adult human are sufficient to biotransform and detoxify around 10 mg of cyanides per hour without exhibiting the symptoms of poisoning. However, exposure to concentrations of 40-100 mg in time frame of 30 minutes usually results in fatal outcome.

In cases of mild poisoning usually the symptoms like chest and throat tightness, nausea, vomiting, muscle weakness and headache are observed. Ingesting larger quantities of seeds and kernels containing cyanogenic glycosides produces symptoms typical to cyanide poisoning, such as fever, mental confusion, visual disturbance, seizures and cyanosis (lack of oxygen in tissues resulting in bluish skin, lips and fingernails). Chronic exposure to cyanide by continuous consumption of toxic plant parts provokes liver damage and neuropathy (pathological changes in the peripheral nervous system).

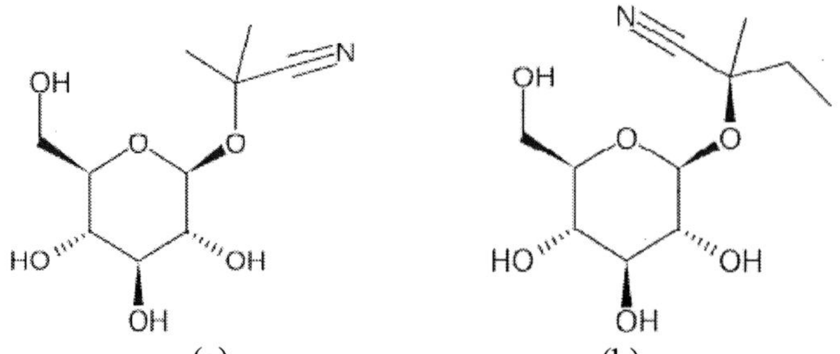

Figure 7. Cyanogenic glycosides in plants. (a) linamarin and (b) lotaustralin.

6. Fatty Acids

6.1. Erucic Acid

Erucic acid is a monounsaturated omega fatty acid (C22 : 1 ω9) which is present in high concentrations in the mustard (*Brassica junca* and *Brassica nigra*) seed oil, rapeseed oil (*Brassica napus*) and the oils of some flowers. Erucic acid has also been found in some marine animal fats.

Concerns regarding erucic acid health effects arise from the fact that this fatty acid has demonstrated marked contribution in the formation of fatty deposits on a heart muscle as well as heart lesions in animal models (de Wildt & Speijers, 1984; Charlton et al., 1975). Fat deposits accumulated on a heart muscle reduce the contractile force of heart muscle. Even not yet confirmed, on the basis of conducted animal studies, it can be expected that humans are also susceptible to myocardial lipidosis resulting from chronic exposure to high levels of erucic acid.

6.2. Phytanic Acid

Branched-chain fatty acids are common constituents of the lipids of bacteria, marine animals and ruminants, where they play a role in increasing the fluidity of lipids. The most common branched chain fatty acids are mono-methyl-branched, but di- and poly-methyl-branched fatty acids are also known. Branched-chain fatty acids like phytanic (3,7,11,15-tetramethyl hexadecanoic) and pristanic (2,6,10,14-tetramethylpentadecanoic) acids have been identified at micromolar levels in the plasma of healthy individuals. Humans can ingest these fatty acids by consuming the meat of ruminants and marine organisms. Furthermore, these fatty acids can also be produced biochemically *in vivo* from ingested plants chlorophyll.

In healthy individuals phytanic acid is metabolized by α-oxidation and is converted to pristanic acid by removing one carbon atom. The individuals with defect enzymes involved in these processes, can not metabolize phytanic acid adequately leading to deposition of phytanic acid and its derivatives in neural myelin layers, blood and tissues. The condition is known as a Refsum's syndrome and is a heritable neurological disorder. The symptoms of this genetic disorder begin in infancy with visual and audial impairments, which eventually develop to blindness and deafness, accompanied with mental and growth retardation (Rake & Saunders, 1966). Other symptoms may include rapid, jerky eye movements, hypotonia (low muscle tone), lack of muscle coordination and facial dimorphism.

6.3. Cyclopropene Fatty Acids

Cyclopropene fatty acids (Figure 8) are naturally present in seeds, leaves, stems and roots of flowering plants belonging to Malvales order, especially Sterculiaceae, Malvaceae, Bombacaceae and Tiliaceae families. The content of these acids in cotton (family Malvaceae) seed oil ranges from 0.6 to 1.2 %.

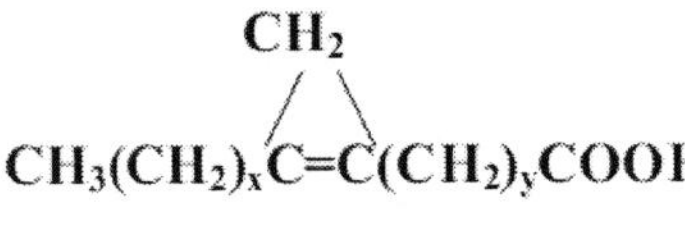

Figure 8. General structure of cyclopropene fatty acids.

Even though experimental date concerning the adverse effects of these acids in humans are not available, animal studies have pointed out the importance of the dietary intake of these fatty acids. The investigations concerning cyclopropene fatty acids impact on health started when it was noticed that pigs fed with the diet rich in cyclopropene fatty acids, such as cotton seed, produce fats with higher melting point then usual. It was also assumed that these fatty acids were responsible for the development of pink and red color in stored eggs. In animal studies in which cyclopropene fatty acids constituted between 10% and 40% of total calorie intake, noticed growth retardation of animals alerted the scientific community and brought in question the influence of these fatty acids on human health (Deshpande, 2002). The studies also revealed impaired reproductive performance and increased risks of gall bladder and liver cancer (Nixon et al., 1977; Hendricks et al., 1980).

7. Hemagglutinins

The substances able to induce agglutination of blood cells can be found in numerous plants, animals and microorganisms and are denoted as hemagglutinins. According to their chemical structure, hemagglutinins are proteins. Different hemagglutinins can provoke clumping of both red blood cells and leukocytes and these processes are initiated by binding of these proteins to carbohydrates on the surface of blood cells. Plant-derived hemagglutinins are denoted as phytohemogglutinins. Independently on their source, all hemagglutinins belong to the lectin class of substances. Lectins are complex proteins which are able to recognize and bind to carbohydrates and sugar-containing substances. The specificity and selectivity of lectins are very high and each lectin binds to specific carbohydrate molecule. In viral infections viruses use their lectins to attach themselves to specific hosts' cells. Different mammalian cells have carbohydrates on their surface and lectin binding provokes their clumping (agglutination). The role of lectins in plants seems to be associated with the storage of nutrients in plant seeds, since upon germination the seed looses most of its lectin. The substances might also play a role in protecting the plants from bacteria and fungi.

High amounts of hemagglutinins are found in different classes of leguminous plants, such as castor bean, jack bean, soybean, kidney beans, green beans and broad beans (*Vicia faba*) and are concentrated in their beans. The jequirity bean (*Abrus precatorius*) has very attractive red and black beans often used to make necklaces. The cases of children poisoning with fatal outcome have been reported after chewing on necklaces made of beans which contained highly toxic lectin component abrin (Gunn, 1969).

Natural phytohemogglutinins (abrin, ricin, robin, and cretin) have been isolated from numerous leguminous plants and were successfully purified to high degree. Purified, the substances are of considerable medical importance and are used for the preparation of antisera and as mitocytes (initiators of cell division). Some researchers also speculate the use of abrin and ricin in the treatment of cancer, by anchoring them to monoclonal antibodies able to recognize malignant cells (Hwang et al., 1984).

Consumption of lectin-containing row beans can cause severe poisoning. The content of hemagglutinins drops significantly with appropriate cooking, however ingestion of as little as few row beans can induce poisoning. The symptoms of poisoning start usually within several hours upon ingestion with nausea, vomiting and diarrhea. For small ingested doses recovery occurs within 5-6 hours of onset symptoms.

Abrin and ricin are very potent phytohemogglutinins naturally found in the seeds of rosary pea and castor oil plant. Ricin comprises about 5 percents of the total protein content of a castor seed, and the amount in a single seed, approximately 250 μg, is sufficient to kill an adult human (Bradberry et al., 2003). These toxic proteins are composed of two subunits bound with the disulphide bridge. One of the protein subunits binds to galactose-containing receptors on a cells surface and other enables the substance to enter the cell. The toxicity of abrin and ricin arise from the fact that after the substances have entered the cell, they further disturb protein synthesis.

Manifestation of poisoning with abrin and ricin depend highly on the exposure dose and route, and are somewhat similar for both phytochemical. The symptoms of poisoning with abrin and ricin occur after several hours or longer (up to several days) upon exposure. The latent period may be quite long because the mechanism of their toxicity comprises indirect route by producing non-functional proteins. After ingesting the substances, nausea and bloody diarrhea are first to be demonstrated and are accompanied with severe dehydratation. (Dickers et al., 2003). Poisoning is accompanied by hemorrhage of the digestive tract, convulsions, and circulatory collapse. Other signs and symptoms may include hallucinations, seizures, and blood in the urine. The condition is marked with heavy sweating and fluid retention in lungs which significantly disturbs breathing. Delayed effects include liver, spleen and kidneys dysfunctions. Treatment of poisoning with phytohemogglutinins includes supportive medical care, such as administration of activated charcoal in recent oral exposures, intravenous fluid administration and different medications.

8. Oxalates

Oxalic acid (HOOC-COOH) is a strong organic acid widely distributed in plant and animal kingdom, with plants containing higher levels of the substance. Being a reactive species, oxalic acid easily binds to minerals like potassium, sodium, calcium, magnesium, iron etc., building the oxalates. Potassium and sodium oxalates are water-soluble, while calcium oxalate crystallizes from water solutions. Calcium oxalate crystals are present in many plants, and even though their exact role in plants is unknown, it is assumed that they are important as high-capacity calcium storage sites.

Edible seeds and leafy plants related to spinach and rhubarb represent human dietary sources high in oxalates. Most nuts, beans, beets, berries and poppy seed are also known for high oxalate content, as well as some spice plants like black pepper and parsley. Orange, prunes, carrots and lentils contain moderate levels of oxalates. Leaves of the tea plant (*Camellia sinensis*) contain among the greatest measured levels of oxalic acid. This, in return, does not contribute significantly to oxalate intake since only small quantity of tea leaves is used for preparing a beverage. Children are advised to reduce chocolate in their diet because of high oxalate content in coca beans.

Oxalates present in diet do not normally pose a serious health risk, however prolonged diet rich in oxalates can cause the obstruction of renal tubules and intestines due to crystallization of calcium oxalate. Calcium oxalate crystallizes in sharp needle-like crystals. Furthermore, high oxalate intake is an important factor contributing to the formation of the kidney stones (Curhan, 1999). Approximately 75 – 80% of all kidney stones are composed predominantly of calcium oxalate. For reasons not yet fully understood, women have a much lower incidence of kidney stones than men. Even though the bioavailability of dietary oxalates is relatively poor, diet low in oxalates is advised for individuals with kidney disorders, gout and rheumatoid arthritis. Interrelationship between dietary calcium and oxalate absorption has also been postulated. Diet rich in oxalates significantly reduces calcium absorption via its complexation in gastrointestinal tract. Reverse is also true and the diet rich in calcium can significantly reduce the risk of kidney stone formation due to reduced oxalate absorption (von Unruh et al., 2004).

Besides being present in many food, nonsoluble calcium oxalate crystals are also found in many ornamental flowering plants like *Anthurium*, *Dieffenbachia*, *Philodendron* and *Zantedeschia* (calla lily) species, and adverse reactions in contact with their stems, roots or leaves have been reported. The stalk of the plant produces the most severe skin reactions in humans due to direct tissue damage by the needlelike crystals of calcium oxalate. Oxalate crystals as well as other plant toxins (bradykinins, enzymes) produce pain and edema in contact with lips, tongue, oral mucosa, eyes, or skin, provoking inflammation. Damaged skin further improves the absorption of other plant toxins.

9. Phenolic Compounds

Plants produce different classes of phenolic compounds, such as p-coumaric, caffeic, ferulic, sinapic and gallic acids and their depside and glycoside derivatives. Flavonoid class of phenolics includes antocyanidines, leucoantocyanidines, flavon, flavanole, flavanone and flavonol subclasses, as well as numerous hydroxyl and metoxyl derivatives of catechin. Tannins are considered more complex polyphenolic compounds with molecular weight above 500, while lignins represent even larger polymers. Some plants like *Ginkgo biloba*, mango and poison ivy produce specific phenolic compounds with long hydrocarbon side chain, while nutmeg (*Myristica fragrans*), sassafras, mayapple, *Derris* and marihuana contain several others specific phenolics as well as other biologically active compounds (Caboni et al., 2004). The roots of *Derris* contain rotenone, a strong phenolic pesticide which is commonly used in fisheries as a piscicide and to destroy parasitic mites on chicken.

Cotton plant contains a polyphenolic aldehyde gossypol that was shown to inhibit several dehydrogenase enzymes. The compound was further studied because it was noticed that high incidence of sterility in some regions of China might be correlated with the consumption of the cotton oil. It was assumed that these findings were linked to gossypol and the substance was further tested as a male oral contraceptive (Coutinho, 2002).

Most of the citrus fruits contain tangeretin bioflavonoid. Due to several recognized health benefits, such as the reduction of the risk of some cancer types and lowering blood cholesterol, the substance is nowdays industrially produced by extracting the peel from citrus fruits (Morley et al., 2007). Tangeretin has also demonstrated promising evidence in protecting nerve cells by increasing the level of dopamine (Datia et al., 2001).

Phlorizin is a naturally occurring compound and dietary constituent found in a numerous fruit trees, such as cherry, apple and mayhaw tree. The substance was initially isolated from the bark of the apple tree. Potent antipyretic properties of the apple bark were recognized long time ago and ground bark was used in the treatment of fever and infectious diseases, particularly malaria (Ehrenkranz et al., 2005). Even though beneficial in some health conditions, phlorizin's demonstrates adverse health impact due to competitive inhibition of glucose reabsorption in renal tubules by affecting the glucose symporters in the proximal renal tubules. This results in glucosuria, i.e. the elevated glucose levels in urine. In addition to acting in urinary tract, the substance also prevents glucose absorption in mucosa of small intestine via inhibition of the sodium–glucose symporters.

Anthraquinones, aromatic organic compounds, occur naturally in some plants, insects and fungi. They represent condensed aromatic structures composed of anthracene and in plants they are most likely to be present as glycosides. Natural anthraquinone derivatives tend to have laxative effects and are used as cathartics (defecation accelerants). Plants containing significant quantities of antraquinones are used as defecation accelerants (cathartics) and include aloe (*Aloe vera*), rhubarb root (*Rheum palmatum*), *Rhamnus* species, senna leaves (*Cassia angustifolia*) and others. Prolonged usage of anthraquinone purgatives damages the nerve endings in the intestinal wall provoking painful colics and bowel sensitivity. Rhein, a representative of plant antraquinones, exhibits the toxicity by inhibiting electron transport in mitochondrial NAD-mediated oxidative processes, and by partial uncoupling of the oxidative phoshorilation (Bironaite & Öllinger, 1997). In addition, the evidence that rhein binds to essential bodily enzymes disturbing their function, also exist.

10. Photosensitizing Agents

Photosensitive reactions in which skin obstruction is observed after exposure to sunlight have been linked to handling or consumption of some plant-derived food. Topical contact with plants containing phototoxic agents has been shown to represent more serious risk to skin damage in comparison to ingestion of such food. Recognized group of phototoxic substances includes furocoumarins. Chemically, furocoumarins are compounds in which the furan ring is fused to coumarin in either linear way as in the case of psoralene (Figure 9) or in an angular manner, such as in angelicine (Figure 10). Naturally, furocoumarins are plant protective agents against wide range of threats, from insects to mammals.

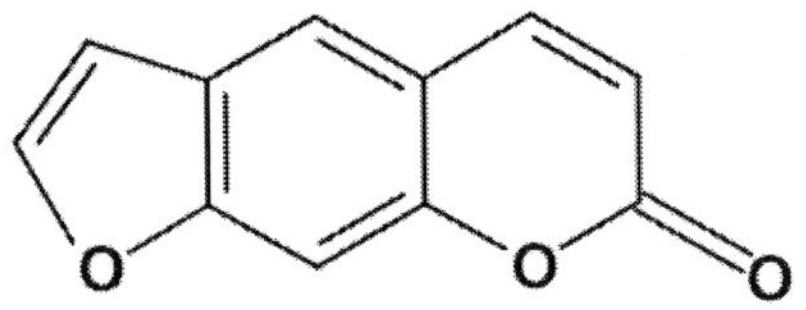

Figure 9. Psoralene.

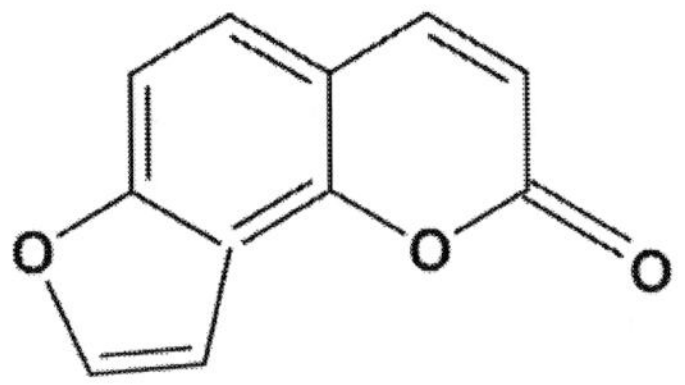

Figure 10. Angelicine.

The effects of natural phototoxic agents have frequently been demonstrated in grazing animals. The animals were sensitive to light, with skin and head edema development accompanied with intense jaundice and accumulation of bile pigments in urine. Affected skin turned brown and hard and conjunctiva and mucosa membrane in mouth become yellow. The offending plants which represent a risk to grazing animals include *Tribulus terrestris*, *Pannicum laevifolium, Pannicum coloratum, Fagopyrum cymosum* and numerous others from the families Vernaceae, Zygophillaceae and Graminae. Many plant pigments such as icterogenin, rehmannic acid, rutin, hypericine, and related fagopyrine, were isolated, characterized and identified as phototoxic agents that were causing toxic reactions in livestock. It is not yet completely elucidated whether all these agents increase the effectiveness of other photosensitizing agents from plants, or act synergistically with them. For example, icterogenin from *Tribulus* plant contributes to the toxicity of phylloerithrine. Phylloerithrine is a rose-red porphyrin end-product of chlorophyll metabolism which is normally excreted in bile, but in combination with icterogenin its excretion is prevented because icterogenin provokes spasic blocking of the bile duct. The phylloerithrine consequently accumulates in the body reaching the phototoxic level (Robey et al., 2006; National Research Council (U.S.), 1973).

Due to prominent photobilogical activity of psoralens together with other substances, they are nowdays used as phototherapeutic agents in the treatment of skin diseases like different types of cutaneous lymphoma, vitiligo and psoriasis (Fitzpatrick et al., 1966). Furocoumarins exhibit also other biological effects. The compounds bergamottin and dihydroxybergamottin, which are produced by citrus fruits, have a high potency of altering the activity of microsomal enzymes, thus, influencing the metabolic biotransformation of natural substances as well as xenobiotics (Švarc-Gajić, 2009).

11. Phytoestrogens

Many plants produce chemicals that mimic biochemical effects of hormones. Phytoestrogens are a plant derived diverse group of naturally occurring non-steroidal compounds that have the ability to act as agonists or antagonists of 17-β-estradiol. Such substances have been identified in more than 300 plant species including grains like wheat and rice, vegetables like beans, carrots, potatoes, soybeans, and fruits (date, cherries, apples, pomegranate), as well as spices like garlic, parsley and anis. Flax seed and soy bean have been identified as food containing among the highest levels of phytoestrogens (Thompson et al., 2006) (Table 6).

Table 6. The content of phytoestrogens in foodstuffs

Food sources	Phytoestrogens content (mg/100g)
Flax seed	379.4
Soy beans	103.9
Sesame seed	8.0
Garlic	0.60
Alfalfa	0.44
Pistachios	0.38
Lentils	0.37
Sunflower seed	0.22
Chestnuts	0.21
Olive oil	0.18
Walnuts	0.14
Almonds	0.13
Hazel nuts	0.11
Green bean	0.11
Peanuts	0.034

The major phytoestrogen chemical groups include isoflavones, flavones, lignans and coumestans (Table 7). Isoflavones are found in high concentration in soy bean and its products, whereas in flax seed lignans are predominant.

Table. 7. Major phytoestrogens

	Phytoestrogen chemical classes			
	Flavones	Isoflavones	Lignans	Coumestans
Compound	Quercetin	Genistein	Secoisolariciresinol	Coumestrol
		Daidzein	Matairesinol	4`-methoxycoumestrol
		Daidzein	Pinoresinol	Repensol
		Formononetin	Lariciresinol	Trifoliol
		Glycitein	Enterodiol	
		Formononetin	Enterolactone	

Feed rich in phytoestrogen-producing plants may negatively influence the reproduction of grazing animals. It is speculated that phytoestrogens might contribute to infertility in the livestock. Animal studies have also demonstrated that genistein and coumestrol deposited in fat tissue of experimental animals and that they stimulated uterine hypertrophy. Furthermore, coumestrol inhibited the gonadotropin function of experimental animals (Medlock et al., 1995). Phytoestrogens pose less serious risk for humans, since usually food rich in phytoestrogens represents only small portion of the diet, and phytoestrogens have several times less potent biochemical activity in comparison to estrogen hormones (Humfrey, 1998). In addition to their estrogenic effects, flavonoid and lignan phytoestrogens exhibit potent antioxidant activity. Other beneficial effects of phytoestrogens include suppression of menopausal symptoms, reduced risk of breast and prostate cancer, as well as possible protection against osteoporosis (Cassidy, 2003).

12. Poisonous Mushrooms

Numerous higher fungi produce toxins which do not degrade even after thermal processing like cooking, boiling, frying or freezing. Poisoning with mushrooms usually occurs when the poisonous species is misidentified with the edible one or in intentional ingestions of hallucinogenic species. Individual specimens of poisonous mushrooms are characterized by variations in toxin content depending on genetics, geographic location, and growing conditions. Besides frequently being a causative agent of alimental intoxications, many mushroom species have also been reported to trigger idiosyncratic adverse reactions resembling allergy. The level of intolerance and the severity of symptoms may significantly differ in individuals due to variations in their susceptibility. Allergy-like adverse reactions are not usually linked to recognized mushroom toxins but to idiosyncratic intolerance to some other mushroom compounds, such as trechalose for example.

Due to vast chemical diversity of mushroom poisons, they are usually classified according to physiological effects produced by them. Protoplasmatic poisons provoke cell destruction eventually resulting in the functional failure of internal organs. This is first seen as impaired functions of liver (elevated billirubin) and kidneys (elevated uric acid, creatinine). Mushroom neurotoxins act primarily on a central nervous system provoking excitement, hallucinations, convulsions and coma. Gastrointestinal disturbances such as abdominal cramping, nausea, vomiting and diarrhea are observed in the cases when mushrooms produce gastrointestinal irritants. Dissulfiram-like mushroom toxins do not pose a serious health risk by themselves, but in combination with alcohol. The symptoms of intoxication might be observed even if alcohol has been consumed 72 hours after mushroom ingestion.

Protoplasmatic mushroom poisons are also called amatoxins or amanitins, because they are produced mostly by Amanita species: *Amanita phalloides*, *Amanita virosa*, *Amanita verna*, but also by some of their relatives and *Galerina autumnalis*. The produced toxins chemically represent cyclic octapeptides. The symptoms of poisoning with amanitins start developing after long latent period (up to 48 hours) in the form of abdominal pain, diarrhea, vomiting, extreme thirst and anuria (inability to urinate). Death occurs in most poisoning cases after approximately 6 days and is due to irreversible liver, kidney, cardiac, and skeletal muscle damage (Hanrahan & Gordon, 1984; Köppel, 1993).

A volatile hydrazine derivative gyromitrin acts as a strong protoplasmic poison and is produced in *Gyromitra esculenta* and *Gyromitra gigas*. The symptoms of poisoning with gyromitrin resemble typical protoplasmatic poisoning. Yet unidentified poison from *Verpa bohemica* produces similar effects as gyromitrin. The latent period in poisoning with orellanine, another protoplasmatic poison produced by *Cortinarius orellanus*, can last up to 14 days. In intoxicated individual's nausea, headache and muscular pains accompany the feeling of unbearable thirst and intensified urination. Besides severe damage to kidneys and liver, inflammatory changes in the intestines occur, requiring several month for full recovery.

Mushroom neurotoxins differ in their structure and can produce different neurological symptoms. Muscarine is an alkaloid produced by several mushroom species, like *Amanita muscaria*, *Inocybe geophylla* and *Clitocybe dealbata*. Poisoning with muscarine is usually revealed soon upon ingestion. Within first half an hour upon ingestion intense salivation, perspiration and lacrimation are observed, followed by intense abdominal pain, diarrhea and blurred vision. The lethal outcomes are rare and the symptoms of poisoning subside within 2 hours (Stallard & Edes, 1989). Ibotenic acid and muscimol exhibit similar toxic effects like muscarine and are produced by *Amanita muscaria* and *Amanita pantherina* species. Muscimol has several times more potent toxicity in comparison to ibotenic acid. Symptoms of poisoning with these toxins start developing within 1-2 hours upon ingestion with abdominal discomfort. Excitability, hyperactivity and delirium follow the initial dizziness and drowsiness. Fatal outcomes are rare in adults, but may happen in children which have ingested large quantities of the poisonous mushroom.

The symptoms of poisoning with mushroom poisons whose primarily mode of action is gastrointestinal distress are similar to protoplasmatic poisoning, however rapid onset of symptoms like, diarrhea, nausea and vomiting make the poisoning with gastrointestinal irritants easily distinguishable from protoplasmatic mushroom poisons. Some of the symptoms may last for several days. Numerous mushrooms like *Chlorophyllum molybdites, Entoloma lividum, Tricholoma pardinum, Omphalotus illudens, Paxillus involutus, Russula emetica, Verpa bohemica, Agaricus arvensis* and *Boletus piperatus* produce gastrointestinal irritants. Fatalities caused by these mushrooms are relatively rare and are associated with dehydration and electrolyte imbalances caused by diarrhea and vomiting.

A numerous mushrooms belonging to genera *Psilocybe, Panaeolus, Copelandia, Gymnopilus, Conocybe*, and *Pluteus*, when ingested, produce a syndrome similar to alcohol intoxication, sometimes accompanied with hallucinations, due to dissulfiram-like compounds that they produce. Thus, specific mushrooms are often intentionally ingested to produce psychotropic effects. The main risk of consuming mushrooms producing dissulfiram-like poisons lies in the fact that these mushrooms may be mistakenly considered as safe and edible. Toxicity of these mushrooms is probable only if consumed with alcohol. Most commonly implicated mushroom in such poisonings is *Coprinus atramentarius* which produces an aminoacid coprine. Coprine metabolite, cyclopropanone hydrate, interferes with ethanol metabolism and blocks the normal biotransformation pathway. Accumulated ethanol metabolites are responsible for the onset symptoms such as flushing, headache, nausea and vomiting. The symptoms last for 2 -3 hours and appear even if the alcoholic beverage has been consumed 72 hours after mushroom ingestion (Chilton, 1994). Psilocin and psilocybin are another compounds that have been isolated from mushrooms and identified as active components producing hallucinations. The symptoms of poisoning with these compounds resemble alcoholic intoxication accompanied with hallucinations. Fatal outcomes in adults are rare and the symptoms of poisoning appear soon upon ingestion and subside within two hours (Stamets, 1996). More severe poisoning cases demonstrate hallucinations with fever, convulsions and coma.

13. Seafood

Many cases of poisoning by seafood, such as crustaces, fish and mussels are reported each day worldwide. Many marine organisms are able to produce venoms which are naturally intendent to protect the animals from predators and are often very toxic to humans too. Other substances representing the health risk to humans, such as biogenic vasoactive amines like tyramine or histamine, are produced by microbial processes during the storage of seafood. The most difficult to predict is the occurrence of toxicants which are initially produced by microorganisms like plankton and algae, and are introduced to other marine species feeding on them. The occurrence of toxin-producing plankton is sporadic and any marine species may represent a potential threat if fed on plankton. The toxins initially produced by plankton are subject of bioaccumulation through the food chain reaching much higher concentrations in tissues of higher marine organisms. On oppose to plankton-derived toxins which can be found in any marine species, the occurrence of venoms is strictly related to specific marine species and the human poisoning occurs usually due to absence or neglectance of the knowledge of the risk that the specific marine species carries.

Fugu dishes, dishes of pufferfish, are highly appreciated and considered a culinary delicacy in Japan. The dishes are normally prepared only by licensed chefs who remove majority of the tetrodotoxin, a toxic substance produced by the fish. Prepared meals might still contain low levels of the toxin even after removal of organs in which the toxin is accumulated provoking the feeling of subtitle tingling in tongue, the feeling the consumer is seeking for. Tetrodotoxin is one of the most potent natural neurotoxins known and, besides produced by puffer fishes, it is also produced by many other venomous organisms such as Amazonian poison arrow frogs. The highest concentrations of the substance is found in fish ovaries and liver, even though in some fish species the toxin can be well distributed in muscle tissue as well. Tetrodotoxin toxicity stems from blocking the conduction of impulses in synapses by increasing the sodium permeability of the membranes. The symptoms of tetrodotoxin poisoning start appearing between 20 minutes to three hours after eating the poisonous pufferfish and begin with vomiting, diarrhea, numbness and tingling in mouth, tongue and lips (Hwang & Noguchi, 2007). Paralyzed, the victim remains completely conscious. Death eventually occurs due to respiratory paralysis.

Ichthyootoxins are the toxins which are stored in fish eggs and are produced by more than 50 species of marine and fresh water fishes. When toxin-containing roe is consumed in meals, severe gastrointestinal disturbances occur, such as cramps, diarrhea and vomiting. The presence of ichthyootoxins has been identified in many fish species, such as the barbell (*Barbus fluviatus*), the pike (*Esox lucius*) and gar (*Lepisosteus* spp.), however probably the most well studied ichthyootoxin is lysophospholipid dinogunellin, isolated from the northern blenny (*Stichaeus grigorjewi*).

Gastrointestinal disturbances triggered by fish consumption can also result from high content of unusual lipid compounds in fish muscles. Fish species producing offending fats such as escolar (*Lepidocybium flavobrunneum*), stromatid fish (*Stromuteus maculatus*), driftfish (*Cubiceps gracilis*) and *Centrolophus* spp usually live in deep tropical waters. Wax esters and diacyl glycerol esters present in muscle tissue of these fishes are responsible for intensified bowel movement, nausea, diarrhea and uncontrollable discharge of rectum after fish consumption.

The poisoning with Japanese ivory mollusk (*Babylonia japonica*) produces both gastrointestinal and neurological symptoms due to antagonism on nicotinic receptors and inhibition of postganglionic transmission by specific toxins found in mollusk (Rechcigl, 1983). The symptoms may be quite severe and the outcome is usually fatal. Toxic component in Japanese ivory mollusk tissue has shown to be surugatoxin (Figure 11). It is not yet clear whether the mollusk produces the toxin itself or the toxicity results from the accumulation of the toxin-producing bacteria in mollusk.

Paralytic shellfish poisoning occurs after consuming mostly the mollusk, but also different species of pufferfish, all containing saxitoxin. Saxitoxin is one of the most potent neurotoxins known and is produced by different species of cyanobacteria (*Aphanizomenon, Anabaena, Lyngbyasp)* and dinoflagellates (*Gymnodinium, Alexandrium, Pyrodinium*). This toxin blocs the sodium channels in synapses causing the paralysis and respiratory failure in intoxicated individuals. Due to some common symptoms, such as the feeling of numbness in tongue and lips in a short time after consuming the food, the weakness and the tingling, paralytic shellfish poisoning can easily be misdiagnosed with the poisoning with other toxins, such as botulism or tetrodotoxin.

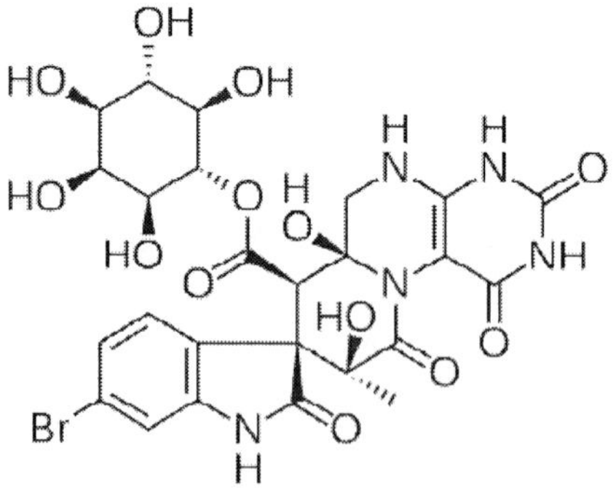

Figure 11. Surugatoxin.

The occurrence of the *Gambierdiscus toxicus* alga is usually limited to tropical waters. This microorganism produces a ciguatoxin (Figure 12) which accumulates mostly in tropical and semitropical bottom-feeding fish species representing, thus, a potential health threat. Ciguatoxin provokes neural and gastrointestinal symptoms which start with nausea, vomiting and diarrhea, followed by parasthesia (the sensation of tingling and pricking in the skin), numbness and hallucinations. The recovery from ciguatera poisoning is very slow and the symptoms may persist for years. Furthermore it was demonstrated that the toxin from intoxicated individuals can be transmitted sexually and is also excreted in human milk representing, thus, a threat to nursing infants (Bagnis et al., 1979; Blythe & De Sylva, 1979).

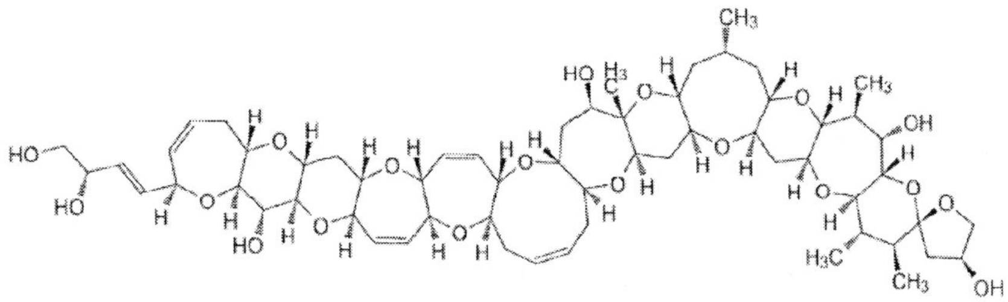

Figure 12.Ciguatoxin.

Saxitoxin and ciguatoxin are the most potent identified poisons produced by dinoflagellates, however many other nonidentified toxic substances found in seafood pose a risk to humans. In poisoning with marine food exact cause of poisoning often remains unelucidated and the substances from different chemical classes might be responsible for the toxicity of sea food (Table 8). Due to chemical diversity of potential marine threats, it is difficult to develop a standardized procedure for controlling the quality of seafood used for human nutrition. The simplest and cheapest possibility is to prepare the seafood extract and to administrate it to experimental mice. More expensive alternative is to use specific bioafinity tests, however such tests are developed only for well established and known toxins such as saxitoxin and ciguatoxin, limiting their application in the general seafood quality control.

Table 8. Some of the identified seafood toxins

Toxin-producing species	Toxin
Puffer fish	Tetrodotoxin
Carp	5-α-cyprinol
Ciguatoxic fish	Cigutoxins, Maitotoxin
Mollusk	Saxitoxin
Pufferfish	Gonyautoxins
Diarrhetic shellfish	Okadaic acid
	Dinophysistoxins, Pectenotoxins
	Yessotoxin
Amnesic shellfish, Anchovies, Sardines	Domoic acid
Ivory shell	Neosurugatoxin, Prosurugatoxin
Gastropod	Tetramine
Abalone	Pyropheophorbide
Japanese annelid	Nereistoxin

14. Spice Plants

Addition of spices to food by humans dates many thousands years BC. In the Middle Age spices were among the most appreciated and luxurious products available in Europe. Besides giving the food specific flavor and enhancing the sensory properties, spices were added to food as a mean of preservation. Many of herbs used as spices produce the substances with strong antimicrobial properties and these were responsible for extending the shelf life of food products when other means of food preservations were unavailable. Spice plants produce many different active substances and besides their use as food components, spices have a long history of their use as aphrodisiacs, stimulants and drugs in folk medicines. Since spices are normally used in relatively small doses in human nutrition, they do not pose a serious health risks to humans, however some evidence linked to specific spice plants is useful to be elaborated.

14.1. Allicin

The plants from *Allium* genus, including garlic, onion and chive, are widely used in many world cuisines and folk medicines owing to their specific flavor, antimicrobial effects and very rich dietary value. Many volatile, mostly sulphur-containing compounds, are responsible for characteristic flavor and odor of these plants, as well as for their lacrimatory properties. Onion, besides containing many enzymes (alinase, arginase, mirosinaze, peroxidase, tyrosinase, desoxyribonuclease) is also rich in vitamins B and C, provitamine A and numerous minerals such as potassium, iron, sulphur, selenium, calcium, phosphorous and others.

Volatile sulphur-containing compounds are produced in the plants from S-substituted cysteine sulfoxide precursors, of which alliin ((+)-S-allyl-Lcysteine sulfoxide) is the most abundant precursor in garlic, reaching the contents up to 2.4 mg/g. The same precursor was also isolated from plants not belonging to *Allium* genus, such as cauliflower, broccoli, cabbage and kohlrabi. By the activity of alliinase, aliin and other sulfoxides are converted in plants to allicin which exhibit strong antimicrobial activity, and disulfides which are responsible for characteristic odor of *Allium* species (Figure 13). This conversation takes place within few seconds after the plant tissue has been damaged and enzymes were activated. This normally occurs by chewing or chopping the *Allium* species. Formed allicin is relatively unstable and is completely inactivated within 16 hours at ambient temperature under the influence of oxygen.

Antimicrobial and insecticidal effects of allicin can be explained by the chemical reaction of the compound with thiol groups of various bacterial enzymes. Some studies have also confirmed that allicin has inhibitory activity on *Helicobacter pylori*, a bacterium responsible for the development of gastric ulcers, as well as on some parasites.

Even though beneficial effects of *Allium* species have been exploited for centuries, some new evidence about the influence of allicin and other related compounds on iodine uptake have alerted the scientific community. Antithyroid activity was confirmed in animal experiments performed with the radioactive iodide for different methyl-, n-propyl- and allyl disulfides, but in normal dietary intake of garlic and onion disruption of thyroid activity is not likely to occur. On the basis of conducted toxicological animal studies the lethal dose (LD_{50}) of allicin for a human of average weight of 70 kg is estimated to be around 21.6 mg (Deshpande, 2002). It is worth mentioning that allicin has been show to be very toxic to pets, causing gastroenteritis and hemolytic anemia.

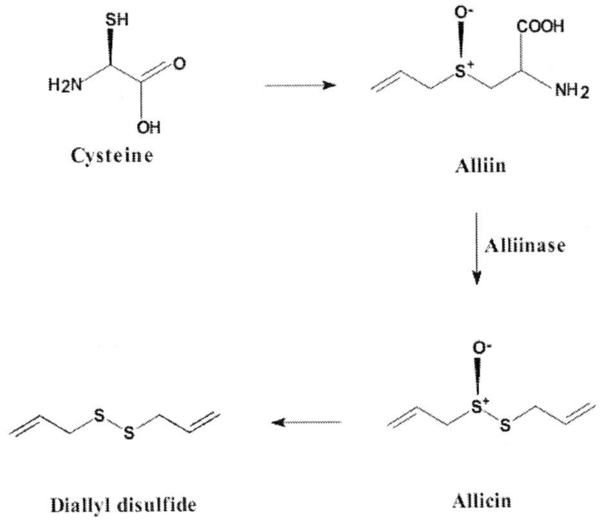

Figure 13. The formation of allicin in vegetables.

14.2. Allyl Isothiocyanate

Allyl isothiocyanate is a pungent organosulphur compound of mustard (*Brassica nigra*, *Brassica juncea*), horseradish, wasabi ("Japanese horseradish"), cabbage and cauliflower. It serves to plants as a protection against herbivores and is stored in the plants in its " inactive ", glucosinolate form sinigrin. Glucosinolate form represents the form of the substance in which glucose moiety is bound to the substance. Allyl isothiocyanate is released by enzymatic activity of mirosinaze enzyme after the plant has been damaged or offended, thus repelling the animals. Similar isothio- compound, benzyl isothiocyanate, is formed by mirosinaze transformation of thioglucoside, glucotropaeolin, found in papaya fruit (*Carica papaya* L.) with seeds having the highest concentrations. In addition to containing pungent components, the leaves and unripe fruits of papaya contain proteolytic enzymes, including papain, chymopapains A and B, and papaya peptidase A. These enzymes, highly concentrated in the plants sap, are responsible for irritating properties of the unripened fruits. Proteolytic potency of papain is nowdays widely used in cosmetic preparations to smoothen the skin.

Normal dietary intake contributes to 50 to 100 ppm of allyl isothiocyanate mostly ingested through vegetables. In humans allyl isothiocyanate has shown to be a strong irritant to skin, eyes and nose. Furthermore it has been demonstrated that it damages mucous membranes. The cases of contact dermatitis when handling horseradish salad were reported and were linked to allyl isothiocyanate. Toxicological studies about the toxicity of allyl isothiocyanate are incomplete, but some animal studies demonstrated that orally taken high doses of the compound over prolonged period provoke stomach ulcers and liver damage.

14.3. Anisatin

The Japanese star anise (*Illicium anisatum*) or Sikimi plant is a tree similar to Chinese star anise (*Illicium verum*) both of which closely resemble anis (*Pimpinella anisum*). Chinese star anis is sometimes used as a cheaper alternative to anis and is widely used in Chinese, Indian and Indonesian cuisine. Even though star anis shouldn't be used for human nutrition due to toxic compounds that it contains, it is used as a less expensive substitute for anise in baking as well as in liquor production. Anis flavor is characteristic and distinctive for numerous liquors like Sambuca, Pastis, Galliano and many types of absinthe. Anethole, an aromatic ether, is the principal anis flavor component and is responsible for the characteristic odor and taste of the listed liquors.

Among all anis species, Japanese star anise is the most dangerous containing several toxic compounds, such as anisatin, safrole, shikimin, sikimitoxin and eugenol, among which anisatin, a convulsant sesquiterpenoid, is the most toxic. Prezizaane-type sesquiterpenes, structurally related to anisatin, have been identified in a number of other *Illicium* species (Kuriyama et al., 2002). Toxic compounds from Japanese star anise are characteristic for that specific anis type and are used to detect adulteration in anis. Consumption of food products prepared with the addition of Japanese star anise can provoke many adverse reactions. Ingestion of the seeds is much more dangerous and provokes inflammation of gastrointestinal and urinary tracts. The symptoms appear 1-6 hours after ingestion and include stomach pain, diarrhea and vomiting, followed by nervous system excitation, seizures and respiratory paralysis. Intoxication with anisatin via dermal absorption is less probable. Due to its pleasant flavor topical use of Japanese star anise preparations is common in folk medicine and is exploited usually without provoking any adverse reactions.

14.4. Asarone

Asarone (4-propenyl-l,2,5-trimethoxybenzene) is a volatile ether, a component of a fragrance oil of some evergreen grass-like plants such as acorus, asarum, calamus and matico. The roots of the plants of *Asarum* genus are sometimes used as a spice because their rhizomes taste like ginger, for what they are often called wild ginger. Besides culinary uses, the extracts of roots and rhizomes of *Asarum* plants have been used in Ayurvedic medicine for centuries due to pronounced pharmacological activity of their ingredients. Asarone, the major active principle of the plants consists of its alpha (*trans*) and beta (*cis*) isomers (Figure 14). Both isomers demonstrate the influence on central nervous system in humans, similarly as reserpine and chlorpromazine (antipsychotics). Asarone has shown to exhibit a potent hypnotic influence, prolonging the sleep and causing hypothermia. Another physiologically active substance that was isolated from asarum plants includes aristolochic acid, whose carcinogenic effects were confirmed in experiments with rats.

Alpha asarone shows a significant capacity to reduce the level of blood lipids, including cholesterol. However, several studies on its toxicity and genotoxicity have revealed that its use may pose a risk to human health. Assays performed on human cell cultures have demonstrated its hepatocarcinogenic and mutagenic character and this were also confirmed in animal studies (Chamorro et al., 1998). Data on how beta asarone is metabolized in humans are very limited and animal toxicological studies indicate hepatotoxicity and cardiotoxicity of beta asarone. Similar results were obtained in experiments in which total extract of the *Asarum* plants was used.

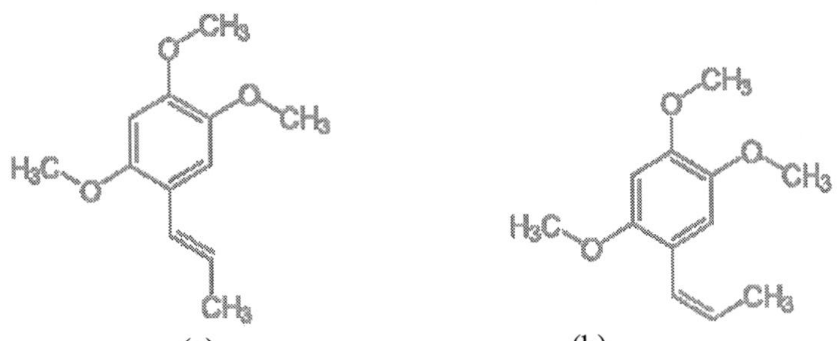

(a) (b)

Figure 14. (a) Alpha and beta (b) asarone.

14.5. Eugenol

Characteristic flavor of clove oil derives from the presence of scent compound eugenol. The compound is also present in cinnamon and other aromatic spices. Due to its pleasant smell the compound is often used in perfume industry. The application of eugenol is very diverse. The compound is used as a component of many pharmaceutical preparations as a UV absorber, insect attractant, as well as an additive in plastic and rubber industry. Eugenol also exhibits strong antiseptic and analgetic properties and deactivates free radicals, acting as an antioxidant. Besides numerous beneficial effects, ingestion of large doses of eugenol, normally via clove oil overdose, can lead to burns in mouth and throat, nausea and strong abdominal pain. Rapid breathing and rapid heartbeat are preceded by seizures and coma. In normal diet the poisoning with eugenol is not probable, but in intentional clove overdosis eugenol may provoke intoxication. Even though not fatal, consumption of the excess of clove via spiced food may produce an unpleasant experience.

14.6. Estragole

Estragole (p-allylanisole, methyl chavicol) is a natural organic compound consisting of a benzene ring substituted with a methoxy and a propenyl groups. The compound is present in essential oils of many spices, such as tarragon (60-75%) , anise (1%), star anise (5-6%), basil (20-30%), bay, marjoram, as well as in culinary herbs like fennel (5-20% of essential oil). Estragol has also been identified in pine oil and terpentine, where it contributes to build-up of the characteristic strong, sweet flavor.

Natural herbal oils containing estragol have widespread applications in folk medicine and aromatherapy and are known to posses a potent local anesthetic activity. Estragole is also used in perfumes and as a food additive for flavoring, however the use of the compound is strictly limited due to the recognized carcinogenic character. Recent concerns about the potential carcinogenicity of estragole had led a number of regulatory bodies to call for restrictions on the use of herbs that contain this constituent.

Experiments conducted *in vitro* have demonstrated that carcinogenesis under the influence of estragole occurs via mutagenic mechanism (Drinkwater et al., 1976). After absorption estragole is metabolized in liver to 1'- hydroxyestragole and several epoxide compounds which are further sulphated in hepatocytes. Formed sulfate conjugates readily bind to DNA provoking carcinogenesis in hepatocytes.

Besides estragole carcinogenicity animal studies conducted with the pure compound revealed other physiological effects. Experiments in mice demonstrated that estragole provokes depolarization of the muscle membrane and that it inhibits some microsomal enzymes (Aline et al., 1995). The finding that estragole and its derivatives exhibit skin whitening effects opened a new perspectives concerning estragole role in dermatology (Yutaka Motoki et al., 2003).

14.7. Glycyrrhizin

Glycyrrhizin is triterpenoid saponin glycoside produced in licorice with pronounced sweet taste. Liquorice *(Glycyrrhiza glabra)* is indigenious to Southern Europe and parts of Asia but is cultivated in many parts of the world. Particularly popular the plant is in Italy, Spain, Netherlands, China and Egypt, where it is used to produce candies, as a sweetener in some soft drinks, for the production of liquors as well as in medicines for masking the unpleasant taste of pharmaceuticals. Due to its sweet taste the substance has been used as a substitute for artificial sweeteners, like aspartame, and was also used as a flavoring in tobacco products. In some countries like Japan, glycyrrhizin is used for the treatment of the liver damage in conditions like liver chyrosis and hepatitis. Experiments conducted on cell cultures have demonstrated that glycyrrhizic acid, which is formed in the body form the glycyrrhizin glycoside, inhibits the growth of several DNA and RNA viruses (Fiore et al., 2008; Numazaki, 2003).

The sweetness of glycyrrhizin glycoside is considered to be 30-50 times stronger in comparison to sucrose and the produced sweet sensation in mouth is somewhat different in comparison to table sugar. After consuming glycyrrhizin the sweet flavor can be felt in mouth for a longer time in comparison to table sugar, but with longer onset. Reported side effects of glycyrrhizin include hypertension and general edema, due to increased retention of sodium and water.

Even though considered as a generally safe, concerns about the safety of glycyrrhizin are primarily due to inhibition of cortisol metabolism and the subsequent stimulation of the mineralocorticoid receptors, provoking the symptoms of hypermineralocorticoidism. Most obvious signs of altered mineralocorticoid signaling include hypokalaemia, low plasma renin and high plasma aldosterone.

14.8. Capsaicin

Capsaicin (8-methyl-*N*-vanillyl-6-nonenamide) is the principle pungent component of chili peppers, belonging to the genus *Capsicum*. There are five species of *Capsicum* peppers, *C. pubescens, C. baccatum, C. annuum, C. frutescens* and *C. chinense* and the hottest chili peppers belong to the *C. chinense* group. Capsaicin, together with other related compounds called capsaicinoids, is produced in the plants as a secondary metabolite to repel herbivores and to protect the plants against fungi. Other capsaicinoids in peppers, less abundant and less pungent in comparison to capsaicin, include dihydrocapsaicine, nordihydrocapsaicin, homodihydrocapsaicin, and homocapsaicin (Figure 15). According to its pungency, dihydrocapsaicine, which contributes to total capsaicinoids content significantly, is very close to capsaicin.

Capsaicin is a strong irritant and it provokes heating sensation in contact with the skin and mucose membranes. The substance can bind to neural receptors from both sides of plasma membrane increasing the permeability of the membrane to cations, especially to calcium, signaling the pain and provoking the release of inflammatory mediators. Even though pain signalization is first observed effect of capsaicin, in prolonged contacts capsaicin provokes the opposite reactions, i.e. the reduced pain sensation. After the capsaicin has been bound to pain receptors, the rush of calcium ions shifts the responsiveness of the receptors to the pain. For these reasons capsaicin is used as an analgetic agent in some pharmaceutical products used to treat pain in conditions like arthritis, diabetic neuropathy and muscle pain. Long-term loss of neural responsiveness to pain under the influence of capsaicin is related to the destruction of neural pain receptors with high doses of capsaicin.

Resiniferatoxin, an extremely potent natural capsaicin analogue found in a cactus-like plant *Euphorbia resinifera*, commonly found in Morocco, mimics the cellular action of capsaicin, while capsazepine, a competitive synthetic capsaicin antagonist, relieves the pain by blocking the current flow between neurons.

Even though beneficial for pain relief, poisoning with capsaicine due to consumption of large doses of chili peppers can cause serious health problems, which usually start with nausea, vomiting, abdominal pain and burning diarrhea. Severe over-exposure to pure capsaicin can result even in death. The lethal dose (LD_{50}) of pure capsaicin in mice after oral administration is estimated to be 18.8 mg/kg for males and 97.4 mg/kg for females (Saito & Yamamoto, 1996).

Mucosal damages after ingesting chili papers have been observed in some studies dealing with capsaicine effects, but could not been firmly linked to sole capsaicin. The evaluation of capsaicin impact on stomach cancer is controversial. Even though the carcinogenic, procarcinogenic, cocarcinogenic, and tumor promotion effects of capsaicine have been reported in animal studies, numerous publications reporting the evidence of its antitumorigenic and anti-tumor promotion effects exist and are in collision with the former ones (Surh & Lee, 1996).

Humans are exposed to capsaicin by ingesting chili pepper or hot food, or topically, by skin contact with chili peppers or chili products. Skin exposure to capsaicin is accompanied with severe burning and stinging pain, while eye exposure produces intense tearing, pain and conjunctivitis. Poisoning with capsaicin is usually treated according to symptoms themselves. Burning sensation of the skin can be reduced by cooling and capsaicin is best removed from the skin with surface active compounds, such as soap or detergency, or with hydrophobic creams and oils. Polar water can not remove hydrophobic capsaicin from the skin, prolonging the contact. In cases when capsaicin has come into contact with eyes and mucose membranes, anesthetics can be administrated to reduce burning sensation. Capsaicin-induced asthma is best treated with bronchodilatators and antihistamines (Goldfrank, 2002).

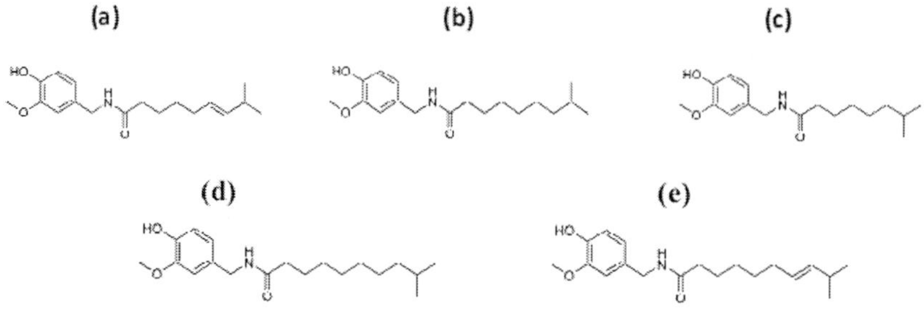

Figure 15. (a) Capsaicin; (b) Dihydrocapsaicine; (c) Nordihydrocapsaicin; (d) Homodihydrocapsaicin; (e) Homocapsaicin.

14.9. Myristicin

Myristicin has been isolated from the nutmeg plant or *Myristica fragrans*, an evergreen tree indigenous to Indonesia, Malasya, Caribbean and some parts of India. Nutmeg plant is used for the production of two spices, nutmeg and mace, as well as for nutmeg butter, jam and nutmeg sweets. The use of nutmeg and mace is very popular in many world cuisines, as a spice or for preparing different dressings, typically for potatoes and meat dishes. Aside from culinary uses, nutmeg has had many other interesting traditional uses in different cultures. It was believed that nutmeg brings luck, especially in gambling. Among the Arabs nutmeg has been used to treat digestive problems and has also been valued as an aphrodisiac. In addition to its aphrodisiac properties, nutmeg oil rubbed on genitals was used to raise the sexual desire. In some cultures nutmeg was used as a sedative, to combat asthma and heart problems or to provoke the abortion.

Myristicin (Figure 16), as a chief aromatic component and active principle of a nutmeg, is not very toxic when consumed in normal diet. In higher doses, however, the substance acts like psychoactive compound probably because myristicin is metabolized via amination to more active methoxymethylenedioxyamphetamine. In high doses myristicin provokes nausea, dehydratation, general body pain, anxiety and convulsions (Gable, 2006). The mechanism of adverse health effects includes the inhibition of monoamine oxidase and prostaglandin synthesis. Prostaglandins are very important physiologically active, hormone-like molecules that are synthetized in the body from fatty acids. They have very complex role in the body, including the regulation of the contraction and relaxation of smooth muscles.

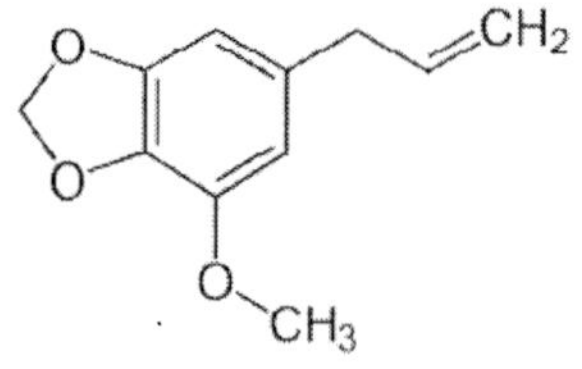

Figure 16. Myristicin.

Myristicin exhibits very potent teratogenic effects and if consumed in high quantities during pregnancy, it can provoke severe fetal malformations. Not of high acute toxicity to humans, myristicin from nutmeg pose a serious threat to domestic animals and pets provoking the lethal outcome even in moderate doses found in dishes prepared with the nutmeg spice.

Safrole is another aromatic component of nutmeg and is also found in high concentrations in *Sassafras* species known for their intense flavor, but banned due to proven carcinogenicity of safrole.

14.10. Piperine

A pungent substance found in plants of Piperaceae family, including black pepper (*Piper nigrum*) and long pepper (*Piper longum*), piperine, has been shown to induce different physiological effects. In traditional approach piperine was used as a folk medicine to treat malaria, ear inflammation, joints pain, liver and lungs diseases, gangrene and many other medical conditions.

Chemically, piperine is composed of the alkali piperidine and piperic acid. The pungency of piperine, similary as capsaicin found in chili pepper, is caused by the activation of ion channels on the pain sensing nerve cells (nociceptors). Piperine derivative, chavicine, accompanies piperine in black pepper and also contributes to peppers pungency. Both pungent substances piperine and chavicine are secondary metabolites of the plants and are stored mostly in the fruits (3 - 7%).

Physiologically active by itself, piperine also demonstrates several marked physiological effects indirectly by affecting the metabolism of other exogenous substances. In general, piperine has pronounced impact on protein transporters located on cell membranes which are responsible for transferring the compounds from one body compartment to another. Most pronounced impact piperine demonstrates by activating aminoacid transporters in intestinal linings. Activated, these transporters can also be exploited by other substances, which, in return, are more efficiently transferred to blood. By this mechanism the absorption of selenium, beta-carotene, vitamins B and sparteine, is significantly improved under the influence of piperine. Furthermore some research postulate that piperine inhibits P protein, the vital protein participating in the transport of the compounds from the innerspace of cells, therefore prolonging the residence time of the compounds in the cells. Conducted studies suggested that piperine inhibits microsomal enzymes involved in the metabolism of xenobiotics, increasing their bioavailability and contributing to their toxicity. For example, piperine enhances the bioavailability of curcumin by 2000% in humans (Shoba et al., 1998). Altered metabolism of compounds under the influence of piperine can significantly influence therapeutic dose of the drugs. Besides increasing the toxicity of some xenobiotics by inhibiting biotransformational enzymes, piperine also exploits another mode. The production of glucuronic acid in gastrointestinal tract is inhibited by piperine. Considering that glucuronic conjugates are among the most important means of toxicant excretion, it is clear that lack of glucuronic acid will contribute to longer residence time of xenobiotics in the body. Other adverse health effects of piperine have been postulated based on animal experiments and *in vitro* studies. The studies suggested that piperine interferes with several crucial reproductive events in mammalian models. (Daware et al., 2000). In conducted studies piperine also induced marked damage to cultured neurons and cultivated astrocytes, demonstrating, thus, the first evidence of piperine neurotoxicity (Unchern et al., 1997). Beneficial effects of piperine include bactericidal, insecticidal and nematocidal effects.

Recently it was discovered that piperine stimulates pigmentation in the skin after exposure to UV light (Faas et al., 2008).

14.11. Umbellulone

The leaves of *Umbellularia californica* (myrtlewood, bay, laurel, pepperwood) are culinary herbs appreciated in Europe and North America and used for seasoning meats, soups, stews and other dishes. Besides very pleasant aroma that the spice gives to dishes, it is believed that the plant posses many beneficial health effects. Historical evidence suggests that dried leaves of laurel have been used for preparing tea to treat chills and fever. All parts of the plant, the leaves, the bark, the fruit and the seeds were used for preparing beverages for treating various medical conditions, including vermin control. Due to strong physiological properties of the *Umbellularia californica* oil, it has been used in some traditional remedies to treat rheumatism, meningitis, nervous disorders, intestinal colics, dyspepsia and inflammation of mucous membranes.

The leaves of laurel contain approximately 0.5 – 4% of an irritating oil, whose principal component is a ketone umbellulone which demonstrates strong fungicidal properties. Umbellulone accounts for 40 – 60 % of the laurel oil and can also be found in the seeds of celery, oak-goal and oil of pyrethrum plants. Other substances present in laurel oil include formic acid, fatty acids, safrole, eugenol, methyeugenol, α-pinene and other aromatic compounds, but it is believed that umbellulone is the most active component of laurel extract. Umbellulone together with other volatile components can cause sneezing, headache, sinus irritation and other severe discomforts. When inhaled, the volatiles from aromatic oil disrupt respiration, heart rate and blood circulation.

15. Other Dangerous Plants and Food Toxins

15.1. Beta-Carotene

Carrots (*Daucus carota*) are vegetables widely used in all world cuisines for preparing salads and dishes. The plant has originally been cultivated in central Asian and Middle Eastern countries. In Europe carrot wasn't a popular vegetable until the Renaissance probably because early varieties had unpleasantly fibrous texture. Today, carrots are highly appreciated dietary source because they are an excellent source of antioxidant compounds, and among the richest vegetable sources of pro-vitamin A. The antioxidant compounds from carrots help protect against cardiovascular diseases and cancer and also promote good vision. One of the carrots' phytonutrients, falcarinol (caratotoxin), has shown strong protection against cancer in animal studies, especially against colon and lung cancers (Harris et al., 1991).

Beta-carotene, as a major nutrient in carrots, belongs to very large group of more than 600 known carotenoids, yellow and red pigments of fruits, vegetables and aquatic organisms. This pro-vitamin is synthetized by numerous plants, fruits and vegetables, such as apricot, carrot, alfa-alfa, mango, sweet potatoes, broccoli, spinach etc. In human body beta-carotene has an important physiological role, acting as a pro-vitamin A and exhibiting strong antioxidant activity. Used topically, as a component of suncreams, beta-carotene reduces skin damage by high-energy UV irradiation.

Apart from being essential and beneficial, this lipid-soluble vitamin may pose a serious health concern when consumed in large excess. In this respect more dangerous are vitamin supplements than a regular diet. Dietary overvitaminosis by vitamin A is also possible when consuming food of an animal origin rich in vitamine A, such as fish liver, and is less probable by consuming food of a plant origin.

Regular diet rich in beta-carotene can cause the reversible skin condition, called carotenodermia, a condition in which a yellowish discoloration of the skin is observed due to accumulated lipophilic beta-carotene retained by the body. Yellowish discoloration of the skin diminishes upon cessation of beta-carotene intake. Much more serious concern regarding adverse health effects of beta-carotene is primarily related to very pronounced teratogenic influence of the compound. Teratogenic changes induced by beta-carotene include fetal brain deformities and damage to other internal organs, cleft palate, spina bifida and others (Thulstrup & Bonde, 2006). Animal studies also revealed other adverse effects of beta-carotene and demonstrated that high intake cessates the growth and provokes the bone anomalies rendering them brittle. Under the influence of high doses of beta-carotene skin changes are very pronounced and include hair loss, eczema and erythema.

The acute poisoning with vitamin A occurs when 2-5 millions I.U. are ingested, even though the cases where the symptoms developed after ingesting much higher contents are known. The signs of acute poisoning appear after 6-8 h following ingestion and they usually start with severe headache, drowsiness, dizziness, nausea and vomiting. After 12-20 h of ingestion changes on the skin, such as reddening and swelling may be observed, and are usually followed by skin peeling (Wiegand et al., 1998). Skin changes are more pronounced in skin areas where the skin is thicker, such as soles of the feet and palms and can persist for weeks.

The symptoms of chronic poisoning with beta-carotene develop in children after several months, whereas in adults symptoms development is much more delayed and the latent period can last from several month to even several years. Chronic exposure to elevated beta-carotene contents may result in headache, blurred vision, hair loss, nose bleeds and reddened gingiva. These symptoms are often accompanied with anemia and enlarged liver and spleen. Human studies demonstrated increased risk of lung cancer and heart disease when consuming more that 20 mg of synthetic beta-carotene per day.

Besides containing high levels of beta-carotene, carrots produce a toxic polyacetylenic alcohol falcarinol or caratotoxin, which besides above-mentioned beneficial effects on cancer development, may also act as a potent nerve poison, depending on the dose. The compound, together with other synthetized substances like falcarindiol, acetylfalcarindiol and falcarinolone, act as antifungal agents in the disease response mechanism of carrots. Acute intravenous toxicity of caratotoxin expressed in terms of LD_{50} in mice is 100 mg/kg (Darbrowski & Sikorski, 2005).

15.2. Bongkrek Acid

The occurrence of bongkrek (or bongkrekic) acid (Figure 17) in food is linked primarily to meals prepared of fermented coconuts. Such meals are traditionally consumed by the population of South-East Asia, especially Indonesia, and the cases of poisoning with bongkrek acid are most common in those parts of the world. Bongkrek acid is produced by microbial activity of the bacterium *Burkholderia gladioli* pathovar *cocovenenans* (earlier *B. cocovenenans*, *Pseudomonas cocovenenans*) and acts as a strong toxin. The process is very closely related to the content of fatty acids in the coconut. For fatty acids contents in coconut below 10% the production of the toxic acid is not notable even if significant growth of bacteria occurs. The fatty acids which are known to stimulate bongkrek acid production include lauric, myristic, oleic and palmitic acids (Garcia et al., 1999). In fermented coconut products besides bongkrek acid another toxin was identified – toxoflavin.

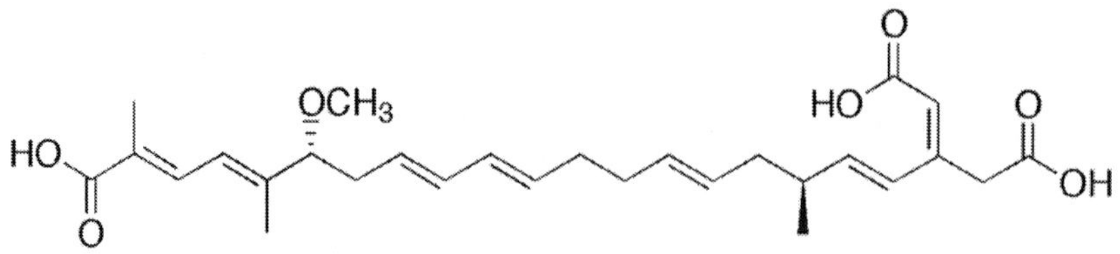

Figure 17. Bongkrek acid.

The toxicity of bongkrek acid arises from the fact that it disturbs the conversion of ADP into ATP in mitochondria, thus compromising the bodies' energy status, disturbing the respiration on a cellular level and provoking the lethal outcome (Henderson & Lardy, 1973). First signs of poisoning with bongkrek acid include severe hyperglycemia, followed with the sharp drop in blood glucose.

15.3. Coumarin

Coumarin (benzopyrone) is a chemical compound found naturally in some plants, such as strawberries, cherries, apricots, cinnamon, tonka beans, lavender, sweet clover and others. Cassia (*Cinnamomum aromaticum*) bark is one of the four components of the cinnamon spice which contributes to high coumarin content in the spice. Chamomile, a common herbal tea, also contains coumarin.

In plants coumarin plays an insecticidal role protecting the plants from various insects. The compound has a very pleasant and distinctive odor and sweet scent, and it has been used as vanilla substitute, as a food additive and ingredient of pharmaceutical products and perfumes.

Naturally occurring coumarin is dangerous only when ingested in high amounts or if consumed during prolonged period of time. In the body the substance acts as a precursor of several anticoagulants, causing blood thinning. Warfarin, a synthetic substance related to natural coumarin, is a common anticoagulant which belongs to the coumarin class and is widely used both as a rodenticide and as a human therapeutic agent. Even though coumarin is not very toxic *per se*, in moldy hay more dangerous dimmer dicoumarol is formed. Formed dicoumarol is a very potent anticoagulant and livestock feeding on moldy hay may suffer from both internal and external bleeding. There are also some concerns regarding potential hepato- and renotoxicity of coumarin. Some beneficial effects of coumarin, such as fungicidal properties and anti-tumor activity have also been reported. Conducted experiments have also revealed that coumarin demonstrates appetite suppressing properties. Some naturally occurring coumarin derivatives including umbelliferone (7-hydroxycoumarin), aesculetin (6,7-dihydroxycoumarin), herniarin (7-methoxycoumarin), psoralen and imperatorin have also demonstrated beneficial health effects and potential anti-cancer and anti-inflammatory activities (Han et al., 2005).

15.4. Finger Cherry

The consumption of indigenious Australian finger-cherry (*Rhodomyrtus macrocarpa*) has been linked to numerous cases of permanent blindness in livestock and children in Australia. After the toxicity of the finger cherry has been recognized the fruit was banned for the consumption by Australian authorities (Ombrain, 1944). The plant is indigenious to Australia and it grows in rainforests in the form of large shrub or small tree, with very hairy evergreen trees. Even though the toxic potency of the plant has been recognized and the consumption of the elongated, finger-like fruits has been banned, some Aborigine tribes still use this fruit as a food. Even thought exact mechanism of toxic action is unknown, the toxic potency of the finger-cherry was linked to the presence of different substituted dibenzofurans, known as rhodomyrtoxins, as well as to different saponins (Johnson, 1981).

15.5. Grayanotoxin

Some species of rhododendrons (*Rhododendron ponticum*, *Rhododendron macrophyllu*, *Rhododendron albiflorum*), as well as other members of Ericaceae family (genera *Azalea*, *Kalmia*) produce a toxic polyhydroxylated cyclic diterpene, grayanotoxin. Depending on the number and the type of functional groups of the cyclic diterpene, there are three types of grayanotoxin. Poisoning with grayanotoxin most often occurs when consuming honey produced of rhododendrons nectar, although the poisoning may also result from ingesting the leaves and flowers of the plants. Several cases of honey poisoning have been reported throughout history. Xenophon (430 - 354 BC), an ancient Greek mercenary, described mass honey poisoning of soldiers in Colchic (the territory of present Georgia) in which the symptoms of severe poisoning cessated after 24 hours, however several soldiers lost their lives. Later-on sporadic cases of honey poisoning have been reported in different parts of the World, Japan, Russia, Balkans and Great Britain. Honey produced from the nectar of yellow jessamine (*Gelsemium sempervirens*) may also be toxic and can induce neurological symptoms, progressive weakness, convulsions, and death due to respiratory failure. The poisoning has been reported in children who have sucked nectar from flowers ingesting in this way a toxic alkaloids of terpenoid, indole and oxindole types produced by *Gelsemium* species. *Kalmia angustifolia* (lambkill) and *Kalmia latifolia* (mountain laurel) are also very toxic and have been used as a mean of suicide by American Indians.

Grayanotoxin binds to the hydrophobic innerspace of the membrane sodium channels on the nerve and muscle cells leaving them in the depolarized, excited state. It has been shown that tetrodotoxin can revert the nerve and muscle cells in their polarized state owing to the fact that tetrodotoxin also binds to sodium channels but on their different parts. By compromising cells membrane potential, in severe cases grayanotoxin can permanently damage the nerves, as well as the cells of heart muscle. Poisoning with grayanotoxin is rarely fatal and usually the symptoms such as dizziness, vomiting, slow heart rate and parasthesia (sensation of tingling, pricking or numbness in the skin) end up within 24 hours (Gunduz et al., 2008). The latent period is dose-dependent and lasts from several minutes to two or more hours, followed by pronounced drop in blood pressure and intense perspiration. Severe intoxications are accompanied with loss of coordination and progressive muscular weakness.

15.6. Kava-Kava

The root of kava-kava (*Piper methysticum*) or kawa, kew, yagona or sakau, is traditionally used in Polynesia, Micronesia, Melanesia and close Pacific regions, to prepare beverages for treating insomnia, stress and anxiety, or during ceremonial occasions such as weddings. Besides sedation, the effects of drinking kava include slight tongue and lip numbing due to the contraction of blood vessels in these areas, talkative and euphoric behavior, calming and a sense of well-being and clear thinking. The strongest effects are produced when the roots of kava-kava plant are chewed or grinded and subsequently ingested. The beverage is prepared by soaking kava-kava powder in hot water with the addition of lecithin, which acts like an emulsifier and helps water extraction of kava active components. After extraction period of approximately half an hour, the water extract is separated from the pulp, producing a ready beverage. In modernized countries the comertial kava beverage is prepared from imported dried, powdered kava-kava roots.

Sedating effects kava-kava owes to more than fifteen identified psychoactive kavalactones. The concentration of kava-kava active components, kavalactones, is the highest in plants root and rhizomes. Kavalactones (Figure 18) kavain, dihydrokavain, methysticin, dihydromethysticin, dihydrokawain, yangonin and desmethoxyyangonin, act by potentiating or changing the level of major neurotransmitters like dopamine, norepinephrine and gamma aminobutyric acid (GABA) in synapses. For these reasons the consumption of beverages prepared from kava-kava root is not recommended for persons with Parkinsonism, as well for those receiving sedative (diazepams) and antidepressant (monoamine oxidase inhibitors) therapy.

In recent years, concerns have been raised about the safety of kava use which prompted the actions of numerous regulatory drug agencies worldwide. Excessive doses of kava-kava may provoke some side effects such as headache, drowsiness, visual disturbances and mouth numbness. In addition, kava-kava extracts act as strong diuretics and disturb clotting processes. Prolonged consumption of kava-kava preparations has been linked to liver and kidney damages, however these findings can not be linked to sole kava-kava influence and are possibly related to the influence of other substances, such as alcohol or drugs, or to preexisting liver pathology (Clough et al., 2003; Center for Food Safety and Applied Nutrition, 2002). In estimating the harmfulness of kava-kava extracts other aspects must be taken into consideration. Some of the kava-kava drinkers chronically used alcohol, so it was unclear whether the liver pathology was concomitant. In other cases the beverage was not prepared from plants roots and included the possibility of pipermethystine hepatotoxicity (Nerurkar et al., 2004). An alkaloid pipermethystine was isolated from stem peelings and leaves of kava-kava, but not from the root, and has demonstrated hepatotoxicity in both *in vitro* and *in vivo* experiments. Flavokavain B, found in the plants' rhizome may also contribute to toxic effects. Other reported side effects of kava-kava include possible allergic reactions and dermopathy, an occurrence of yellowish, scaly skin in chronic kava-kava consumers (Ernst, 2002). Effects on the skin that kava-kava produces were used by ancient Hawaiians to renew the skin rendering it beautiful.

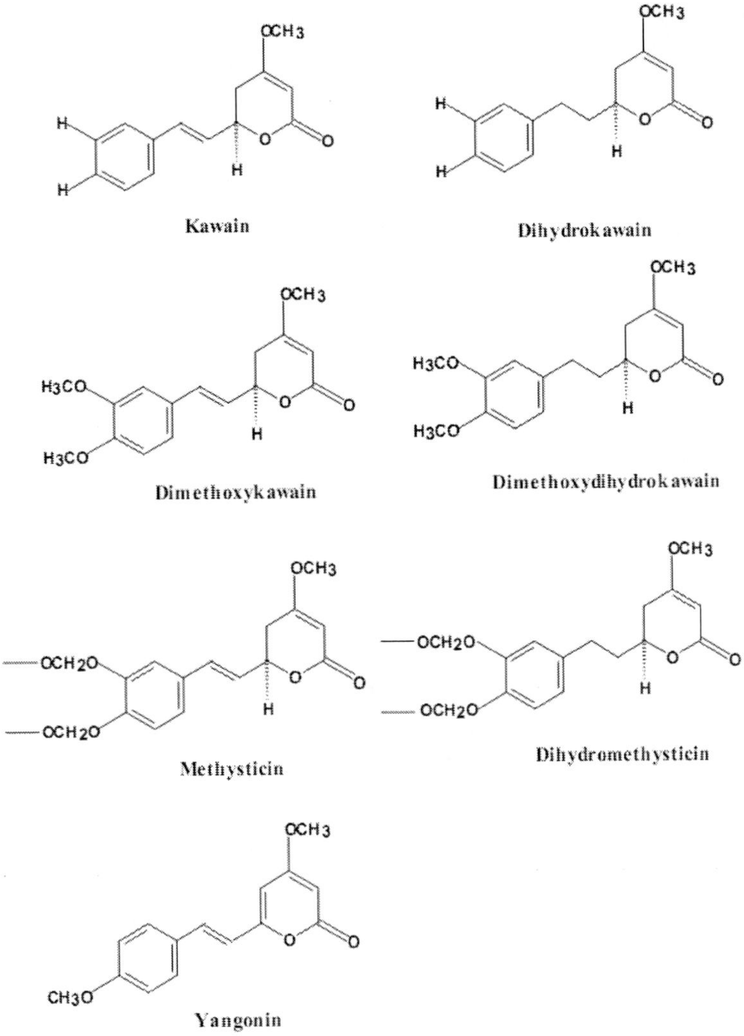

Figure 18. Major kavalactones.

15.7. Miracle Fruit

The miracle fruit (*Synsepalum dulcificum*) which grows in tropics, produces berries which, when consumed, alter the responsiveness of taste receptors rendering sour food like lime and lemon, sweet.

Even though the exact mechanism of the modulation of the receptors responsiveness is unclear, it is assumed that the glycoprotein from the berries, miraculin, binds to taste buds and changes the shape of sweetness receptors, making them responsive to acids. The effects of miraculin last for at least 30 minutes and longer. Even though the fruit itself has a very subtle sweet taste, the attempts were made to commercialize the fruit by isolating miraculin and producing a low-calorie sweetener, however this was prevented by FDA which classified miraculin as a food additive. Another protein with similar taste-modifying properties, curculin, was isolated from Malaysian fruit (*Curculigo latifolia*) but on oppose to miraculin, curculin itself has a sweet taste up to several hundreds to thousands times more strong than sucrose. Also, mixture of proteins (thaumatins) isolated from katemfe fruit (*Thaumatococcus daniellii*) from West Africa exhibit pronounced sweet taste, up to 2000 times stronger in comparison to sucrose, as well as flavor modifying properties. The sweet taste of miraculin, curculin and thaumatins is build-up gradually and last longer in comparison to sucrose, leaving a sweet aftertaste. All these proteins, miraculin, curculin and thaumatins are heat sensitive and they loose their taste-altering properties upon heating.

Today different miracle fruit products can be found on the market. Miracle fruit is sold in the form of tablets, granules, candies and similar fun products. The fruit has found its role in specialized parties where the principal idea of the party is to consume different sour and bitter food after consuming the miracle fruit. These parties, as much as they offer fun and unique experience, also pose a serious risk of developing stomach ulcers due to ingestion of large quantities of food aggressive to stomach. In this game offending prosperities of very acidic or hot food, like chili, pickles, limes, pepper etc., are completely masked due to altered taste signals, compromising the consumers' health.

15.8. Persin

Avocado (*Persea americana*) naturally produces fungicidal and insecticidal substance which has been shown to trigger allergic reactions in humans. The active substance, persin (Figure 19), has been isolated from both the fruit and the leaves of avocado plant, and was identified only recently, revealing that the chemical structure of the compound is similar to linoleic acid. Persin also pose a serious risk to domestic animals, causing gastrointestinal disturbance and respiratory distress. The compound has also been shown to cause arrhythmia and mastitis in numerous animal species (Oelrichs et al., 1995).

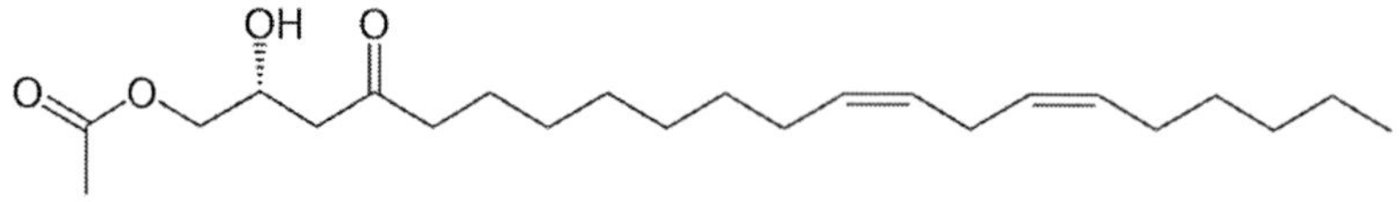

Figure 19. A fatty-acid like persin isolated from avocado.

Medical uses of persin include its application in the treatment of breast cancer. Furthermore, the substance has been shown to boost the effects of popular breast cancer drugs, affecting the steroid hormone receptors and increasing the susceptibility of the tumor cells to the drug (Roberts et al., 2007).

15.9. Pokeweeds

The pokeweeds or pokeberry, from the genus *Phytolacca*, are indigenious to North America, South America, East Asia and New Zealand. The plant grows up to 3 m and produces dark berries. The plant is toxic to mammals due to the presence of the alkaloid phytolaccine, a resin phytolaccotoxin, and a saponin phytolaccigenin, present in all parts of the plant, but mostly concentrated in the root. Berries and leaves can become edible after appropriate preparing which includes double boiling of the leaves and cooking of berries. Dark berries of pokeweeds attract the birds, however birds remain unaffected by the toxins because the berries pass the digestive tract of the birds intact due to very hard outer shell. Regardless the recognized toxicity of the plant, the leaves of the pokeweeds are widely used in America for salad preparation or are prepared as spinach, after they have been cooked for several times in order to reduce the toxin content. Prepared leaves are also canned and sold as a ready product. Ingested uncooked parts of pokeweed cause nausea, vomiting, persistent diarrhea and severe stomach cramping. In severe poisoning cases death occurs due to respiratory arrest after the episodes of muscle weakness and spasms, and episodes of severe convulsions.

15.10. Sassafras

Sassafras species (*Sassafras albidum, Sassafras hesperia, Sassafras randaiense*) are medium-sized, moderately fast growing, aromatic trees with three distinctive leaf shapes. The root bark of sassafras is used for the production of aromatic oil by steam distillation. Characteristic fragrance of sassafras oil derives from the principal component safrole which constitutes up to 80% of the root bark oil. Safrole has also been isolated from a camphor oil and variety of spices such as cinnamon, nutmeg, pepper and basil. The compound has also been found in the oils of *Asarum arifolium, Asarum Blumei*, wormseed oil, Japanese staranise oil, in the common staranise oil, in the oils of ylang-ylang and laurel.

In the past, different parts of sassafras trees were used for various medicinal purposes, such as to treat gonorrhea and to make tea with anticoagulant properties. Sassafras root bark has been used as carminative (substance combating flatulence) at doses of 10 g and insect bites and stings have been treated with extracts to relieve symptoms. Other external uses of sassafras included treatment of eye inflammation, rheumatism, gout, sprains, swelling and cutaneous eruptions. Culinary uses of sassafras included tea preparation, the production of spice made of dried and ground sassafras leaves, and preparation of specific types of stews, as well as the production of a typical American root bear. Before FDA has banned sassafras, the use of sassafras oil in tobacco, soap and perfume industries owing to its specific pleasant fragrance was widespread. Today sassafras products have been withdrawn due to recognized adverse health effects.

Several animal studies have demonstrated that safrole and its naturally occurring isomer isosafrole (4-propenyl-1,2-methylenedioxybenzene) produce liver tumors in experimental animals (Kapadia et al., 1978) and induce several hepatic microsomal enzymes including cytochrome P-488, cytochrome P-450 and biphenyl hydroxylase (Duke, 1989). Regarding its carcinogenic character and taking into account the safety factor of 100, it is estimated that the dose of 0.66 mg of safrole per kg of body weight is considered dangerous in humans (Bisset, 1994). Another fact supporting the statement about the dangerous character of sassafras is the increased incidence of esophageal cancer that has been noted in areas with habitual sassafras consumption as well as confirmed hepatotoxicity of safrole. Besides being a cancer-causing agent, acute poisoning with high doses of safrole can induce vomiting, stupor and hallucinations. The compound has been shown to be able to cause abortion, diaphoresis (profuse sweating), and dermatitis (Duke, 1989).

References

Aline, A; Albuquerque, C; Sorenson, AL; Leal-Cardoso, JH. Effects of essential oil of *Croton zehntneri*, and of anethole and estragole on skeletal muscles. *Journal of Ethnopharmacology*, 1995, Vol. 49, Issue 1, 41-49.

Aronow, L; Kerdel-Vegas, F. Seleno-Cystathionine, a Pharmacologically Active Factor in the Seeds of *Lecythis ollaria*: Cytotoxic and Depilatory Effects of Extracts of *Lecythis ollaria*. *Nature*, 1965, 205, 1185-1186.

Asano, N; Kato, A; Matsui, K; Watson, AA; Nash RJ; Molyneux, RJ; Hackett, L; Topping, J; Winchester, B. The effects of calystegines isolated from edible fruits and vegetables on mammalian liver glycosidases. *Glycobiology*, 1997, Vol. 7, 1085-1088.

Bagnis, RA; Kuberski, T; Langier, S. Clinical observations on 3009 cases of ciguatera (fish poisoning) in the south pacific. *American Journal of Tropical Medicine and Hygiene*, 1979, Vol. 286, 1067-1073.

Bentley, KW. β-phenylethylamines and the isoquinoline alkaloids. *Natural Product Reports*, 2001, Vol. 18, Number. 2, 148–170.

Bironaite, D; Öllinger, K. The hepatotoxicity of rhein involves impairment of mitochondrial functions. *Chemico-Biological Interactions*, 1997, Vol. 103, Issue 1, 35-50.

Bisset, N. *Sassafras lignum*. Herbal Drugs and Phytopharmaceuticals. Stuttgart, Germany: CRC Press; 1994, 455-456.

Blythe, DG; De Sylva, DP. Mother's milk turns toxic after fish feast. *Journal of the American Medical Association*, 1979, 265, 2339-2344.

Bolton, S; Null, G; Caffeine: Psychological Effects, Use and Abuse. *Orthomolecular Psychiatry*, 1981, Vol. 10, Number 3, 202-211.

Bradberry, SM; Dickers, KJ; Rice, P; Griffiths, GD; Vale, JA. Ricin poisoning. *Toxicological Reviews*, 2003, 22, 65–70.

Caboni, P; Sherer, T; Zhang, N; Taylor, G; Na, H; Greenamyre, J; Casida J. Rotenone, deguelin, their metabolites, and the rat model of Parkinson's disease. *Chemical Research in Toxicology*, 2004, Vol. 17, Number 11, 1540–1548.

Cassidy, A. Potential risks and benefits of phytoestrogen-rich diets. *International Journal for Vitamines and Nutritional Research*, 2003, Vol. 73, Number 2, 120-126.

Center for Food Safety and Applied Nutrition. Kava-Containing Dietary Supplements May Be Associated with Severe Liver Injury, 2001. United States Food and Drug Administration.

Chamorro, G; Garduño, L; Martínez, E; Madrigal, E; Tamariz, J; Salazar, M. Dominant lethal study of α-asarone in male mice. *Toxicology Letters*, 1998, Vol. 99, Issue 2, 15, 71-77.

Charlton, KM; Corner, AH; Davey, K; Kramer, JK; Mahadevan, S; Sauer, FD (1975). Cardiac lesions in rats fed rapeseed oils. *Canadian Journal of Computational Medicine*, 1975, Vol. 39, Number 3, 261–269.

Cheeke, PR. Endogenous toxins and mycotoxins in forage grasses and their effects on livestock. *Journal of Animal Science*, 1995, 73, 909–918.

Cheeke, PR. *Pyrrolizidine alkaloids in natural toxicants in feeds, forages, and poisonous plants*. Danville, Illinois: Interstate Publishers; 1998, 338-352.

Chilton, WS. The chemistry and node of action of mushroom toxins. In: Spoerke, DG; Rumack, BH, editors. *Handbook of mushroom poisoning,* 2nd ed. Boca Raton, Florida: CRC Press; 1994: 165-231.

Clough, AR; Bailie, RS; Currie B. Liver function test abnormalities in users of aqueous kava extracts. *Journal of Toxicology- Clinical Toxicology*, 2003, Vol. 41, Number 6, 821–829.

Colegate, SM; Dorling, PR, *Plant-Associated Toxins: Agricultural, Phytochemical and Ecological Aspects*. Wallingford, UK: CAB International; 1994.

Copani, A; Canonico, PL; Nicoletti, F. β-N-Methylamino-l-alanine (l-BMAA) is a potent agonist of 'metabolotropic' glutamate receptors. *European Journal of Pharmacology*, 1990, 181, 327–328.

Coutinho, FM. Gossypol: a contraceptive for men. *Contraception*, 2002, Vol. 65, Number 4, 259–263.

Curhan, GC. Epidemiologic evidence for the role of oxalate in idiopathic nephrolithiasis. *Journal of Endourology*, 1999, Vol. 13, Number 9, 629-631.

Darbrowski WM; Sikorski, ZE. *Toxins in Food.* CRP Press LLC, 2005.

Datia, KP; Christidou, M; Widmer, WW; Harcharan, RK; Dexter, DT. Tissue distribution and neuroprotective effects of citrus flavonoid tangeretin in a rat model of Parkinson's disease. *Neuroreport*, 2001, Vol. 12, Number 17, 3871-3875.

Daware, MB; Mujumdar, AM; Ghaskadbl, S. Reproductive toxicity of Piperine in Swiss albino mice. *Planta Medica*, 2000, Vol. 66, Number 3, 231-236.

Dawson, DA; Rinaldi, AC; Poch, G. Biochemical and toxicological evaluation of agent-cofactor reactivity as a mechanism of action for osteolathyrism. *Toxicology*, 2002, Vol. 177, Number 2-3, 267-284.

de Wildt, DJ; Speijers, GJ. Influence of dietary rapeseed oil and erucic acid upon myocardial performance and hemodynamics in rats. *Toxicology and. Applied Pharmacology*, 1984, Vol. 74, Number 1, 99–108.

Deshpande, SS. *Handbook of food toxicology*. NewYork: Marcel Dekker; 2002.

Dickers, KJ; Bradberry, SM; Rice, P; Griffiths, GD; Vale, JA. Abrin poisoning. *Toxicological Reviews*, 2003, Vol. 22, Number 3, 137–142.

Drinkwater, NR; Miller, EC; Miller, JA, Pitot, HC. Hepatocarcinogenicity of estragole (1-allyl-4-methoxybenzene) and 1'-hydroxyestragole in the mouse and mutagenicity of 1'-acetoxyestragole in bacteria. *Journal of the National Cancer Institute*, 1976, Vol. 57, Number 6, 1323-1331.

Duke, J. *Sassafras albidum* (Nutt.). *CRC Handbook of Medicinal Herbs*. Boca Raton, Florida: CRC Press, Inc.; 1989, 430–431.

Ehrenkranz, JR; Lewis, NG; Kahn, CR; Roth, J. Phlorizin: a review. *Diabetes/Metabolism Research and Reviews*, 2005, Vol. 21, Issue 1, 31-38.

Ernst, E. Safety concerns about kava. *Lancet*, 2002, Vol. 359, Number 9320, 1865-1869.

Faas, L; Venkatasamy, R; Hider, RC; Young, AR.; Soumyanath, A. *In vivo* evaluation of piperine and synthetic analogues as potential treatments for vitiligo using a sparsely pigmented mouse model. *British Journal of Dermatology,* 2008, Vol. 158, 941-944.

Farran, MT; Darwish, AH; Uwayjan, MG; Sleiman, FT; Ashkarian, VM. Vicine and Convicine in Common Vetch (*Vicia sativa*) Seeds Enhance β-Cyanoalanine. *International Journal of Toxicology,* 2002, 21, 201-209.

Feng, PC; Patrick, SJ. Studies of the action of hypoglycine-a, a hypoglycemic substance. *British Journal of Pharmacology and Chemotherapy*, 1958, Vol. 13, Number 2, 125–130.

Fiore, C; Eisnhut, M; Krausse, R. Antiviral effect of Glycyrrhiza species. *Phytotherapeutic Research*, 2008, Vol. 22, 141-148.

Fitzpatrick, TB; Arndt, KA; el Mofty, AM; Pathak, MA. Hydroquinone and Psoralens in the Therapy of Hypermelanosis and Vitiligo. *Archives of Dermatology,* 1966, 93, Number 5, 589-600.

Gable, RS. The toxicity of recreational drugs. *American Scientist,* 2006, 94, 206–208.

Garcia, RA; Hotchkiss, JH; Steinkraus, KH. The effect of lipids on bongkrekic (Bongkrek) acid toxin production by *Burkholderia cocovenenans* in coconut media. *Food Additives and Contaminants*, 1999, 16, 63-69.

Goldfrank, LR. *Goldfrank's Toxicologic Emergencies*. 7th edition. New York: McGraw-Hill; 2002.

Gunduz, A; Turedi, S; Russell, RM; Ayaz, FA. Clinical review of grayanotoxin/mad honey poisoning-past and present. *Clinical Toxicology*, 2008, Volume 46, Issue 5, 437 – 442.

Gunn, CR. *Abrus precatorius*: Pretty but poisonous. *Science*, 1969, 164, 245–246.

Han, S; Zhou, V; Pan, S; Liu, Y; Hornsby, M; McMullan, D; Klock, HE; Haugen, J; Lesley, SA; Gray, N; Caldwell, J; Gu, XJ. Identification of coumarin derivatives as a novel class of allosteric MEK1 inhibitors. *Bioorganic and Medicinal Chemistry Letters*, 2005, Vol. 15, Number 24, 5467-5473.

Hanrahan JP; Gordon MA. Mushroom poisoning. Case reports and a review of therapy. *The Journal of the American Medical Association (JAMA)*, 1984, Vol. 251, Number 8, 1057–1061.

Harborne, JB. Cyanogenic glucosides and their function. In: *Phytochemical ecology.* London: Academic Press; 1972, 104-123.

Harris, RA; Key, TJ, Silcocks, PB; Bull, D; Wald, NJ. A case-controlled study of dietary carotene in men with lung cancer and in men with other epithelial cancers. *Nutrition and Cancer*, 1991, Vol. 15, 63-68.

Henderson, PJ; Lardy, HA. Bongkrekic acid: An Inhibitor of Adenine Nucleotide Translocase of Mitochondria. *Journal of Biological Chemistry*, 1970, Vol. 245, Number 6, 1319-1323.

Hendricks, JD; Sinnhuber, RO; Loveland, PM; Pawlowski, NE; Nixon, JE. Hepatocarcinogenicity of glandless cottonseeds and cottonseed oil to rainbow trout (*Salmo gairdnerii*). *Science,* 1980, Vol. 208, Number 4441, 309 – 311.

Howard, AS; Michael, JP. Simple Indolizidine and quinolizidine alkaloids. In: Brossi, A, editor. *The Alkaloids*. New York: Academic Press; 1986; 183–308.

Humfrey, CD. Phytoestrogens and human health effects: weighing up the current evidence. *Natural Toxins*, 1998, Vol. 6, Number 2, 51-59.

Hwang, DF; Noguchi, T. Tetrodotoxin poisoning. *Advances in Food and Nutritional Research*, 2007, 52, 141–236.

Hwang, KM; Foon, KA; Cheung, PH; Pearson, JW; Oldham, R. Selective antitumor effect on L10 hepatocarcinoma cells of a potent immunoconjugate composed of the A chain of abrin and a monoclonal antibody to a hepatoma-associated antigen. *Cancer Research,* 1984, 44, 4578-4586.

Il, HP; Falke, HE; Prinsen, MK; Willems, MI. Acute and subacute toxicity of tyramine, spermidine, spermine, putrescine and cadaverin in rats. *Food and chemical toxicology*, 1997, Vol. 35, Number 3-4, 337-348.

Iskit, AB; Sungur, A; Gedikoglu, G; Guc, MO. The effects of bosentan, aminoguanidine and L-canavanine on mesenteric blood flow, spleen and liver in endotoxaemic mice. *European Journal of Pharmacology*, 1999, Vol. 379, 73-80.

Johnson, RW. Obituary: Selwyn Lawrence Everist 1913-1981. *Australian Weeds*, 1981, Vol 1, Number 2, 42-49.

Kapadia, GJ; Chung, EB; Ghosh, B; Shukla, YN; Basak, SP; Morton JF; Pradhan, SN. Carcinogenicity of some folk medicinal herbs in rats. *Journal of the National Cancer Institute*, 1978, 60, 683-686.

Kisby, GE; Ellison, M; Spencer, PS. Content of the neurotoxins cycasin (methylazoxymethanol ß-D-glucoside) and BNLAA (ß-N-methylamino-L-alanine) in cycad flour prepared by Guam Chamorros. *Neurology*, 1992, 42, 1336-1341.

Köppel, C. Clinical symptomatology and management of mushroom poisoning. *Toxicon*, 1993, Vol. 31, Number 12, 1513–1540.

Kravić, S; Suturović, Z; Švarc-Gajić, J; Stojanović, Z; Pucarević, M. Determination of *trans* fatty acids in foodstuffs by gas chromatography-mass spectrometry after simultaneous microwave assisted extraction-esterification. *Journal of the Serbian Chemical Society*, 2010, Vol 73, Number 6, 803-813.

Kravić, S; Marjanović, N; Suturović, Z; Švarc-Gajić, J; Stojanović, Z; Pucarević, M. Determination of *trans* fatty acids in Serbian shortenings by gas chromatography mass spectrometry. *Acta Alimentaria*, 2010 in press.

Kuriyama, T; Schmidt, TJ; Okuyama, E; Ozoe, Y. Structure-activity relationships of secoprezizaane terpenoids in gamma-aminobutyric acid receptors of houseflies and rats. *Bioorganic and Medical Chemistry,* 2002, 10, 1873–1881.

Liaudet, L; Feihl, F; Rosselet, A; Markert, M; Hurni, JM; Perret, C. Beneficial effects of L-canavanine, a selective inhibitor of inducible nitric oxide synthase, during rodent endotoxaemia. *Clinical Science.* 1996, Vol. 90, Number 5, 369-377.

Makkar, HPS; Siddhuraju, S; Becker, K. *Plant Secondary Metabolites*. Vol. 393, Totowa, New Jersey: Humana Press; 2007, 41-46.

Medlock, KL; Branham, WS; Sheehan, DM. The effects of phytoestrogens on neonatal rat uterine growth and development. *Proceedings of the Society for Experimenal Biology and Medicine*, 1995 Vol. 208, Number, 3, 307-313.

Michael, JP. Simple indolizidine and quinolizidine alkaloids. In: Cordell, G, editor. *The Alkaloids*, Chemistry and Pharmacology. New York: Academic Press; 2001; 91–258.

Morley, KL; Ferguson, PJ; Koropatnick, J. Tangeretin and nobiletin induce G1 cell cycle arrest but not apoptosis in human breast and colon cancer cells. *Cancer Letters*, 2007, Vol. 251, Number 1, 168-178.

National Research Council (U.S.). Food Protection Commitee. *Toxicants occuring naturally in food.* Washington; National Academy of Sciences, 1973.

Nerurkar, PV; Dragull, K; Tang, CS. *In Vitro* Toxicity of Kava Alkaloid, Pipermethystine, in HepG2 Cells Compared to Kavalactones. *Toxicological Sciences*, 2004, 79, 106-111.

Nixon, JE; Eisele, TA; Hendricks. JD; Sinnhuber, RO. Reproduction and Lipid Composition of Rats Fed Cyclopropene Fatty Acids. The Journal of Nutrition, 1977, Vol. 104, Number 4, 574 – 583.

Numazaki K. Glycyrrhizin therapy for viral infections. *African Journal of Biotechnology*, 2003, Vol 2, Number 10, 392-393.

Nunn, PB; Ponnusamy, M. β-N-Methylaminoalanine (BMAA): Metabolism and metabolic effects in model systems and in neural and other tissues of the rat *in vitro*. *Toxicon*, 2009, Volume 54, Issue 2, Pages 85-94.

Oelrichs, PB; Ng, JC; Seawright, AA; Ward, A; Schäffeler, L; MacLeod JK. Isolation and identification of a compound from avocado (*Persea americana*) leaves which causes necrosis of the acinar epithelium of the lactating mammary gland and the myocardium. *Natural Toxins*, 1995, Vol.3, Number 5, 344-349.

Ombrain, AD. Sudden blindness after eating finger cherries (*Rhodomyrtus macrocarpa*). *Medical Journal of Australia*, 1944, 2, 263-270.

Orane, LA; Maurice, BR; Jose, JC. Ackee (*Blighia sapida*) hypoglycine A toxicity : Dose response assessment in laboratory rats. *Food and chemical toxicology*, 2006, Vol. 44, Number 2, 207-213.

Osweiler GD. Strychnine poisoning. In: Kirk RW, editor. *Current Veterinary Therapy*. Philadelphia: WB Saunders; 1983, 98 -100.

Rake, M; Saunders, M. Refsum's disease: a disorder of lipid metabolism. *Journal of Neurology, Neurosurgery and Psychiatry*. 1966, Vol. 29, Number 5, 417–422.

Rechcigl, M. *CRC handbook of naturally occurring food toxicants*. Boca Raton, Florida: CRC Press; 1983.

Roberts, CG; Gurisik, E; Biden, TJ; Sutherland, RL; Butt, AJ. Synergistic cytotoxicity between tamoxifen and the plant toxin persin in human breast cancer cells is dependent on Bim expression and mediated by modulation of ceramide metabolism. *Molecular Cancer Therapeutics,* 2007, Vol. 6, Number 10, 2777-2785.

Robey, RW; Fetsch, PA; Polgar, O; Dean, M; Bates, SE. The livestock photosensitizer, phytoporphyrin (phylloerythrin), is a substrate of the ATP-binding cassette transporter ABCG2. *Research in Veterinary Science*, 2006, Vol. 81, Issue 3, Pages 345-349.

Rosenthal, GA. Metabolism of L-canavanine and L-canaline in leguminous plants. *Plant Physiology,* 1990, 94, 1-3.

Rosenthal, GA. *Plant non-protein amino and imino acids: biological, biochemical, and toxicological properties*. Boston: Academic Press; 1982.

Rubenstein, ET; McLaughlin, RC; Winant, A; Sanchez, M; Eckart, KM; Krasinska, A; Chien, A. Azetidine-2-carboxylic Acid in the Food Chain. *Phytochemistry,* 2008, Vol. 70, Number 1, 100 -104.

Saito A; Yamamoto M. Acute oral toxicity of capsaicine in mice and rats. *Journal of Toxicology Science,* 1996, Volume 21, Number 3, 195-200.

Sharma, RP; Salunkhe, DK. Solanum glycoalkaloids. In: Cheeke, PR, editor. *Toxicants of Plant Origin*, Vol. 1. Boca Raton, Florida: CRC Press; 1989, 179-236.

Shoba, G; Joy, D; Joseph, T; Majeed, M; Rajendran, R; Srinivas, PS. Influence of piperine on the pharmacokinetics of curcumin in animals and human volunteers. *Planta Medica,* 1998, Vol. 64, Number 4, 353–356.

Stallard, D; Edes, TE. Muscarinic poisoning from medications and mushrooms. *Postgraduate Medicine,* 1989, 85, 341-345.

Stamets, P. *Psilocybin Mushrooms of the World.* Berkeley, California: Ten Speed Press; 1996.

Su, DR; Tang, DG; Xu, JW; Zhang, X. 1992. Determination and extraction of Levodopa in legume of *Mucuna cochinchinensis. Tiaran Chanwu Yanji Yu Kairfa*, 1992, Vol. 4, Number 4, 27–30.

Surh, YJ; Lee, SS. Capsaicin in hot chili pepper: carcinogen, co-carcinogen or anticarcinogen? *Food Chemical Toxicology*, 1996, Vol. 34, Number 3, 313-316.

Suturović, Z; Švarc-Gajić, J; Marjanović, N; Kravić, S. Development of a chronopotentiometric stripping method for the determination of selenium in mixed diets. *Food Chemistry*, 2005, 92, 771-776.

Švarc-Gajić, J; Suturović, Z; Marjanović, N; Kravić, S. Determination of As(III) and As(V) in oilseeds by chronopotentiometric stripping analysis: Development of a method. *Molecular Nutrition and Food Research*, 2005, 49, 337-342.

Švarc-Gajić, J; Suturović, Z; Marjanović, N; Kravić S. Determination of mercury by chronopotentiometric stripping analysis using glassy carbon vessel as a working electrode. *Electroanalysis*, 2006, 18, 513-516.

Švarc-Gajić, J; Stojanović, S; Suturović, Z; Marjanović N; Kravić; S. Determination of α-tocopherol in cosmetic products by chronopotentiometry. *Analytical Letters*, 2008, Vol. 41, Number 12, 2153-2161.

Švarc-Gajić, J; Stojanović, Z; Suturović, Z; Marjanović N; Kravić, S. Direct mercury determination in natural waters by chronopotentiometric stripping analysis in macroelectrode process vessel. *Desalination*, 2009a, 249, 253-259.

Švarc-Gajić, J; Stojanović, Z; Marjanović, N; Suturović, Z; Kravić, S. Sulphide as an internal standard for selenium determination by chronopotentiometric stripping analysis. *Journal of International Scientific Publications: Materials, Methods and Technologies,* 2009b, Volume 3, Number 1, 199 - 210.

Švarc-Gajić, J. *General Toxicology*. New York: Nova Science Publishers; 2009.

Švarc-Gajić, J; Stojanović, Z. Electrocatalytic determination of histamine on a nickel-film glassy carbon electrode, *Electroanalysis*, 2010, Vol. 22, Number 24, 2931-2939.

Švarc-Gajić, J; Stojanović, Z. Determination of histamine in cheese by chronopotentiometry on a thin film mercury electrode. *Food Chemistry*, 2011, 124, 1172–1176.

Takahata, H; Momose, T. Simple indolizidine alkaloids. In: Cordell, G, editor. *The Alkaloids.* San Diego: Academic Press; 1993; 189–256.

Thompson, LU; Boucher, BA; Lui, Z; Cotterchio, M; Kreiger, N. Phytoestrogen content of foods consumed in Canada, including isoflavones, lignans and coumestan. *Nutrition and Cancer*, 2006, Vol. 54, Number 2, 184-201.

Thulstrup, AM; Bonde, JP. Maternal occupational exposure and risk of specific birth defects. *Occupational Medicine*, 2006, 56, 532-543.

Unchern, S; Saito, H; Nishiyama, N. Selective cytotoxicity of piperine on cultured rat hippocampal neurons in comparison with cultured astrocytes : The possible involvement of lipid peroxidation. *Biological and pharmaceutical bulletin*, 1997, Vol. 20, Number 9, 958-961.

Vachvanichsanong, P; Lebel, L. Djenkol beans as a cause of hematuria in children. *Nephron*, 1997, Vol. 76, Number 1, 39-42.

von Unruh, GE; Susanne, V; Tilman Sauerbruch, T; Hesse, A. Dependence of Oxalate Absorption on the Daily Calcium Intake. *Journal of the American Society of Nephrology*, 2004, 15, 1567-1573.

Wiegand, UW, Hartmann, S, Hummler H. Safety of vitamin A: recent results. *International Journal of Vitamin and Nutrition Research,* 1998, Vol. 68, Number 6, 411-416.

Wilmarth, KR; Froines JR. *In Vitro* and *In Vivo* Inhibition of Lysil Oxidase by Aminopropionitriles. *Journal of Toxicology and Environmental Health*, 1992, Vol. 37, Number 3, 411-423.

Yutaka Motoki, Y; Fujita, S; Fujihara, Y; Okada, Y; Nomura, M. Skin Whitening Effects of Estragole Derivatives. *Journal of Oleo Science*, 2003, Vol. 52, Number 9, 495-498.

Zhao, B; Moochhala, SM; Tham S. Biologically active components of *Physostigma venenosum*. *Journal of Chromatography B*, 2004, Vol. 812, Number 1-2, 183-192.

In: Nutritional Insights and Food Safety
Editor: Jaroslava Švarc-Gajiæ
ISBN: 978-1-61122-130-5

Chapter III

Nitrate and Nitrite Contents of Fresh Vegetable Samples: A Review

Manuela Correia[1], Maria Beatriz Prior Pinto Oliveira[2] and Cristina Delerue-Matos[1]
[1]REQUIMTE, Instituto Superior de Engenharia do Porto, Rua Dr. António Bernardino de Almeida, 431, 4200-072 Porto, Portugal
[2]REQUIMTE, Serviço de Bromatologia, Faculdade de Farmácia, Universidade do Porto, Rua Aníbal Cunha, 164, 4099-030 Porto, Portugal

Abstract

Fresh vegetables should constitute an important part of balanced diets and have long been associated to beneficial health effects. Nevertheless, some natural constituents of plant materials, such as nitrates, are still in the centre of an interesting debate concerning their effect on human health. The purpose of this study is to review the levels of nitrate and nitrite reported for fresh vegetable samples. The latest developments regarding nitrate and nitrite effects on human health, legislation and maximum levels, analytical methodologies for both extraction and analysis, the effects of storage and technological processing on analytes' contents and the dietary intake of nitrate and nitrite from vegetable sources are also discussed.

Introduction

The World Health Organization (WHO) recommends a consumption of at least 400 g or five portions a day of fruits and vegetables (excluding tubers) (WHO, 2003). There is general consensus that eating fruits and vegetables is an important component of a healthy diet, if consumed in sufficient amounts, with potential beneficial health effects, as demonstrated in studies describing the relationship between fruits, vegetables and health. However, concerns related to the presence certain compounds, such as nitrate, allergens, mycotoxins, contaminants and pesticide residues in vegetables have been raised (Bottex et al., 2008).

Nitrate is present in food naturally, or may be present as a result of the use of fertilizers on crops, or from its use as a preservative (European Commission 1998). Green leafy vegetables, particularly lettuce and spinach, naturally contain higher levels of nitrates than other foods and are one of the main sources of nitrates in the diet (Santamaria, 2006).

The nitrate levels in vegetables are influenced by factors including the biological properties of the plant culture, (day)light intensity, type of soil, temperature, humidity, frequency of plants in the field, plant maturity, vegetation period, harvesting time, size of the vegetable unit, storage time and source of nitrogen (Tamme et al., 2006). Nitrogen fertilization and light intensity have been identified as the major factors that influence nitrate content in vegetables (Gruda, 2005; Santamaria, 2006).

Nitrogen fertilizers play an important role in crop yield and quality. Nitrate is often the major source of nitrogen available to higher plants, especially to vegetables. Nitrate uptake and distribution in crops is of major importance with respect to both environmental concerns and the quality of crop products (Chen et al., 2004).

Although most of the higher plants are capable of reducing nitrate in both roots and shoots, nitrate is reduced more efficiently in leaves than in roots because of the readily available reductants, energy and carbon skeletons produced by photosynthesis, which are dependent on plant species (Chen et al., 2004). This is also true for most leafy vegetables. Nitrate taken up by a plant is either reduced or stored in the vacuoles or transported in the xylem transpiration stream to the leaf for reduction, and most is stored in the vacuole until released for reduction in the cytosol (Chen et al., 2004). Since nitrate reductase (NR) is assumed to be the rate-limiting step for nitrate assimilation, and is an inducible enzyme, there is a close relationship between NR activity (NRA) and nitrate concentration in plants. Furthermore, nitrate induces the expression of both the uptake and reduction systems. Thus it can be seen that nitrate accumulation might be regulated by many factors, such as plant growth, endogenous nitrate, and nitrate uptake and reduction (Chen et al., 2004).

Generally, nitrate-accumulating vegetables belong to the families of Brassicaceae (rocket, radish, mustard), Chenopodiaceae (beetroot, Swiss chard, spinach) and Amarantaceae; but also Asteraceae (lettuce) and Apiaceae (celery, parsley) include species with high nitrate contents (Santamaria, 2006). The differing nitrate reductase activity, as well as the differing degree of nitrate absorption and transfer in the plant may be responsible for the varying capacities of vegetable species to accumulate nitrate (Santamaria, 2006). A classification of vegetables according to their nitrate content has been presented by Santamaria (2006) and is shown in Table 1.

Nitrate is stored mainly in the vacuole where it functions as an osmotic ion that might (i) compensate for low levels of organic solutes, (ii) be available for assimilation, and (iii) serve as a reservoir to sustain growth processes during subsequent periods when the external nitrogen supply becomes limiting (Chen et al., 2004). Nitrate content differs in the various parts of a plant. The vegetable organs can be listed by decreasing nitrate content as follows: petiole > leaf > stem > root > inflorescence > tuber > bulb > fruit > seed (Santamaria, 2006).

Nitrate concentrations in vegetables increase with increasing nitrate concentrations in nutrient solutions used in hydroponic production, however, for higher concentrations tested, there may be a decrease in nitrate concentrations in the vegetable tissues (Chen et al, 2004; Wang et al., 2009). Li et al. (2003) indicated that for field conditions a linear relation was found between the nitrate concentration in Chinese cabbage and the nitrate fertilizer applied to the soil. This difference may be mainly due to the fact that when plants are grown under field conditions soil nitrate concentration is often lower than the values used in the study reported by Wang et al. (2009).

Table 1. Classification of vegetables according to nitrate content (mg kg^{-1} fresh matter) (Santamaria, 2006)

Nitrate content (mg kg-1 fm)	Vegetable
Very low (< 200)	Artichoke, asparagus, broad bean, Brussels sprouts, eggplant, garlic, onion, green bean, melon, mushroom, pea, pepper, potato, summer squash, sweet potato, tomato, watermelon
Low (200-500)	Broccoli, carrot, cauliflower, cucumber, pumpkin, 'puntarelle' chicory
Middle (500-1000)	Cabbage, broccoli rab, dill, Savoy cabbage, turnip
High (1 000-2500)	Celeriac, Chinese cabbage, endive, fennel, kohlrabi, leaf chicory, leek, parsley
Very high (> 2500)	Celery, chervil, cress, lamb's lettuce, lettuce, radish, red beetroot, rocket, spinach, Swiss chard

The nitrate and nitrite content is of interest to governments and regulators owing to the possible implications for health and also for food quality control purposes. Nitrate is present in most types of food, usually at low concentrations, but vegetables, and in particular green leafy vegetables and beetroot, typically contain higher nitrate concentrations than other foods (Ysart et al., 1999b; Santamaria, 2006). For these reasons, the determination of nitrate and nitrite in food has received increased attention and several recent studies have addressed the dietary exposure of human population to these compounds (Thomson et al., 2007; Menard et al., 2008).

According to literature, the primary dietary sources of nitrate and nitrite include vegetables, processed and cured meat, fish and poultry (to which nitrite has been added), and possibly water, especially if there is runoff or contamination by nitrate from agricultural sources. Plant foods are the primary sources of nitrate (80-95%), while processed and cured meat are the primary sources of nitrite (Pennington, 1998; Ximenes et al., 2000).

Recent researches suggest that dietary nitrate may have beneficial effects based on the hypothesis that nitric oxide (NO) formed in the stomach from dietary nitrate has antimicrobial effects on gut pathogens and a role in host defense (Santamaria, 2006).

Although vegetables are one of the major sources of dietary exposure to nitrate, numerous studies have reported that the consumption of vegetables decreases the incidences of cancer. This is mainly due to antioxidant compounds (ascorbate, tocopherol, β-carotene, phenol compounds, indole) that suppress the formation of carcinogenic agents like nitrosamines (Chung et al., 2003). Therefore it has been argued that naturally occurring nitrates in foods are not toxic, which is one of the reasons for the absence of regulations controlling nitrates in vegetables in some countries (Chung et al., 2003).

1. Nitrate and Nitrite Effects on Human Health and their Relation to Vegetable Composition

Nitrate is in the centre of an interesting debate concerning its effects on human health. Nitrate *per se* is a compound of low toxicity but it is currently accepted that its metabolites may produce a number of health effects. However, the chemistry of dietary nitrate metabolism in humans is complex (Ysart et al., 1999b). Upon ingestion, free nitrate is rapidly absorbed from the gastrointestinal tract, after which approximately 20 – 28 % of an oral dose is actively secreted into saliva. In the oral cavity, part of the secreted nitrate is reduced to nitrite by nitrate reducing bacteria. About 4 – 8 % of the dietary nitrate is reduced to nitrite (van Velzen et al., 2008). This value can reach up to 20% for individuals with a high rate of conversion (Thomson et al., 2007).

In the stomach, nitrite is acidified leading to the formation of a number of reactive intermediates including *N*-nitrosamines (Ysart et al., 1999b; Yordanov et al., 2001; Santamaria, 2006). These have been related to an increased risk of gastric, esophageal, nasopharyngeal, and bladder cancers (Choi et al., 2007). Recent studies suggest that when nitrate is consumed as part of a normal diet containing vegetables, other bioactive substances concomitantly consumed, such as the antioxidant vitamin C, can reduce the amount of nitrosamine formed by up to half (EFSA, 2008).

Methemoglobinemia is another health hazard attributed to nitrite, a condition where reduced iron (Fe^{2+}) in hemoglobin is oxidized by nitrite to Fe^{3+}, thus reducing the total oxygen carrying capacity of the blood (Santamaria, 2006). Young infants are more susceptible to methemoglobinemia because, as concluded by McKnight et al. (1999): (i) young infants have a higher gastric pH (pH > 4); (ii) there are low concentrations of reducing agents, such as, ascorbic acid; (iii) the methemoglobin reductase system is not mature (Du et al., 2007).

The human stomach normally contains high levels of bioactive NO. In humans, NO can be generated by the nitrate both from exogenous nitrate intake and endogenous synthesis (Du et al., 2007). It was suggested that the total nitrite in saliva would generate about only one tenth of the NO that is actually measured in the stomach (McKnight et al. 1999), indicating that other NO generation pathways should exist. It was considered that the endogenous NO was synthesized from NO synthetase acting on L-arginine (Moncada & Higgs 1993), and this NO generation pathway was defined as the endogenous pathway (Du et al., 2007).

The past decade has witnessed a significant increase in the interest of biologists in NO. This highly reactive species, first considered only a noxious air pollutant, is an important mediator in a wide range of physiological and pathological events. Vasodilatation, neurotransmission, blood pressure, host defense, mucus secretion and gastric motility, and programmed cell death are among the many processes in which NO plays a role (Moncada et al., 1991; Wu & Thiemermann, 1996; Viuda-Martos et al., 2009). On the other hand, nitrite and nitrate are the oxidative products of nitric oxide, and usually serve as indexes of NO content in biological fluids, including serum, plasma, urine, and cell supernatants (Wang & Mazza, 2002).

From the 1980s, many studies have already demonstrated the signal transduction function of NO, which is an effective vasodilator agent and platelet aggregation inhibitor (McKnight et al. 1999; Du et al., 2007). Therefore, NO deficiency will cause many diseases, such as arteriosclerosis, diabetes, low blood pressure, and coagulation diseases (Coss et al. 2004). In addition, it has been reported that macrophage could produce nitrate when suffering from the toxicity of bacterial compounds, and that once macrophages were attacked by toxic elements, they release NO to increase the phagocytosis before the NO was converted to nitrite and nitrate. Later, De Groote and Fang (1995) found that the phagocytosis would be impaired if NO synthesis was inhibited, demonstrating the important antibacterial role of NO during stress induction (Du et al., 2007).

Numerous studies conducted over the past 20 years have shown that diets rich in fruits and vegetables are associated with lower risk of cardiovascular diseases and certain forms of cancer, but the mechanisms behind this protection are not completely understood. Recent epidemiological studies suggest a cardioprotective action afforded specifically by green leafy vegetables (Lundberg et al., 2006). Fresh vegetables have low nitrite accumulation and plenty of protective antioxidants, which can decrease the incidence of cancer (Du et al., 2007).

The evidence for nutritional prevention of diseases by some flavonoids has been obtained from a variety of interdisciplinary studies including epidemiological studies, distribution of some flavonoids in human organs and tissues, supplementation studies, and studies with small animals and humans (Wang & Mazza, 2002). Such effects have been ascribed, in part, to non-nutritive but potentially bioactive secondary metabolites in fruits, vegetables, herbs, spices, teas, and wines. For example, simple phenolic compounds (hydroxybenzoic acid and hydroxycinnamic acid derivatives) and polyphenolic flavonoids are ubiquitous in plant-based foods. Many have numerous potential anti-atherogenic properties including the modification of lipid profiles, vasodilatory effects and the ability to prevent the oxidation of low-density lipoproteins (Ostertag et al., 2010).

The first bioavailability study of nitrates from vegetables in humans has been presented by van Velzen et al. (2008). This study shows that nitrates from vegetables, whether cooked or uncooked, is absorbed very effectively, resulting in an absolute nitrate bioavailability of around 100%. In the conditions used in the study, there was no significant increase of plasma nitrite concentrations (van Velzen et al., 2008).

2. Legislation and Maximum Levels Regarding Nitrate and Nitrite in Vegetables

In response to potential adverse health effects of nitrate and nitrite, maximum nitrate levels for some vegetables were set in the European Commission Regulation (EC) No 1881/2006. These range from 2000 mg kg^{-1} for frozen spinach to 4500 mg kg^{-1} for fresh lettuce (excluding iceberg type lettuce; grown under cover and harvested from 1st October to 31st March) (Table 2). These different values reflect a trend for higher levels of nitrate in vegetables during winter, as well as in vegetables grown under glass/plastic cover. Thus, light intensity has an important effect on the nitrate level in vegetables.

No nitrate standards for vegetables have been introduced in the USA (Santamaria, 2006). In China, a suggested maximum level for nitrate in vegetables of 3100 mg kg^{-1} has been established (Santamaria, 2006) and the tolerance limit for nitrite is 4 mg kg^{-1} (Zhou et al., 2000).

Table 2. Maximum levels for nitrate (mg kg^{-1} fm) according to European Commission Regulation (EC) No. 1881/2006

	Foodstuffs	Maximum levels (mg NO_3 kg^{-1} fm)	
1.1	Fresh spinach (*Spinacia oleracea*)	Harvested 1 October to 31 March	3000
		Harvested 1 April to 30 September	2500
1.2	Preserved, deep-frozen or frozen spinach		2000
1.3	Fresh Lettuce (*Lactuca sativa L.*) (protected and open-grown lettuce) excluding lettuce listed in point 1.4	Harvested 1 October to 31 March:	
		lettuce grown under cover	4000
		lettuce grown in the open air	4500
		Harvested 1 April to 30 September:	
		lettuce grown under cover	3500
		lettuce grown in the open air	2500
1.4	Iceberg-type lettuce	Lettuce grown under cover	2500
		Lettuce grown in the open air	2000
1.5	Processed cereal-based foods and baby foods for infants and young children		200

3. Nitrate Contents in Fresh Vegetables

According to literature, vegetables were shown to contain nitrates at varying levels ranging from 1 to 10 000 mg kg^{-1}. A value of 10 800 mg kg^{-1} has been reported for a celery sample grown using hydroponic cultivation method (Zhong et al., 2002). Recently, the European Food Safety Authority (EFSA, 2008) has published the data on nitrate levels in vegetables regarding 41 969 analytical results from 20 European Union (EU) Member States and Norway. There was a large variation in median concentrations of nitrate in different vegetables from as low as 1 mg kg^{-1} (peas and Brussels sprouts) to 4800 mg kg^{-1} (rucola, *Eruca sativa*). Less than 5% of all samples were reported as being below the limit of detection (LOD) for nitrate (EFSA, 2008).

The factors leading to the difference of nitrate contents in different vegetables are complex, and a number of studies on the mechanism of nitrate accumulation have been done, mainly on the nitrate uptake rate, nitrate reductase activity, and growth rate, which are closely related to carbon metabolism. Moreover, there is always significant variance of nitrate content among different genotypes, and sometimes it can even reach several folds, such as in the case of spinach (Du et al., 2007). Most of the studies suggest that the imbalance between nitrate uptake and reduction should be the fundamental factor for nitrate accumulation. In addition, once the increment of nitrate accumulation is stronger than its growth, growth lag would strengthen the nitrate accumulation through nutrient enrichment (Du et al., 2007).

The time of the day the plants were harvested was shown to have a significant effect on the variability of nitrate levels in lettuce, although with no consistent temporal trends (Weightman et al., 2006). Other studies failed to detect a significant relationship between nitrate levels and time of harvest within the day (Reinink, 1991).

Nitrate contents of organic and conventional vegetables may differ significantly and some studies suggest that organic farming has the potential of reducing nitrate levels in vegetables products. However, the literature also reports inconsistent or not significant differences in nitrate content in conventional and organically grown crops (Merino et al., 2006). In Belgium, the mean nitrate contents of organic and conventional products were significantly different, 1703 mg kg^{-1} and 2637 mg kg^{-1}, respectively (Pussemier et al., 2006). On the other hand, in a study conducted in Italy, organically grown vegetables contained significantly higher contents of nitrate than conventionally cultivated products (De Martin & Restani, 2003). When comparing organic and conventional vegetables, a major difficulty is due to the numerous confounding factors (growing conditions, soil type, etc.). These factors add to the difficulty in differentiating whether a potential added value of organic over conventional vegetables is due to a difference in composition or not (Hoefkens et al., 2009).

Even among different samples of the same vegetable varieties, the range of concentrations may be large (Tamme et al., 2006; Thomson et al., 2007; Prasad & Chetty, 2008). Variations within site for plants growing in the same plot can be explained by differences in soil mineral nitrogen, and individual plant growth in response to localized areas of soil compaction, or variability in soil pH (Weightman et al., 2006).

Potato (*Solanum tuberosum*) is classified among vegetables with low nitrate content. However, because of the large amounts consumed, it can contribute greatly to the daily intake of nitrate in the diet (Santamaria, 2006). This is the reason for the increasing attention being paid to potato nitrate content (Ysart et al., 1999). To date, no official limits for nitrate content of potato have been set in the EU, although several countries have put forward the proposal of guidelines. In Germany, for instance, only tubers with less than 200 mg NO_3 kg^{-1} fresh weight are accepted (Santamaria, 2006), and in Poland there is a maximum limit of 183 mg NO_3 kg^{-1} fresh weight (Ierna, 2009). As discussed before for vegetables in general, the amount of nitrates in tubers has been shown to vary with the cultivar, maturity of the tubers and their size, type and amount of nitrogen fertilizers, weather, site and storage conditions (Ierna, 2009).

The results reported in recent literature for the nitrate contents of some fresh vegetables are presented in Table 3. These vegetables were selected based on legislation (lettuce, spinach), dietary importance (potato) and available information, particularly from National Monitoring Programs.

Table 3. Nitrate contents (mg kg^{-1}) in selected fresh vegetables described in some recent studies

Vegetable	Year reported	Author	Country	Nitrate (mg kg^{-1}) Mean	Min.	Max.	No of samples	Notes
Beetroot	1999	Ysart et al.	UK	1211	224	1877	4	UK total diet study, 1997
	2001	Yordanov et al.	Bulgaria	451.6			1	
	2008	Menard et al.	France	644.3	-	1141	3	Green cabbage (2000-2006)[a]
Broccoli	2000	Ximenes et al.	Brasil	566				
	2007	Thomson et al.	New Zealand	97.1	37.2	204.4	8	November - December, 2003; 2 urban regions
	2008	Menard et al.	France	442.4	< LOD	1131	7	(2000-2006)[a]; 14.3 % of the samples < LOD
	2009	Leszczyńska et al.	Poland	277.7			1	

Table 3. (Continued)

Vegetable	Year reported	Author	Country	Nitrate (mg kg^{-1})			No of samples	Notes
				Mean	Min.	Max.		
Brussels sprouts	2008	Menard et al.	France	24.1	< LOD	78	4	(2000-2006)[a]; 25 % of the samples < LOD
	2009	Leszczyńska et al.	Poland	37.6			1	
Cabbage	1999	Ysart et al.	UK	338	26	1523	16	UK total diet study, 1997
	1999	Fytianos and Zarogiannis	Greece	209	19.6	414	10	
	2002	Zhong et al.	China	1530	26	2670		North China (1998-1999)
	2003	Chung et al.	Korea	730	29	1498	15	Winter (November – March), 1998
				722	1	1788	25	Summer (April – October), 1998
	2006	Tamme et al.	Estonia	437	74	1138	168	(2003-2004)[a]
	2006	Sušin et al.	Slovenia	881	112	1864	52	(1996-2002)[a]
	2007	Thomson et al.	New Zealand	241	88	503	8	November - December, 2003; 2 urban regions
	2008	Menard et al.	France	498	-	1855	16	Green cabbage (2000-2006)[a]; 6.3% of the samples < LOD
	2008	Prasad and Chetty	Fiji	1425			6	"English cabbage", SD = 732 mg kg^{-1} (2006)
Carrot	1999	Ysart et al.	UK	97	11	566	20	UK total diet study, 1997
	2001	Yordanov et al.	Bulgaria	123.1			1	
	2003	Chung et al.	Korea	373	6	971	15	Winter (November – March), 1998
				282	1	1158	25	Summer (April – October), 1998
	2006	Tamme et al.	Estonia	148	< 30	525	202	(2003-2004)[a]
	2006	Sušin et al.	Slovenia	264	7	1042	65	(1996-2002)[a]
	2007	Thomson et al.	New Zealand	42.6	< 3.6	211.7	8	November - December, 2003; 2 urban regions
	2008	Menard et al.	France	120.7	< LOD	861	185	(2000-2006)[a]; 16.2 % of the samples < LOD
	2009	Chetty and Prasad	Fiji	91.3	81.0	100	6	
Cauliflower	1999	Ysart et al.	UK	86	34	164	8	UK total diet study, 1997

Vegetable	Year reported	Author	Country	Nitrate (mg kg^{-1})			No of samples	Notes
				Mean	Min.	Max.		
	2000	Zhou et al.	China	497	448	556	3	Beijing City (1979-1981)
	2006	Tamme et al.	Estonia	287	104	404	3	(2003-2004) [a]
	2009	Leszczyńska et al.	Poland	171.2			1	
Lettuce	1999	Fytianos and Zarogiannis	Greece	282	8	808	12	
	1999	Ysart et al.	UK	1051	85	3857	22	UK total diet study, 1997
	1999	Ysart et al.	UK	1085	50	3209	131	UK (1996 – 1997); outdoor lettuce
	2000	Ximenes et al.	Brazil	1420	-	-	1	
	2000	Zhou et al.	China	896	580	1454	6	Beijing City (1979-1981)
	2001	Yordanov et al.	Bulgaria	570			1	
	2003	Chung et al.	Korea	1933	247	3283	15	Winter (November – March), 1998
				2728	884	4488	25	Summer (April – October), 1998
	2003	De Martin and Restani	Italy	1473	< LOD	3270	177	(1996-2002)
	2006	Tamme et al.	Estonia	2167	397	3230	14	(2003-2004) [a]
	2006	Sušin et al.	Slovenia	1074	21	3986	151	(1996-2002) [a]
	2006	Weightman et al.	UK	838	-	-	60	Goodison var., open field, September 2003
				1352	-	-	60	Iceberg var., open field, September 2003
	2006	Merino et al.	Sweden	2684*	58	5406	159	Fresh lettuce, under covered fields (1996-2005) [a]
				826*	442	2038	14	Fresh lettuce, organic farming (1996-2005) [a]
				931*	94	2298	71	Iceberg lettuce (1996-2005) [a]
	2007	Thomson et al.	New Zealand	1160	61	2495	18	November - December, 2003; 2 urban regions
	2008	Menard et al.	France	1974	< LOD	5600	579	(2000-2006) [a]; 1.9 % of the samples < LOD
	2008	Pham et al.	France	-	377	3240	10	
	2008	Prasad and Chetty	Fiji	1297			6	SD = 348 mg kg^{-1} (2006)

Table 3. (Continued)

Vegetable	Year reported	Author	Country	Nitrate (mg kg^{-1}) Mean	Min.	Max.	No of samples	Notes
	2010	Correia et al.	Portugal	1156			1	
Parsley	2001	Yordanov et al.	Bulgaria	3			1	
	2002	Öztekin et al.	Turkey	1204			1	
	2006	Tamme et al.	Estonia	966	674	1588	4	(2003-2004) [a]
	2008	Menard et al.	France	1980	-	4300	16	(2000-2006) [a]; 6.3 % of the samples < LOD
Potato	1999	Ysart et al.	UK	155	3	1077	180	UK total diet study, 1997
	2001	Yordanov et al.	Bulgaria	40			1	
	2002	Zhong et al.	China	164	31.5	714	26	North China (1998-1999)
	2003	Chung et al.	Korea	294	2	977	15	Winter (November – March), 1998
				546	34	5521	25	Summer (April – October), 1998
	2006	Tamme et al.	Estonia	94	< 30	360	449	(2003-2004) [a]
	2006	Sušin et al.	Slovenia	158	2	704	202	(1996-2002) [a]
	2007	Thomson et al.	New Zealand	94.2	42.8	175.2	8	November - December, 2003; 2 urban regions
	2008	Menard et al.	France	191.8	< LOD	730	167	(2000-2006) [a]; 4.2 % of the samples < LOD
	2009	Chetty and Prasad	Fiji	110.8	102.9	119.8	6	
Spinach	1999	Ysart et al.	UK	1631	266	2834	13	UK total diet study, 1997
	1999	Ysart et al.	UK	1900	50	4650	34	UK (1996 – 1998)
	1999	Fytianos and Zarogiannis	Greece	1250	545	3760	10	
	2000	Ximenes et al.	Brazil	528	-	-	1	
	2000	Zhou et al.	China	2358	239	3872	35	Beijing City (1979-1981)
	2001	Yordanov et al.	Bulgaria	860			1	
	2002	Öztekin et al.	Turkey	2820			1	
	2003	Chung et al.	Korea	3334	427	7439	15	Winter (November – March), 1998
				4814	195	7793	25	Summer (April – October), 1998
	2003	De Martin and Restani	Italy	1757	< LOD	3720	23	(1996-2002)

Vegetable	Year reported	Author	Country	Nitrate (mg kg^{-1})			No of samples	Notes
				Mean	Min.	Max.		
	2005	Jaworska (2005a)	Poland	900				SD = 264 mg kg^{-1}; New Zealand spinach
	2006	Tamme et al.	Estonia	2508	2508	2508	1	(2003-2004)[a]
	2006	Merino et al.	Sweden	1747*	47	5975	63	Fresh spinach (1996-2005)[a]
	2007	Thomson et al.	New Zealand	722	73	1138	8	November - December, 2003; 2 urban regions
	2008	Menard et al.	France	1682	-	8700	266	(2000-2006)[a]; 3.4 % of the samples < LOD
Turnip	2000	Ximenes et al.	Brazil	2098	-	-	1	
	2000	Zhou et al.	China	2127			1	Beijing City (1979-1981)
	2006	Tamme et al.	Estonia	307	64	1062	58	(2003-2004)[a]
	2008	Menard et al.	France	657	-	2128	42	(2000-2006)[a]

SD: standard deviation; var.: variety; a National monitoring programme; * Value refers to median.

3.1. Nitrate Levels Variation within Season

Seasonal differences, statistically significant at the 5% level, in nitrate concentrations were observed by Ysart et al. (1999b) for potato, lettuce, carrot, cauliflower and onion. Nitrate concentrations in potatoes were lowest during the summer period (104 mg kg^{-1}) compared with spring, autumn and winter periods. Concentrations in lettuce (608 mg kg^{-1}) and carrots (19 mg kg^{-1}) were lower in the spring period than in the autumn and winter periods. For cauliflowers, nitrate concentrations were higher in the spring and summer periods than in the autumn and winter periods. Nitrate concentrations in onions were greatest in the autumn period (Ysart et al., 1999b).

In a different study, Ysart et al. (1999a) concluded that nitrate concentrations in UK-grown protected lettuce were influenced by the season with summer-grown crops having lower levels than those grown in the winter (mean of 2382 and 3124 mg kg^{-1}, respectively). Weather conditions also affected concentrations in protected lettuces with long hours of sunshine and low rainfall associated with low nitrate levels (Ysart et al., 1999a). Accordingly, Tamme et al. (2006) reported that the nitrate content of lettuce samples from Estonia was lower in summer than in winter (1952 and 3024 mg kg^{-1}, on average, respectively).

For the potato varieties used in the study by Ierna (2009), higher nitrate content in winter-spring than in summer–autumn crop was found.Regarding the nitrite contents, Chung et al. (2003), found that there was no significant difference in nitrite levels of vegetables harvested between the summer and the winter.

4. Nitrite Contents in Fresh Vegetables

It is commonly assumed that the nitrite levels in fresh leafy vegetables are usually less than 2 mg kg^{-1} (Santamaria, 2006). It has been shown that nitrite concentrations in fresh, uninjured, well-stored vegetables are extremely low, possibly because the nitrite reductase activity rate is in equilibrium with one of the nitrate reductase enzymes under proper storage conditions (Chung et al., 2004). Nitrite concentrations may increase dramatically via microbiological reduction of nitrate in vegetables while the nitrate content decreases during storage at ambient temperature. Under refrigerated storage, however, nitrite accumulation tended to be inhibited but may take place (Chung et al., 2004; Prasad & Chetty, 2008). Under frozen storage, nitrite accumulation was inhibited. Therefore, a poor storage could probably result in bacterial growth which can contribute to the increasing accumulation of high nitrite levels (Chung et al., 2004).

Although the number of results reported for the nitrite contents of fresh vegetables is considerably lower than those reported for nitrate, the data on Table 4 regarding nitrite levels described in some different studies, show that contents higher than 2 mg kg^{-1} have been reported. Values < 4.77 mg kg^{-1} were reported for cabbage (Zhong et al., 2002). For lettuce, a maximum value of 25 mg kg^{-1} was presented by Menard et al. (2008) and for spinach a maximum of 220 mg kg^{-1} was reported. For spinach, although 92% of the 112 samples showed nitrite levels < LOD, the estimate of the average nitrite concentration reported is 10.17 – 18.88 mg kg^{-1} (Menard et al., 2008).

Fytianos and Zarogiannis (1999) reported nitrite values in the range 0.8 – 8.5 mg kg^{-1} in spinach, with a mean value of 4.0 mg kg^{-1}. In vegetables of Estonian origin, the content of nitrites, assessed by a National Monitoring Program (2003 – 2004), was lower than 5 mg kg^{-1} (Tamme et al., 2006).

According to Amr and Hadidi (2001), nitrite levels in vegetables grown in Jordan ranged from non-detectable levels in open-field-grown cauliflower, to a maximum level of 4.3 mg kg^{-1} in greenhouse-grown squash.

In many studies regarding the nitrate contents of fresh vegetables, the contribution of nitrite is disregarded considering its lower level when compared to nitrate. Therefore the results reported for nitrate in these studies are in fact the sum of nitrite and nitrate levels (Ximenes et al., 2000; Prasad & Chetty, 2008).

Although these results are not discussed by the authors, high nitrite levels (>2 mg kg^{-1}, the traditionally admitted quantity for nitrite in fresh vegetables) may be due to the microbial reduction of nitrates to nitrites under room temperature or even under refrigeration. Considering this possibility, the techniques used in nitrate assessment in commercial vegetable samples should account for the different contributions of both nitrate and nitrite.

Table 4. Nitrite contents (mg kg-1) in fresh vegetables described in some recent studies

Vegetable	Year reported	Author	Country	Nitrite (mg kg^{-1})			No of samples	Notes
				Mean	Min.	Max.		
Beetroot	2001	Yordanov et al.	Bulgaria	1.54			1	
Broccoli	2007	Thomson et al.	New Zealand	3.7	< 3.33	18	8	November - December,

Vegetable	Year reported	Author	Country	Nitrite (mg kg^{-1}) Mean	Min.	Max.	No of samples	Notes
								2003; 2 urban regions
	2008	Menard et al.	France	< LOD			2	(2000-2006)[a]
	2009	Leszczyńska et al.	Poland	1.9			1	
Brussels sprouts	2008	Menard et al.	France	< LOD			1	(2000-2006)[a]
	2009	Leszczyńska et al.	Poland	2.28			1	
Carrot	2007	Thomson et al.	New Zealand	< LOD			8	November - December, 2003; 2 urban regions LOD = 3.33 mg kg^{-1}
	2008	Menard et al.	France	< LOD			84	(2000-2006)[a]
Cabbage	2001	Yordanov et al.	Bulgaria	1.02			1	
	2002	Zhong et al.	China	0.472	< LOD	4.77	23	North China (1998-1999)
	2003	Chung et al.	Korea	0.4	< LOD	3.6	15	Winter (November – March), 1998
				0.3	< LOD	2.2	25	Summer (April – October), 1998
	2006	Sušin et al.	Slovenia	0.2	LOQ	0.4	52	(1996-2002)[a]; LOQ = 0.16 mg kg^{-1}; 79/151 < LOQ
	2007	Thomson et al.	New Zealand	< LOD			8	November - December, 2003; 2 urban regions LOD = 3.33 mg kg^{-1}
	2008	Menard et al.	France	< LOD			7	Green cabbage (2000-2006)[a]
Carrot	2001	Yordanov et al.	Bulgaria	0.82			1	
	2003	Chung et al.	Korea	0.5	< LOD	1.8	15	Winter (November – March), 1998
				0.2	< LOD	2.9	25	Summer (April – October), 1998
	2006	Sušin et al.	Slovenia	0.2	< LOQ	0.4	65	(1996-2002)[a]; LOQ = 0.16 mg kg^{-1}; 54/65 samples < LOQ
Cauliflower	2008	Menard et al.	France	< LOD			4	(2000-2006)[a]
	2009	Leszczyńska et al.	Poland	3.49			1	

Table 4. (Continued)

Vegetable	Year reported	Author	Country	Nitrite (mg kg^{-1})			No of samples	Notes
				Mean	Min.	Max		
Lettuce	2000	Zhou et al.	China	0.21	0.01	0.45	6	Beijing City (1979-1981)
	2001	Yordanov et al.	Bulgaria	3.04			1	
	2003	Chung et al.	Korea	0.6	< LOD	2.9	15	Winter (November – March), 1998
				0.7	< LOD	4.6	25	Summer (April – October), 1998
	2006	Sušin et al.	Slovenia	0.3	LOQ	1.4	151	(1996-2002) [a]; LOQ = 0.16 mg kg^{-1}; 47/52 samples < LOQ
	2007	Thomson et al.	New Zealand	< LOD			18	November - December, 2003; 2 urban regions LOD = 3.33 mg kg^{-1}
	2008	Menard et al.	France	0.10-6.25[b]		25	259	(2000-2006) [a]; 99.6% of the samples < LOD
Parsley	2008	Menard et al.	France	< LOD			7	(2000-2006) [a]
Potato	2001	Yordanov et al.	Bulgaria	0.66			1	
	2002	Zhong et al.	China	1.59	0.1	4.9	26	North China (1998-1999)
	2003	Chung et al.	Korea	0.6	< LOD	2.7	15	Winter (November – March), 1998
				0.3	< LOD	3.4	25	Summer (April – October), 1998
	2006	Sušin et al.	Slovenia	1.2	< LOQ	7.6	202	(1996-2002) [a]; LOQ = 0.16 mg kg^{-1}; 13/202 samples < LOQ
	2007	Thomson et al.	New Zealand	< LOD			8	November - December, 2003; 2

Vegetable	Year reported	Author	Country	Nitrite (mg kg^{-1})			No of samples	Notes
				Mean	Min.	Max		
	2008	Menard et al.	France	< LOD			2	urban regions (2000-2006) [a]
Spinach	1999	Fytianos and Zarogiannis	Greece	4.0	0.8	8.5	12	
	2000	Zhou et al.	China	0.27	< LOD	0.73	6	Beijing City (1979-1981)
	2001	Yordanov et al.	Bulgaria	7.44			1	
	2003	Chung et al.	Korea	0.5	< LOD	1.8	15	Winter (November – March), 1998
				1.2	< LOD	5.1	25	Summer (April – October), 1998
	2005	Jaworska (2005a)	Poland	0.34				SD = 0.16; New Zealand spinach
	2007	Thomson et al.	New Zealand	< LOD			8	November - December, 2003; 2 urban regions LOD = 3.33 mg kg^{-1}
	2008	Menard et al.	France	10.17-18.88 [b]		220	112	(2000-2006) [a]; 92% of the samples < LOD
Turnip	2000	Zhou et al.	China	< LOD			1	Beijing City (1979-1981)
	2008	Menard et al.	France	< LOD			13	(2000-2006) [a]

LOD: Limit of detection; SD: Standard deviation; var.: variety; a National monitoring programme; b Lower and upper bounds for the estimate of the average concentration; * Value refers to median

5. Effects of Storage and Technological Processing on Nitrate and Nitrite Contents

The levels of nitrate and nitrite contents in raw plant material is not in direct proportion to their actual uptake, as both initial handling of the vegetables (washing and peeling) and cooking techniques may affect the final levels of these compounds (Leszczyńska et al., 2009).

During the storage period, the content of nitrites in frozen spinach products, previously cooked in boiling water for 4 minutes, increased by 27-42% but did not exceed 1 mg kg^{-1} (Jaworska, 2005b).For a set of fresh leafy vegetables whose initial nitrate contents ranged between 1297 and 5658 mg kg^{-1}, Prasad and Chetty (2008) concluded that boiling reduces nitrate content by 47–56% whereas frying in Soya bean oil elevates nitrate content by as much as 159–307%. No significant change was observed in nitrate content after baking. The deep-freezing of the selected leafy vegetables shows that nitrate content fluctuates slightly from the original nitrate values over a seven day period (Prasad & Chetty, 2008).

Regarding the results for root vegetables, Chetty and Prasad (2009) report that boiling reduces the nitrate content in these fresh vegetables by 23.3 – 42.6%, while frying in soya bean oil elevates nitrate contents from 204.5 – 299.1%.

Leszczyńska et al. (2009) studied the effects of some processing methods on nitrate and nitrite changes in cruciferous vegetables. Both blanching and boiling of the cruciferous vegetables caused a significant decrease of the total amount of nitrate but, at the same time, no unequivocal changes in the nitrite level (Leszczyńska et al., 2009).

According to Kmiecik et al. (2004), the blanching of dill (*Anethum graveolens* L.) induced considerable reductions of the contents of nitrates and nitrites. This concerned whole plants to a greater degree than leaves. Freezing did not affect the level of the analyzed compounds in frozen products, with the exception of non-blanched whole plants in which the level of nitrites significantly rose in relation to the raw material.

6. Dietary Intake of Nitrate and Nitrite from Vegetable Sources

The nitrate and nitrite contents of the vegetables contribute to the dietary exposure to nitrate and nitrite. This exposure has been assessed in some recent studies and the results are occasionally compared to the acceptable daily intake (ADI) values. An ADI for nitrate of 0-3.7 mg NO_3^- kg^{-1} body weight (bw), equivalent to 222 mg NO_3^- per day for a 60 kg adult, has been set by the Joint Expert Committee of the Food and Agriculture (JEFCA) of the United Nations/World Health Organization (WHO) and the European Commission's Scientific Committee on Food (SCF). For nitrite, the JEFCA and the SCF have proposed an ADI of 0-0.07 and 0-0.06 mg NO_2- kg^{-1} bw, respectively (Santamaria, 2006).

Penington (1998) discussed several approaches to estimating dietary exposure to nitrate and nitrite and reported some estimates of nitrate and/or nitrite in daily diets from 1973-1997. Intake values can differ to a large extent, depending on the method used for the estimation of additives and contaminants intake from food (Pennington, 1998; Tamme et al., 2006). Dietary intake assessment can be considered as a two-step process consisting of collecting and evaluating food composition data, and combining these data with food consumption data (Hoefkens et al. 2009).

Regarding nitrate, the mean total daily intake per person in Europe ranges between 50 and 140 mg and in the USA about 40 – 100 mg (Tamme et al., 2006). A comparison of the intake of nitrate and nitrite from vegetables in different countries, with a special focus on recent reports, is shown in Table 5.

Dietary exposures to nitrate for the general UK population estimated from the 1997 Total Diet Study were similar to those from previous UK Total Diet Studies and to those in other European countries. Dietary exposures to nitrates of consumers of vegetables (including those who eat above average amounts of vegetables) were below the ADI (Ysart et al., 1999).

Table 5. Comparison of the intake of nitrate and nitrite from vegetables in different countries (mg person^{-1} day^{-1}) using a basis of 60 kg body weight

Country	Year report	Author	Vegetable consumption (g day^{-1})	Nitrate intake (mg day^{-1})	Nitrite intake (mg day^{-1})	% ADI nitrate	% ADI nitrite	Notes
China	2002	Zhong et al.	444	422.8	0.68	219		North China; nine vegetables that account for 80% of the total consumption in the north Chinese diet
Denmark	1999	Petersen and Stolze	142	38.9	0.091			
England	1999	Ysart et al.	233	36		69		Green vegetables + potatoes + other vegetables
Egypt	1998	Saleh et al.	159	296	-	116 (F) 140 (M)		($NO_2^- + NO_3^-$); Total diet study
France	2008	Menard et al.	67.1			27	<0.05-33.3	Children (3-14 year-old), excluding potatoes n = 1018
			110.8	90	1.2-2.4	24.3	<0.05-16.7	Adults (>15 year-old), n = 1474; excluding potatoes
Korea	2003	Chung et al.	104.4	181.6	0.12			Chinese cabbages only
Italy	2003	De Martin and Restani	34.1	65.8	-	29.8		Adults; includes the 5 most consumed vegetables, supposed to provide most of the nitrate intake in the typical Italian diet
			8.5	14.5		19.6		Children (4-6 years, bw = 20kg); includes the 5 most consumed vegetables, supposed to provide most of the nitrate intake in the typical adult Italian diet
Estonia	2006	Tamme et al.	376	58		26		Adults, Consumption Survey National Board of Statistics

Table 5. (Continued)

Country	Year report	Author	Vegetable consumption (g day^{-1})	Nitrate intake (mg day^{-1})	Nitrite intake (mg day^{-1})	% ADI nitrate	% ADI nitrite	Notes
			226	30		40		Children (4-6 year-old), 2 kindergarten menu consumption survey
			198	26		52		Children (1-3 year-old), recommended infant menu
New Zealand	2007	Thomson et al.	231	42	0.48	16	13	Adults; food and water combined.
New Zealand	2004			31.2	0.54			Total diet, additives plus vegetables, 2004

The total intake calculated from nine vegetables that account for 80% of the total consumption in the North Chinese diet was 422.8 mg day^{-1} for nitrates and 0.68 mg day^{-1} for nitrites (Zhong et al., 2002). In New Zealand, the mean dietary exposure to nitrates from food and water combined was estimated to be 16% of the ADI, with a median exposure level of 9% of the ADI. Approximately 1% of exposure scenarios resulted in daily dietary exposures above the ADI for nitrates (Thomson et al., 2007). The most significant contributors were potatoes (32%) and lettuce (29%). The mean dietary exposure to exogenous nitrite was about 13% of the ADI, excluding endogenous conversion of nitrate. If a contribution from the conversion of dietary nitrate to nitrite was considered, the ADI was exceeded 10% of the time for an average conversion rate (5%) and 50% of the time for individuals with high conversion rate (20%) (Thomson et al., 2007).

In Estonia, reported low levels of nitrates in vegetables and in infant foods were probably related to the lower use of fertilizers in this country. The results showed that cabbage and potato were the main sources of nitrate intake (Tamme et al., 2006).

Nitrate dietary exposure in France averaged 40% of the ADI for adults and 51-54% for children (Menard et al., 2008). The major contributors were, for adults and children, respectively, vegetables (24 and 27% of ADI), potatoes (5 and 11% of ADI) and water (5 and 5% of the ADI). Nitrite dietary exposure averaged 33-67% of the ADI for adults and 67-133% for children. This was the first French estimate of the dietary exposure to nitrate and nitrite based on concentrations analyzed in foods (13657 analyses in foods and 6870 analyses in water) (Menard et al., 2008).

Based on the average consumption of selected vegetables and cured meat in Australia, the estimated dietary intake for nitrate and nitrite for Australians were 267 and 5.3 mg/adult/day, respectively (Hsu et al., 2009). Although great differences exist in diary habits and water quality between different countries, vegetables are still the major source of nitrate intake (Du et al., 2007).

In the study "Risk-benefit health assessment of food - Food fortification and nitrate in vegetables", Bottex et al. (2008) have used diets database (WHO, 2006) as well as consumption information supplied by 11 European Member States and Norway. The figures viewed overall gave a highest (97.5th percentile) daily intake of ''most vegetables'' just below 400 g/day. This amount, taking a conservative approach, is similar to the WHO recommendation that the daily intake of fruit and vegetables should be about 400 g/day. For the risk assessment, for the base case, it was assumed that all of the 400 g were consumed in the form of vegetables. In addition high consumer intakes also have to be considered, such as the potato intake in Ireland (771 g/day). The highest reported level of leafy vegetable (lettuce) consumption in EU is from Spain, approximately 133 g/day, which is about 1/3 of the 400 g base case vegetable total intake (Bottex et al., 2008). For nitrate intake the main driver is not the amount of vegetables eaten, but the type of vegetable and nitrate level which is the determining factor together with variables such as the production type, light, fertilizer use, and temperature (EFSA, 2008; Bottex et al., 2008).

Vegetarians consume up to 10 times more nitrate than non-vegetarians, and a typical Mediterranean diet, for example, is likely to contain considerably more nitrate than the average Western diet (Lundberg et al., 2006).

The knowledge of the nitrate and nitrite metabolisms in humans and their toxicological effects must be improved to better characterize the risk of dietary exposure to nitrate and nitrite present in food (Menard et al., 2008). Case-control studies examining dietary intake of nitrate and the risk of gastric cancer have consistently found a negative association (Kelley & Duggan, 2003). In such studies, vegetable intake has been consistently related to a decreased risk of gastric cancer. Nitrate intake was probably an index of vegetable intake what can explain the negative association. Recent case-control studies have all reported a weak, statistically non-significant increased risk of gastric cancer for high vs. low nitrite intake. Nitrite intake may be related to the consumption of preserved meat, typically high-salt foods, what can also contribute to an increased risk of gastric cancer. It is interesting to note that a diet high in nitrite does not appear to confer an increased risk if that diet is also high in antioxidants from fruits and vegetables (Kelley & Duggan, 2003).

7. Analytical Methodologies for Both Extraction and Analysis

A variety of analytical methods have been developed for the determination of nitrate and applied to the analysis of food and agriculture products, including: high-performance liquid chromatography (Dennis et al., 1990; Cheng & Tsang, 1998; Hsu et al., 2009), ion chromatography (De Martin & Restani, 2003), spectrophotometry (ISO, 1984; Pinho et al., 1998; Zatar et al., 1999), polarography (Ximenes et al., 2000), potentiometry with ion selective electrode (Tamme et al., 2006; Wilhelm et al., 2000), capillary electrophoresis (Jimidar et al., 1995; Öztekin et al., 2002; Merusi et al., 2010), electron paramagnetic resonance spectrometry (Yordanov et al., 1999). GC/MS coupled with ^{15}N-labeled analogue as an internal standard is generally considered the most accurate and effective technique for the quantification of both nitrite and nitrate in biological fluids (Wang & Mazza, 2002).

A review of the strategies employed to facilitate the detection, determination and monitoring of nitrate and/or nitrite has been presented in a very interesting review by Moorcroft et al. (2001).

Spectroscopic methods are by far the most widely used for nitrate/nitrite determination due to the excellent limits of detection obtained and facile assay-type protocols. A broad range of techniques have been evaluated, including UV/VIS, chemiluminescence, fluorimetric, IR, Raman, and molecular cavity emission protocols (Moorcroft et al., 2001).

While the compositional complexities offered by real world media often preclude the direct UV determination of either nitrate or nitrite, such an approach does serve as a principal detection system in a host of chromatographic and electrophoretic systems (Moorcroft et al., 2001).

The most common approach to the detection of nitrite however is undoubtedly the Griess Assay. First developed in 1879, it has found numerous applications for both nitrate and nitrite analysis. The assay typically relies on the diazotization of a suitable aromatic amine by acidified nitrite with the subsequent coupling reaction providing a highly colored azo chromophore from which the concentration of nitrite can be assessed (Moorcroft et al., 2001). The most common arrangement utilizes sulphanilamide and *N*-(1-naphthyl)ethylenediamine as the target amine and coupler, respectively, with the product of the reaction detected at 540 nm. Sulphanilic acid, nitroaniline and *p*-aminoacetophenone have been used as the target amine with phenol, 1-naphthol, 1-naphthol-4-sulphonate, 1- amino naphthalene and 1,3-diaminobenzene investigated as potential coupling agents. The reaction can be used directly for the determination of nitrite, but nitrate requires the incorporation of a reduction step prior to detection (Moorcroft et al., 2001).

Nevertheless, regarding the nitrate/nitrite determination in vegetable samples, this methodology requires steps of extraction, clarification and reduction of nitrate to nitrite that turns it time consuming (Ximenes et al., 2000; Pham et al., 2008).

A new UV-spectrophotometric method for the determination of nitrates in vegetables has been presented by Pham et al. (2008), based on deconvolution of UV spectra.

In the polarographic method proposed by Ximenes et al. (2000) nitrate is determined through an electroactive complex formed in a cobalt (II)-thiocyanate-acid solution in the presence of nitric oxide generated by the reduction of nitrate outside the polarographic cell (Ximenes et al., 2000).

FIA with colorimetric analysis of nitrate/nitrite in different matrices has proved to be an inexpensive technique (Prasad & Chetty, 2008).

A method for the simultaneous determination of chloride, nitrate and sulphate in vegetable samples by single-column ion chromatography has been proposed by Zhou and Guo (2000). The ion chromatographic method is fast, allows the direct determination of the nitrate ions, is suitable for all leafy vegetables, with excellent analytical performance as regard to precision and repeatability. The drawbacks include higher limits of detection than in other analytical methods, and the need for specific equipment that is not available in all laboratories (De Martin & Restani, 2003).

Capillary electrophoresis (CE) has been proposed as a powerful technique for anions' analyses, since it permits fast analyses and low running cost (Merusi et al., 2010). Jimidar et al. (1995) have determined the nitrate amounts in vegetable samples using capillary electrophoresis with the indirect detection method. Marshall and Trenerry (1996) have proposed a direct detection method for the simultaneous determination of nitrites and nitrates in a variety of foodstuffs. The simultaneous detection of the two analytes by capillary electrophoretic methods depends on the slowing down or reversal of the electroosmotic flow by buffer additives. As buffer additives, commercially available reagents of unknown composition or cationic surfactants are commonly used (Öztekin et al., 2002). Nitrates and nitrites have a very similar electrophoretic mobility, but low pH can selectively reduce the mobility of nitrites compared to that of nitrates, since nitrites at low pH are not completely dissociated (Merusi et al., 2010).

Determination of the concentration of nitrate by means of potentiometric sensors such as ion-selective electrodes (ISE) is also possible. Among the advantages of this competitive technique are easy use, low coast, portability, wide linear range of measured concentrations, rapid response, low detection limit (about 10^{-5} mol L^{-1} NO_3^-) and time-efficiency. Moreover, in contrast to optical methods, solution color or turbidity does not affect the results of measurements (Mourzina et al. 2003).

GC/MS analysis can be used for the determination of nitrate and nitrite in biological fluids and cell cultures, after derivatization using α-bromo-2,3,4,5,6- pentafluorotoluene (PFB-Br) (Tsikas, 2000; Moorcroft et al, 2001). Briefly, a nitrite containing sample or matrix is mixed with acetone and PFB-Br and incubated at 50°C for 60 min. After derivatization, samples are cooled to room temperature, and acetone is evaporated under a nitrogen stream. The reaction products are extracted from the remaining aqueous phase by vortex mixing with toluene for GC/MS analysis (Tsikas, 2000).

Regarding the extraction of nitrate and nitrite from vegetable samples, hot water is generally added to homogenized portions, considering the high solubility of these ions in water. Precipitation of the proteins is usually accomplished by the addition of solutions of potassium hexacyanoferrate (II) and zinc acetate. Activated charcoal may also be included in this protocol (Thomson et al., 2007). The precipitate is subsequently removed by filtration. Filtered extracts can be purified by solid phase extraction when the nitrate determination is performed using ion chromatography and UV detection at 214 nm (Ysart et al., 1999b; De Martin & Restani, 2003; Chang et al., 2003).

The use of an additional re-suspension stage including enzymatic hydrolysis using α-amylase digestion may be necessary when analysing certain types of food products (bread, miscellaneous cereals and potatoes) (Ysart et al., 1999b).

Merino et al. (2006) used hot water (50 – 60°C) to extract the nitrates from vegetable samples and the test solution was treated with acetonitrile to remove suspended material prior to analysis by ion chromatography with UV detection at 205 nm.

In some studies using flow-injection-analysis, fresh samples are homogenized with water, centrifuged and the supernatant is used for nitrate determination after Cd-catalysed reduction to nitrite (Chen et al., 2004). Homogenization with water (50°C), filtration and dilution are used for extracting nitrates and nitrites from meat products and vegetables prior to capillary electrophoresis analysis (Öztekin et al., 2002). This procedure has also been used for nitrate and nitrite determination using HPLC (Chung et al., 2004) and ion chromatography (Zhong et al. 2002).

Regarding the use of potentiometry with ion selective electrode, nitrates were extracted from homogenized vegetables or vegetable juices using a $KAl(SO_4)_2$ solution (Tamme et al., 2006).

Prasad and Chetty have compared two extraction techniques for nitrate analysis from different types of vegetables, namely, extraction using activated carbon and alkaline extraction. The activated carbon extraction has been preferred for leafy vegetables (Prasad &

Chetty, 2008) and root vegetables (Prasad & Chetty, 2009), in combination with FIA and colorimetric detection.

Conclusion

Although food is required to be safe, there can be risk factors associated with the consumption of some vegetables containing naturally compounds with potential deleterious effects e.g. anti-nutrients or allergens. On the beneficial side, with regard to vegetable consumption there is general agreement that their content of macronutrients (e.g. fibre), micronutrients (e.g. vitamins), and bioactive substances results in an overall health benefit (WHO, 2005; Bottex et al., 2008).

Leafy vegetables, contain naturally high levels of nitrates which together with its metabolites, nitrites and nitric oxide, have not only physiological and potential beneficial roles in the body, but also potential for adverse effects. Therefore, both aspects need to be balanced in relation to the consumption of vegetables, as part of the conclusions of the EFSA Scientific Panel on Contaminants in the Food chain (EFSA, 2008; Bottex et al., 2008). However, according to actual knowledge, the ingestion of vegetables is supposed to be beneficial for the population nevertheless its nitrate and nitrite contents.

References

Amr, A; Hadidi, N. Effect of cultivar and harvest date on nitrate (NO_3) and nitrite (NO_2) content of selected vegetables grown under open field and greenhouse conditions in Jordan. *Journal of Food Composition and Analysis*, 2001, 14, 59-67.

Bottex, B; Lou, J.; Dorne, CM; Carlander, D; Benford, D; Przyrembeld, H; Heppner, C; Kleiner, J; Cockburn, A. Risk-benefit health assessment of food - Food fortification and nitrate in vegetables. *Trends in Food Science and Technology*, 2008, 19, S113-S119.

Chen, BM; Wang, ZH; Li, SX; Wang, GX; Song, HX; Wang, XN. Effects of nitrate supply on plant growth, nitrate accumulation, metabolic nitrate concentration and nitrate reductase activity in three leafy vegetables. *Plant Science*, 2004, 167, 635–643.

Cheng, CF; Tsang, CW. Simultaneous determination of nitrite, nitrate and ascorbic acid in canned vegetable juices by reverse-phase ion-interaction HPLC. *Food Additives and Contaminants: Part A*, 1998, 15, 753-758 .

Chetty, AA; Prasad, S. Flow injection analysis of nitrate-N determination in root vegetables: Study of the effects of cooking. *Food Chemistry*, 2009, 116, 561-566.

Choi, SY; Chung, MJ; Lee, SJ; Shin, JH; Sung, NJ. N-nitrosamine inhibition by strawberry, garlic, kale, and the effects of nitrite-scavenging and N-nitrosamine formation by functional compounds in strawberry and garlic. *Food Control*, 2007, 18, 485–491.

Chung, JC; Chou, SS; Hwang, DF. Changes in nitrate and nitrite content of four vegetables during storage at refrigerated and ambient temperatures. *Food Additives and Contaminants*, 2004, 21, 317–322.

Chung, SY; Kim, JS; Kim, M; Hong, MK; Lee, JO; Kim, CM; Song, IS. Survey of nitrate and nitrite contents of vegetables grown in Korea. *Food Additives and Contaminants*, 2003, 20, 621-628.

Correia, M; Barroso, A; Barroso, MF; Soares, D; Oliveira, MBPP; Delerue-Matos, C. Contribution of different vegetable types to exogenous nitrate and nitrite exposure. *Food Chemistry*, 2010, 120, 960-966.

Coss, A; Cantor, KP; Relf, JS; Lynch, CF; Ward, MH. Pancreatic cancer and drinking water and dietary sources of nitrate and nitrite. *American Journal of Epidemiology*, 2004, 159, 693-701.

De Groote, MA; Fang, FC. NO inhibitions: antimicrobial properties of nitric oxide. *Clinical Infectious Diseases*, 1995, 21, 162-165.

De Martin, S; Restani, P. Determination of nitrates by a novel ion chromatographic method: occurrence in leafy vegetables (organic and conventional) and exposure assessment for Italian consumers. *Food Additives and Contaminants*, 2003; 20, 787-792.

Dennis, MJ; Key, PE; Papworth, T; Pointer, M; Massey, RC. The determination of nitrate and nitrite in cured meat by HPLC/UV. *Food Additives and Contaminants: Part A*, 1990, 7, 455-461.

Du, ST; Zhang, YS; Lin, XY. Accumulation of nitrate in vegetables and its possible implications to human health, *Agricultural Sciences in China*, 2007, 6, 1246-1255.

EFSA (European Food Safety Authority). (2008). Nitrate in vegetables. Scientific opinion of the panel on contaminants in the food chain. *EFSA Journal*, 689, 1e79, Available from http://www.efsa.europa.eu/EFSA/Scientific_Opinion/contam_ej_689_nitrate_en.pdf

European Commission, 1998, Reports of the Scientific Committee for Food (Thirty-eight Series). Opinion on Nitrates and Nitrite (Luxembourg: Office for the Official Publications of the European Communities), 1-33.

European Commission. Commission Regulation (EC) No. 1881/2006 of 19 December 2006 setting maximum levels for certain contaminants in foodstuffs. *Official Journal of the European Union,* 2006, L 364 20.12.2006, 5-24.

Fytianos, K; Zarogiannis, P. Nitrate and nitrite accumulation in fresh vegetables from Greece. *Bulletin of Environmental Contamination and Toxicology*, 1999, 62, 187-192.

Gruda, N. Impact of environmental factors on product quality of greenhouse vegetables for fresh consumption. *Critical Reviews in Plant Sciences*, 2005, 24, 227–247.

Hoefkens, C; Sioen, I; De Henauw, S; Vandekinderen, I; Baert, K; De Meulenaer, B; Devlieghere, F; Van Camp, J. Development of vegetable composition databases based on available data for probabilistic nutrient and contaminant intake assessments. *Food Chemistry*, 2009, 113, 799-803.

Hsu, J; Arcot, J; Lee, NA. Nitrate and nitrite quantification from cured meat and vegetables and their estimated dietary intake in Australians. *Food Chemistry*, 2009, 115, 334-339.

Ierna, A. Influence of harvest date on nitrate contents of three potato varieties for off-season production. *Journal of Food Composition and Analysis*, 2009, 22, 551-555.

ISO 6635:1984 (E). Fruits, vegetables and derived products – Determination of nitrite and nitrate content – Molecular absorption spectrometric method. International Organization for Standardization, Geneve, Switzerland.

Jaworska, G. Content of nitrates, nitrites and oxalates in New Zealand spinach. *Food Chemistry*, 2005a, 89, 235-242.

Jaworska, G. Nitrates, nitrites, and oxalates in products of spinach and New Zealand spinach. Effect of technological measures and storage time on the level of nitrates, nitrites, and oxalates in frozen and canned products of spinach and New Zealand spinach. *Food Chemistry*, 2005b, 93, 395-401.

Jimidar, M; Hartmann, C; Cousement, N; Massart, DL. Determination of nitrate and nitrite in vegetables by capillary electrophoresis with indirect detection. *Journal of Chromatography A*, 1995, 706, 479-492.

Kelley, JR; Duggan, JM. Gastric cancer epidemiology and risk factors. *Journal of Clinical Epidemiology*, 2003, 56, 1-9.

Kmiecik, W, Lisiewska, Z; Słupski, J. Effects of freezing and storing of frozen products on the content of nitrates, nitrites, and oxalates in dill (*Anethum graveolens* L.). *Food Chemistry*, 2004, 86, 105-111.

Lala, PK; Orucevic, A. Role of nitric oxide in tumor progression: lessons from experimental tumors. *Cancer and Metastasis Reviews*, 1998, 17, 91-106.

Leszczyńska, T; Filipiak-Florkiewicz, A; Cieślik, E; Sikora, E; Pisulewski, PM. Effects of some processing methods on nitrate and nitrite changes in cruciferous vegetables. *Journal of Food Composition and Analysis*, 2009, 22, 315-321.

Li, JL; Chen, XP; Li, XL; Zhang, FS. Effect of N fertilization on yield, nitrate content and N apparent losses of Chinese cabbage. *Acta Pedologica Sinica*, 2003, 40, 261-6.

Lundberg, JO; Feelisch, M.; Björne, H; Jansson, EA; Weitzberg, E. Cardioprotective effects of vegetables: Is nitrate the answer? *Nitric Oxide*, 2006, 15, 359-362.

McKnight, GM; Smith, LM; Drummond, RS; Duncan, CW; Golden, M; Benjamin, N. Chemical synthesis of nitric oxide in the stomach from dietary nitrate in humans. *Gut*, 1997, 40, 211-214.

Marshall, PA; Trenerry, VC. The determination of nitrite and nitrates in foods by capillary ion electrophoresis. *Food Chemistry*, 1996, 57, 339-345.

Menard, C; Heraud, F; Volatier, JL; Leblanc, JC. Assessment of dietary exposure of nitrate and nitrite in France. *Food Additives and Contaminants*, 2008, 25, 971–988.

Merino, L; Darnerud, PO; Edberg, U; Åman, P; Castillo, MDP. Levels of nitrate in Swedish lettuce and spinach over the past 10 years. *Food Additives and Contaminants*, 2006, 23, 1283-1289.

Merusi, C; Corradini, C; Cavazza, A; Borromei, C; Salvadeo, P. Determination of nitrates, nitrites and oxalates in food products by capillary electrophoresis with pH-dependent electroosmotic flow reversal. *Food Chemistry*, 2010, 120, 615-620.

Moncada, S; Palmer, RM; Higgs, EA. Nitric oxide: Physiology, pathophysiology, and pharmacology. *Pharmacological Reviews*, 1991, 43, 109- 142.

Moncada, S; Higgs, A. L-arginine-nitric oxide pathway. *New England Journal of Medicine*, 1993, 329, 2002-2012.

Moorcroft, MJ; Davis, J; Compton, RG. Detection and determination of nitrate and nitrite: a review. *Talanta*, 2001, 54, 785–803

Mourzina, YG; Ermolenko, YE; Yoshinobu, T; Vlasov, Y; Iwasakic, H; Schöning, MJ. Anion-selective light-addressable potentiometric sensors (LAPS) for the determination of nitrate and sulphate ions. *Sensors and Actuators B*, 2003, 91, 32-38.

Ostertag, LM; O'Kennedy, N; Kroon, PA; Duthie, GG; de Roos, B. Impact of dietary polyphenols on human platelet function – A critical review of controlled dietary intervention studies. *Molecular Nutrition and Food Research*, 2010, 54, 60–81.

Öztekin, N; Nutku, MS; Erim, FB. Simultaneous determination of nitrite and nitrate in meat products and vegetables by capillary electrophoresis. *Food Chemistry*, 2002, 76, 103-106.

Pennington, JAT. Dietary exposure models for nitrates and nitrites. *Food Control*, 1998, 9, 385-395.

Pham, HN; Benitez, A; Hommet, F; Bombe, D; Schoefs, O.; Pauss, A. A new quantitative and low-cost determination method of nitrate in vegetables, based on deconvolution of UV spectra. *Talanta*, 2008, 76, 936–940.

Pinho, O; Ferreira, IMPLVO; Oliveira, MBPP; Ferreira, MA. FIA evaluation of nitrite and nitrate contents of liver pâtés. *Food Chemistry*, 1998, 62, 359-362.

Prasad, S; Chetty, AA. Nitrate-N determination in leafy vegetables: Study of the effects of cooking and freezing. *Food Chemistry*, 2008, 106, 772-780.

Pussemier, L; Larondelle, Y; Van Peteghem, C; Huyghebaert, A. Chemical safety of conventionally and organically produced foodstuffs: a tentative comparison under Belgian conditions. *Food Control*, 2006, 17, 14-21.

Reinink, K. Genotype × environment interaction for nitrate concentration in lettuce. *Plant Breeding*, 1991, 107, 39-49.

Saleh, ZA; Brunn, H; Paetzold, R; Hussein, L. Nutrients and chemical residues in an Egyptian total mixed diet, *Food Chemistry*, 1998, 63, 535-541.

Santamaria, P. Nitrate in vegetables: toxicity, content, intake and EC regulation (Review), *Journal of the Science of Food and Agriculture*, 2006, 86, 10-17.

Sušin, J; Kmecl, V; Gregorčic, A. A survey of nitrate and nitrite content of fruit and vegetables grown in Slovenia during 1996-2002. *Food Additives and Contaminants*, 2006, 23, 385-390.

Tamme, T; Reinik, M; Roasto, M; Juhkam, K; Tenno, T; Kiis, A. Nitrates and nitrites in vegetables and vegetable-based products and their intakes by the Estonian population. *Food Additives and Contaminants*, 2006, 23, 355-361.

Thomson, BM; Nokes, CJ; Cressey, PJ. Intake and risk assessment of nitrate and nitrite from New Zealand foods and drinking water, *Food Additives and Contaminants*, 2007, 24, 113-121.

Tsikas, D. Simultaneous derivatization and quantification of the nitric oxide metabolites nitrite and nitrate in biological fluids by gas-chromatography/mass spectrometry. *Analytical Chemistry*, 2000, 72, 4064-4072.

van Velzen, AG; Sips, AJAM; Schothorst, RC; Lambersa, AC; Meulenbelt, J. The oral bioavailability of nitrate from nitrate-rich vegetables in humans. *Toxicology Letters*, 2008, 181, 177–181.

Viuda-Martos, M; Fernández-López, J; Sayas-Barbera, E; Sendra, E; Navarro, C; Pérez-Álvarez, JA. Citrus co-products as technological strategy to reduce residual nitrite content in meat products. *Journal of Food Science*, 2009, 74, Nr. 8, 2009, R93-R100.

Wang, HJ; Wu, LH; Tao, QN; Miller, DD; Welch, RM. Glutamine nitrogen and ammonium nitrogen supplied as a nitrogen source is not converted into nitrate nitrogen of plant tissues of hydroponically grown pak-choi (*brassica chinensis* L.), *Journal of Food Science*, 2009, 74, T21-T23.

Wang, J and Mazza, G. Quantification of nitrite in the presence of anthocyanins using Griess and GC/MS assays. *Journal of Food Biochemistry*, 2002, 26, 339-354.

Weightman, RM; Dyer, C; Buxton, J; Farrington, DS. Effects of light level, time of harvest and position within field on the variability of tissue nitrate concentration in commercial crops of lettuce (*Lactuca sativa*) and endive (*Cichorium endiva*). *Food Additives and Contaminants*, 2006, 23, 462-469.

WHO (World Health Organization). (2003). Diet, nutrition and the prevention of chronic diseases. Report of the joint WHO/FAO expert consultation. Technical Report Series, No. 916. Available from http://www.who.int/dietphysicalactivity/publications/trs916/download/en/index.html

Wilhelm, WW; Arnold, SL; Schepers, JS. Using a nitrate specific ion electrode to determine stalk nitrate-nitrogen concentration. *Agronomy Journal*, 2000, 92, 186-189.

Wu, Cc; Thiemermann, C. Biological control and inhibition of induction of nitric oxide synthase. *Methods Enzymology*, 1996, 268, 408-420.

Ximenes, MIN; Rath, S; Reyes, FGR. Polarographic determination of nitrate in vegetables. *Talanta*, 2000, 51, 49-56.

Yordanov, ND; Novakova, E; Lubenova, S. Consecutive estimation of nitrate and nitrite ions in vegetables and fruits by electron paramagnetic resonance spectrometry. *Analytica Chimica Acta*, 2001, 437, 131-138.

Ysart, G; Clifford, R; Harrison, N. Monitoring for nitrate in UK-grown lettuce and spinach. *Food Additives and Contaminants: Part A*, 1999a, 16, 301-306.

Ysart, G; Miller, P; Barrett, G; Farrington, D; Lawrance, P; Harrison, N. Dietary exposures to nitrate in the UK. *Food Additives and Contaminants*, 1999b, 16, 521-532.

Zatar, NI; Abu-Eid, MA; Eid, AF. Spectrophotometric determination of nitrite and nitrate using phosphomolybdenum blue complex. *Talanta*, 1999, 50, 819-826.

Zhong, W; Hu, C; Wang, M. Nitrate and nitrite in vegetables from north China: content and intake, *Food Additives and Contaminants*, 2002, 19, 1125-1129.

Zhou, M; Guo, D. Simultaneous determination of chloride, nitrate and sulphate in vegetable samples by single-column ion chromatography. *Microchemical Journal*, 2000, 65, 221-226.

Zhou, ZY; Wang, MJ; Wang, JS. Nitrate and nitrite contamination in vegetables in China, *Food Reviews International*, 2000, 16, 61-76.

In: Nutritional Insights and Food Safety
Editor: Jaroslava Švarc-Gajiæ
ISBN: 978-1-61122-130-5

Chapter IV

Inorganic Food Contaminants

Žarko Kevrešan
Institute for Food Technology – FINS; Bulevar cara Lazara 1;
21 000 Novi Sad; Serbia

Abstract

This chapter gives the overview of major inorganic food contaminants, encompassing chemical and physical contaminants, as well as radionucleides, and elaborates the mechanisms of their introduction into the food chain further explaining their fate. The sources of most frequent inorganic toxicants are elaborated as well as some toxicological aspects, including the availability from food sources and most evident poisoning symptoms. In addition, the significance of safety management systems during food processing, such as HACCP, and risk analysis important in improving the food safety are described. The most commonly used analytical methods for the determination of inorganic contaminants in foodstuffs are presented as well by this chapter.

Introduction

The term inorganic contamination of food usually implies (a) heavy metals and metalloids, such as lead (Pb), cadmium (Cd), mercury (Hg) and arsenic (As), main anions – fluoride (F^-), nitrate (NO_3^-) and nitrite (NO_2^-) (b) radionuclides - cesium - $^{134/137}Cs$, strontium - ^{90}Sr, iodine - ^{131}I, carbon - ^{14}C, hydrogen - ^{3}H, sulphur - ^{35}S, and potassium - ^{40}K, (c) excess concentrations of essential elements (copper (Cu), chromium (Cr), F, molybdenum (Mo), nickel (Ni), selenium (Se), zinc (Zn) and tin (Sn) which in elevated concentrations can be potentially hazardous to human health, and (d) particles of metals, send, stones, bones, wood or other foreign material.

1. Origin of Inorganic Food Contaminants

Inorganic contaminants in food generally originate from several different sources including agricultural activities, industrial or household processing and migration from package during the storage of final food products. The ways of introduction and migration of inorganic contaminants throughout the food chain differ for physical contaminants which are represented as inorganic particles occurring in food products, and chemical contaminants, which are chemically incorporated in the matrix of food products.

1.1. Physical Contamination

Physical contamination of food products includes: stones, send, pips, bones, twigs, hair, pieces of machinery used during food production. This type of food contamination implies particles that usually enter the food chain as a result of human error, presence of pests or accidents with machinery or equipment. Physical contamination in foodstuffs is often easily spotted and perceived during food consumption, and thus usually do not result in serious hazards for consumers health but, however, results in consumers disgust and rejection of consumed food products in which contamination is registered or suspected.

Physical contamination can occur at any stage of food production chain and its prevention is possible only by careful monitoring of all steps of food production process.

1.2. Chemical Contamination

Chemical inorganic contamination includes cation (metals, metalloids and radionucleides) and anion (fluorides, nitrates etc.) contamination. During last decades the paths and mechanisms of introduction of different inorganic chemical contaminants into the food chain have been the topic of interest of numerous authors and some of the most important findings related to this subject are presented bellow.

The predominant route of entrance of inorganic contaminants into the food chain arises during plant cultivation. During vegetation plants absorb macro- and micronutrients from the soil. Soils, depending on their origin, can naturally be rich in some highly toxic elements. Some of the contaminants, especially soluble ones, are present in soil solution in high concentration. For example, cadmium content in soils originating from crustal rocks was determined to vary from 1 to 90000 $\mu g\ kg^{-1}$ (Page et al., 1981; Cook & Freny, 1988; Kabata-Pendias & Pendias, 1992) and for the soils that overlay some sedimentary rocks the content of several hundreds of mg of As per kg of soil was reported (Peterson et al., 1981).

Besides natural occurrence, elevated concentrations of inorganic contaminants in soil can also be a result of human activities. It was established that elevated concentrations of arsenic in soil can be the consequence of coal burning in power stations (Wickstrom, 1982) while cadmium contamination of rice in Japan was linked to the contaminated fields (Asami, 1991). Soils can also be polluted by other industrial activities such as ore melting or battery production. Abundant traffic is significant source of soil pollution with lead (Chow, 1970). As one of the most studied pollutants, it was tracked that lead reaches food chain as a result of combustion of lead containing petrol additives, smelting and other anthropogenic activities (Alloway, 1990). Regardless the route by which lead finds its way to the soil, it mainly occurs in upper layers of soil profiles due to its intensive sorption by soil (Cartwright et al., 1977; Gulson et al., 1981; Merry et al., 1983). Having in mind anthropogenic sources of environmental pollution, intensive agriculture itself can significantly contribute to soil pollution. For example arsenic is extensively used as a constituent of insecticides, herbicides and defoliants (McLaughlin et al., 1999) while mercury is introduced into the soil as a constituent of fungicides, fertilizers, limestone, natural gypsum and manure (Andersson, 1979). Avoidance of soil pollution by some inorganic contaminants, for example cadmium, is somewhat impossible to achieve. Namely, cadmium is present practically in all phosphate fertilizers as an impurity (McLaughlin et al., 1999).

Besides through soil, inorganic contaminants can enter the food chain via atmospheric deposits. The deposits of inorganic contaminants accumulate in soil when persistent emission source is encountered, while single emissions of different contaminants usually leads to foliar uptake of the emitted toxic elements by food and pasture plants. Some specific inorganic contaminants, such as fluoride, can be introduced into the environment by volcanic emissions (WHO 2000). Main persistent sources of fluorides are industrial emissions particularly ones that burn coal. Also, endemic fluoride pollution in some areas occurs due to the burning of coal (Ten Brink et al., 1988) or firing bricks or tiles (Chen et al., 1993). Regarding anionic contaminants, beside fluoride, nitrates and nitrites represent the contaminants of major interest. Due to their high solubility in water their natural concentrations in soil are very low. In intensive agricultural production the utilization of fertilizers and, especially, the use of nitrogen fertilizers, represent the main anthropogenic source of nitrates. All nitrates that are not taken up by plants or microorganisms are washed out from soil.

Radionuclides are naturally present in the environment. Radionuclides like $^{134/137}Cs$, ^{90}Sr, ^{131}I, ^{14}C, ^{3}H, ^{35}S, and ^{40}K are mobile circulating in the environment and finding its way to enter the food chain mostly via plants due to their similarity with essential elements (Zitouni, 2007). The natural sources of radionucleides are cosmic and gamma rays from earth that continuously produce radioactivity in the environment. In addition, radionuclides are, due to planned or accidental discharges, dispersed in environment through atmospheric deposits. Furthermore it has been reported that waste disposal sites are important sources of ^{14}C, ^{36}Cl, ^{99}Tc, ^{129}I, ^{137}Cs, ^{237}Np and their daughters, as well as $^{239,240,242}Pu$ and its daughters (Naito & Smith, 1998). Incidental contamination of the environment, such as incident on Chernobyl nuclear power plant, can significantly impact the food production.

Availability of inorganic contaminants in food plants from soil depends on many factors, some of which include the soil properties, e.g. pH value, amount of clay, amount and type of organic compound in soil, redox potential, textural class of soil, and the presence of microorganisms. For example, radiocaesium is strongly bound to clay minerals present in soil being unavailable to plants and other organisms (Cornell, 1993; Dumat et al., 1997). By influencing the factors which determine the availability, agricultural practice can affect the available/unavailable ratio of toxic metals and radionuclides.

Ion pumps as a part of cell membranes of root cells utilized by terrestrial plants for the intake of inorganic nutrients from soil are semi selective. Besides the specificity and selectivity of plant transporters, elements of similar chemical properties to plant nutrients can inhibit their uptake by competing in plant root mechanisms. For example, arsenate is absorbed via same transport system naturally used for phosphorous (Mehang et al., 1994) while selenium exploits the same route as sulphur (Mayland et al., 1989; Läuchli, 1993). On oppose to mercury for which the uptake by plants is relatively low despite good availability in soil, cadmium is readily absorbed by roots and at low concentrations it does not influence the root metabolism significantly (US EPA, 1993). Due to this fact cadmium can be transported to aboveground parts and to plant fruits and seeds influencing the safety of edible parts. Except being taken up from the soil and transported within plants, some inorganic contaminants like lead can enter the food chain through above ground parts of food/feed plants contaminated with atmospheric deposits or dust (Chamberlain, 1983; Thornton & Jones, 1984).

Uptake of toxic metals by terrestrial plants is often considered as entering point of many inorganic food contaminants in food chain and thus is the subject of many studies oriented to different metals, concentrations, species, genotypes and translocation rates (Kevrešan & Petrović, 2003; Petrović et al., 1998). Alternatively, inorganic contaminants can enter the food chain from different environmental compartments, for example from fresh water plants that are also able to uptake the toxic metals from rivers and canals (Pajević et al., 2002), or through food animals via feed additives containing dangerous elements like e.g. arsenic. Small, localized incidents occurring quite frequently, for example by consuming the seeds treated with mercuric fungicides (Bakir at al., 1973), can also be considered as entering point of inorganic contaminants into the food chain.

2. Distribution of Inorganic Contaminants in Agricultural Products

In the case when inorganic contaminants are taken up by food plants from soil the main portion of inorganic contaminants remain in root and plant organs that were in direct contact with the soil. On the other hand, depending on the plant type, fruits can be the most important edible parts of plants and thus when considering the contamination of food plants by inorganic contaminants, the focus has to be on the transport of inorganic contaminants to edible parts of plants. Some contaminants such as arsenic are toxic to plants at low concentrations and their accumulation in roots causes plant injury preventing further transport to aboveground parts (Peterson et al., 1981; O'Neill, 1990).

Beside uptake from soil, foliar uptake can also be significant source of plant contamination. For example, it was shown that foliar uptake of ^{134}Cs and its transport to fruits in grapes is dominant process compared to direct deposition (Carini et al., 1996).

Cadmium concentration in plant food can vary widely. In general, the highest concentrations of cadmium are present in roots followed by steams and leaf and the lowest amounts are registered in fruits and seeds (Kevrešan et al., 2004). In this respect oilseeds are exception containing high levels of cadmium and thus being often regulated individually concerning cadmium content.

In food animals one of the most important factors that influence the content of heavy metals in animal products is the life span of the animal. Animals with long life span such as horses, older cattle and game, can accumulate some inorganic contaminants. When exposed to feed contaminated with toxic metals, long-lived animals accumulate metals in blood, bones and meat. The edible organs where the highest concentrations of metals are expected are kidneys and liver (Janković et al., 2008; Sharma et al.,. 1982). Despite the fact that game usually is not a part of regular daily diet it is important to mention that it can be contaminated with lead, cadmium and other contaminants (Janković et al., 2008; Tojagić et al., 2004). Considering toxic metal content meat from intensively produced animals, especially ones with short life span, represents low risk (Pavlović et al., 2001; Janković et al., 2008).

Nitrates and nitrites are utilized regularly as additives in cured meat products. Nitrates in meat react with myoglobin and produce nitrosyl myoglobin which provides desirable color altering lightness and redness of meat products (Bloukas et al., 1999). Microbiological and biochemical processes normally undergoing in meat products convert nitrate into nitrite. Nitrite has a bacteriostatic or growth-inhibiting effects on bacteria, and is particularly effective in inhibiting the spores of *Clostridium botulinum*, hence, preventing the production of its toxin. On the other hand there are serious health concerns about the presence of nitrates in food as they can be metabolized to potentially carcinogenic N-nitroso compounds. Maximum amount of nitrates permitted to be added to meat products is 150 mg/kg resulting in average of 5 to 40 mg/kg of nitrites in the products, wich is usually bellow the maximum permitted amount (50 mg/kg).

3. Mechanisms of Toxicity of Inorganic Contaminants in Human

Inorganic contaminants display a wide variability in their toxicological profile and in the mechanisms of their toxicity. Arsenic toxicity, for example, is different for organic and inorganic compounds. Inorganic arsenic (As(III) and As(IV)) is considered to be more hazardous to human health, although organic arsenic is more frequently present in food, mainly in seafood, and is readily absorbed by human body. On contrary to arsenic, mercury is considered to be more toxic for humans in its organic form, most dangerous of which is methyl mercury (von Burg & Greenwood, 1991). Due to low uptake and transport of mercury to above-ground parts of food plants the main risk of mercury entrance into the food chain arises from the seafood (Hapke, 1991). Absorption of mercury by humans depends predominantly on its chemical properties. Organic mercury compounds, particularly methyl-mercury are due to their high bioavailability almost completely absorbed from the food, thus being more toxic than inorganic mercury compounds. Upon absorption of methyl-mercury it reaches its target bodily system, i.e. central nervous system. Elemental mercury is not absorbed well in intestines, while mercury vapors are efficiently and rapidly absorbed through lungs. Some inorganic compounds of mercury are more toxic than elemental mercury. In human body mercury exhibits the properties of cumulative poison. Absorbed inorganic mercury is deposited in kidneys causing severe kidney damage and failure (Reilly, 2007).

Dietary cadmium is relatively poorly absorbed and only 6% of the element taken by food enters the systematic circulation (Reilly, 2007). Initially absorbed cadmium causes nausea, vomiting and stomach cramp. Long-term exposure to cadmium can cause irreversible kidney damage affecting the renal tubular functions. In extreme cases cadmium toxicity leads to osteomalacia and bone fractures (Itai Itai disease) (McLaughlin et al., 1999; Friberg et al., 1986; Fox, 1988; Nordberg, 1996).

Acute dietary lead poisoning is very rear and easily recognized by the group of symptoms including general weakness, malaise and gastrointestinal problems (Rossi et al., 1990). Poisoning with lead affects many systems in human body, but main target of lead is the bone marrow affecting the hemoglobin synthesis (Pagliuca et al., 1990). Chronic, low-level lead poisoning is not easily recognized because of non characteristic symptoms such as tiredness and mild anemia. Chronic, low level poisoning of children with lead interferes their neurophysiological development (Pocock et al., 1994).

Soluble forms of fluoride are almost completely absorbed in gastrointestinal tract. Only 50% of absorbed fluoride is eliminated through healthy kidneys (Ekstrand et al., 1977). Fluoride present in blood tends to deposit in bones more rapidly in children then in adults (Heifetz & Horowitz, 1986). In stomach fluorides react with gastric acid and produce hydrofluoric acid, causing vomiting, diarrhea, abdominal pains, cardiac arrhythmias and tetanic contractures due to hypocalcaemia (McIvor, 1987, 1990).

4. Management of Inorganic Contaminants

Exposure assessment is one of the key parts of the process of risk assessment to inorganic contaminants. Only intake of toxicologically significant amounts can lead to adverse health effects. As stated by Kroes et al. (2002) exposure assessment to contaminants from food should besides estimating the consumption patterns of certain foodstuffs include the quantitative determination and evaluation of contaminants in individual foods and diets, including their fate during food processing in different stages of food production. Incorporating Hazard Analysis Critical Control Points (HACCP) allows the assessment of the risk and estimation of hazards severity, which may be associated with the used raw materials, their processing and the distribution system. HACCP plans ensure that product safety is sustainable (Baker, 1995). According to Notermans et al. (1995) an important aspect of the hazard analysis critical control point (HACCP) system is the specification of criteria with setting the critical limits which ensure that the activities at a specified critical control point (CCP) are under control.

Due to ever-improving analytical capabilities, very low levels of unexpected chemicals including toxic elements can now be detected in foods although these may be toxicologically insignificant (Felter et al., 2009). Certain limitations of the risk assessment approaches currently used to establish the pathway and frequency of food contamination can lead to uncertainties which can either cause an over- or underestimation of real intakes (Kroes et al., 2002). As claimed by Marvin et al. (2009) there is a need for early identification of emerging food safety issues in order to prevent them from developing into health risks. Various methods and procedures which can be used for early identification of safety issues including the monitoring of the occurrence of specific hazards within the food supply, or the incidences of food-borne diseases, as well as the combination of these data with other data or with expert opinions, enable pro-active operating by pre-defining indicators for hazards and follow-up measures based on HACCP principles.

The assessment of food production chain concerning the risk management and critical control points for inorganic contaminants including heavy metals (As, Pb, Hg and Cd) and send and stone traces, has been presented by Mastilović et al. (2009a, 2009b). The main conclusion concerning chemically incorporated inorganic contamination, graphically presented by Figure 1, is that there are no procedures or processing operations for the removal of these risks from the product once they have been brought into the production chain either in the form of contaminated agricultural products, additional raw materials, additives, and packaging materials, or as the contamination from equipment or used chemicals. Risk management of possible contamination sources in agricultural production and processing on one side, and prevention of entering of contamination into the food production chain on the other side, anticipates the definition of the critical control points wherever significant quantities of new materials are introduced into the food production chain. Food processing procedures result in dilution of contaminant concentration, when contaminated ingredient is only part of the final product (e.g. wheat germ as ingredient of fine bakery products), or its concentration, when the most contaminated part of starting raw material becomes the final product.

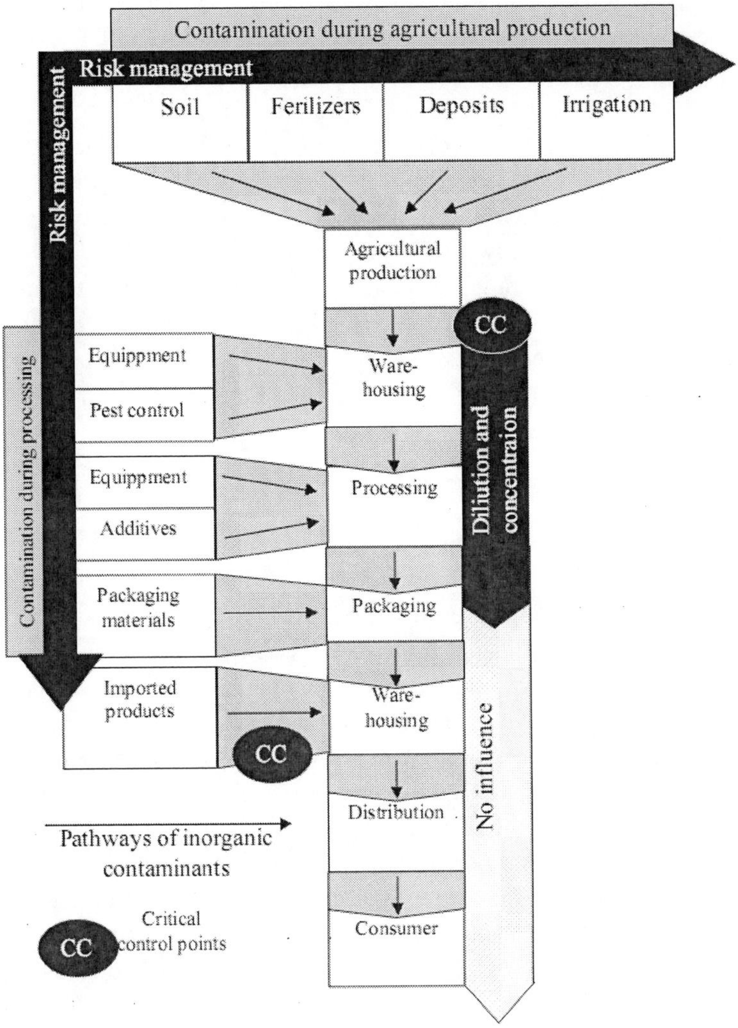

Figure 1. Possible entering points of inorganic contaminants into the food and their control points (Mastilović et al., 2009).

5. Determination of Inorganic Contaminants in Food

The first step in the determination of inorganic contaminants in food is adequate sample preparation. Except for liquid matrices, this step generally involves the elimination of organic matter by dry or wet ashing procedure or extraction of the analyte from food. Slurries, oils and crystals are suitable substrates for extraction procedures but in general, for the determination of inorganic contaminants in food ashing procedure is used. Advantages of dry ashing procedure are simplicity and the possibility of having large samples, up to 25 g (Zhang et al., 2000). Main disadvantage of ashing procedure is the possibility of loss of volatile analytes due to the high temperatures implied in the preparation process. Wet ashing, especially in closed vessel, overcomes the problem of analyte loss but limits the weight of the sample.

Upon digestion inorganic contaminants in foodstuffs are detected by AAS (flame AAS, cold vapor generation, hydride generation or electro thermal AAS), ICP (AES or MS), or by implying spectrophotometric or electroanalytical methods, neutron activation analysis and recently, atomic fluorescence spectrometry (Montoro & Vèlez, 2004)

Some modifications on analytical instruments allow introduction of unprepared (undigested) food samples. Obvious advantage of direct sample analysis is the avoidance of risk caused by sample preparation but disadvantages are small sample size, micro-weighing, sample homogeneity and necessity of instrument calibration. Instrumental determination of cadmium has been done using tungsten boat furnace sample cuvette technique to generate cadmium vapor, which was quantified by ICP-MS (Okamoto, 1999) and electrothermal atomic absorption (Dakuzaku et al., 2001).

Conclusion

Inorganic contaminants are present in environment naturally or are introduced as a consequence of human activity, representing a threat to human health by contaminating food products. There are many entering points of inorganic contaminants into the food chain. Absorption of inorganic contaminants from soil through plant roots is considered to be the most important entering point. Inorganic contaminants enter the human diet through contaminated food plants or are introduced in meat and meat products by contaminated feed.

Step forward in food safety management was made by introducing the Hazard Analysis and Critical Control Points (HACCP) system which enables prevention of entrance and spreading of contaminants in the food chain, especially important from the aspect of inorganic chemical contamination which, on oppose to easily removable physical contamination, cannot be eliminated once it has appeared in the food chain. Development of analytical capabilities for detecting of extremely low concentrations of inorganic contaminants contributes to the reduction of risk that inorganic contamination carries for human health and overall food safety.

References

Alloway, B.J. Cadmium. In: Alloway, B.J. (Ed.), *Heavy Metals in Soils*. Glasgow: Blackie and Son, 1990; 100-121.

Andersson, A. Mercury in Soil. In: Nriagu, J.O., (Ed.), *The Biogeochemistry of Mercury in the Environment*, Amsterdam: Elsevier; 1979; 79-102.

Asami, T. Cadmium pollution of soils and human health in Japan, in: Låg, J., (Ed.), *Human and Animal Health in Relation to Circulation Processes of Selenium and Cadmium*, Oslo: Norwegian Academy of Science and Letters, 1991, 115-125.

Baker D. A. Application of modelling in HACCP plan development. *International Journal of Food Microbiology*, 1995, 25, 251-261.

Bakir, F.; Damluji, S.; Amin-Zaki, L.; Murtadha, L.; Khalidi, A.; AlRawi, N.; Tikriti, S.; Dhakhir, H.; Clarkson, T.W.; Smith, J.; Doherty, R. Methylmercury poisoning in Iraq. An Interuniversity Report. *Science*, 1973, 181, 230-241.

Bloukas, J. G.; Arvanitoyannis, I. S.; Siopi, A. A. Effect of natural colourants and nitrites on colour attributes of frankfurters. *Meat Science*, 1999, 52, 257-265.

Carini,F.; Anguissola Scotti, I.; Montruccoli, M.; Silva S. ^{134}Cs foliar contamination of vine: translocation to grapes and transfer to wine, in: *Proceedings of the International Symposium on Radioecology Ten Years Terrestrial Radioecological Research following the Chernobyl Accident*. Vienna: Austrian Soil Science Society and Federal Environment Agency; 1996; 163-169.

Cartwright, B.C.; Merry, R.H.; Tiller, K.G.. Heavy metal contamination of soils around a lead smelter at Port Pirie, South Australia. *Australian Journal of Soil Research*, 1977, 15, 69-81.

Chappel, W.R.; Abernathy, C.O.; Cothern, C.R.. *Arsenic Exposure and Health*. Northwood: Science and Technology Letters; 1994

Chen, Y.; Lin, M.; He, Z.; Xie, X.; Liu, Y.; Xiao, Y.; Zhou, J.; Fan, Y.; Xiao, X.; Xu, F. Air pollution-type fluorosis in the region of Pingxyang, Jiangxi, People's Republic of China. *Archives of environmental health*, 1993, 48, 246–249.

Chow, T.J. 1970. Lead accumulation in roadside soil and grass. *Nature* 225, 295-296.

Cook, P.J.; Freney, R.J. Sources of cadmium in agriculture, In: Simpson, J., Curnow, B. (Eds.), *Cadmium Accumulations in Australian Agriculture*. National Symposium, Canberra, 1-2 March 1988, Australian Govt. Publ. Service, Canberra. 1988, 4-19.

Cornell, R.M. Adsoption of caesium on minerals: a review. *Journal of Radioanalytical and Nuclear Chemistry*, 1993, 171, 483-500.

Dakuzaku, C. S.; Freschi, G.P.G.; Moraes, M.de; Nobrega, J. A. ; Gomes Neto, J. A. Direct determination of arsenic in sugar by GFAAS with transversaly heated atomizer and longitudinal Zeemman-effect background correction. *Atomic Spectroscopy*, 2001, 22, 271-275.

Dumat, C.; Cheshire, M.V.; Fraser, A.; Shand, C.; Staunton, S. The effect of removal of soil organic matter and iron on the adsorption of radiocaesium. *European Journal of Soil Science*, 1997, 48, 675-683.

Ekstrand, J.; Alván, G.; Boréus, L. O.; Norlin A. Pharmacokinetics of fluoride in man after single and multiple oral doses. *European journal of clinical pharmacology*, 1977, 12, 311–317.

Felter S.; Lane R.W.; Latulippe M.E.; Llewellyn G.C.; Olin S.S.; Scimeca J.A.; Trautman T.D. Refining the threshold of toxicological concern (TTC) for risk prioritization of trace chemicals in food. *Food and Chemical Toxicology*, 2009, 47, 2236-2245.

Fox, M.R.S. Nutritional factors that may influence bioavailability of cadmium. *Journal of Environmental Quality*, 1988, 17, 175-180.

Friberg, L.; Elinder, C.G.; Kjellstrom, T.; Nordberg, G. Cadmium and Health: *A Toxicological Appraisal. Vol. II. Effects and Response*. Boca Raton, FL, USA: CRC Press, 1986.

Gulson, B.L.; Tiller, K.G.; Mizon, K.J.; Merry, R.H. Use of lead isotopes in soils to identify the source of lead contamination near Adelaide South Australia. *Environmental Science and Technology*, 1981, 15, 691-696.

Hapke, H.J. Metal accumulation in the food chain and load of feed and food. In: Merian, E. (Ed.), *Metals and Their Compounds in the Environment. Occurrence, Analysis and Biological Relevance*. Weinheim: VCH; 1991; 469-479.

Heifetz, S.B.; Horowitz, H.S. The amounts of fluoride in self-administered dental products: safety considerations for children. *Pediatrics*, 1986, 77, 876–882.

Kabata-Pendias, A.; Pendias, H. *Trace Elements in Soils and Plants*, Baton Raton, FL. USA: CRC Press; 1992.

Kevrešan S.; Ćirin-Novta, V.; Kuhajda, K.; Kandrač, J.; Petrović, N.; Grbović, Lj.; Kevrešan, Ž. Alleviation of cadmium toxicity by naphthenate treatment. *Biologia Plantarum*, 2004, 48, 453-455,

Kevrešan, Ž.č Petrović, N. Effect of different cadmium concentrations on cadmium retranslocation into the reproductive organs in pea of different ages. *Central European Journal of Occupational and Environmental Medicine*, 2003, 9, 322-326.

Kleter G.A.; Groot M.J.; Poelman M.; Kok E.J.; Marvin H.J.P. Timely awareness and prevention of emerging chemical and biochemical risks in foods: Proposal for a strategy based on experience with recent cases. *Food and Chemical Toxicology*, 2009, 47, 992-1008.

Kroes R.; Müller D.; Lambe J.; Löwik M. R. H.; Klaveren J.; Kleiner J.; Massey R.; Mayer S.; Urieta I.; Verger P.; Visconti A. Assessment of intake from the diet. *Food and Chemical Toxicology*, 2002, 40, 327-385.

Läuchli, A. Selenium in plants: uptake, functions and environmental toxicity. *Botanica Acta*, 1993,106, 455-468.

Marvin, H.J:P.; Kleter, G.A.; Frewer, L.J.; Cope, S.; Wentholt, M.T.A.; Rowe, G. A working procedure for identifying emerging food safety issues at an early stage: Implications for European and international risk management practices. *Food Control*, 2009, 20, 345-356.

Mastilović, J.; Kevrešan, Ž.; Janić Hajnal, E.; Novaković, A.; Radusin, T. Occurence and risk managment of main toxic elements in food production chain. *Food processing, quality and safety*, 2009, 36, in press.

Mayland, H.F.; James, L.F.; Panter, K.E.; Sonderegger, J.L.. Selenium in seleniferous environments. In: Jacobs, L.W. (Ed.), *Selenium in Agriculture and the Environment*. Madison, WI. USA: Soil Sci. Soc. Am. Spec. Pub. No. 23. ASA, SSSA, 1989; 15-50.

McIvor, M.E. Sudden cardiac death from fluoride intoxication: the role of potassium. *Annals of emergency medicine*, 1987, 16, 777–781.

McIvor, M.E. Acute fluoride toxicity: pathophysiology and management. *Drug safety*, 1990, 5, 79–85.

McLaughlin, M.J.; Parker, D.R.; Clarke, J.M. Metals and micronutrients – food safety issues. *Field Crops Research*, 1999, 60, 143-163.

Meharg, A.A. Integrated tolerance mechanisms: Constitutive and adaptive plant responses to elevated metal concentrations in the environment. *Plant Cell and Environment*, 1994, 17, 989-993.

Merry, R.H.; Tiller, K.G.; Alston, A.M. Accumulation of copper, lead and arsenic in Australian orchard soils. *Australian Journal of Soil Research*, 1983, 21, 549-561.

Montoro, R.; Vélez, D. Detecting metal contamination. In: Watson, D.H. (ed.) *Pesticide, veterinary and other residues in food. Cambridge*, England: CRC Press, Woodhead Publishing; 2004; 610–640.

Naito, M.; Smith G. Revised Sets of Example Assessment Contexts, BIOMASS Theme 1, Task group 3, Note 1, Version 1.0, 1998.

Nordberg, G. Human cadmium exposure in the general environment and related health risks - a review. In: *Sources of Cadmium in the Environment.* Paris: Organisation for Economic Co-Operation and Development; 1996; 94-104.

Notermans, S.; Gallhoff, G.; Zwietering, M.H.; Mead G.C. The HACCP concept: specification of criteria using quantitative risk assessment. *Food Microbiology*, 1995, 12, 81-90.

Okamoto, Y. Furnace-fusion system for the direct determination of cadmium in biological samples by inductively coupled plasma atomic emission spectrometry using tungsten boat furnace–sample cuvette technique. *Journal of Analytical Atomic Spectrometry*, 1999, 14, 1767 – 1770.

Page, A.L.; Bingham, F.T.; Chang, A.C.; Cadmium. In: Lepp, N.W. (Ed.), *Effect of Heavy Metal Pollution on Plants. Vol. 1: Effects of Trace Metals on Plant Function*. London: Applied Science; 1981; 77-109.

Pagliuca, A.; Mufti, G.J.; Baldwin, D.; Lestas, A. N.; Wallis, R. M.; Bellingham, A. J. Lead poisoning: clinical, biochemical and haematological aspects of a recent outbreak, *Journal of Clinical Pathology*, 1990, 43, 277-281.

Pajević, S.; Vučković, M.; Stanković, Ž.; Krstić, B.; Kevrešan, Ž.; Radulović, S. The content of some macronutrients and heavy metals in aquatic macrophytes of three ecosystems connected to the Danube in Yugoslavia. *Archiv für Hydrobiologie. Supplementband: Large rivers*, 2002, 13, 73-83.

Pavlović, A.; Kevrešan, Ž.; Kelemen-Mašić, Đ.; Mandić., A.: Micro and toxic elements in skin meat and gills of grass carp (*Ctenopharyngodon idella*). *Proceedings of the 8th symposium of analitical and environmental problems*, Szeged, Hungary, October 2001, 117-121.

Peterson, P.J.; Benson, L.M.; Zieve, R. Metalloids. In: Lepp, N.W. (Ed.), *Effect of Heavy Metal Pollution on Plants, Vol. 1.* London: Applied Science Publ; 1981; 279-342.

Petrović, N.; Kastori, R.; Sekulić, P.; Kevrešan, Ž. Effect of Cr and Ni on the accumulation and distribution of mineral elements in young sugar beet plants. *Zemljište i biljka*, 1998, 47, 17-29.

Pocock, S.J.; Smith, M.; Baghurst, P. Environmental lead and children's intelligence: a systematic review of epidemiological evidence, *British Medical Journal*, 1994, 309, 1189-1197.

Reilly, C. Pollutants in Food — Metals and Metalloids. in: *Mineral Components in Foods*, Szefer, P.; Nriagu, J.O., (Eds) CRC Press,Taylor Francis Group, London New York, 2007, 363-388.

Rossi, E.; Costin, K.A.; Garcia-Webb, P. Effects of occupational lead exposure lymphocyte enzymes involved in haem biosynthesis, *Clinical Chemistry*, 1990, 36, 1980-1983.

Sharma, R.P.; Street, J.C.; Shupe, J.L. Translocation of lead and cadmium from feed to edible tissues of swine. *Journal of Food Safety*, 1982, 4, 151-163.

Ten Brinka, H.M.; Janssena, A.J.; Slaninaa, J. Plume wash-out near a coal-fired power plant: measurements and model calculations. *Atmospheric environment,* 1988, 22, 177–188.

Tojagić, S.; Kevrešan, Ž.; Jokanović, M.: (in Serbian: Some quality indicators of vineyard snail meat (*Helix pomatia*)) Neki pokazatelji kvaliteta mesa vinogradarskog puža (*Helix pomatia*). *Veterinarski glasnik*, 2004, 58, 157-161.

US EPA, Standards for the use or disposal of sewage sludge; final rules (40 CFR Parts 257, 403 and 503). *Fed. Reg.,* 1993, 58, 9248-9415.

von Burg, R.; Greenwood, M.R.. Mercury. In: Merian, E. (Ed.), *Metals and Their Compounds in the Environment, Occurrence, Analysis and Biological Relevance.* Weinheim: VCH; 1991; 1045-1088.

WHO Chapter 6.5 Fluorides In: *Air Quality Guidelines - Second Edition*, Copenhagen, Denmark: WHO Regional Office for Europe; 2000.

Wickstrom, G., Arsenic emission from the Novaky power station, Work Environ. *Health*, 1982, 9, 2.

Zhang, D.; Li, C.; Yang, L.; Sun, H. Determination of cadmium in flour by atom trapping flame atomic absorption spectrometry using derivative signal processing. *Analytica Chimica Acta*, 2000, 405, 185-190.

Zitouni, OD. Pollutants in Food — Radionuclides. In: Mineral Components in Foods, Szefer. P.; Nriagu, J.O.; (eds.) Taylor Francis Group, London New York: CRC Press; 2007; 389-411.

In: Nutritional Insights and Food Safety
Editor: Jaroslava Švarc-Gajiæ

ISBN: 978-1-61122-130-5

Chapter V

Persistent Organic Pollutants (POPs)

Ernest Vončina
Institute for public health, Prvomajska 1, 2000 Maribor, Slovenia

Abstract

Persistent organic pollutants (POPs) are heterogeneous class of compounds sharing common properties such as long persistency and global transport throughout the environment, adverse effects on humans and biodiversity and bioaccumulation throughout the food chain. Being chemicals of a global concern it is of utmost importance to monitor these chemicals in the environment and foodstuffs, especially in respect to their bioconcentration in food like fish, meat and dairy products. This chapter describes the most important persistent organic pollutants that can be found in food describing the routes of their entrance into environment and effects they produce in humans. In addition, some regulatory aspect and analytical procedures used for their monitoring in food products are presented.

Introduction

Persistent organic pollutants (POPs) encompass different chemical classes of compounds (Table 1) with some common characteristics such as persistency, global transport through the environment and high toxicity to humans and wildlife. The compounds belonging to POPs class were detected in remote areas where their use or production is excluded, indicating that they are able to spread through great distances via air, water flora and fauna severely affecting human health and environment. Some pesticides, like those belonging to organochlorine class (DDT, dieldrin) can also be classified as POPs. Other organochlorine contaminants, which fall into the group of persistent organic pollutants, include chlorinated hydrocarbons such as polychlorinated dibenzo-p-dioxins (PCDDs), polychlorinated dibenzofurans (PCDFs) and dioxin-like polychlorinated biphenyls (PCBs). These are three groups of compounds which are also referred to as dioxin-like compounds. By circulating in the environment for a long time and being highly lipophilic (log Kow >5), POPs can concentrate in the food of animal origin (milk, meat, eggs) reaching high levels and posing a risk to consumers. Concentrations of these compound increase along the food chain reaching concentration factors up to 100 000 (Švarc-Gajić, 2009).

Table 1. Compounds which are for the present classified as POPs

Aldrin	Dieldrin	Mirex	Hexachlorbenzene
Chlordane	Dioxins (PCDD)	Furans (PCDF)	Heptachlor
DDT	Endrin	PCBs	Toxafene

The persistency of organic pollutants in the environment significantly depende on the type of compound, the environmental compartment and environmental conditions. In average half lives of majority of compounds that fall within the group of POPs is the longest in soil and sediments, reaching 6 month, and being shorter in waters (2 month). The compounds are most efficiently degraded under the influence of UV light, thus the half lives are the shortest in air and are about 2 days.

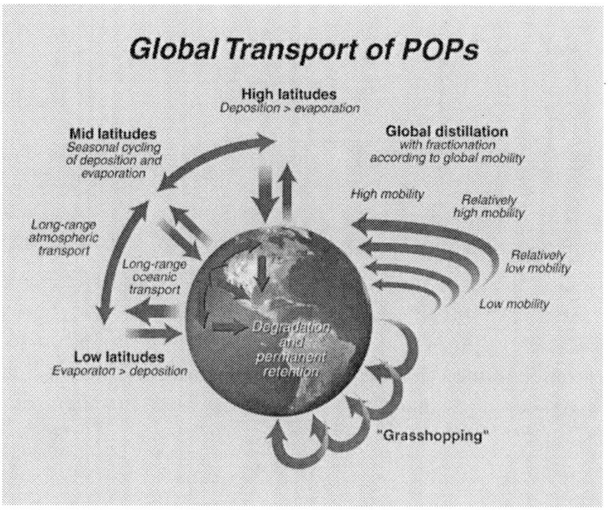

Figure 1. The transport of POPs through environment (courtesy of Stockholm Environment Institute-York).

POPs move around the world by a process called "global transport" (Figure 1). They appear in places where they have never been used or produced because POPs evaporate in regions with warm climate and settle beck down in colder regions. Their vapors travel by air currents of the atmosphere. When the vapors cool, they settle on the land and water. POPs move thousands of miles from the warmer latitudes of the Earth, where they are produced, to the cooler latitudes at the North Pole and South Pole.

Long-term uptake of POPs can have adverse effects in organisms such as carcinogenesis, endocrine disruptions, effects on immune system and negative developmental impacts. Physico-chemical properties of these compounds result in their ability to bioaccumulate and biomagnify in higher trophic organisms. More than 90% of the POP body burden in humans and other mammals is accumulated via food.

1. Polychlorinated Dibenzo-p-Dioxins (PCDD) and Polychlorinated Dibenzofurans (PCDF)

Compounds belonging to this class are chlorinated aromatic ethers where an oxygen atom binds two benzene rings. Usually they are labeled with PCDD/PCDF or in short, dioxins. They contain chlorine homologs with one to eight chlorine atoms and so it is possible for dioxins to obtain 75 positional isomers and for furans 135 positional isomers. Most toxic are compounds with chlorine atom at 2,3,7,8-position. Beside chlorinated dibenzo-p-dioxins and dibenzofurans also mixed bromo-chloro compounds appear because of increasing use of brominated compounds as flame retardants. Structure formula of polychlorinated dibenzo [b,e] [1,4] dioxins or dibenzo-p-dioxins (PCDD) and polychlorinated dibenzofurans (PCDF) and their systematic numbering using IUPAC nomenclature is shown in Figure 2.

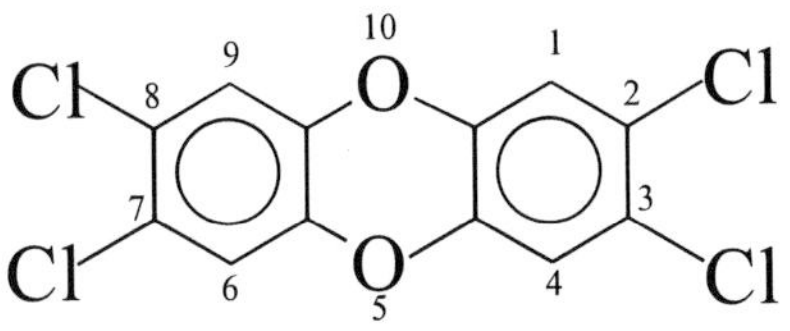

2,3,7,8-TCDD

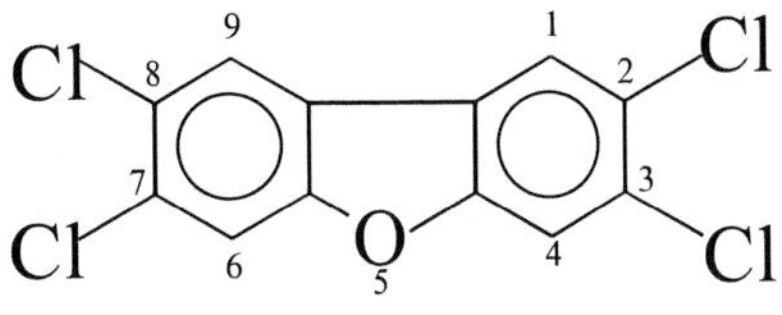

2,3,7,8-TCDF

Figure 2. Structure of tetra halogenated 2,3,7,8-tetrachloro dibenzo-p-dioxin (2,3,7,8-TCDD) and 2,3,7,8-tetrachloro dibenzofuran (2,3,7,8-TCDF) with systematic numbering using IUPAC nomenclature.

1.1. Physical and Chemical Properties

Polychlorinated dibenzodioxins and dibenzofurans, especially most investigated 2,3,7,8-tetrachloro dibenzodioxin (TCDD), are compounds which have many unpleasant properties. It is worth noting that chlorinated dioxins and furans are never target of syntheses and that their intentional use is not known. Usually they are just side products arising during synthesis of other compounds and originating from different thermal processes. They have extremely toxic effects to all live beings. From 210 dioxins and furans seventeen congeners with chlorine atom at position 3,7,8 are extremely toxic. They are extremely persistent and their half lives in soil are from 10 to 12 years. They are poorly soluble in water and they are enough volatile for spreading into environment. Their solubility in water is in the range from several ng/L to several μg/L at 25 °C. These compounds have high biological concentration factors. Being lipophilic compounds their partition coefficients in n-octanol/water are high. Logarithmic values are dependent on number of chlorine atoms and log Kow are ranging from 4.3 to 8.26, depending on the congener. The persistency of dioxins combined with their high lipophilicity make them great candidates for bio-accumulation in living organisms. Bioconcentration factors are very high and range between 100.000 and 300.000. According to number of chlorine atoms in a molecule they are classified into moderately volatile compounds. Their melting points are in the range from 100 °C to 330 °C and boiling points are from 315 °C to

510 ° C. Thermodynamically PCDD/PCDF are very stable compounds. They can be formed in low temperature range between 250 ° C and 300 ° C during thermal processes. At temperatures of incomplete incineration between 300 ° C and 600 ° C dioxins are always found in gases and ash emission from waste incineration. The chemical properties of dioxins and polychlorinated biphenyls with low water solubility, high stability and semi-volatility, favour their long-range transport in the environment, making them detectable in remote areas like in the arctic air, water and organisms.

1.2. Sources Of Dioxins (PCDD/PCDF)

Dioxins are not intentionally produced, but are formed as by-products or impurities of several different industrial processes such as chemical, paper and metal industries. They are also produced by most combustion processes, incineration of municipal and hazardous waste and small scale burning. Fossil energy production, traffic, and their industrial sources both in Central Europe and in the countries around the Baltic Sea also contribute to dioxin emission. Dioxins enter the Baltic Sea as air fallout when transported from land-based sources and via the multitude of waterways. The waterway pollution by dioxins in past could be attributed to a large extent to some chemical and forest industries, where chlorine was used in large amounts for pulp bleaching until the early 1990s.

1.3. Dioxins as Environmental, Food and Feed Pollutants

The main problem with dioxins is their unique chemical stability. Once ingested by living organisms dioxins are stored in the fatty tissues for a long time. Because they accumulate, their concentrations increase as they move up in the food chain. Thus top predators and humans are exposed to the highest levels of contamination. It is not easy to determine the overall pathways of dioxins in the environment. These vary geographically depending on their sources and data are not always available for different areas and species.

Nowadays dissemination of PCDD/F in the environment is designated almost entirely to anthropogenic sources. Exceptions are possible and natural thermal processes like wood and grass fires and volcanoes eruptions also contribute to dioxins emission in the environment. Something still holds: „Dioxins are present from the time when the use of fire was discovered". Formation of PCDD/PCDF on fly ash in temperature range of 250-400 ° C after burning zone of furnace represent the main part of all dioxin emissions from municipal and dangerous waste burning facilities.

2. Polychlorinated Biphenyls (PCBs)

The polychlorinated biphenyls (PCBs) are a group of chemical substances which can contain chlorine, namely from 1-10 chlorine atoms per molecule. There are 209 substances of this kind. PCBs with different number of chlorine atoms are called "congeners", and with the same chlorine content but at different positions, "isomers". The industrial production of PCBs started in 1929 and reached a maximum in the year 1970. PCBs are no longer manufactured in Europe and in the US. The industrially produced PCB mixtures are colourless liquids. Viscosity, chemical stability and lipophilicity are practically the same as for dioxins. The PCBs are very persistent in the environment and are associated with the organic components of soils, marine sediments and biological tissues, in which they accumulate and then enter the food chain. They are distributed in the environment due to long range atmospheric transport and have been detected in the fatty tissues of animals and humans even in remote areas.

3. Principle of Toxic Equivalency Factors (TEF)

Reported dioxin measurements are difficult to compare because different methods might be used. The quantities reported are also presented in different ways (by dry weight, wet weight, lipid weight etc.) and cannot be readily compared. Furthermore, dioxins are a mixture of different compounds (congeners) with varying levels of toxicity.

International principle of Toxic Equivalency Factors (TEF) was developed and accepted with the main goal to asses the possibility for determination of toxicity and risk assessment for different persistent organic compounds. Using TEF principle the international comparison of different studies of dioxins, PCBs, polychlorinated naphtalenes and other POPs can be achieved. The concept of Toxic Equivalency Factors is based on the fact that dioxin like compounds has common principle of acting, namely by bonding to »Ah-receptor«. This is receptor in mammals for bonding compounds of planar aromatic hydrocarbons. To 29 planar aromatic hydrocarbons significant toxicity was assigned by World Health Organization (WHO) (Van den Berg et al., 1998). The toxicity of compounds was evaluated in comparison to dioxin congener 2,3,7,8-TCDD on the basis of their toxicological data. TEF was determined for every compound in respect to 2,3,7,8-tetrachlorodibenzodioxin, which has TEF value 1 (Table 2). By multiplying Toxic Equivalency Factors of individual compounds with their concentrations toxic equivalents (TEQ) can be calculated which can be used for risk assessment, for calculation of Tolerable Daily Intake (TDI), for international comparison etc.

Table. 2. Toxic Equivalency Factors (TEFs) for PCDDs, PCDFs and dioxin-like PCBs for humans and mammals

Compound	WHO-TEF	Compound	WHO-TEF
2378-TCDD	1	Non-ortho PCBs	
12378-PeCDD	1	PCB 77	0. 0001
123478-HxCDD	0.1	PCB 81	0. 0001
123678-HxCDD	0.1	PCB 126	0. 1
123789-HxCDD	0.1	PCB 169	0. 01
1234678-HpCDD	0.01		
OCDD	0.0001	Mono-ortho PCBs	
		PCB 105	0. 0001
2378-TCDF	0.1	PCB 114	0. 0005
12378-PeCDF	0.05	PCB 118	0. 0001
23478-PeCDF	0.5	PCB 123	0. 0001
123478-HxCDF	0.1	PCB 156	0. 0005

Table. 2. (Continued)

Compound	WHO-TEF	Compound	WHO-TEF
123678-HxCDF	0.1	PCB 157	0.0005
234678-HxCDF	0.1	PCB 167	0.00001
123789-HxCDF	0.1	PCB 189	0.0001
1234678-HpCDF	0.01		
1234789-HpCDF	0.01		
OCDF	0.0001		

According to planar structure only few from 209 possible PCBs are chemically related to planar PCDD/PCDF. They are named "dioxin like PCBs", as they have the same toxic properties and they are acting in the same way as dioxins. Also their toxicity and biological activity are affected by the number and position of the chlorine atoms, as substitution in the ortho position hinders the rotation of the rings. PCBs without ortho substitution are generally referred to as coplanar and all others as non-coplanar. Coplanar PCBs can bind to the Ah receptors and may exert additional effects, which are not observed with non-coplanar PCBs.

For PCDD/Fs and PCBs, Toxic equivalency (TEQ) calculations were carried out using the WHO-98 toxicity equivalency factors (TEF). It was assumed that non-detected isomer concentrations would be equal to one half of the respective limit of detection (LOD) (ND = ½ LOD) (EC No 1883/2006).

4. The Toxicity of Persistent Organic Pollutants

The toxicity of persistent organic pollutants (POPs) is well known and it is also known that dietary intake is the major route of human exposure to most POPs. In recent years, concern on dietary intake of POPs and other organic environmental contaminants has much increased. Dietary intake of these pollutants is of special interest in children, who in relation to their body weights consume greater quantities of food than adults. From the toxicological point of view it is clearly evident that there is a difference in longevity of nonpersistent and persistent chemicals in the human body (Barr et al., 2005).

Nonpersistent chemicals pass quickly through body after their absorption, distribution and metabolism. On contrary it is evident that persistent chemicals like dioxins and PCBs metabolize and eliminate very slowly and compounds are well distributed among tissues. Their concentrations in tissue are in equilibrium with blood concentrations.

4.1. Effects in Humans

Acute dioxin exposures in humans may result in severe skin lesions, altered liver function and lipid metabolism, general weakness associated with drastic weight loss, depression of the immune system and endocrine and nervous system abnormalities. Long term exposure leads to increased dioxin levels in fatty tissues and may have adverse developmental effects in children. Furthermore prolonged exposure to this chemical increase the incidence of carcinogenesis and other diseases. Dioxins have attracted national and international attention and are the focus of many international conventions and agreements on persistent organic pollutants, which call for prohibitions on their use, and the prevention or limitation of emissions.

A studies of dioxin blood serum levels of residents of some regions in US revealed that the TEQ values are increasing through the whole life as a result of the concentration of quantities resulting from previous manufacturing operations and waste menagement practices (Patterson et al. 2004). Monitoring programme of POPs among different European countries through their content in human milk revealed that concentrations of different POPs are decreasing, but that the content of polybrominated diphenylethers are increasing exponentially in human milk (Lunden et al. 1998, Noren et al. 2000). In general, due to strict legislation aimed to protect the environment, the concentrations of POPs are lowering in food and feed.

4.2. Human Intake

About 90% of the human intake of dioxins comes from fatty food including fish. The most significant food sources of dioxins and dioxin like PCBs are dairy products, fresh water fish and milk, followed by meat, marine fish and eggs. The dioxins in food originate from background pollution of the natural food and the fodder the animals consume, but isolated point sources may also play a role in food contamination. The potential dangers to human health relate to the carcinogenic risk and other harmful effects (skin lesions and dark spots on the skin), which can be produced once exposure exceeds a certain threshold. Neuro behavioral effects and immune-system deficiencies can even be seen at markedly lower levels of exposure.

Measures to restrict human exposure to dioxins through food intake have been taken at international level. The United States with 90 other countries and the European Community signed the treaty, known as the Stockholm Convention, in 2001 and agreed to reduce or eliminate the production, use, and/or release of 12 key POPs. The EU has set limits for the maximum dioxin content of various types of food. The tolerable weekly intake (TWI) of 14 pg TEQ/kg/week was recommended.

In 1998, the WHO proposed a Tolerable Daily Intake for dioxins and "dioxin-like" compounds in the range of 1-4 pg WHO-TEQ/kg body weight/day. The non-carcinogenic risks derived from exposure to PCDD/Fs and "dioxin-like" PCBs trough the diet was calculated by dividing the total daily intake by the WHO-TDI. Estimated risk for children resulted in a range of 2.0-7.9 pg WHO-TEQ/kg body weight/day, a range significantly higher than that obtained for adults (0.3-1.4 pg WHO-TEQ/kg body weight/day), which in turn is within the WHO-TDI. For potential carcinogenic effects, risk is expressed as the probability of suffering cancer over the lifetime.

5. Regulations and Actions Designed to Decrease POPs Levels

The Stockholm Convention is an essential tool which meets challenges and is used to create and maintain a POPs-free future worldwide. In 1995, the Governing Council of the United Nations Environment Programme (UNEP) called for global action to be taken on POPs, which are defined as "chemical substances that persist in the environment, bio-accumulate through the food web, and pose a risk of causing adverse effects to human health and the environment". Following this, the Intergovernmental Forum on Chemical Safety (IFCS) and the International Programme on Chemical Safety (IPCS) prepared an assessment of the 12 worst offenders, known as the dirty dozen. The negotiations for the Convention were completed on 23 May 2001 in Stockholm. The convention entered into force on 17 May 2004 with ratification by an initial 128 parties and 151 signatories.

The European Union has adopted several Directives which deal with polluting sectors and sources as well as a comprehensive legislative framework regulating chemicals and products. One key element in the EU policy is the "Communication on a Community Strategy for Dioxins, Furans and Polychlorinated Biphenyls" adopted by the European Commission in 2001. The strategy entails an integrated and systematic approach to reduce the presence of these substances in the environment and the identification of short, medium, and long term actions, particularly with regard to establishing maximum limits in food and fodder. The European Commission is committed to protect both human and animal health and welfare, which can be affected by the presence of residues and contaminants in food and feed.

For many residues (pesticides, veterinary drugs) and contaminants (e.g. dioxins, PCBs, PAHs, heavy metals, mycotoxins, processing contaminants) in food and/or feed, legislation has been established in which maximum limits (MRLs) have been set. European legislation commits the Member States to enforce compliance of food and feed with MRLs. Therefore, national monitoring and control plans, and EU coordinated monitoring programs have been established. As part of these programs, samples are taken at various stages in the food chain and analyzed in laboratories. To ensure the quality and comparability of the data generated by laboratories involved in the official monitoring and surveillance, a hierarchically structured system of Community Reference Laboratories (CRLs), National Reference Laboratories (NRLs) and Official Field Laboratories (OFLs) has been established. The concept of the European Union Reference Laboratories (EU-RLs) and National Reference Laboratories (NRLs) is laid down in the Regulation (EC) No. 882/2004 of the European Parliament and of the Council. The overall objective of the CRLs and NRLs is to improve the quality, accuracy and comparability of the results at the official control laboratories.

According to Regulation (EC) No. 882/2004 the EU-Reference Laboratories are responsible for:

- Providing NRLs with details of the analytical methods, including reference methods
- Organization of proficiency tests for NRLs
- Development and validation of new analytical methods
- Coordinating practical arrangements needed to apply new analytical methods and to inform NRLs on advances in this field
- Organization of workshops and training of laboratories in the Member States

- Performing analyses in case of disagreement between Member States
- Providing scientific and technical assistance to the Commission
- Providing the Commission with a work programme and an annual activity report
- Assisting NRLs of third countries

Quality control (QC) and quality assurance (QA) are important factors in sampling and analysis. Any method performance must be verified through control tables where optimal operational ranges are defined, and the periodical analysis of certified reference materials, own laboratory reference materials, and blind or divided samples should be included in routine QA/QC. The inter-calibration exercises are an essential component in quality assurance of the results and are deemed indispensable in the implementation of a regional laboratory network. A recommendation would be that at least once a year such an intercalibration study is performed for each matrix and persistent organic pollutant of interest in accredited laboratories.

The European Union Reference Laboratory for Dioxins and PCBs in Feed and Food is located at the CVUA Freiburg, Germany. The services of the CRL is available to National Reference Laboratories (NRLs) within the EU-Member States.

6. Analytical Methods for Determining POPs

Modern instruments of high resolution gas chrommatography hyphenated to high resolution mass spectrometry (HRGC/ HRMS) can test food samples for the presence of dioxins and other POPs in the low femtogram range. Even difficult sample types with heavy matrix effects can be successfully analyzed. The high-resolution gas chromatography and high-resolution mass spectrometry method, which is capable of increased levels of sensitivity, selectivity, detection and long-term robustness, has been recognized as the most effective analytical technique for this application. The EPA as well as many European regulatory bodies require the use of the HRGC/HRMS method as an obligatory standard method for determination of PCDD/PCDF, PCBs and other POPs with TEFs quantification. Solely isotope dilution HRMS is recommended. Using HRGC/HRMS, the system delivers confirmatory analyses that ensure compliance with worldwide regulations, making it an ideal test method to ensure that public health is safeguarded from the threat of dioxin contamination.

Among numerous methods for determination of different POPs two methods are most important, namely EPA Method 1613 and Method 1668.

EPA Method 1613, Revision B: Tetra- through Octa-Chlorinated Dioxins and Furans by Isotope Dilution HRGC/HRMS. Method is assigned for determination of PCDD/PCDF and PCBs in biological samples like tissues, serum or plasma, human milk and also in food with high fat content. The food samples designated by the method include vegetables with high oil content and food of animal origin (animal tissues, milk and milk products eggs, etc.) The GC/MS portions of this method are to be performed only by analysts experienced with HRGC/HRMS or under the close supervision of such qualified persons. Each laboratory that uses this method must demonstrate the ability to generate acceptable results. This method is "performance-based." The laboratory is permitted to modify the method in order to improve performance or to overcome interferences, improve the sensitivity, accuracy or precision of the results; provided that all performance criteria defined by the EPA method are met.

EPA Method 1668, Revision A: This method is intended for the determination of 12 polychlorinated biphenyls (PCBs) designated as toxic by the World Health Organization (WHO) and the remaining 197 PCBs, approximately 125 of which are resolved adequately on an SPB-octyl gas chromatographic column to be determined as individual congeners. The remaining approximately 70 congeners are determined as mixtures of isomers (co-elutions). The 12 PCBs designated as toxic by WHO (toxic, also known as dioxin-like PCBs; DL-PCBs) are determined by the isotope dilution quantitation technique. The remaining congeners are determined by the internal standard quantitation technique. The detection limits and quantitation levels in this method are usually dependent on the level of interferences and laboratory background levels rather than instrumental limitations. This method is "performance-based." The laboratory is permitted to modify the method in order to improve performance or to overcome interferences, to improve the sensitivity, accuracy or precision of the results; provided that all performance criteria defined by the EPA method are met.

Prior analyzing real sample the capabilities of HRGC/HRMS instruments in the analysis of dirty matrix samples must be tested. This test is performed by setting the mass spectrometer in the multiple ion detection (MID) mode at a resolution of 10,000 (10% valley definition). FC43 is used as a reference compound to provide the inherent lock and calibration masses. These reference masses are monitored scan to scan to ensure the highest mass precision, stability, and ruggedness necessary for routine target compound analysis on an HRMS. For all native dioxin congeners, as well as for their specific 13C labeled internal standards, one quantification mass and one ratio mass are implemented in the MID setup.

Analysis of blank sample of corresponding reference matrix performed through whole analytical procedure should confirm that there is no contamination. Blank test of corresponding reference matrix through the whole analytical procedure should show that throughout analytical procedure contamination is avoided and that concentration levels of blank samples are low enough and can permit determination at LOQ level. Interferences in gas chromatographic analysis can originate from solvents, reagents, glassware or organic compounds present in extract. Every compound which causes response on detector at retention time of determined compound is source of interference. Critical parameters are concentration levels of PCBs, especially owing to worldwide spreading of these compounds in the environment.

6.1. Sample Preparation

Sophisticated chromatographic techniques used in determination of dioxins and dioxin-like food contaminants require thorough purification of food extracts. For cleaning samples different techniques can be used: re-extraction using acids/bases, size exclusion chromatography (SEC), adsorption column chromatography using aluminium oxide or silica gel (neutral, acid or alkaline), Florisil or activated carbon as well as preparative HPLC. SEC is used for elimination of interferences with high molecular mass, which could damage GC columns and cause interferences during mass spectrometric scanning. Acid, neutral and alkaline silica gel, aluminium oxide, and Florisil can be used for elimination of non polar and polar interferences. Aluminium oxide and Florisil are used for elimination of chlorinated diphenylethers, which are the main interfering compounds during analysis. Carbon distributed on diatomeic earth, such as Celit, or directly Carbopack C, can be used for elimination of non polar interferences. Separation is performed according to planarity of substances. Planar compounds like dioxins and dioxin like PCBs are strongly retained on carbon column.

References

Approval of EPA Method 1613 for Analysis of Dioxins and Furans in Wastewater. Available from http://www.epa.gov/waterscience/methods/method/dioxins/1613-fs.html#method 1613.

Barr, DB; Wang, R; Needham, LL. Biologic Monitoring of exposure to environmental chemicals through the life stage: Requirements and issues for consideration for the National Children's study. *Environ. Health Perspect* 2005, 113(8), 1083-1091.

Berg, van den M; Birnbaum, L.; Bosveld, A.T.C.; Brunstrom, B.; Cook, P.; Feeley, M.; Giesy, J.P.; Hanberg, A.; Hasegawa, R.; Kennedy, S.W.; Kubiak, T.; Larsen, J.C.; Leeuwen, van F.X.R.; Liem, A.K.D.; Nolt, C.; Peterson, R.E.; Poellinger, L.; Safe, S.; Schrenk, D.; Tillitt, D.; Tysklind, M.; Younes, M.; Waern, F.; Zacharewski, T. Toxic equivalency factors (TEFs) for PCBs, PCDDs, PCDFs for humans and wildlife. *Environ. Health Perspect*, 1998, 106(12), 775-792.

Commission decision No 2006/130/EC of 10 February 2006 amending Decision 98/536/EC establishing the list of National Reference laboratories for the detection of residues (notified under document number C(2006) 330.

Commission regulation (EC) No 776/2006 of 23 May 2006 amending Annex VII to Regulation (EC) No 882/2004 of the European Parliament and of the Council as regards Community Reference Laboratories.

Council Directive 96/23/EC of 29 April 1996 on measures to monitor certain substances and residues thereof in live animals and animal products and repealing Directives 85/358/EEC and 86/469/EEC and Decisions 89/187/EEC and 91/664/EEC, *Official Journal L* 125 , 23/05/1996 P. 0010 – 0032

Decision 2002/657/EC, Performance criteria, other requirements and procedures for analytical methods.

Dioxin exposure and health. Available at http://ec.europa.eu/environment/dioxin/index.htm.

Environmental Protection Agency, Office of Water, Method 1613 (Revision B): Tetra- through Octa-Chlorinated Dioxins and Furans by Isotope Dilution HRGC/HRMS.

Environmental Protection Agency, Office of Water, Method 1668 (Revision A): Chlorinated Biphenyl Congeners in Water, Soil, Sediment, and Tissue by HRGC/HRMS. Available at http://chm.pops.int/Portals/0/docs/publications/sc_factsheet_001.pdf

EPA. 2,3,7,8-Tetrachlorodibenzo-p-Dioxin (2,3,7,8,-TCDD). Available from http://www.epa.gov/ttn/atw/hlthef/dioxin.html.

European Union Reference Laboratory for Dioxins and PCBs in Feed and Food. Dioxins and PCBs. Available from http://www.crl-freiburg.eu/dioxin/functions.html.

http://europa.eu.int/comm/environment/dioxin/index.htmwww.helcom.fi4

http://europa.eu.int/comm/food/food/chemicalsafety/contaminants/dioxins_en.htmDG

Linhardt, DL; Recalculation of u.s. background dioxin blood serum levels significance to tittabawassee river residents. 2005. Available from http://www.trwnews.net/Documents/Dioxin/ld_recalc_bkdgrnd_levels.pdf.

Lunden A, Noren K. Polychlorinated naphthalenes and other organochloride contaminants in Swedish human milk. *Archives of Environmental Contamination and Toxicology*, 1998, 34, 414–423.

Needham, LL. The Exposure - Effect Continuum: Emphasis on Biomonitoring. 2006. Available from www.isesweb.org/About/Docs/WesolowskiPresentation-Needham_2006.ppt.

Noren K, Meironyte D. Certain organochlorine and organobromine contaminants on Swedish human milk in perspective of past 20–30 years. *Chemosphere,* 2000, 40, 1111–1123.

Patterson, DG; Canady, R; Wong, LY; Lee, R; Turner, W; Caudill, S; Needham, L; Henderson, A. Age Specific Dioxin TEQ Reference Range, *Organohalogen Compounds,* 2004, Vol 66, 2878-2883.

Regulation (EC) No 1883/2006 of the European parliament and of the council of 19 December 2006, Laying down methods of sampling and analysis for the official control of levels of dioxins and dioxin-like PCBs in certain foodstuffs, *Official Journal of the European Union L* 364/32, 20.12.2006.

Regulation (EC) No 882/2004 of the European parliament and of the council of 29 April 2004 on official controls performed to ensure the verification of compliance with feed and food law, animal health and animal welfare rules, *Official Journal of the European Union L* 191, 28.5.2004, P 01-52.

Stockholm Convention on Persistent Organic Pollutants 2001. Available from http://chm.pops.int/Countries/StatusofRatification/tabid/252/language/en-US/Default Aspx

Švarc-Gajić, J. General Toxicology, Nova Science Publishers: New York, 2009.

In: Nutritional Insights and Food Safety
Editor: Jaroslava Švarc-Gajiæ
ISBN: 978-1-61122-130-5

Chapter VI

Pesticides

Tijana Zeremski Škorić, Petar Sekulić and Jordana Ninkov
Institute of Field and Vegetable Crops, Maksima Gorkog 30, 21 000 Novi Sad, Serbia

Abstract

Pesticides are an integral part of agriculture today, but their use can lead to residues in food which have been linked to a wide spectrum of human health hazards. The determination and monitoring of pesticide residues in food has become an increasingly essential requirement for consumers, producers and authorities responsible for food quality control. Maximum residue limits (MRLs) are defined as the upper legal levels of a pesticide residue in or on food or feed which result from agricultural practices.

Very low concentrations fixed as maximum residue limits (MRLs) have fostered the development of powerful sensitive and selective analytical methods to meet the requirements for analyzing pesticide residues in food samples. Fresh fruit and vegetables are an important part of a healthy diet, as they are a significant source of vitamins and minerals. But because fruits and vegetables are consumed raw or semi-processed, they are expected to contain higher pesticide residue levels than other food groups like milk or meat. Levels of pesticide residues in fruits and vegetables depend to a great extent on the method of growing (conventional, greenhouse or organic production) and the part of the year (season) in which they were produced. Food processing techniques such as washing, peeling, cooking etc. have been found to significantly reduce the pesticide residues in fruits and vegetables.

Introduction

The Food and Agriculture Organization of the United Nations (FAO) has defined a pesticide as a substance or mixture of substances intended for preventing, destroying or controlling any pest, including vectors of human or animal diseases, unwanted species of plants or animals causing harm or otherwise interfering with the production, processing, storage, transport, or marketing of food, agricultural commodities, wood and wood products or animal feedstuffs, or substances which may be administered to animals for the control of insects, arachnids or other pests in or on their bodies. Also included in the FAO definition are substances intended for use as plant growth regulators, defoliants, desiccants, or agents for thinning of fruits or preventing the premature fall of fruits, and substances applied to crops either before or after harvest to protect the commodity from deterioration during storage or transport (FAO, 2002).

After the World War II, chemical pesticides have become the most important consciously-applied form of pest management. First-generation pesticides, such as arsenic and hydrogen cyanide, were highly toxic compounds. Their use was largely abandoned, because they were either too ineffective or too toxic. Second-generation pesticides mostly included synthetic organic compounds.

Today, more than 140,000 tonnes of pesticides are used during food and agricultural commodities production in the EU each year. Grapes, citrus fruits and potatoes are the three most intensively pesticide-treated food crops in the EU and all receive over 6 kg/ha of pesticides (EUROSTAT, 2007).

The pesticides currently in use include a wide variety of chemicals with great differences in the mode of action, metabolism and toxicity to humans. Owing to their pest-destroying properties, pesticides are required in worldwide food production, but they inevitably remain present in vegetable and animal food as residues (Harris et al., 2000).

Pesticide residues in foods have been linked to a wide spectrum of human health hazards, ranging from short-term impacts such as headaches and nausea to chronic impacts like cancer, reproductive harm, and endocrine disruption. Chronic health effects may occur years after even minimal exposure to pesticides in the environment. Such effects may also result from pesticide residues ingested through food and water (Barnett, 1997; JMPR, 2004). It is speculated that about 30% of human cancers are caused by low exposure to initiating carcinogenic contaminants in the diet (Tricker & Preussmann, 1990).

1. Major Groups of Conventional Pesticides

There are three major groups of conventional pesticides that are used in agriculture today: organophosphate, chlorinated and carbamate pesticides.

1.1. Organochlorine Pesticides

Organochlorine pesticides have been used extensively in past decades. The first important representative of this group was dichlorodiphenyltrichloroethane, or DDT. DDT was developed in the 1940s and was used as an insecticide against a very wide range of insect pests (ATSDR, 2002), spread of malaria, typhus and other diseases. DDT is a long-lasting, toxic chemical which builds up in the tissues of living organisms (Braune et al., 2005). Gamma-HCH (hexachlorocyclohexane), which is more commonly known as lindane, is the second most important member of the group of chlorinated pesticides (ASTDR 2005).

Due to their toxicity, low biodegradability and great stability, organochlorine pesticides are considered among the most dangerous contaminants in the environment. Organochlorine pesticides are characterized by high lipid solubility and high persistency and hence tend to accumulate in fatty tissue.

The production and use of chlorinated pesticides have been restricted or even banned for some decades in most countries. However, chlorinated pesticides are still widespread in the environment because of their extreme stability and probable indiscriminate use in the past (Concha-Grana et al. 2006; Manirakiza et al. 2002). Some of these pesticides have been included as persistent organic pollutants (POPs) in the Stockholm Convention of 2001 (UNEP, 2006, Ritter et al., 1995), which is a global treaty to protect human health and the environment from these compounds. Dichlorodiphenyltrichloroethane (DDT), hexachlorobenzene (HCB), chlordane and hexachlorocyclohexane (HCH) are all banned organochlorine pesticides.

Exposure to organochlorine pesticides can occur in several ways, but the primary exposure route to people in the developed nations (where organochlorines are no longer used) is through contaminated food. The most commonly contaminated foods typically include oily fish and food of animal origin such as fatty meat and dairy products. Once in the body, organochlorines tend to accumulate in fatty tissues and can remain there for years (Covaci et.al., 2002a, Alawi et al., 1999). During pregnancy, organochlorine residues can be transferred in uterus to the developing fetus via the placental blood supply (Sala et al., 2001). For example, organochlorine pesticides have been found in amniotic fluid, human placentas, fetuses, and maternal and umbilical cord blood (Jaraczewska et al., 2006, Covaci et al., 2002b, Foster et al., 2000, Kanja et al., 1992).

1.2. Organophosphorus Pesticides

Organophosphorus pesticides have been used extensively as insecticides, fungicides and animal pesticides for more than four decades. The most commonly used such pesticides are dichlorvos, dimethoate, malathion, and monocrotophos. Organophosphate pesticides have higher acute toxicities than chlorinated pesticides, but they have an advantage of being more rapidly degraded in the environment. Their toxicological effects are mostly due to the inhibition of acetylcholinesterase in the nervous system, resulting in respiratory, myocardial and neuromuscular transmission impairment (Goh et al., 1990).

1.3. Carbamates

Carbamates and ureas are an important pesticide group. They are used as herbicides (phenylureas, sulfonylureas, phenylcarbamates and alkylthiocarbamates), insecticides (benzoylureas, methylcarbamates and oximethylcarbamates), or fungicides (dithiocarbamates, alkylenebisdithiocarbamates and benzimidazolecarbamates) in different crops for the purposes of controlling weeds, pests, and diseases in agriculture. Some of these pesticides may persist in the soil and water long after their application, so their residues may be found in food produced on contaminated soil or in fish living in contaminated water. For the carbamates, it has been established that they inhibit acetylcholinesterase by carbamylation, resulting in a spectrum of acute cholinergic effects (Pope, 1999). Dithiocarbamates exposure can result in neuropathology, thyroid toxicity and developmental toxicity to the central nervous system of laboratory animals (US EPA, 2001).

2. Pesticide Residues in Fruits and Vegetables

Fresh fruit and vegetables are an important part of a healthy diet, as they are a significant source of vitamins and minerals. According to the World Health Organization (WHO), fruits and vegetables account for an average of 30% of an individual's food consumption by weight and are the most consumed food group (WHO, 2003). Furthermore, because fruits and vegetables are consumed raw or semi-processed, they are expected to contain higher pesticide residue levels than other food groups like milk or meat (USFDA, 2006). It is also important to note that fruit and vegetables are traded worldwide and the list of pesticides that might have been applied in their agricultural production is usually not known which makes residue detection and analysis more complicated (Stan, 2000). Also, fruit and vegetables that are imported from developing countries may contain residues of pesticides which are banned in the USA and EU countries due to their toxicity. For example, in a study performed by Juraske et al. (2009), the herbicide paraquat, which is banned in Switzerland, was found in residual concentrations in bananas and pineapples imported from Brazil and India, where paraquat is not banned (Juraske et al. 2009).

Although most of the organochlorine pesticides have been banned for decades in different parts of the world, their residues still appear as pollutants in food as well as in the environment. Organochlorine pesticides are highly lipophilic compounds, but their presence in carrots, cabbages, potatoes, cucumbers, spinaches, lettuces and other crops has been widely reported in the literature (Lichtenstein, 1959; White, 2001; Schroll & Scheunert, 1992; Mattina et al., 2000; Gonzales et al., 2005). In those studies vegetables were grown in soils treated with the insecticides up to 5-20 years earlier. Organochlorine pesticides were detected in almost all edible tissues but in concentrations below MRLs (Mansour et al. 2009).

In developing countries, due to widespread misuse of pesticides, some of which are banned in the USA and EU because of their toxicity, it is possible that vegetables might contain residues in concentrations sufficient to increase health risks. This has been the case with the insecticide methyl-parathion, the use of which has been banned in the USA and EU. Increased concentrations of this chemical were detected in vegetables produced in Ghana and India (Darko & Akoto, 2008; Bhanti & Taneja, 2007).

Levels of pesticide residues in fruits and vegetables depend in a great extent on the method of growing (conventional, greenhouse or organic production) and the part of the year (season) in which they were produced. Vegetables produced in greenhouses tend to have more residues compared to organically and conventionally grown ones (Mansour et al. 2009). Greenhouse conditions may favor the spread of plant pathogenic diseases and insect pests that require excessive use of pesticides, which in turn are protected from rapid degradation due to lack of direct sunlight. Variations of pesticide residues in vegetables grown in different seasons have been well documented. For instance, low temperatures, short day duration, and rain in the winter season, are reported as factors causing an increase in pesticide residues in vegetables grown in the winter when compared to those grown in the other seasons (Mansour et al. 2009; Bhanti & Taneja 2007).

2.1. Monitoring of Pesticide Residues in Food

The determination of pesticide residues in food has become an increasingly essential requirement for consumers, producers and authorities responsible for food quality control. It is the responsibility of the government authorities to register and set the maximum residue limits (MRLs) to regulate their concentration in foods (Fong et al., 1999). MRLs encourage food safety by restricting the concentration of a permitted residue in a commodity and by limiting the type of commodity in which such residue is allowed. EU Directives established different MRLs that are adapted in each member state for each pesticide within each food group (European Commission, 1991, 2005; Martin-Plaza, 2005). The establishment of MRL is based on good agricultural practice data for food derived from commodities. MRLs are not toxicological limits but must be toxicologically acceptable. Exceeded MRLs are strong indicators of violations of good agricultural practices. If the MRLs are exceeded, comparisons of the exposure with acceptable daily intakes (ADIs) will then indicate whether or not there is a possible chronic or acute health risk, respectively. ADI is defined as the amount of a pesticide, in mg/kg body weight, which can be ingested, on a daily basis, during a lifetime without causing adverse health effects.

Taking into account ADI parameters, it is unlikely that a consumer would be exposed to levels exceeding MRLs of pesticides during all his life. However, the most important problem is to actually determine if there is any risk related to an accidental consumption of a commodity with a level of pesticide residues superior to the MRL. Only a small proportion of pesticides are likely to give rise to acute effects via the food chain, namely some groups of insecticides, a few fungicides and certain herbicides. Although many molluscides and rodenticides have the potential to be acutely toxic, they are unlikely to represent a hazard in food (Mars, 2000; Harris et al., 2000). Similarly, reports of acute clinical poisoning by residues seem to be unusual in comparison with occupational intoxication. Moreover reports of adverse effects following exposure to residues from foods that were treated with pesticides in accordance with respective approval standards are very rare (Nasreddine & Parent-Massin, 2002).

In EU member states, monitoring of pesticide residues in various food commodities has been in place since 1996 and the results have been published in the form of an Annual Report (CEC 2008). In 2007, in accordance with Regulation (EC) No 396/2005, the task of preparing the Annual Report on Pesticide Residues has been transferred to the European Food Safety Authority (EFSA) (EFSA 2009). In 2007, a total of 74,305 samples of about 350 different food commodities were analyzed for pesticide residues. In total, 354 different pesticides were found in measurable quantities in fruit and vegetables, while in cereals residues of 72 different pesticides were observed. 96.01% of the samples analyzed were compliant with the legal Maximum Residue Levels (MRLs). In 3.99% of the samples the legal limits were exceeded for one or more pesticide. Over the years, the percentage of samples with residues above the MRL increased from 3.0% in 1996 to 5.5% in 2002/2003. Since 2003, there has been a decrease, with 3.99% of the samples being non-compliant in 2007. The percentage of samples of fruit, vegetables and cereals with multiple residues has increased over the years from 15.4% in 1997 to 27.7% in 2006. In 2007, the percentage of samples with multiple residues decreased slightly (in 26.2% of the samples two or more pesticide residues were detected). The crops with the highest rates of MRL exceedance were oats (3.8%), peaches (3.4%), strawberries, and lettuce (2.9% each). The crops which contained the most frequently detectable levels of pesticide residues were strawberries, apples, peaches and lettuce (66%, 60.9%, 47.1%, and 44.9%, respectively (EFSA 2009).

In developing countries, however, management and regulation of pesticide use in crop production is often inadequate due to lack of resources, weak import controls, poor storage and stock management, lack of training and education on appropriate pesticide use and widespread misuse of pesticides (Waichman et al., 2007). Due to high demands in farm production and low perception of the toxic effects of pesticide residues in food, some farmers do not wait long enough for the residues to wash off after spraying before harvesting. Increased use of pesticides, therefore, results in the occurrence of residues and metabolites in food commodities (Darko & Akoto, 2008; Bhanti & Taneja, 2007; Mansour et al. 2009). The second very important problem is that some pesticides (e.g. methyl parathion, paraquat and phorate) already banned in the USA and EU countries due to their toxicity and persistence, are still in use in developing countries.

2.2. The Effect of Food Procesing

Food processing techniques such as washing, peeling, cooking etc. have been found to significantly reduce the pesticide residues in fruits and vegetables. Holland et al. (1994) and Kaushik et al. (2009) established that there was reduction of pesticide residue levels due to processing techniques in most of the food materials except where the material was concentrated like in juicing of fruits and pressing or extraction of oil from vegetable seeds. These authors suggested that the effects of food processing on pesticide residue levels may be influenced by the physical location of the pesticide residue as well as by the physico-chemical properties of the pesticide such as solubility, volatility, hydrolytic rate constants, water–octanol partition coefficient and thermal degradation. Other food processing studies provide basic information on the reduced levels of residues in passing from the raw agricultural product to a processed food commodity. A measure for this reduction is the processing factor, which is defined as the residue level in the processed product divided by the residue level in the raw agricultural commodity. The average processing factor established on the basis of several studies (Fernandez-Cruz et al. 2004; Boulard et al. 2005; Chavarri et al. 2005; Caldas et al. 2006; Zhang et al., 2007) is 0.31 for residues in washed products, 0.17 for peeled products, and 0.13 for cooked products.

2.3. Organically Produced Fruit and Vegetables

Chemophobia is the commonest reason for the public to choose organic food assuming that such food is free of synthetic pesticides. Subsequently, this has resulted in an increasing demand for organic production of different varieties of vegetables, fruits, milk products and cereals in many parts of the world. Organic agriculture has developed rapidly during the last decade and governments have encouraged the development of this tillage practice, mainly in developed countries. Organic farms are distinguished from all other forms of farming (including conventional agriculture) by the rejection of soluble minerals as fertilizer and synthetic pesticides in favor of natural ones (Trewavas, 2004). Most organic farms are supposed to remain small and self-sufficient, whereas conventional farms are increasing in size as a result of economic pressures. However, organic food contains pesticide traces, although the amounts are lower than in conventional products (Trewavas, 2004; Gonzales et al., 2005, Mansour et al. 2009). Sometimes the presence of residues in fruits and vegetables may indicate illegal use of pesticides, but in most cases the residues originate from soils used for crop production. For example, Gonzales et al. (2005) reported residues of organochlorine pesticides in organically produced leafy vegetables that were grown in soils treated with insecticides 20 years earlier. The other very important source of pesticide contamination in organic farming is spray drift from neighboring crops. A study on pesticides in cucumber fruits produced under different farming systems (conventional, greenhouse, organic) revealed that more than 50% of the samples contained methamidphos, an insecticide used in cotton production in measurable concentrations but below MRLs.

3. Analytical Methods for Pesticide Residues

Monitoring of pesticide residues in food is one of the most important aspects in minimizing potential hazards to human health. Therefore, periodical monitoring of pesticide residues in food samples is very important to guide the food producers, especially vegetable and fruit growers, on the judicial use of pesticides in the interest of public health. The very low concentrations fixed as MRLs have fostered the development of powerful sensitive and selective analytical methods to meet the requirements for analyzing pesticide residues in food samples. The development of multi-residue methods, which allows proper control of a large number of pesticides in a single analysis, is basically the main strategy applied. However, the different classes and physico-chemical properties of pesticides make the development of methodologies which cover all the analytes under study difficult. Sometimes, different sample treatment methodologies are necessary (Gilbert-Lopez et al., 2009).

The selection of sample preparation methodology is highly dependent on both analyte and sample nature. In relation to the later, sample preparation methods are developed taking into consideration the fat content, where the limit between "fatty" and "non-fatty" food matrices is usually set at 2–5%. Non-fatty foods of plant origin represent the most frequently analyzed samples for pesticide residues. Among this group, special attention is paid to fruits and vegetables that are mostly consumed raw or after minimum postharvest processing. In addition, fruits and vegetables represent the main ingredients in products intended for infants and small children ("baby food") in which pesticide residues are specially strictly regulated and monitored (Commision directive, 2006). For these matrices (i.e. tomato, lettuce, apples, etc.) comprehensive, straightforward and reliable methods can be found in the literature (Martín-Plaza, 2005). In contrast, the analysis of pesticide residues in fatty vegetable matrices is still a challenging issue, because of the inherent complexity of the matrix (Gilbert-Lopez et al., 2009).

Numerous analytical methods for determining organohalogenated, organophosphorous and organonitrogen pesticides residues in various foods have been published. Most of them are based on gas chromatography (GC) with electron-capture (ECD), nitrogen–phosphorous (NPD) and flame photometric detection (FPD) when pesticide molecules have functional groups giving a response in those detectors (Albero et al., 2003). Nowadays, gas chromatography with a mass spectrometric detector (GC–MS) is preferred due to its high selectivity and sensitivity (Pugliese et al., 2004; Tadeo et al., 2004). Pesticides with low volatility or thermal instability are determined by high performance liquid chromatography (HPLC) coupled with diode-array (DAD), fluorescence and mass spectrometry detection (Garrido, et al., 2004; Kovalczuk et al., 2006, Lacina et al. 2010). Application of enzyme-linked immunosorbent assays (ELISA) in the determination of pesticides has also been reported (Belleville et al., 2004; Kolosova et al., 2004). Dithiocarbamates are poorly soluble in common solvents (e.g. mancozeb, propineb, zineb) and are sometimes also poorly soluble in water (e.g. mancozeb, maneb, metiram, propineb, thiram, zineb, ziram). They are thermolabile and unstable in aqueous solutions, and sometimes their molecular weight is unknown, because they are actually polymers (e.g. manozeb, maneb, metiram, propineb, zineb) (Vettorazzi et al., 1995). Analysis of dithiocarbamates has been the subject of numerous studies. Usually they are quantified by spectrophotometry and head space gas chromatography (HS-GC) analysis of the carbon disulphide (CS_2) formed during an acidic treatment of dithiocarbamate residues in a reducing media (Kessari & Gupta, 1998; Sharma et al., 2005).

References

Agency for Toxic Substances and Disease Registry (ATSDR). Public Health Statement for DDT, DDE, and DDD (2002,September) Available from: http://www.atsdr.cdc.gov/ toxprofiles/phs35.html.

Agency for Toxic Substances and Disease Registry (ATSDR) (2005). Public Health Statement for Hexachlorocyclohexane (August 2005) Available from: http://www.atsdr.cdc.gov/toxprofiles/phs43.html.

Albero, B; Sanchez-Brunete, C; Tadeo JL. Determination of organophosphorous pesticides in fruit juices by matrix solid-phase dispersion and gas chromatography. *Journal of Agricultural Food Chemistry,* 2003, 51, 6915– 6921.

Alawi, MA; Tamimi, S; Jaghabir, M. Storage of organochlorine pesticides in human adipose tissues of Jordanian males and females. *Chemosphere,* 1999, 38, 2865-2873.

Barnett, JB. Effects of organic solvents and pesticides on immune system parameters. In Massaro EJ, editor. *Handbook of human toxicology.* Boca Raton, FL: CRC Press; 1997; 853–924.

Belleville, E; Dufva, M; Aamand, J; Bruun, L; Clausen, L; Christensen, CBV. Quantitative microarray pesticide analysis. *Journal of Immunological Methods,* 2004, 286, 219–229.

Bhanti, M; Taneja, A. Contamination of vegetables of different seasons with organophosphorus pesticides and related health risk assessment in northern India. *Chemosphere,* 2007, 63-68.

Braune, BM; Outridge, PM; Fisk, AT; Muir, DC; Helm, PA; Hobbs, K; Hoekstra, PF; Kuzyk, ZA; Kwan, M; Letcher, RJ; Lockhart, WL; Norstrom, RJ; Stern, GA; Stirling, I. Persistent organic pollutants and mercury in marine biota of the Canadian Arctic: an overview of spatial and temporal trends. *Science of the Total Environment*, 2005, 351-352, 4-56.

Boulaid, M; Aguilera, A; Camacho, F; Soussi, M; Valverde, A. Effect of household processing and unit-to-unit variability of pyrifenox, pyridaben, and tralomethrin residues in tomatoes. *Journal of Agricultural and Food Chemistry,* 2005, 53, 4054–4058.

Caldas, E.D; Tressou, J; Boon, PE. Dietary exposure of Brazilian consumers to dithiocarbamate pesticides – a probabilistic approach. *Food and Chemical Toxicology*, 2006, 44, 1562–1571.

Commission of the European Communities (CEC). Monitoring of pesticide residues in products of plant origin in the European Union, Norway, Iceland and Liechtenstein. (2008, november, 20). Available from: http://ec.europa.eu/food/fvo/specialreports/pesticide_residues/report_2006_en.pdf.

Commission directive 2006/125/EC of 5 December 2006 on processed cerealbased foods and babyfoods for infants and young children. Official *Journal of European Union* L339/16 (December 6, 2006) and subsequent updates (Council decision of 9 October 2007).

Concha-Graña, E; Turnes-Carou, MI; Muniategui-Lorenzo, S; López-Mahía, P; Prada-Rodríguez, D; Fernández-Fernández, E. Evaluation of HCH isomers and metabolites in soils, leachates, river water and sediments of a highly contaminated area. *Chemosphere*, 2006, 64, *588-595.*

Covaci, A; de Boer, J; Ryan, JJ; Voorspoels, S; Schepens, P. Distribution of organobrominated and organochlorinated contaminants in Belgian human adipose tissue. *Environmental Research*, 2002a, 88, 210-218.

Covaci, A; Jorens, P; Jacquemyn, Y; Schepens, P; Distribution of PCBs and organochlorine pesticides in umbilical cord and maternal serum. *Science of the Total Environment*, 2002b, 298, 45-53.

Chavarri, MJ; Herrera, A; Arino, A. The decrease in pesticides in fruit and vegetables during commercial processing. *International Journal of Food Science and Technology*, 2005, 40, 205–211.

Darko, G; Akoto, O. Dietary intake of ogranophosphorus pesticide residues through vegetables from Kumasi, Ghana. *Food and Chemical Toxicology*, 46, 3703-3706.

European Commision Regulation (EC) No 396/2005 of the European Parliament and of the council of 23 February 2005 on maximum residue levels of pesticides in or on food and feed of plant and animal origin and amending Council Directive 91/414/EC (2003)

European Commision Council Directive of 15 July 1991 (91/414/EEC) concerning the placing of plant protection products on the market *Official Journal* L 230 , 19/08/1991, 1 -32.

EUROSTAT. The use of plant protection products in the European Union, European Commission (2007). Available from: http://epp.eurostat.ec.europa.eu/cache/ITY_OFFPUB/KS-76-06-669/EN/KS-76-06-669-EN.PDF

European Food Safety Authority (EFSA). (2009): 2007 Annual Report on Pesticide Residues according to Article 32 of Regulation (EC) No 396/20051 (2009). Available from: http://www.efsa.europa.eu/en/scdocs/scdoc/305r.htm.

Fernàndez-Cruz, ML; Villarroya, M; Llanos, S; Alonso-Prados, JL; Garcìa-Baudìn, JM. Field-incurred fenitrothion residues in kakis: comparison of individual fruits, composite samples, and peeled and cooked fruits. *Journal of Agricultural and Food Chemistry*, 2004, 52, 860–863.

Food and Agriculture Organization of the United Nations (FAO). International Code of Conduct on the Distribution and Use of Pesticides (2002). Available from:

http://www.fao.org/WAICENT/FAOINFO/AGRICULT/AGP/AGPP/Pesticid/Code/Downlod/code.pdf

Fong, WG; Moye, HA; Seiber, JN; Toth, JP. *Pesticide residues in foods, methods, techniques and regulations.* 1 edition. New York, NY: John Wiley and Sons; 1999.

Foster, W; Chan, S; Platt L; Hughes, C. Detection of endocrine disrupting chemicals in samples of second trimester human amniotic fluid. *Journal of Clinical Endocrinology and Metabolism*, 2000, 85, 2954-2957.

Garrido, FA; Martínez, VJL; Lopez, LT; Cortes, AS; Martínez, SI. Monitoring multi-class pesticide residues in fresh fruits and vegetables by liquid chromatography with tandem mass spectrometry. *Journal of Chromatography A*, 2004, 1048, 199–206.

Gilbert-López, B; García-Reyes, JF; Molina-Díaz, A. Sample treatment and determination of pesticide residues in fatty vegetable matrices: A review. *Talanta*, 2009, 79, 109-128.

Goh, KT; Ong, KH; Tan, IK; Yew, FS. Acute organophosphorus food poisoning caused by contaminated green leafy vegetables. *Archives of Environmental Health,* 1990, 45, 180–184.

Gonzales, M; Miglioranza, KSB; de Moreno, JEA; Moreno, VJ. Evaluation of conventionally and organically produced vegetables for high lipophilic organochlorine pesticide (OCP) residues. *Food and Chemical Toxicology*, 2005, 43. 261-269.

Harris, CA; Mascall, JR:, Waren, SF; Crossley, SJ. Summary report of the International Conference on Pesticide Residues Variability and Acute Dietary Risk Assesment. *Food Additives and Contaminants*, 2000, 17, 481-485.

Holland, PT; Hamilton, D; Ohlin, B; Skidmore, MW; Effects of storage and processing on pesticide residues in plant products. *Pure and Applied Chemistry*, 1994, 66, 335–356.

Jaraczewska, K; Lulek, J; Covaci, A; Voorspoels, S; Kaluba-Skotarczak, A; Drews, K; Schepens, P. Distribution of polychlorinated biphenyls, organochlorine pesticides and polybrominated diphenyl ethers in human umbilical cord serum, maternal serum and milk from Wielkopolska region, Poland. *Science of the Total Environment*, 2006, 372, 20-31.

JMPR Guidance on the establishment of acute reference doses. In: *Pesticide residues in food* – 2004. Report of the JMPR 2004, FAO plant production and protection paper, 2004,.78, FAO, Rome, 3–9.

Juraske, R; Mutel, CL; Stoessel, F; Hellweg, S. Life cycle human toxicity assessment of pesticides: Comparing fruit and vegetable diets in Switzerland and the Unated States. *Chemosphere,* 2009, 77, 939-945.

Kovalczuk, T; Jech, M; Poustka, J; Hajšlová, J. Ultra-performance liquid chromatography mass spectrometry: a novel challenge in multiresidue pesticide analysis in food. *Analytica Chimica Acta,* 2006, 577, 8–17.

Kolosova, AY; Park, JH; Eremin, SA; Park, SJ; Kang, SJ; Shim, WB. Comparative study of three immunoassays based on monoclonal antibodies for detection of the pesticide parathion-methyl in real samples. *Analytica Chimica Acta*, 2004, 511, 323–331.

Kessari, R; Gupta, VK. A sensitive spectrophotometric method for the determination of dithiocarbamate fungicide and its application in environmental samples. *Talanta*, 1998, 45, 1097–1102.

Kanja, LW; Skaare, JU; Ojwang, SB; Maitai, CK. A comparison of organochlorine pesticide residues in maternal adipose tissue, maternal blood, cord blood, and human milk from mother/infant pairs. *Archives of Environmental Contamination and Toxicology*, 1992, 22, 21-24.

Kaushik, G; Satya, S; Naik, SN. Food processing a tool to pesticide residue dissipation – a review. *Food Research International*, 2009, 42, 26–40.

Lacina, O; Urbanova, J; Poustka, J; Hajslova, J. Identification/quantification of multiple pesticide residues in food plants by ultra-high-performance liquid chromatography-time-of-flight mass spectrometry. *Journal of Chromatography A*, 2010, 1217, 648-659.

Mansour, S; Belal, M; Abou-Arab, AAK; Gad, MF. Monitoring of pesticides and heavy metals in cucumber fruits produced from different farming systems. *Chemosphere,* 2008, *75,* 601-609.

Mars, TC. The health significance of pesticide variability in individual commodity items. *Food Additives and Contamination*, 2000, 17, 487–490.

Martín-Plaza, L. European Union legislation on pesticide residues. In: Fernández-Alba, AR, editor. Chromatographic-Mass Spectrometric Food nalysis for Trace determination of Pesticide Residues, Comprehensive Analytical Chemistry, vol. 43, The Netherlands: Elsevier; 2005; 39-74.

Manirakiza, P; Covaci, A; Nizigiymana, L; Ntakimazi, G; Schepens, P. Persistent chlorinated pesticides and polychlorinated biphenyls in selected fish species from Lake Tanganyika, Burundi, Africa *Environmental Pollution,* 2002, 117, 447.

Nasreddine, P; Parent-Massin, D. Food contamination by metals and pesticides in the European Union. Should we worry? *Toxicology Letters*, 2002, 127, 29-41.

Pugliese, P; Moltó, JC; Damiani, P; Marín, R; Cossignani, L; Mañes, J. Gas Chromatographic evaluation of pesticide residue contents in nectarines after non-toxic washing treatment. *Journal of Chromatography A*, 2004, 1050, 185–191.

Pope, CN. Organophosphorus pesticides: do they all have the same mechanism of toxicity? *Journal of Toxicology and Environmental Health Part B*, 1999, 2, 161–181.

Ritter, L; Solomon, KR; Forget, J; Stemeroff, M; O'Leary, C. Persistent organic pollutants. (1995). Available from: http://www.chem.unep.ch/POPS/ritter/en/ritteren.pdf.

Sharma, VK; Aulakh, JS; Malik, AK. Fourth derivative spectrophotometric determination of fungicide thiram (tetramethyldithiocarbamate) using sodium molybdate and its application. *Talanta*, 2005, 65, 375–379.

Sala, M; Ribas-Fito, N; Cardo, E; de Muga, ME; Marco, E; Mazon, C; Verdu, A; Grimalt, JO; Sunyer, J. Levels of hexachlorobenzene and other organochlorine compounds in cord blood: exposure across placenta. *Chemosphere*, 2001, 43, 895-901.

Stan, HJ. Pesticide residue analysis in foodstuffs applying capillary gas chromatography with mass spectrometric detection State-of-the-art use of modified DFG-multimethod S19 and automated data evaluation. *Journal of Chromatography A*, 2000, 892, 347–377.

Tadeo, JL; Sánchez-Brunete, C; Albero, B; González, L. Analysis of Pesticide Residues in Juice and Beverages. *Critical Reviews in Analytical Chemistry*, 2004, 34, 121–131.

Tricker, AR; Preussmann, R. Chemical food contaminants in the initiation of cancer. *Proceedings of the Nutrition Society*, 1990, 49, 133-144.

Trewavas, A. A critical assessment of organic farming and food assertions with particular respect to the UK and the potential environmental benefits of no-till agriculture. *Crop Protection*, 2004, 23, 757– 781.

UNEP (United Nations Environment Program). Persistent Organic Pollutants (POPs). (2006). Available from: http://www.chem.unep.ch/pops.

US Environmental Protection Agency (EPA). The Determination of Whether Dithiocarbamate Pesticides Share a Common Mechanism of Toxicity. 2001, December, 1. Available from: http://www.epa.gov/oppsrrd1/cumulative/dithiocarb.pdf.

USFDA (United States Food and Drug Administration), 2006. US Food and Drug Administration: Total Diet Study. Market baskets 1991–1993 through 2003– 2004.

Vettorazzi, G; Almeida, WF; Burin, GJ; Jaeger, RB; Puga, FR; Rahde, AF. International safety assessment of pesticides: Dithiocarbamates, pesticides, ETU and PTU. A review and update. *Teratogenesis Carcinogenesis and Mutagenesis*, 1995, 15, 313–317.

Waichman, AA; Eve, E; Nina, NCS. Do farmers understand the information displayed on pesticide product labels? A key question to reduce pesticides exposure and risk of poisoning in the Brazilian Amazon. *Crop Protection*, 26, 576-583.

WHO (World Health Organization), 2003. Regional *per Capita* Consumption of Raw and Semi-Processed Agricultural Commodities.

Zhang, ZY; Liu, XJ; Hong, XY. Effects of home preparation on pesticide residues in cabbage. *Food Control*, 2007 18, 1484–1487.

In: Nutritional Insights and Food Safety
Editor: Jaroslava Švarc-Gajiæ
ISBN: 978-1-61122-130-5

Chapter VII

Occurrence of Polycyclic Aromatic Hydrocarbons and Seafood Safety

Maria João Ramalhosa[a,b], Simone Morais[a], Cristina Delerue-Matos[a], and Maria Beatriz Prior Pinto Oliveira[b]
[a]Requimte, Instituto Superior de Engenharia do Porto, Rua Dr. António Bernardino de Almeida 431, 4200-072 Porto, Portugal
[b]Requimte, Serviço de Bromatologia, Faculdade de Farmácia, Universidade do Porto, Rua Aníbal Cunha, 164, 4099-030 Porto, Portugal

Abstract

Human health is largely determined by diet. A recommendable diet should be able to provide sufficient nutrients containing low levels of pathogenic microorganisms, as well as chemical contaminants. Fish constitutes an important source of proteins, minerals, vitamins and unsaturated essential fatty acids (PUFAs), especially omega-3 PUFAs. Epidemiological studies have shown over time certain beneficial effects of fish consumption in the prevention of coronary heart diseases. In contrast to the potential health benefits of dietary fish intake, an issue of concern related with frequent fish consumption is the risk derived from exposure to chemical pollutants.

Polycyclic aromatic hydrocarbons (PAHs) are ubiquitous environmental pollutants and some of them are human genotoxic carcinogens. PAHs are produced mainly by high-temperature reactions, such as incomplete combustion and pyrolysis of fossil fuels and biomasses. In the past decade, PAHs were under evaluation by the International Programme on Chemical Safety (IPCS), the Scientific Committee on Food (SCF) and by the Joint FAO/WHO Expert Committee on Food Additives (JECFA). They concluded that research must be focused on the following 16 PAHs in Food: benz(a)anthracene, benzo(b)fluoranthene, benzo(j)fluoranthene, benzo(k)fluoranthene, benzo(g,h,i)perylene, benzo(a)pyrene, chrysene, cyclopenta(cd)pyrene, dibenz(a,h)anthracene, dibenzo(a, e)pyrene, dibenzo(a,h)pyrene, dibenzo(a,i)pyrene, dibenzo(a,l)pyrene, indeno(1,2,3-cd)pyrene, 5-methylchrysene and benzo(c)fluorene. Excluding smokers and occupationally exposed populations, most individuals are exposed to PAHs predominantly from dietary sources. In the marine environment, PAHs are bioavailable to species via the food chain, as waterborne compounds and from contaminated sediments.

As lipophilic compounds they can easily cross lipid membranes and have the potential to bioaccumulate in aquatic organisms. Benzo(a)pyrene is regarded as a marker of the genotoxic and carcinogenic PAHs and maximum levels had been set for diverse categories of fish products. Although for most people finfish and shellfish represent only a small part of the total diet, the contribution of this food group to the daily intake of PAHs in some individuals may be comparatively important.

In this chapter, the contemporary contributions regarding the contents of PAHs in seafood will be reviewed.

Introduction

Polycyclic aromatic hydrocarbons (PAHs) are a large class of ubiquitous organic pollutants. PAH release from natural or anthropogenic sources (Beg et al., 2009). Volcanic eruptions, forest and prairie fires are among the major natural sources of PAHs in the atmosphere. Anthropogenic PAHs are mainly formed as a result of pyrolytic processes, including automobile exhaust and tire degradation, industrial emission from catalytic cracking, petroleum refining, chemical manufacturing, air blowing for asphalt, cooking coal, domestic heating emission from coal, oil, gas and wood refuse incineration, biomass burning, power generation and vehicle emission (Siddiqi et al., 2009). PAHs consist of two or more fused aromatic rings in linear, angular or clustered arrangements (Alomirah et al., 2009) being identified more than 100 PAHs (IPCS, 1998). PAHs with two rings are more soluble in water and more volatile than PAHs with three rings or more, which have low solubility's in water and low vapor pressure. As molecular weight increases, solubility and vapor pressure decrease but the carcinogenicity of PAHs increases and they become more toxic and lipophilic. According to different health and environmental protection organizations, such as the International Agency for Research on Cancer (IARC) and the United States Environmental Protection Agency (US EPA), several PAHs have mutagenic, carcinogenic and endocrine disrupting properties (IARC, 1983; IARC, 2002; IARC, 2008; EPA, 1986). In particular, benzo(a)pyrene has been identified as being highly carcinogenic (Table 1). The US EPA has promulgated 16 unsubstituted PAHs as priority pollutants (EPA, 1986) which are commonly quantified for purposes of evaluating potential health effects in humans (Table 1).

In the past decade, PAHs were evaluated by the International Programme on Chemical Safety (IPCS), the Scientific Committee on Food (SCF) and by the Joint FAO/WHO Expert Committee on Food Additives (JECFA). Excluding smokers and occupationally exposed populations, most individuals are exposed to PAHs predominantly from dietary sources (Domingo et al., 2007; Domingo, 2007a; Alomirah et al., 2009). Food can be contaminated from environmental sources (air, soil or water), industrial food processing (smoking, heating and drying processes that allow combustion products to come into direct contact with food) and from certain home cooking practices (e.g. grilling, roasting and smoking). In the marine environment, PAHs are bioavailable to species via the food chain, as waterborne compounds and from contaminated sediments. Of these three possible routes of PAH absorption, uptake of waterborne PAHs across the gills is considered to be the most significant.

Table 1. Carcinogenicity of the 16 PAHs, commonly evaluated in human health risk assessment, according to IARC and EPA classification systems

Compound	Chemical structure	Abbreviation	Classification IARC[a]	EPA[b]	TEF[c]
Naphthalene	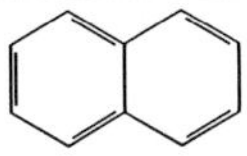	Naph	2B	C	not available
Acenaphthylene	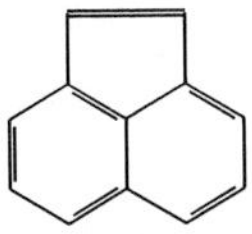	Acl	not available	D	0.001
Acenaphthene	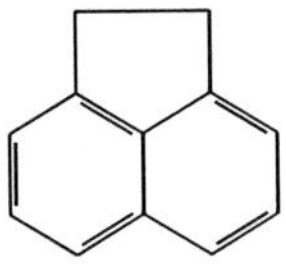	Ace	3	not available	0.001
Fluorene	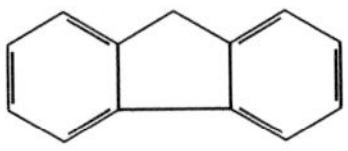	Flu	3	D	0.001
Phenanthrene	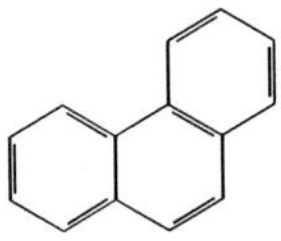	Phe	3	D	0.001
Anthracene	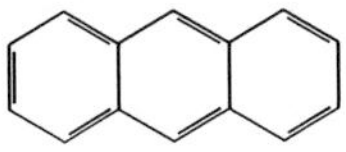	Ant	3	D	0.01
Fluoranthene	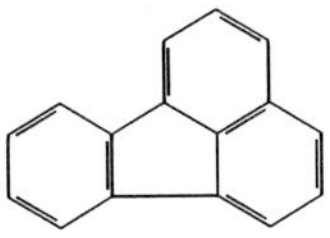	Fln	3	D	0.001
Pyrene	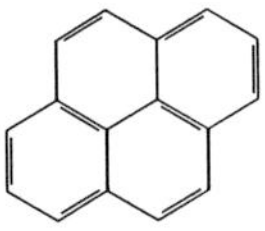	Pyr	3	D	0.001
Benz(a)anthracene	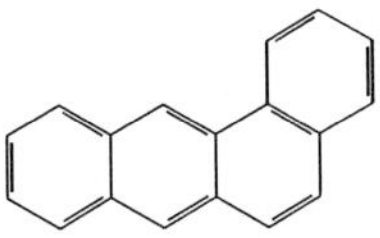	B(a)A	3	B_2	0.1
Chrysene	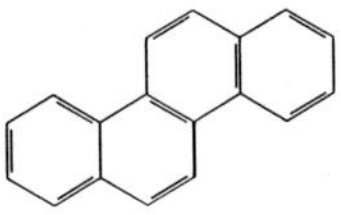	Chry	2A	B_2	0.1
Benzo(b)fluoranthene	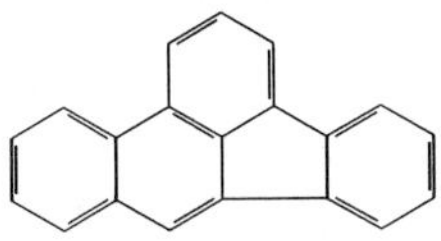	B(b)F	2B	B_2	0.1
Benzo(k)fluoranthene	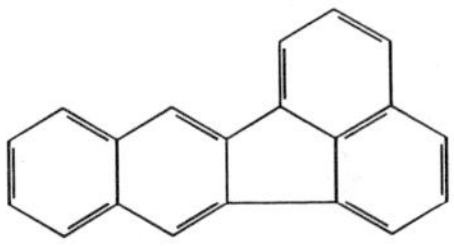	B(k)F	2B	B_2	0.1

Table 1. (Continued)

Compound	Chemical structure	Abbreviation	Classification IARC[a]	EPA[b]	TEF[c]
Benzo(a)pyrene	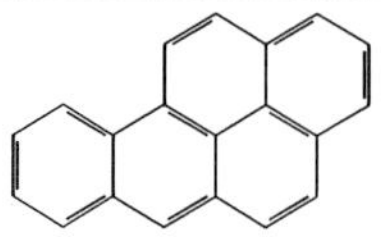	B(a)P	1	B_2	1
Dibenz(a,h)anthracene	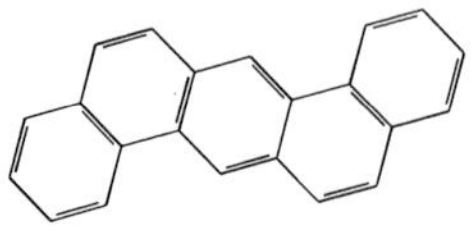	DB(a,h)A	2A	B_2	5
Benzo(g,h,i)perylene	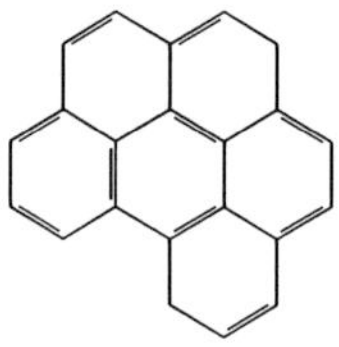	B(g,h,i)P	3	D	0.01
Indeno(1,2,3-cd)pyrene	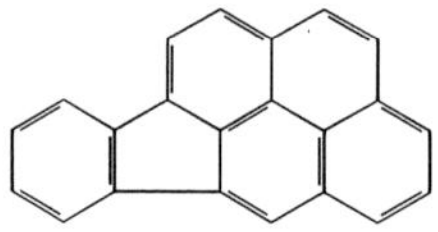	InP	2B	B_2	0.1

[a](IARC, 1983; IARC, 2002; IARC, 2008): Group 1 - carcinogenic to humans; Group 2A - probably carcinogenic to humans; Group 2B - possible carcinogenic to humans; Group 3 - unclassifiable as to carcinogenetic in humans; Group 4 - probably not carcinogenic to humans.

[b](EPA, 1986): Group A - human carcinogens; Group B - probable human carcinogens (B_1: based on limited evidence of carcinogenicity in humans and sufficient evidence of carcinogenicity in animals; B_2: based on sufficient evidence of carcinogenicity in animals); Group C - possible human carcinogens; Group D - not classifiable as to human carcinogenicity; Group E - evidence of non-carcinogenicity for humans.

[c]Toxicity Equivalency Factor (TEF): estimation based on the relative potency to benzo(a)pyrene (Nisbet and LaGoy, 1992).

PAHs uptake always depends on their bioavailability as well as the physiology of the organisms (Meador et al., 1995). As lipophilic compounds they can easily cross lipid membranes and have the potential to bioaccumulate in aquatic organisms. Bioaccumulation, therefore, is a result of the different uptake and elimination processes of the compounds combined with metabolic clearance (biotransformation) (Verweij et al., 2004). In aquatic food chains, fish have the best capacity to metabolize PAHs, crustaceans are intermediate, and mollusks have the poorest metabolic capacity. PAHs biotransformation occurs in many aquatic organisms, but it is most effective in the liver of fish (van der Oost et al., 2003). PAHs are easily metabolized by the phase I enzymes such as oxygenase system, to more hydrophilic products like phenols, dihydrodiols, quinones and epoxides (Lech & Vodicnik, 1985; Sijm et al., 1989). Reported half-lifes of parental PAHs in rainbow trout range from 1 day for acenaphtylene to 9 days for phenanthrene (Meador et al., 1995). Some of the PAHs can be excreted directly as unconjugated metabolites in bile (via the gallbladder), but most PAHs will be excreted after conjugation by phase II enzymes (Vermeulen et al., 1992). Due to efficient metabolism even in contaminated areas, only low to moderate PAH concentrations are typically found in finfish. Although for most people, finfish and shellfish represent only a small part of the total diet, the contribution of this food group to the daily intake of PAHs in some individuals may be comparatively important (Domingo et al., 2007; Domingo, 2007a; Domingo, 2007b).

This chapter reports the latest information published over the years of 2000 to 2009 about the detected PAH concentrations in fish and fishery products (muscle meat of finfish; bivalve mollusks; crustaceans; cephalopods; smoked fish and smoked fishery products). Only studies concerning edible marine products that were available to consumers were considered in order to assess their status of contamination and the public health risks.

1. Seafood Consumption and Nutrition

Dietary habits are among the major society concerns, and the quality and amount of the nutrients ingested is considered fundamental for good health and well being. Among the products available, seafood is currently considered one of the most interesting. Fish and shellfish are nutritious and highly essential in a balanced diet, being an important source of proteins, liposoluble vitamins and also lipids of high biological value (long chain polyunsaturated fatty acids) (Chow, 2008). The American Heart Association (AHA) suggests that patients without or with documented cardiovascular disease eat, respectively, a variety of fish (preferably oily) at least twice a week, or to consume about 1 g of eicosapentaenoic acid plus docosahexaenoic acid per day, preferably from oily fish (Kris-Etherton et al., 2002, 2003). These recommendations are based on a large body of evidence from epidemiologic and controlled clinical studies. Seafood also contains most of the 90 natural elements (Causeret, 1962; Lall, 1995) being an important source of essential minerals (iron, copper, zinc, iodine, manganese, selenium and fluorine). The largest concentrations of structural elements correspond to carbon, hydrogen, nitrogen, oxygen and sulphur followed by chlorine, potassium, phosphorus, sodium, magnesium and calcium (Lall, 1995; Oehlenschläger, 1997). Thus, all over the world, fish is assuming an enormous importance and its consumption is increasing. World apparent *per capita* fish consumption has steadily increasing from an average of 9.9 kg in the 1960s, 11.5 kg in the 1970s, 12.5 kg in the 1980s, 14.4 kg in the 1990s, reaching 16.4 kg in 2005 (FAO, 2009). Capture fisheries and aquaculture supplied the world with about 110 million tonnes of food fish in 2006, providing an apparent *per capita* supply of 16.7 kg (live weight equivalent). 77% of world fish production was used for direct human consumption. Almost all of the remaining 33 million tonnes was destined for non-food products, in particular fishmeal and fish oil (FAO, 2009). In 2006, 48.5% of the fish for human consumption was in live and fresh form, which is often the most preferred and highly priced product. 54% (77 million tonnes) of the world's fish production underwent some form of processing. 74% (57 million tonnes) of this processed fish was used for direct human consumption in frozen, cured and prepared or preserved form, and the rest for non-food uses (FAO, 2009). Freezing is the main method of processing fish for food use, accounting for 50% of total processed fish for human consumption in 2006, followed by prepared and preserved (29%) and cured fish (21%). Fish products production have diversified significantly in the last two decades, particularly into high-value fresh and processed products, fuelled by changing consumer tastes and advances in technology, packaging, logistics and transport (FAO, 2009).

In 2006, overall, fish provided more than 2.9 billion people with at least 15% of their average *per capita* animal protein intake (7.6% in North and Central America, more than 11% in Europe, around 19% in Africa, nearly 21% in Asia and about 19% in the low-income food-deficit countries including China). Although the attributes of fish attract a more health conscious consumers, the safety and nutritional benefits related to fish consumption have become an increasing public health concern in recent years. Pollution and environmental issues have further focused people´s attention on contamination problems. The Scientific Statement of the AHA (Kris-Etherton et al., 2002, 2003) also indicates that finfish and shellfish is potentially a major source of human exposure to various environmental contaminants (Domingo et al., 2007; Domingo, 2007a). Consumers enforce expectations for enhanced safety.

2. Risk Assessment of PAHs in Food

The EFSA Panel on Contaminants in the Food Chain (CONTAM Panel) explored a toxic equivalency factor (TEF) approach in the risk characterization of the PAH mixtures in food. This panel concluded that the TEF approach is not scientifically valid because of the lack of data from oral carcinogenicity studies on individual PAHs, their different modes of action and the evidence of poor predictivity of the carcinogenic potency of PAH mixtures based on the currently proposed TEF values (EFSA, 2008a). Therefore the CONTAM Panel concluded that the risk characterization should be based upon the PAHs for which oral carcinogenicity data were available, i.e. for benzo(a)pyrene and the other PAHs that were measured in the two coal tar mixtures used in the carcinogenicity studies of Culp et al. (1998): benz(a)anthracene, benzo(b)fluoranthene, benzo(k)fluoranthene, benzo(g,h,i)perylene, chrysene, dibenz(a, h)anthracene and indeno(1,2,3-cd)pyrene. Based on the currently available data relating to occurrence and toxicity, the assumption that benzo(a)pyrene is a good indicator of any PAH contamination in food was proved dubious and the CONTAM Panel concluded that these eight PAHs (PAH8) and the sum of benzo(*a*)pyrene, chrysene, benz(a)anthracene and benzo(b)fluoranthene (PAH4), are currently the only possible indicators of the carcinogenic potency of PAHs in food, with PAH8 not providing much added value compared to PAH4 (EFSA, 2008).

A "margin of exposure" (MOE) approach has been developed and is now recommended by the European Food Safety Authority (EFSA, 2007a, 2007b, 2008) and the World Health Organization (WHO, 2006, 2008) as the preferred method of risk assessment of genotoxic and carcinogenic PAHs. MOE is defined as the ratio of a chosen point of departure (POD; EPA, 1999) on a dose-response curve to a human exposure estimate (MOE = POD/Exposure). There is a broad agreement that the lower the MOE, the greater is the concern. EFSA's Scientific Committee advocated that, in general, an MOE of 10,000 or higher, if based on the benchmark dose chosen at a 10% incidence above the control (BMDL10; user-friendly software for modeling the benchmark dose is available from the EPA 2008; Barlow & Schlatter, 2009) from an animal study, and taking into account overall uncertainties in the interpretation, would be of low concern from a public health point of view and might be reasonably considered as a low priority for risk management actions (EFSA, 2005; Barlow & Schlatter, 2009). This opinion was based on species differences and human variability in toxicokinetics and toxicodynamics, human variability in cell cycle control and capacity for DNA repair, and the fact that the POD is an effect level. Furthermore, the Committee also indicated that such a judgment is ultimately a matter for the risk managers and that an MOE of that magnitude or above should not preclude the application of risk management measures to reduce human exposure (Barlow & Schlatter, 2009). Particular MOE values or range of values have been further debated without, so far, any consensus (Barlow et al., 2006; Barlow & Schlatter, 2009).

3. Legislation Regarding PAHs in Seafood

The Scientific Committee on Food and the Joint FAO/WHO Expert Committee on Food Additives, regarding the genotoxic and carcinogenic PAHs, concluded that the evaluation has to be focussed on the following 16 PAHs in food: benz(a)anthracene, benzo(b)fluoranthene, benzo(j)fluoranthene, benzo(k)fluoranthene, benzo(g,h,i)perylene, benzo(a)pyrene, chrysene, cyclopenta(cd)pyrene, dibenz(a,h)anthracene, dibenzo(a,e)pyrene, dibenzo(a,h)pyrene, dibenzo(a,i)pyrene, dibenzo(a,l)pyrene, indeno(1,2,3-cd)pyrene, 5-methylchrysene and benzo(c)fluorine (EFSA, 2008a). Considering disparities caused by different maximum levels (ML) for PAHs in food in several Member States, the European Commission set harmonized ML for benzo(a)pyrene for the first time in 2005 by Commission Regulation (EC) No. 208/2005 amending Regulation (EC) No. 466/2001 as regards PAHs. Benzo(a)pyrene was chosen because Scientific Committee on Food concluded that this compound can be used as a marker for the occurrence and genotoxic and carcinogenic effects of PAHs in food, based on examinations of its profiles in food and on evaluation of a carcinogenicity study of two coal tar mixtures in mice (EFSA, 2008a). Following a recommendation on investigation into levels of PAHs in certain foods (Commission Regulation (EC) No. 208/2005), eighteen Member States submitted almost 10,000 results for PAH levels in different food commodities. Products tested covered a broad range of food categories with an emphasis on fish and seafood, meat and meat products, fat and oils, and food supplements (EFSA, 2008a). An evaluation of these data performed by the European Food Safety Authority (EFSA) in June 2007 and updated in June 2008 demonstrated that benzo(a)pyrene could be detected in about 50% of the samples. In decreasing order, the highest concentrations of benzo(a)pyrene were found in food supplements, mollusks, olive pomace oil, spices, smoked fish, smoked meat and cocoa butter (EFSA, 2008b).

However, in about 30% of all the samples other carcinogenic and genotoxic PAHs were detected despite testing negative for benzo(a)pyrene. Of the individual PAHs, chrysene was most commonly found in the samples negative for benzo(a)pyrene with the highest level of 242 μg/kg (EFSA, 2008a). Moreover, the data on occurrence and relative proportions of other carcinogenic PAHs than benzo(a)pyrene in food were considered insufficient by the Commission for setting further ML. Maximum levels for benzo(a)pyrene are especially set for foodstuffs containing fats and oils and foods where environmental pollution or smoking and drying processes might cause high levels of contamination. The maximum levels for benzo(a)pyrene in seafood species are presented in Table 2.

Table 2. Maximum levels (ML) for benzo(a)pyrene in edible marine species as laid down in Commission Regulation (EC) No. 1881/2006

Foodstuff	Maximum level (µg/kg wet weight)
Bivalve mollusks	10.0
Crustaceans, cephalopods, other than smoked. The maximum level applies to crustaceans, excluding the brown meat of crab and excluding head and thorax meat of lobster and similar large crustaceans (Nephropidae and Palinuridae).	5.0
Muscle meat of smoked fish and smoked fishery products, excluding bivalve mollusks. The maximum level applies to smoked crustaceans, excluding the brown meat of crab and excluding head and thorax meat of lobster and similar large crustaceans (Nephropidae and Palinuridae).	5.0
Muscle meat of fish, other than smoked fish	2.0

4. PAHs Levels in Muscle Meat of Finfish other than Smoked

Of the 16.4 kg of seafood *per capita* available for consumption in 2005, about 74% came from finfish. Marine finfish species provided more than 47 million tonnes, of which 20.0 million tonnes were demersal fish, 19.9 million tonnes were pelagic species and 7.6 million tonnes were unidentified marine fish. Demersal fish are among the main species preferred by consumers in Northern Europe and in North America (FAO, 2009).

Commission Regulation (EC) 1881/2006 specifies a maximum level of 2.0 µg/kg of benzo(a)pyrene in muscle meat of fish other than smoked fish (Table 2). The maximum level set in the legislation applies to fresh fish. In this section, contributions published over the years of 2000 to 2009 regarding the contents and distribution of PAHs in finfish will be reviewed. Published results related with finfish species were firstly classified according to their ecological characteristics, namely, pelagic, bathypelagic, benthopelagic, demersal and reef-associated. Overall, available information covers 14 pelagic, 1 bathypelagic, 34 benthopelagic, 34 demersal and 18 reef-associated species. The mean benzo(a)pyrene, PAH8 (the sum of benzo(a)pyrene, benz(a)anthracene, benzo(b)fluoranthene, benzo(k)fluoranthene, benzo(g,h,i)perylene, chrysene, dibenz(a,h)anthracene and indeno(1,2,3-cd)pyrene) and total PAH concentrations reported for the fish samples, as well as the corresponding estimated daily intakes, are shown in Tables 3-6. The compounds mainly included in the analyses were the US Environmental Protection Agency's 16 priority pollutants. Alomirah et al. (2009) quantified the highest number of PAHs (23), including also in their study benzo(c)phenanthrene, benzo(j)fluoranthene, 7,12-dimethylbenz(a)anthracene, 3-methyl-cholenthrene, dibenzo(a,h)pyrene, dibenzo(a,i)pyrene and dibenzo(a,l)pyrene. Edible portions of fish from unpolluted locations generally do not contain detectable levels, or higher than maximum level, of benzo(a)pyrene. Environmental pollution seems to be the main influencing factor. All pelagic (Table 3), benthopelagic (except for Japanese gizzard shad *(Nematalosa japonica)*; Table 4), demersal (Table 5) and reef-associated (except for Dusky spinefoot (*Siganus luridus*); Table 6) finfish species collected from Egypt (Great Bitter Lakes; El Temsah Lake; Alexandria coast and Abu Qir Bay) exceeded the maximum level established for benzo(a)pyrene reaching maximum values of 2510 µg/kg (Spanish mackerel

(Scomberomorus commerson)), 4310 μg/kg (Common two-banded seabream (*Diplodus vulgaris*)), 358 μg/kg (Sole (*Solea solea*)) and 32900 μg/kg (Shrimp scad (*Alepes djedaba*)), respectively for the diverse ecological classifications. Other particular geographic regions had some benthopelagic (1 specie) and demersal aquatic organisms (5 species) that showed high contents of benzo(a)pyrene, namely Cotonou lagoon, République du Bénin (Tilapia (*Tilapia sp.*), Bay of Auha, Kuwait (Yellow Finned Black Seabream (*Acanthopagrus latus*); Klunzinger's mullet (*Liza klunzingeri*); Tongue sole (*Cynoglossus arel*)), Kuwait city, Kuwait (Yellow Finned Black Seabream (*Acanthopagrus latus*), Guanabara Bay, Brazil (Kneeled mullet (*Mugil lisa*) and Siokolo Fishing Settlement, Nigeria (Nagahanadai (*Pseudanthias elongatus*)).

Al-Hassan et al. (2003) analyzed twelve species of edible fish from the same region, the Arabian Gulf. Their study involved pelagic (River shad (*Hilsa ilisha*)), benthopelagic (Silvery Pomfret (*Pampus argenteus*) and Tiger-toothed croaker (*Otolithes argenteus*)), demersal (Yellow Finned Black Seabream and Greenback mullet (*Liza subviridis*)) and reef-associated (Greasy Grouper (*Epinephelus tauvina*) and Grouper (*Epinephelus areolatus*)) fish. They concluded that all these marine organisms carried a noticeable concentration of PAHs. Based upon the data presented by these authors, the bioaccumulation trend for the Arabian Gulf is: reef-associated > demersal > benthopelagic > pelagic (Al-Hassan et al., 2003). Said (2007) observed a similar pattern of variation. He concluded that PAHs levels in the different fish species may be associated with ecological niches and fish habits (Said, 2007). In his study, the species that generally had the highest PAH concentrations were a reef-associated, carnivorous fish and thus subjected to near-shore discharges (Shrimp scad (*Alepes djedaba*)) (Said, 2007; Table 6). Some of the other less contaminated species, e.g. Spanish mackerel (*Scomberomorus commerson*) and European barracuda (*Sphyraena sphyraena*), were pelagic (Said, 2007). Generally, uptake of PAHs by fish can occur through bioconcentration from water and/or bioaccumulation from diet and/or suspended sediments (Meador et al., 1995).

Fish take up PAHs mainly in the dissolved form. PAHs residence time depends on the metabolic ability of organism but usually fish can rapidly convert up to 99% of the PAHs to metabolites within 24 h of uptake, changing the pattern and the concentrations in the several tissues (Lech & Vodicnik, 1985; Sijm et al., 1989; van der Oost et al., 2003; Said, 2007). PAH distributions and contents in organisms vary according to species, their location in the water column (i.e., pelagic and benthic organisms), length of exposure and their feeding mode. Fish living in the reef-associated environments (reef-associated fish), close to or lying on the bottom (demersal) and living in the water column but associated with the sea floor (benthopelagic) have an increased pollutant exposure since PAHs tend to accumulate in bottom sediments/reefs and may constitute a continuous source to aquatic organisms. Pelagic and bathypelagic species which live in the open seas or oceans have a lower exposure to PAHs, principally to the higher molecular weight PAHs. In general, PAHs preferentially partition from surface water to more hydrophobic organic media such as sediments/reefs with high organic carbon. However, the two- and three-ring PAHs, such as naphthalene and phenanthrene, have lower molecular weights and octanol-water coefficients (Kow) than the larger PAHs, partition to surface water and are available for uptake by biota (Varanasi, 1989). The higher molecular weights PAHs remain in the sediments (Hellou et al., 1994, 1995; Means, 1998).

The considerable variation in levels of PAHs among the same species in different environments (e.g the benthopelagic Common two-banded seabream from Egypt and Spain,

Table 4, as well as the demersal Sole also from Egypt and Spain, Table 5) and between different species in the same location, highlights the important role of ecological and physiological factors in concentrating pollutants. A global analysis of the published studies indicates that:

- PAHs composition pattern in finfish is dominated by higher percentages of 2 and 3 rings PAHs (DouAbul et al. 1997; Baumard et al., 1999; Deb et al., 2000; Al-Hassan et al., 2003; Bordajandi et al., 2004; Llobet et al., 2006; Cheung et al., 2007; Liang et al., 2007; Perugini et al., 2007a; Said, 2007; Varlet et al., 2007a; Malik et al., 2008; Soclo et al., 2008; Beg et al., 2009);

- Concentrations of the most toxic PAHs in muscle of bottom fish are typically (excluding high polluted geographic areas) near or below the limits of detection, because they are readily metabolized to intermediates or form conjugates that pass into the bile (Varanasi, 1989; Deb et al., 2000). This metabolism depends on the specific species (within the same species also influenced by age and gender), route and duration of exposure, environmental factors (e.g., salinity, temperature, etc.), and also the presence of other xenobiotics that could influence their transformation (Varanasi, 1989).

On the basis of the sum of the determined genotoxic and carcinogenic (PAH8) and total PAHs, the most contaminated fish species found were the pelagic Keeled mullet (*Liza carinata*) from Egypt with 12760-543900 μg/kg for PAH8 and 15160-728900 μg/kg for total PAHs (Table 3). The less contaminated was the demersal Silver hake (*Merluccius bilinearis*), from Estonia (Yurchenko & Molder, 2005), with non-detectable contents of PAHs.

Using a body weight of 70 kg and the *per capita* consumption of finfish in 2005 (12.2 kg; FAO, 2009), the values obtained for benzo(a)pyrene contaminant intake estimation in adults reach a maximum of 1.2 μg/kg body weight (b.w.) per day (Spanish mackerel; Table 3) for pelagic, 2.06 μg/kg b.w. per day (Common two-banded seabream; Table 4) for benthopelagic, 3.24 μg/kg b.w. per day (Nagahanadai; Table 5) for demersal and as much as 15.7 μg/kg b.w. per day (Shrimp scad (*Alepes djedaba*); Table 6) for reef-associated fish. Benzo(a)pyrene estimated daily intake can not be calculated for the unique bathypelagic reported specie. Using PAH8, to evaluate the intake of PAHs classified as probable/possible human carcinogens, and total PAHs, the highest contributor to the dietary exposure was found as Keeled mullet (6.09 to 260 and 7.24 to 348 μg/kg b.w. per day, respectively, for estimated PAH8 and total PAHs intakes; Table 3).

Fatty fish, such as anchovies, sardine, herring, chub mackerel, salmon and tuna, are recommended for cardiovascular disease prevention by many authoritative groups including the American Heart Association due to their highest concentration in eicosapentaenoic acid and docosahexaenoic acid per serving among food sources. Available information concerning these marine species indicates that they should not cause adverse health effects for consumers, when eaten in moderation, since benzo(a)pyrene levels were well below the maximum level. Maximum estimated daily intake of PAH8 and total PAHs were found as 0.0103 μg/kg b.w. per day and 0.0192 μg/kg b.w. per day, respectively, for tuna (*Thunnus thynnus*) from Kuwait (Al-Omair & Helaleh, 2004; Table 3). These results are in the same order of magnitude than those determined in the survey performed across European countries for PAH levels in different food commodities (EFSA 2008b).

The median dietary exposure was calculated both for mean and high dietary consumers and varied between 0.0039 μg/kg b.w. per day and 0.0065 μg/kg b.w. per day, respectively for benzo(a)pyrene alone, and 0.0288 μg/kg b.w. per day and 0.0513 μg/kg b.w. per day, respectively for PAH8. The two highest contributors to the dietary exposure in the 10,000 products analyzed were cereals and cereal products, and seafood and seafood products (EFSA, 2007c).

Using the published data within the period of 2000 to 2009, dependence between benzo(a)pyrene concentration, PAH4 and PAH8 *versus* total amount of PAHs was evaluated and quadratic correlation coefficients of 0.24, 0.97 and 0.96 were obtained for pelagic species, 0.034, 0.10 and 0.99 for benthopelagic, 0.977, 0.993 and 0.986 for demersal and 0.18, 0.57 and 0.74 for reef-associated fish. The number of points was insufficient to analyze the bathypelagic group. As indicated by the EFSA Panel on Contaminants in the Food Chain (EFSA, 2008a), PAH4 and PAH8 seem to be clearly better indicators than benzo(a)pyrene for the occurrence of PAHs in muscle meat of fish other than smoked fish. There was almost no correlation between benzo(a)pyrene content and the total amount of PAHs in pelagic, benthopelagic and reef-associated fish.

5. PAHs Levels in Fresh Bivalve Mollusks

Of the 16.4 kg of fish *per capita* available for consumption in 2005, mollusks supplied about 2.0 kg *per capita* (FAO, 2009). Commission Regulation (EC) 1881/2006 specifies a maximum level of 10.0 μg/kg for benzo(a)pyrene in fresh bivalve mollusks (Table 2).

The relevant information concerning PAH levels detected in bivalve mollusks all over the world during 2000 to 2009 is presented in Table 7. The number of PAHs that were detected in mollusks varied between 8 and 16 in the studies that characterized the recommended set of 16 PAHs. Law et al. (2000) and Gagnon et al. (2004) determined 17 PAHs in Mediterranean mussel (*Mytilus galloprovincials*) collected from Wadden Sea, The Netherlands, and 22 PAHs in soft-shell clam (*Mya arenaria*) from St. Lawrence River, Canada, respectively. Overall, mainly all samples had detectable amounts of benzo(a)pyrene with the exception of Mediterranean mussel samples from Central Adriatic and Ionian Seas (Italy), Blue mussel (*Mytilus edulis*) samples from Scotland, and some clam species (*Chamelea sp. and Tapes sp.*) from Huelva, Spain.

Table 3. Concentrations (µg/kg of wet weight unless indicated otherwise) of benzo(a)pyrene (B(a)P), genotoxic and carcinogenic PAHs (PAH8) and total PAHs (∑PAHs), as well as estimated daily intake (µg/kg body weight per day) of B(a)P, PAH8 and ∑PAHs in pelagic and bathypelagic finfish

Species	Location, Region	n PAHs	Fish meat (x10³ µg/kg)			Intake (µg/kg body weight per day)			Ref.
			B(a)P	PAH8	∑PAHs	B(a)P	PAH8	∑PAHs	
Allice (*Alosa fallax lacustris)*	Lake Iseo, Italy	16	b)	b)	1.30	a)	a)	0.624	Binelli and Provini, 2004
Anchovy *(Engraulis encrasicholus)*	Catalonia, Spain	16	0.0000750	0.000879	0.00680	0.0000358	0.000420	0.00324	Llobet et al., 2006
Atlantic horse mackerel *(Trachurus trachurus)*	Oporto, Portugal	16	ND	ND	0.00255	a)	a)	0.00122	Ramalhosa et al., 2009
Atlantic mackerel (*Scomber scombrus)*	Central Adriatic Sea, Italy	16	ND	0.000290-0.00149	0.00167-0.332	a)	0.000138-0.000711	0.000796-0.158	Perugini et al., 2007a
	Tyrrhenian Sea, Italy	11	ND	0.00244-0.0245	0.00555-0.0326	a)	0.00117-0.0117	0.00265-0.0156	Perugini et al., 2007b
	Catalonia:, Spain	16	0.000117	0.00230	0.00940	0.0000559	0.00109	0.00449	Llobet et al., 2006
Blue whiting c) (*Micromesistius Poutassou)*	Central Adriatic Sea, Italy	16	ND	0.000330-0.0675	0.00130-0.209	a)	0.000158-0.0322	0.000620-0.0997	Perugini et al., 2007a
	Tyrrhenian Sea, Italy	11	ND	0.00585-0.0134	0.00865-0.0281	a)	0.00279-0.00642	0.00413-0.0135	Perugini et al., 2007b
Chub mackerel *(Scomber japonicus)*	Oporto, Portugal	16	ND	ND	0.00406	a)	a)	0.00194	Ramalhosa et al., 2009
European barracuda *(Sphyraena sphyraena)*	Alexandria coast, Egypt	16	1.90	6.15	8.26	0.908	2.93	3.94	Said, 2007
Golden grey mullet *(Liza aurata)*	Great Bitter lakes/El Temsah lake, Egypt	16	ND-1.53	28.2-47.5	147-157	≤0.733	13.5-22.7	70.2-75.1	Said and El Agroudy, 2006
Hilsa shad *(Tenualosa ilisha)*	Kuwait city, Kuwait	23	ND	0.00110 d)	0.0165 d)	a)	0.000525	0.00788	Alomirah et al., 2009
Keeled mullet *(Liza carinata)*	Great Bitter lakes/ El Temsah lake, Egypt	16	ND-2.03	12.8-544	15.2-729	≤0.967	6.09-260	7.24-348	Said and El Agroudy, 2006
River shad	Arabian Gulf	14	ND	ND	1.33	a)	a)	0.0635	Al-Hassan et al.,

Species	Location, Region	n PAHs	Fish meat (x10^{3} µg/kg)			Intake (µg/kg body weight per day)			Ref.
			B(a)P	PAH8	∑PAHs	B(a)P	PAH8	∑PAHs	
(*Hilsa ilisha*)									2003
Sardine (*Sardina pilchardus*)	Catalonia, Spain	16	0.0000730	0.000712	0.00530	0.0000349	0.000340	0.00253	Llobet et al., 2006
	Catalonia, Spain	16	0.0000400	0.000870	0.0177	0.0000191	0.000415	0.00848	Perelló et al., 2009
	Oporto, Portugal	16	ND	ND	0.00522	a)	a)	0.00249	Ramalhosa et al., 2009
Spanish mackerel (*Scomberomorus commerson)*	Alexandria coast, Egypt	16	2.51	2.92	3.86	1.20	1.39	1.85	Said, 2007
Swordfish (*Xiphias gladius)*	Catalonia, Spain	16	0.000135	0.00230	0.00600	0.0000645	0.00110	0.00286	Llobet et al., 2006
Tuna (*Thunnus thynnus)*	Kuwait	16	ND	0.0215	0.0403	a)	0.0103	0.0192	Al-Omair and Helaleh, 2004
	Catalonia , Spain	16	0.0000400	0.00116	0.0156	0.0000191	0.000554	0.00743	Perelló et al., 2009
	Catalonia, Spain	16	0.0000730	0.000674	0.00400	0.0000349	0.000322	0.00191	Llobet et al., 2006
	Tyrrhenian Sea, Italy	11	ND	0.00585-0.0134	0.00865-0.0281	a)	0.00279-0.00642	0.00413-0.0135	Perugini et al., 2007b

n - number of PAHs analyzed; ND – not detected; a) can not be estimated; b) value not specified in the article, but indicated that it is lower than the maximum level; c) blue whiting is a bathypelagic fish; d) the concentrations reported in µg/kg dry weight were multiplied by the conversion factor indicated by the authors to obtain the concentrations in µg/kg wet weight

Table 4. Concentrations (µg/kg of wet weight unless indicated otherwise) of benzo(a)pyrene (B(a)P), genotoxic and carcinogenic PAHs (PAH8) and total PAHs (∑PAHs), as well as estimated daily intake (µg/kg body weight per day) of B(a)P, PAH8 and ∑PAHs in benthopelagic finfish

Species	Location, Region	n PAHs	Fish meat (x10^{2} µg/kg)			Intake (x10^{-2} µg/kg body weight per day)			Ref.
			B(a)P	PAH8	∑PAHs	B(a)P	PAH8	∑PAHs	
African sicklefish (*Drepane Africana)*	Cotonou lagoon, République du Bénin	12	0.00352 a)	0.0183 a)	0.0586 a)	0.0168	0.0874	0.280	Soclo et al., 2008
Bighead carp (*Aristichthys nobilis)*	Hong Kong, China	16	ND	0.00130-0.00540	0.0284-0.0390	b)	0.00620-0.0258	0.135-0.186	Cheung et al., 2007
	Pearl River Delta, China	16	ND	<0.000100-0.0292	0.240-0.740	b)	<0.000478-0.139	1.15-3.53	Kong et al., 2005

Table 4. (Continued)

Species	Location, Region	n PAHs	Fish meat (x10^2 μg/kg)			Intake (x10^{-2} μg/kg body weight per day)			Ref.
			B(a)P	PAH8	∑PAHs	B(a)P	PAH8	∑PAHs	
Bleak (*Alburnus alburnus alborella)*	Lake Iseo, Italy	16	c)	c)	16.2	b)	b)	77.4	Binelli and Provini, 2004
Blotched snakehead *(Channa maculata)*	Hong Kong, China	16	ND	0.00510-0.00980	0.0784-0.146	b)	0.0243-0.0468	0.374-0.697	Cheung et al., 2007
Carp (*Cyprinus carpio)*	Lake Iseo, Italy	16	c)	c)	17.5	b)	b)	83.3	Binelli and Provini, 2004
Chub (*Leuciscus cephalus)*	Lake Iseo, Italy	16	c)	c)	8.10	b)	b)	38.7	Binelli and Provini, 2004
Common two-banded seabream *(Diplodus vulgaris)*	Alexandria cost, Egypt	16	43.1	50.8	57.4	206	243	274	Said, 2007
	Huelva, Spain	16	ND	ND	0.657	b)	b)	3.14	Bordajandi et al., 2004
	Abu Qir Bay, Egypt	16	0.325	11.5	15.1	1.55	54.8	72.1	El Deeb et al., 2007
Crucian carp *(Carassius auratus)*	Pearl River Delta, China	16	ND	<0.000100-0.0254	0.116-0.740	b)	<0.000478-0.121	0.554-3.53	Kong et al., 2005
Farmed Atlantic and Chinook salmon (*Salmo salar and Oncorhynchus tshawytscha)*	Pacific Coast	20	ND	0.00130	0.0830	b)	0.00620	0.397	Easton et al., 2002
Grey mullet *(Mulgil cephalus)*	Hong Kong, China	16	ND	0.00270-0.00630	0.0477-0.123	b)	0.0129-0.0301	0.228-0.588	Cheung et al., 2007
Herring *(Clupea harengus)*	Estonia	6	ND	ND	ND	b)	b)	b)	Yurchenko and Molder, 2005
Japanese gizzard shad *(Nematalosa japonica)*	Great Bitter lakes, Egypt	16	ND	160-162	194-197	b)	759-774	930-937	Said and Agroudy, 2006
Mandarin fish *(Siniperca kneri)*	Hong Kong, China	16	ND	0.00140-0.00820	0.0157-0.128	b)	0.00669-0.0391	0.0751-0.612	Cheung et al., 2007
Mandarin fish/ fresh water grouper *(Siniperca chuatsi)*	Pearl River Delta, China	16	ND	<0.000100-0.0694	0.554-1.31	b)	<0.000478-0.331	2.65-6.24	Kong et al., 2005
Mozambique tilapia *(Oreochromis mossambicus)*	Hong Kong, China	16	ND	0.00360-0.00860	0.0528-0.0547	b)	0.0172-0.0411	0.252-0.261	Cheung et al., 2007
	Pearl River Delta,	16	ND	<0.000100-	0.0191-	b)	<0.000478-	0.0915-	Kong et al., 2005

Species	Location, Region	n PAHs	Fish meat (x10^{2} µg/kg)			Intake (x10^{-2} µg/kg body weight per day)			Ref.
			B(a)P	PAH8	∑PAHs	B(a)P	PAH8	∑PAHs	
	China			0.0230	0.621		0.110	2.97	
Mozambique tilapia (*Sarotherodon mossambicus)*	Mai Po Marshes Nature Reserve, China	15	ND	0.00200-0.0130 a)	0.423-0.446 a)	b)	0.00955-0.0621	2.02-2.13	Liang et al., 2007
Mud carp *(Cirrhinus molitorella)*	Hong Kong, China	16	ND	0.00330-0.0145	0.0363-0.0818	b)	0.0158-0.0693	0.173-0.391	Cheung et al., 2007
Nile tilapia *(Oreochromis niloticus niloticus)*	Egypt/Kuwait	23	ND	0.0151 a)	0.523 a)	b)	0.0721	2.50	Alomirah et al., 2009
Pigsnout grunt *(Pomadasys rogerii)*	Cotonou lagoon, République du Bénin	12	ND	0.0129 a)	0.0512 a)	b)	0.0616	0.244	Soclo et al., 2008
Rainbow trout *(Oncorhynchus mykiss)*	Aquaculture, South of Italy	11	ND	0.540	1.95	b)	2.57	9.30	Visciano et al., 2008
Redbelly tilapia *(Tilapia zilli)*	El Temsah lake, Egypt	16	ND-2.90	140-202	140-202	≤13.8	669-967	669-967	Said and El Agroudy, 2006
Salmon *(Salmo salar)*	Reared in Norway, France	19	<0.000200	c)	c)	<0.000952	b)	b)	Varlet et al., 2007
	Catalonia, Spain	16	0.00108	0.00864	0.0600	0.00516	0.0413	0.286	Llobet et al., 2006
Silvery Pomfret *(Pampus argenteus)*	Arabian Gulf	14	ND	ND	17.8	b)	b)	84.8	Al-Hassan et al., 2003
	Kuwait city, Kuwait	23	ND	0.00384-0.00768 a)	0.124-0.341 a)	b)	0.0183-0.0367	0.592-1.63	Alomirah et al., 2009
Small snakehead *(Channa asiatica)*	Hong Kong, China	16	ND	0.00570-0.00950	0.106-0.130	b)	0.0272-0.0454	0.506-0.620	Cheung et al., 2007
Spotted snakehead *(Channa punctatus)*	Gomti river, India	16	ND	ND-0.110	0.129-0.349	b)	≤ 0.526	0.614-1.67	Malik et al., 2008
Tiger-toothed croaker *(Otolithes argenteus)*	Arabian Gulf	14	ND	ND	30.6	b)	b)	146	Al-Hassan et al., 2003
Tigertooth croaker *(Otolithes rubber)*	Kuwait city, Kuwait	23	ND	ND-0.00264 a)	0.0950-0.156 a)	b)	≤ 0.0126	0.454-0.745	Alomirah et al., 2009
Tilapia *(Tilapia sp.)*	Cotonou lagoon, République du Bénin	12	0.0120 a)	0.0221 a)	0.0914 a)	0.0573	0.106	0.436	Soclo et al., 2008
Tilapia fish (*Oreochromis aureus)*	Lake Timsah, Egypt	13	0.0690-0.969	1.10-3.27	1.12-15.9	0.330-4.63	5.26-15.6	5.33-75.9	Mostafa, 2002

Table 4. (Continued)

Species	Location, Region	n PAHs	Fish meat (x10^2 µg/kg)			Intake (x10^{-2} µg/kg body weight per day)			Ref.
			B(a)P	PAH8	∑PAHs	B(a)P	PAH8	∑PAHs	
Wild Chinook, Chum and Sockeye salmon d) (*Oncorhynchus tshawytscha, Oncorhynchus keta and Oncorhynchus nerka)*	Pacific Coast	20	ND	0.000600	0.130	b)	0.00286	0.620	Easton et al., 2002
Yellow croaker *(Pseudosciaena crocea)*	Hong Kong, China	16	ND	0.165-0.662	0.535-1.15	b)	0.789-3.16	2.55-5.49	Cheung et al., 2007

n - number of PAHs analyzed; ND – not detected; a) the concentrations reported in µg/kg dry weight were multiplied by the conversion factor indicated by the authors to obtain the concentrations in µg/kg wet weight; b) cannot be estimated; c) value not specified in the article, but indicated that it is lower than the maximum level; d) values for each fish species are not specified by the authors; sockeye salmon is a pelagic fish.

Table 5. Concentrations (µg/kg of wet weight unless indicated otherwise) of benzo(a)pyrene (B(a)P), genotoxic and carcinogenic PAHs (PAH8) and total PAHs (∑PAHs), as well as estimated daily intake (µg/kg body weight per day) of B(a)P, PAH8 and ∑PAHs in demersal finfish

Species	Location, Region	n PAHs	Fish meat (x10^3 µg/kg)			Intake (x10^{-1} µg/kg body weight per day)			Ref.
			B(a)P	PAH8	∑PAHs	B(a)P	PAH8	∑PAHs	
Bleeker's grouper *(Epinephelus bleekeri)*	Hong Kong, China	16	ND	0.00204-0.00366	0.0376-0.0458	a)	0.00975-0.0175	0.179-0.219	Cheung et al., 2007
Bogue (*Boops boops*) Pandora (*Pagellus* erythrinus) Rainbow wrass (*Coris julis)* Rock goby (*Gobius paganellus*) Scorpion fish (*Scorpaena scrofa*), Spotted	Campi Flegrei Bay, Italy	16	b)	b)	0.00500-0.812 0.00500-0.414	a)	a)	0.0239-3.88 0.0239-1.98	Amodio-Cocchieri et al., 2003

Species	Location, Region	n PAHs	Fish meat (x10^{3} µg/kg)			Intake (x10^{-1} µg/kg body weight per day)			Ref.
			B(a)P	PAH8	∑PAHs	B(a)P	PAH8	∑PAHs	
weever c) (*Trachinus araneus*)									
Cassava croaker (*Pseudotolithus senegalensis*)	Cotonou lagoon, République du Bénin	12	0.000356 d)	0.00115 d)	0.00442 d)	0.00170	0.00549	0.0211	Soclo et al., 2008
Catfish (*Clarias fuscus*)	Hong Kong, China	16	ND	0.000870-0.00181	0.00910-0.0248	a)	0.00415-0.00863	0.0434-0.118	Cheung et al., 2007
Croaker (*Micropogonias furnieri*) Kneeled mullet e) (*Mugil lisa*)	Guanabara Bay, Brazil	16	0.0000100-0.00310	0.00123-0.0943	0.00282-0.279	0.0000478-0.0148	0.00588-0.450	0.0135-1.33	da Silva et al., 2007
European eel (*Anguilla anguilla*)	Vaccarès lagoon, France	16	b)	b)	2.37-90.5 f)	a)	a)	11.3 - 432	Roche et al., 2002
European hake (*Merluccius merluccius*)	Catalonia, Spain	16	0.0000690	0.000552	0.00320	0.000330	0.00264	0.0153	Llobet et al., 2006
	Catalonia, Spain	16	0.0000400	0.000550	0.00606	0.000191	0.00263	0.0289	Perelló et al., 2009
European hake (*Merluccius merluccius*)	Tyrrhenian Sea, Italy	11	ND	0.00280-0.00714	0.00300-0.0120	a)	0.0134-0.0341	0.0144-0.0574	Perugini et al., 2007b
	Central Adriatic Sea, Italy	16	ND	0.000440-0.0407	0.00666-0.222	a)	0.00210-0.194	0.0318-1.06	Perugini et al., 2007a
European seabass (*Dicentrarchus labrax*)	Oporto, Portugal	16	ND	0.000770	0.0146	a)	0.00368	0.0695	Ramalhosa et al., 2009
Golden African snapper (*Lutjanus fulgens*)	Cotonou lagoon, République du Bénin	12	0.000364 d)	0.00392 d)	0.00812 d)	0.00174	0.0187	0.0388	Soclo et al., 2008
Golden threadfin bream (*Nemipterus virgatus*)	Hong Kong, China	16	ND	0.00396-0.0292	0.0406-0.118	a)	0.0189-0.139	0.194-0.563	Cheung et al., 2007
Grass carp (*Ctenopharyngodon idellus*)	Pearl River Delta, China	16	ND	<0.0000100-0.00608	0.0103-0.123	a)	<0.0000478-0.0290	0.0491-0.586	Kong et al., 2005

Table 5. (Continued)

Species	Location, Region	n PAHs	Fish meat (x10^3 μg/kg)			Intake (x10^{-1} μg/kg body weight per day)			Ref.
			B(a)P	PAH8	∑PAHs	B(a)P	PAH8	∑PAHs	
	Hong Kong, China	16	ND	0.000150-0.000350	0.00396-0.00409	a)	0.000716-0.00167	0.0189-0.0196	Cheung et al., 2007
Greenback mullet *(Liza subviridis)*	Arabian Gulf	14	ND	ND	2.43	a)	a)	11.6	Al-Hassan et al., 2003
Hake (*Merluccius merluccius)* Sardine g) (*Sardinna sp.)*	Catalonia, Spain	16	0.000235	0.00219	0.00789	0.00112	0.0104	0.0377	Falcó et al., 2003
Klunzinger's mullet *(Liza klunzingeri)*	Bay of Auha/Kuwait, Kuwait	16	0.0150-0.223 h)	0.0320-0.809 h)	1.08-7.20 h)	0.0716-1.06	0.153-3.86	5.16-34.4	Beg et al., 2009
	Kuwait city, Kuwait	23	ND	ND	0.0177 d)	a)	a)	0.0845	Alomirah et al., 2009
Nagahanadai *(Pseudanthias elongatus)*	Siokolo Fishing Settlement, Nigeria	16	6.78	80.9	100	32.4	386	478	Anyakora et al., 2005
Perch (*Perca fluviatilis)*	Lake Iseo, Italy	16	b)	b)	0.542	a)	a)	2.59	Binelli and Provini, 2004
Pike (*Esox lucius)*	Lake Iseo, Italy	16	b)	b)	0.945	a)	a)	4.52	Binelli and Provini, 2004
Red mullet *(Mullus barbatus)*	Central Adriatic Sea, Italy	16	ND	0.00152-0.0102	0.00441-0.0363	a)	0.00726-0.0486	0.0211-0.173	Perugini et al., 2007a
Rice field eel *(Monopterus albus)*	Hong Kong, China	16	ND	0.000590-0.00124	0.00831-0.0113	a)	0.00282-0.00741	0.0397-0.0539	Cheung et al., 2007
Silver hake	Estonia	6	ND	ND	ND	a)	a)	a)	Yurchenk

Species	Location, Region	n PAHs	Fish meat (x10^3 µg/kg)			Intake (x10^{-1} µg/kg body weight per day)			Ref.
			B(a)P	PAH8	∑PAHs	B(a)P	PAH8	∑PAHs	
(Merluccius bilinearis)									o and Molder, 2005
Sobaity seabream *(Sparidentex hasta)*	Kuwait city,Kuwait	23	ND	ND	0.00766 d)	a)	a)	0.0366	Alomirah et al., 2009
Sole *(Solea solea)*	Catalonia, Spain	16	0.0000790	0.000632	0.00250	0.000377	0.00302	0.0119	Llobet et al., 2006
	Abu Qir Bay, Egypt	16	0.358	0.929	1.77	1.71	4.43	8.41	El Deeb et al., 2007
	Huelva, Spain	16	ND	ND	0.0714	a)	a)	0.341	Bordajandi et al., 2004
Striped Red mullet *(Mullus surmuletus)*	Tyrrhenian Sea, Italy	11	ND	0.00375-0.0123	0.00925-0.0274	a)	0.0179-0.0588	0.0442-0.131	Perugini et al., 2007b
	Catalonia, Spain	16	0.0000800	0.000640	0.00310	0.000382	0.00306	0.0148	Llobet et al., 2006
Tench (*Tinca tinca)*	Lake Iseo, Italy	16	b)	b)	0.427	a)	a)	2.04	Binelli and Provini, 2004
Tongue sole (*Cynoglossus arel)*	Bay of Auha/Kuwait, Kuwait	16	0.395-1.85 h)	0.599-4.83 h)	4.42-15.0 h)	1.89-8.85	2.86-23.1	21.1-71.7	Beg et al., 2009
Tongue sole *(Cynoglossus robustus)*	Hong Kong, China	16	ND	0.00464-0.0164	0.0377-0.145	a)	0.0222-0.0781	0.180-0.693	Cheung et al., 2007
Yellow Finned Black Seabream *(Acanthopagrus latus)*	Arabian Gulf	14	0.720	2.40	4.11	3.44	11.5	19.6	Al-Hassan et al., 2003
	Hong Kong, China	16	ND	0.00653-0.0122	0.0570-0.0671	a)	0.0312-0.0583	0.272-0.321	Cheung et al., 2007
	Bay of Auha/Kuwait, Kuwait	16	0-0.399 h)	0.0520-1.11 h)	2.55-5.77 h)	≤1.91	0.248-5.31	12.2-27.5	Beg et al., 2009

Table 5. (Continued)

Species	Location, Region	n PAHs	Fish meat (x10^3 µg/kg)			Intake (x10^{-1} µg/kg body weight per day)			Ref.
			B(a)P	PAH8	∑PAHs	B(a)P	PAH8	∑PAHs	
	Kuwait city,Kuwait	23	ND	0.000576-0.00180 d)	0.0183-0.0593 d)	a)	0.00275-0.00859	0.0874-0.283	Alomirah et al., 2009

n - number of PAHs analyzed; ND – not detected; a) cannot be estimated; b) value not specified in the article, but indicated that it is lower than the maximum level; c) values for each fish species are not specified by the authors; pandora is a benthopelagic fish; rainbow wrass is a reef-associated fish; d) the concentrations reported in µg/kg dry weight were multiplied by the conversion factor indicated by the authors to obtain the concentrations in µg/kg wet weight; e) values for each fish specie are not specified by the authors; f) concentration expressed in µg/kg dry weight; g) values for each fish specie are not specified by the authors; sardine is a pelagic fish; mussels were analysed too; h) concentration expressed in µg/kg lipid weight.

Table 6. Concentrations (µg/kg of wet weight unless indicated otherwise) of benzo(a)pyrene (B(a)P), genotoxic and carcinogenic PAHs (PAH8) and total PAHs (∑PAHs), as well as estimated daily intake (µg/kg body weight per day) of B(a)P, PAH8 and ∑PAHs in reef-associated finfish

Species	Location, Region	n PAHs	Fish meat (x10^3 µg/kg)			Intake (x10^{-1} µg/kg body weight per day)			Ref.
			B(a)P	PAH8	∑PAHs	B(a)P	PAH8	∑PAHs	
Bartail flathead *(Platycephalus indicus)*	Hong Kong, China	16	ND	0.000530-0.000650	0.0356-0.0385	a)	0.00253-0.00310	0.170-0.184	Cheung et al., 2007
Bigeye *(Priacanthus macracanthus)*	Hong Kong, China	16	ND	0.000450-0.00197	0.0155-0.0683	a)	0.00215-0.00937	0.0740-0.326	Cheung et al., 2007
Doublebar Bream (*Acanthopagrus bifasciatus)*	Gulf coast, Saudi Arabia	6	b)	0.0201	0.0201	a)	0.0960	0.0960	Al-Saleh and Al-Doush, 2002
Dusky spinefoot *(Siganus luridus)*	Great Bitter lakes/El Temsah lake, Egypt	16	ND	6.00-81.3	6.00-115	a)	28.6-388	28.6-547	Said and El Agroudy, 2006
Emperors (*Lethrinus miniatus*)	Gulf coast, Saudi Arabia	6	b)	0.0139	0.0139	a)	0.0663	0.0663	Al-Saleh and Al-Doush, 2002
Goldspotted rabbitfish *(Siganus punctatus)*	Hong Kong, China	16	ND	0.00168-0.00278	0.0181-0.0248	a)	0.00804-0.0132	0.0863-0.118	Cheung et al., 2007
Greasy Grouper or Brown Spotted Grouper	Arabian Gulf	14	ND	ND	2.63	a)	a)	12.6	Al-Hassan et al., 2003

Species	Location, Region	n PAHs	Fish meat (x10^{3} µg/kg)			Intake (x10^{-1} µg/kg body weight per day)			Ref.
			B(a)P	PAH8	∑PAHs	B(a)P	PAH8	∑PAHs	
(Epinephelus tauvina)	Gulf coast, Saudi Arabia	6	b)	0.00627	0.00627	a)	0.0300	0.0300	Al-Saleh and Al-Doush, 2002
Grouper *(Epinephelus areolatus)*	Arabian Gulf	14	ND	12.8	18.1	a)	61.2	86.3	Al-Hassan et al., 2003
Haffara seabream *(Rhabdosargus haffara)*	Great Bitter lakes/El Temsah lake, Egypt	16	ND-1.60	ND-76.7	ND-76.7	≤7.66	≤366	≤366	Said and El Agroudy, 2006
Javelin grunter *(Pomadasys kaakan)*	Kuwait city, Kuwait	23	ND	0.000240-0.000600 c)	0.0157-0.0228 c)	a)	0.00115-0.00286	0.0750-0.109	Alomirah et al., 2009
Little tuna *(Euthynnus alleferatus)*	Alexandria coast, Egypt	16	5.69	6.81	6.94	27.2	32.5	33.1	Said, 2007
Marbled spinefoot *(Siganus rivulatus)*	Great Bitter lakes/El Temsah lake, Egypt	16	ND-0.650	ND-51.1	ND-179	≤ 3.10	≤ 244	≤ 856	Said and El Agroudy, 2006
Orange-spotted grouper *(Epinephelus coioides)*	Kuwait city, Kuwait	23	ND	0.000168-0.000768 c)	0.00958-0.0230 c)	a)	0.000802-0.00367	0.0457-0.110	Alomirah et al., 2009
	Hong Kong, China	16	ND	0.00115-0.00318	0.0302-0.0502	a)	0.00549-0.0152	0.144-0.240	Cheung et al., 2007
Shrimp scad *(Alepes djedaba)*	Alexandria coast, Egypt	16	32.9	35.4	35.7	157	169	170	Said, 2007
Silvery Grunt *(Pomadasys Kaakan)*	Arabian Gulf	14	ND	ND	2.25	a)	a)	10.7	Al-Hassan et al., 2003
Snapper *(Lutjanus sp.)*	Great Bitter lakes, Egypt	16	ND-0.286	32.5-42.3	32.5-68.2	≤ 1.37	155-202	155-326	Said and El Agroudy, 2006
Snubnose pompano *(Trachinotus blochii)*	Hong Kong, China	16	ND	0.0126-0.0176	0.0487-0.0672	a)	0.0602-0.841	0.233-0.321	Cheung et al., 2007
White-spotted spinefoot *(Siganus canaliculatus)*	Gulf coast, Saudi Arabia	6	b)	0.0112	0.0112	a)	0.0535	0.0535	Al-Saleh and Al-Doush, 2002

n - Number of PAHs analyzed; ND – not detected; a) cannot be estimated; b) not determined; c) the concentrations reported in µg/kg dry weight were multiplied by the conversion factor indicated by the authors to obtain the concentrations in µg/kg wet weight.

The concentrations of benzo(a)pyrene for all samples of Mediterranean mussels were below the maximum level except for those from Tyrrhenian Sea, Italy (13.5 μg/kg; Perugini et al., 2007b) and, Istanbul Strait and Marmara Sea, Turkey (Karacik et al., 2009). Istanbul Strait has been affected by urbanization, harbor activities, ship traffic, commercial fishing and by the pollutants entering from the Black Sea basin. In this study, both sediments and mussels contained high amount of PAHs. The most important contributors to PAH burdens in mussels were phenanthrene, benzo(b)fluoranthene, benzo(j)fluoranthene, fluoranthene, chrysene, pyrene, benz(a)anthracene and fluorine (Karacik et al., 2009). In Tyrrhenian Sea (Perugini et al., 2007b), 71.4% of mussels collected in winter exceeded the ML fixed for the benzo(a)pyrene, whereas all samples collected in summer reported values lower than this limit. The value obtained ranged from 44.5 to 212.3 μg/kg of fresh weight and appear particularly high if compared with some other data reported for Mediterranean areas (Law et al., 2000; Storelli & Marcotrigiano, 2001; Orbea et al., 2002; Llobet et al., 2006; Perugini et al., 2007a). This pattern of contamination could depend on the proximity of the sampling site to the filled in area and the presence of particularly contaminated sediments and materials dumped during landfill. Furthermore, it is important to consider that Pozzuoli Bay belongs to the Campi Flegrei volcano-tectonic system and represents the northern margin of a volcanic caldera. Its geology is very dynamic and related to an intense and relatively recent volcanic activity, displayed by underwater gas emissions and seismic movements (Romano et al., 2004).

The average concentration of benzo(a)pyrene in Blue mussels is generally much below ML; however, samples taken from Loch Leven, Scotland may contain as much as 795 μg/kg (McIntosh et al., 2004). The Blue mussel can accumulate PAHs in high concentrations without apparent detrimental effects and as such have been used extensively as indicator organisms (Topping et al., 1997). McIntosh et al. (2004) clearly observed, during 2000/2001 and 2001/2002 in mussels from the Kinlochleven and Ballachulish farms (Scotland), the seasonal cycle in PAHs concentration. The increase in PAH contents in mussels over late autumn and winter was consistent with the uptake of PAHs and deposition in the lipid rich tissue laid down during gamete maturation. Decreasing of PAH levels during spring was the result of a number of factors including loss of lipid rich tissue during spawning (McIntosh et al., 2004). Oysters (*Crassostrea* sp.), from Estuary of Urdaibai/Plentzia, Spain, show the same trend, and in winter PAHs content (208–218 μg/kg) was 3.5–7 times higher than in summer (31–59 μg/kg) (Orbea et al., 2002).

Clams (*Strombus tricornis* and *Venerupis decussata*) and gastropods (*Munes Sp.*) from Lake Timsah, Egypt, were found to be contaminated with benzo(a)pyrene concentrations of 14.8-114 and 24.8-284 μg/kg, respectively (Mostafa, 2002; Table 7). The residues were determined in either shells and in tissues (edible portion). The concentrations of total and carcinogenic PAHs were significantly higher in tissues than shells in both clams and gastropods. But these species are often prepared by the local population by boiling; thereby the residues of PAHs in the shells go to the soup. The residues of total and carcinogenic PAHs in tissues of gastropods were significantly higher than those in tissues of clams. This increase could be contributed to that the shells of clams are smoother than those of gastropods which may reduce the accumulation of PAHs in the clams.

Wedge shell *(Donax trunculus)* samples, also from Egypt (El Deeb et al., 2007), presented benzo(a)pyrene contents higher than the maximum level (Table 7).

Various studies have shown that bivalves are excellent sentinels for monitoring of bioavailable contaminants, such as PAHs for marine trends analyses (Oros et al., 2007). Mostafa et al. (2002) detected different residues of the total PAHs in different sizes of bivalve samples being significantly higher in big weight samples than small and medium one, respectively. However, there was no significant differences between big and medium samples in carcinogenic PAH residues. Fluorene, phenantherene, anthrathene, and chrysene were mostly absent in all tested samples (Mostafa et al., 2002).

Table 7. Concentrations (μg/kg of wet weight unless indicated otherwise) of benzo(a)pyrene (B(a)P), genotoxic and carcinogenic PAHs (PAH8) and total PAHs (∑PAHs), as well as estimated daily intake (μg/kg body weight per day) of B(a)P, PAH8 and ∑PAHs in bivalve mollusks

Species	Location, Region	n PAHs	Fish meat (x 10 μg/kg)			Intake ($x10^{-3}$ μg/kg body weight per day)			Ref.
			B(a)P	PAH8	∑PAHs	B(a)P	PAH8	∑PAHs	
Blue mussel (*Mytilus edulis)*	Loch Leven, Scotland	16	ND-79.5	a)	30.0-826	≤ 62.2	b)	23.5-646	McIntosh et al., 2004
	Cotonou lagoon, République du Bénin	12	0.0770 c)	1.21 c)	5.61 c)	0.0603	0.947	4.39	Soclo et al., 2008
Blue mussel (*Mytilus trossulus)*	Baltic sea, Poland	14	0.0280-0.238	0.611-1.98	0.864-2.97	0.0219-0.186	0.478-1.55	0.676-2.33	Potrykus et al., 2003
Clam (*Chamelea sp.)*	Huelva, Spain	16	ND	ND	4.04	b)	b)	3.16	Bordajandi et al., 2004
Clam (*Mya arenaria)*	St. Lawrence river, Canada	22	a)	a)	a)	b)	b)	b)	Gagnon et al., 2004
Clam (*Strombus tricornis)*	Lake Timsah, Egypt	13	2.71	4.87	4.91	2.12	3.81	3.84	Mostafa, 2002
Clam (*Tapes decussates)*	Catalonia, Spain	16	0.0197	0.276	2.15	0.0154	0.216	1.68	Llobet et al., 2006
Clam (*Tapes sp.)*	Huelva, Spain	16	ND	ND	5.23	b)	b)	4.09	Bordajandi et al., 2004
Clam (*Venerupis decussata)*	Lake Timsah, Egypt	13	1.48-11.4	11.5-20.5	13.5-23.7	1.16-8.88	9.00-16.0	10.5-18.6	Mostafa, 2002
Gastropod (*Munes sp)*	Lake Timsah, Egypt	13	2.48-28.4	9.62-77.8	11.0-84.8	1.94-22.2	7.53-60.9	8.59-66.4	Mostafa, 2002

Although the contamination is widespread, it varies greatly with geographic location, species, size, gender, *etc*. Normally, bivalve mollusks are filter-feeding organisms that retain particles larger than 4 μm and are exposed to both dissolved and particulate forms of PAHs present in the water column, which concentrate in their lipid tissue. Mussels absorb lower molecular weight PAHs through interstitial filtered water, whereas heavier weight PAHs are absorbed through the digestive system (Perugini et al., 2007b). Depuration, which is applied to clean the alimentary tract of live bivalve mollusks, does not significantly decrease the pollution with PAHs (Stołyhwo & Sikorski, 2005). In contrast to fish, their metabolic activity is low, so an equilibrium is reached between the PAH levels accumulated and those present in the marine environment.

The species that showed the highest total concentrations of PAHs were collected from stations affected by stronger human activities (industrial fallout, urban wastewaters, and contaminants transported via riverside discharge). In general and considering the total (∑PAHs) and carcinogenic PAHs (PAH8), the biota originating from Loch Leven (Scotland), Abu Qir Bay and Lake Timsah (Egypt), Campi Flegrei Bay (Italy) and from Istanbul Strait/Marmara Sea (Turkey) show the higher bioaccumulation pattern. From a human health perspective it is important to assess whether PAHs pose a risk, especially in regions where fish provides a cheap and readily available source of protein. The median dietary exposure was calculated by assuming that a 70 kg individual will consume 2.0 kg/year *per capita* (world mollusks *per capita* consumption in 2005, FAO, 2009). Samples taken from these polluted waters may promote a benzo(a)pyrene, PAH8 (the sum of benzo(a)pyrene, benz(a)anthracene, benzo(b)fluoranthene, benzo(k)fluoranthene, benzo(g,h,i)perylene, chrysene, dibenz(a,h)anthracene and indeno(1,2,3-cd)pyrene) and total PAHs dietary intake as much as 0.0622, 0.0609 and 0.646 µg/kg body weight per day, respectively (Table7). Both low-risk groups (adolescents and adults) and high-risk groups (pregnant mothers and children) should consume bivalve mollusks in moderation since large consumption pattern may result in increased health risks.

Using the published data, dependence between the benzo(a)pyrene concentration, PAH4 and PAH8 *versus* the total amount of PAHs was evaluated. In contrast with the other set of data, benzo(a)pyrene *vs* PAH8 and benzo(a)pyrene *vs* total PAHs were found to be linear (quadratic correlation coefficient of 0.67 and 0.91, respectively; coefficient of 0.35 for PAH4 *versus* ∑PAHs). R^2 values above 0.5 indicate that there is a reasonable goodness of fit for the linear regression (EFSA, 2007c).

6. PAHs Levels in Crustaceans, Cephalopods, other than Smoked

Of the 16.4 kg of fish *per capita* available for consumption in 2005, about 1.6 kg consisted of crustaceans and 0.5 kg of cephalopods (FAO, 2009). Marine species consumption differs among countries, and within countries it differs among segments of society. These differences reflect consumer preferences, availability, product developments, prices and levels of disposable income. Cephalopods are mainly consumed in Mediterranean and Asian countries whereas the consumption of crustaceans, being high-priced commodities, is concentrated mainly in affluent economies. However, as a result of the increased production of shrimps and prawns from aquaculture and the consistent decrease in their price, *per capita* availability of crustaceans increased more than threefold, from 0.4 to 1.6 kg between 1961 and 2005 (FAO, 2009).

Commission Regulation (EC) 1881/2006 specifies a maximum level of 5.0 µg/kg for benzo(*a*)pyrene in crustaceans and cephalopods other than smoked (Table 2). The reported values during the period of 2000 to 2009 for these two categories are summarized in Table 8.

Most of the species are less contaminated than 5 μg/kg, although far higher concentrations were found in Crabs (*Portunus pelagicus* from Egypt (Mostafa, 2002) and *Carcinus maenas* from Spain (Orbea et al., 2002)) and occasionally in Tiger prawn ((*Penaeus japonicus*) from Egypt; (El Deeb et al., 2007). In about 57% of the analyzed samples, benzo(a)pyrene was not detected but other carcinogenic and genotoxic PAHs were present reaching a maximum total value (PAH8) of 113 μg/kg (*ca.* 88% of the sum of all determined PAHs) in European flying squid (*Todarodes sagittatus*) from Tyrrhenian Sea, Italy (Table 8). In the samples positive for benzo(a)pyrene, the highest PAH8 was attained, in decreasing order, in crabs, prawns, shrimps, squids and cuttlefish. The much higher concentrations of PAHs in crabs could be contributed to the nature of their bodies which helps to accumulate, and their very limited ability to carry out metabolic transformation of PAHs (Mostafa, 2002).

Table 8. Concentrations (μg/kg of wet weight unless indicated otherwise) of benzo(a)pyrene (B(a)P), genotoxic and carcinogenic PAHs (PAH8) and total PAHs (∑PAHs), as well as estimated daily intake (μg/kg body weight per day) of B(a)P, PAH8 and ∑PAHs in crustaceans and cephalopods

Species	Location, Region	n PAHs	Fish meat (x 10 μg/kg)			Intake ($x10^{-3}$ μg/kg body weight per day)			Ref.
			B(a)P	PAH8	∑PAHs	B(a)P	PAH8	∑PAHs	
Blue and red shrimp *(Aristeus antennatus)*	Tyrrhenian Sea, Italy	11	ND	0.293 - 0.906	0.598-1.93	a)	0.183 - 0.567	0.374-1.21	Perugini et al., 2007b
Blue crab *(Portunus pelagicus)*	Lake Timsah, Egypt	13	32.6-99.0	127-374	132-377	20.4-62.0	79.2-234	82.6-236	Mostafa, 2002
Crab *(Carcinus maenas)*	Estuary of Urdaibai/Plentzia, Spain	14	0.0300-2.47	0.240-15.0	0.940-22.2	0.0188-1.55	0.150-9.36	0.589-13.9	Orbea et al., 2002
Cuttlefish *(Sepia esculenta)*	Huelva, Spain	16	ND	ND	2.18	a)	a)	0.427	Bordajandi et al., 2004
	Catalonia, Spain	16	0.00740	0.0629	0.300	0.00145	0.0123	0.0587	Llobet et al., 2006
European flying squid *(Todarodes sagittatus)*	Central Adriatic Sea, Italy	16	ND	0.00500-0.0200	0.117-7.64	a)	0.000978-0.00391	0.0229-1.49	Perugini et al., 2007a
	Tyrrhenian Sea, Italy	11	ND	0.379-11.3	1.11-12.8	a)	0.0742-2.20	0.217-2.50	Perugini et al., 2007b
European squid *(Loligo vulgaris)*	Catalonia, Spain	16	0.00790	0.0632	0.300	0.00155	0.0124	0.0587	Llobet et al., 2006

Published information concerning PAH levels in cephalopods is scarce. Only four studies characterizing three species, namely European flying squid (*Todarodes sagittatus)*, European squid (*Loligo vulgaris)* and Cuttlefish (*Sepia esculenta*), from Italy and Spain were found (Bordajandi et al., 2004; Llobet et al., 2006; Perugini et al., 2007a, 2007b). Benzo(a)pyrene was only detected in European squid and cuttlefish species well below the maximum level.

Although being carnivorous, feeding mainly on small fish, crustaceans and other cephalopods, squids live pelagically which may limit exposure to the higher molecular weight PAHs (≥ 4 rings) that remain mainly in the sediments (Baird et al., 2007; Means, 1998). These results are in agreement with a case study performed in Catalonia, Spain, about the health risks arising from the dietary intake of chemical contaminants through consumption of edible marine species (Domingo, 2007a). Both cuttlefish and squid (and the finfish sole (*Solea solea*)) showed the lowest mean total concentrations of PAHs. Using a body weight of 70 kg and the *per capita* consumption of crustaceans (1.6 kg) and cephalopods (0.5 kg) in 2005 (FAO, 2009), the values obtained for contaminant intake estimation in adults of benzo(a)pyrene varied between 1.55×10^{-6} μg/kg b.w. per day (for European squid) and 6.20×10^{-2} μg/kg b.w. per day (for crabs). Using PAH8 to evaluate the intake of PAHs classified as probable/possible human carcinogen, and total PAHs, the two highest contributors to the dietary exposure were Blue crab and Tiger prawn from Egypt.

Using the published data within the period of 2000 to 2009, dependence between benzo(a)pyrene concentration, PAH4 and PAH8 *versus* total amount of PAHs was evaluated and quadratic correlation coefficients of 0.9739, 0.9957 and 0.9884 were obtained, respectively. It is interesting to notice that as indicated by the EFSA Panel on Contaminants in the Food Chain (EFSA, 2008), PAH4 and PAH8 are slightly better indicators than benzo(a)pyrene for the occurrence of PAHs in crustaceans and cephalopods.

7. PAHs Levels in Smoked Fish and Smoked Fishery Products

Fish is one of the most versatile food commodities and can be utilized in a great variety of ways and product forms. It is usually distributed as live, fresh, chilled, frozen, heat-treated, fermented, dried, smoked, salted, pickled, boiled, fried, freeze-dried, minced, powdered or canned, or as a combination of two or more of these forms. However, fish can also be preserved by many other methods (FAO, 2009). Smoking is one of the oldest methods of food preservation and is still widely used in fish processing. In Europe, about 15% of the total amount of fish for human consumption is offered on the market in the form of smoked products.

Commission Regulation (EC) 1881/2006 specifies a maximum level of 5.0 μg/kg for benzo(a)pyrene in muscle meat of smoked fish and smoked fishery products, excluding bivalve mollusks (Table 2). The maximum level applies to smoked crustaceans, excluding the brown meat of crab and excluding head and thorax meat of lobster and similar large crustaceans (*Nephropidae and Palinuridae*).

The concentration of benzo(a)pyrene was below the maximum level of 5.0 μg/kg for all smoked fishes, with the exception of hot-smoked mackerel (*Scomber scombrus*) from Thessaloniki market, Greece (Iliadis et al., 2004) (Table 9). Iliadis et al. (2004) compared the levels of benzo(a)pyrene, fluoranthene and perylene in cold and in hot smoked fishes of the same origin. The amount of the above PAHs was higher in the hot-smoked mackerel samples (9.2±0.01, 7.8±0.03 and 9.4±0.14 μg/kg for benzo(a)pyrene, fluoranthene and perylene, respectively) than in the cold-smoked mackerel samples (2.1±0.07, 4.3±0.04 and 7.2±0.05 μg/ They concluded that the type of smoking process affected the production of all three PAHs, since the production of these compounds is influenced by temperature. Yurchenko and Molder (2005) observed the same pattern of variation. In this work, the level of six PAHs (benzo(a)pyrene, benz(a)anthracene, benzo(k)fluoranthene, benzo(b)fluoranthene, benzo(g,h, i)perylene and indeno(1,2,3-cd)pyrene) was determined in 84 samples of hot-smoked fish (mackerel, bream, trout, salmon, herring, herring in tomato sauce, silver hake, cod, burbot, Sea perch, Pike, Sprat, Sprats in tomato sauce (Table 9)), 13 samples of cold-smoked fish (mackerel, salmon and herring (Table 9)), in 32 smoked samples in oil (Sprats (Table 9)) and 11 samples of fresh fish (Herring & Silver hake) purchased from Estonian market. In samples of fresh fish, the level of PAHs was not detected.

In 20 of 84 samples of commercially hot-smoked fish, the concentration of benzo(a)pyrene exceeded 1 μg/kg (maximum level established in Estonia for smoked fish; The Decision of the Government of the Republic of Estonia, 2000).

The levels of PAHs in fresh and cold-smoked fish were lower than in hot-smoked fish samples. The highest PAHs levels were found in samples of smoked sprats in oil (12.4 μg/kg). The temperature of the smoke is < 35°C during cold-smoking. In hot-smoking, the process may be carried out in different stages, during which the temperature of the smoke ranges from about 50–100°C and that in the centre of the product may reach up to 85°C (Stolyhwo & Sikorski, 2005). The composition of the smoke and the conditions of processing affect the sensory quality, shelf life, and wholesomeness of the product. Traditional smoking technique involves treating of pre-salted, whole or filleted fish with wood smoke. The smoke is produced by smouldering shavings or sawdust of certain kind of wood (beech, hickory, oak) in the oven directly below the hanging fish. Furthermore, the smoke could be added in the smoking chamber from external smoke generators under controlled conditions of temperature and air access. During this combustion undesirable compounds can be formed, mainly the polycyclic aromatic hydrocarbons. PAHs contamination of smoked foods can be significantly reduced by replacing direct smoking, in which smoke is developed inside the smoking chamber where fish are located, with indirect smoking, by an external smoke generator, or by the use of liquid smoke flavorings, produced from condensed smoke. These flavourings agents are generally smoke extracts, filtered and separated from the resinous material that contains most of the PAHs. The liquid smoke flavourings are produced according to the Commission Regulation (EC) No. 2065/2003 of the European Parliament and of the Council of 10 November 2003 on smoke flavourings used or intended for use in or on food (Commission Regulation (EC) No. 2065/2003), which provides the adoption of appropriate provisions concerning source materials used for the production of smoke flavourings and reaction conditions under which they are prepared (Visciano et al., 2008). A lowering of the PAHs content in products smoked with this type of flavoring has been reported by some authors (Gomaa et al., 1993; Chen and Lin, 1997; Visciano et al., 2008) and by the EFSA (EFSA 2007c).

PAH amounts of different samples appear not strictly related to the different smoking technologies applied. For smoked Trout (*Oncorhynchus mykiss*) and Herring (*Clupea harengus*) (Table 9), the differences between samples of the same specie (of different provenance) are bigger than those among samples of different groups. Visciano et al. (2008) characterised the PAH levels of farmed rainbow trout processed by traditional flue gas smoking and by liquid smoke flavourings.

Table 9. Concentrations (μg/kg of wet weight unless indicated otherwise) of benzo(a)pyrene (B(a)P), genotoxic and carcinogenic PAHs (PAH8) and total PAHs (∑PAHs), as well as estimated daily intake (μg/kg body weight per day) of B(a)P, PAH8 and ∑PAHs in smoked finfish

Species	Location, Region	n PAHs	Fish meat (x 10 μg/kg)			Intake (x10-4 μg/kg body weight per day)			Ref.
			B(a)P	PAH8	∑PAHs	B(a)P	PAH8	∑PAHs	
Atlantic Bonito (Sarda sarda)	Black Sea, Turkey	1							Duyar et al., 2008
Smoking with mixed woods			0.0220	0.0220	0.0220	0.215	0.215	0.215	
Smoking with apple wood			0.00880	0.00880	0.00880	0.0861	0.0861	0.0861	
Burbot (Lota lota) Hot-smoked	Estonia	6	0.0330	0.378	0.378	0.323	3.70	3.70	Yurchenko and Molder, 2005
Cod (Gadus ogac) Hot-smoked	Estonia	6	0.00500	0.309	0.309	0.489	3.02	3.02	Yurchenko and Molder, 2005
Herring (Clupea harengus) Cold-smoked	Estonia	6	ND	ND	ND	a)	a)	a)	Yurchenko and Molder, 2005
Direct and indirect smoking	Denmark	27	< 0.00800-0.390	b)	3.40 - 139	<0.0783-3.82	a)	33.3-136	Duedahl-Olesen et al., 2006
Hot-smoked	Estonia	6	0.0720	0.548	0.548	0.705	5.36	5.36	Yurchenko and Molder, 2005
Herring in tomato sauce (Clupea harengus) Hot-smoked	Estonia	6	0.0810	0.667	0.667	0.793	6.53	6.53	Yurchenko and Molder, 2005
Mackerel (Scomber scombrus) Cold-smoked	Estonia	6	ND	ND	ND	a)	a)	a)	Yurchenko and Molder, 2005

The following compounds, anthracene, fluoranthene, pyrene, benz(a)anthracene, chrysene, benzo(b)fluoranthene, benzo(k)fluoranthene and benzo(g,h,i)perylene were detected in all samples and no significant difference ($p > 0.05$) was found between processed samples by the two different smoking techniques, except for chrysene and benzo(b)fluoranthene (Visciano et al., 2008). It is interesting to notice that the levels determined by these authors in aquacultured trout, reaching 54.1 μg/kg for genotoxic and carcinogenic PAHs (the maximum concentration found in all published data concerning smoked samples) and 182 μg/kg for total PAHs, are much higher than the reported values in other studies concerning trout (ranging from not detected to 3 μg/kg for PAH8 and from 3 to 103 μg/kg for total PAHs) (Moret et al., 1999; Yurchenko & Molder, 2005; Duedahl-Olesen et al., 2006).

The highest value of total PAHs was found in Herring collected during a survey performed in 2004 in Denmark attaining a maximum value of 1390 μg/kg in some samples (Duedahl-Olesen et al., 2006). This result is comparably higher than the obtained by Yurchenko and Molder (Yurchenko & Molder, 2005) from Estonian Herring smoked and processed in several ways (Table 9).

Although the contents of benzo(a)pyrene in smoked fish are, on average, not higher than the limit set by different national and World regulations, the intake of benzo(a)pyrene, PAH8 and total PAHs from the several smoked species presented in Table 9 were calculated for a 70 kg person. The estimates were based on data for Europe (15% of 16.4 kg *per capita* consumption of seafood, 2005) since world *per capita* consumption of this type of processed products was not found. The dietary exposure by the general population may attain 90 μg/kg b.w. per day for benzo(a)pyrene alone (hot-smoked Mackerel from Greece; Iliadis et al., 2004), 529 μg/kg b.w. per day for PAH8 (farmed and traditionally flue gas smoked Rainbow trout from Italy; Visciano et al., 2008) and as large as 13600 μg/kg b.w. per day for total PAHs (Herring from Denmark; Duedahl-Olesen et al., 2006), respectively.

A comparison was also made between benzo(a)pyrene levels and PAH4, PAH8, as well as total PAH contents. By decreasing order, the best fits for the three linear regression tested, with benzo(a)pyrene as the independent variable, were observed for PAH4 (quadratic correlation coefficient of 0.66), PAH8 (quadratic correlation coefficient of 0.42) and total PAHs (quadratic correlation coefficient of 0.11). Based on the data collected in this chapter that correspond to distinct seafood categories (finfish, bivalve mollusks, crustaceans, cephalopods, smoked fish and smoked fishery products), it seems that benzo(a)pyrene represents very poorly PAH contamination in smoked fish and smoked fishery products. Comparatively with the other groups, an additional source of PAHs contamination may be introduced in the raw material by the smoking process. The control of some important parameters such as smoke generation, temperature, time, distribution, humidity and circulation rate, can contribute to the minimization of PAHs contamination, especially when traditional smoking techniques are applied.

8. Analytical Methods for Determination of PAHs in Seafood

PAHs are typically present in the environment and in foodstuff as mixtures. The composition of these mixtures can vary, depending on the source of pollution, the type of sample or even the time between pollution and measurement (Karsten, 2002; Srogi, 2007). The complex mixture of these similar molecules makes detailed analysis of PAH contaminations often difficult, and various approaches are described in the literature (Ali & Cole, 2002; Martinez et al., 2004; Pensado et al., 2005; Navarro et al., 2006; Tudorache & Bala, 2007; Duedahl-Olesen & Ghorbani, 2008; Castro et al., 2009; Hyötyläinen, 2009). Research is carried out in PAHs extraction, separation and specific detection. At present, there is still a lack of officially approved methods that would solve the difficulties associated with quantitative isolation of PAHs from the food material, clean-up of the extract without significant loss of the analyte, separation of all individual PAHs contained in the purified extract, detection of the separated components, unequivocal identification of the PAHs, and quantification of the identified compounds. In particular, methods do not include many of the dibenzopyrenes or 5-methylcrysene selected by The Scientific Committee on Food and the Joint FAO/WHO Expert Committee for evaluation in food.

During sampling and preparation, precautions shall be taken to avoid any changes in composition of the sample. Containers shall be rinsed with high purity acetone or hexane before use to minimize the risk of contamination. Wherever possible, apparatus and equipment coming into contact with the sample shall be made of inert materials such as aluminum, glass or polished stainless steel. Plastics such as polypropylene or polytetrafluoroethylene (PTFE) shall be avoided because PAHs can adsorb onto these materials (EFSA, 2007c). Furthermore, losses of PAHs may occur in samples exposed to light and high temperatures during sample collection and storing, or due to their reaction with other matrix substances during a long-term storage.

Efficiency of PAHs extraction depends upon the polarity of the solvent, on the nature of the matrix, and on the preparation of the sample (Hyötyläinen, 2009). PAHs recovery can be high when samples are totally soluble in the organic solvents used for extraction, e.g., some dairy products. However, in fish, although PAHs accumulate preferentially in the lipid tissue, they diffuse also into the muscles, where they may be bound by some structural elements (Stołyhwo & Sikorski, 2005). From the analytical point of view, isolation of fat-soluble analytes, such as PAHs from biological matrices, often involves the hydrolysis of lipids by an alkaline saponification before the extraction of analytes (Jánska et al., 2006; Perugini et al., 2007a, 2007b; Visciano et al., 2008; Alomirah et al., 2009). Traditionally, Soxhlet extraction has been used for solid samples and liquid-liquid extraction for aqueous samples. However, these techniques have inherent disadvantages, for example the large volumes of organic solvents required. They are also time-consuming and involve multistep processes that have always the risk of loss of some analytes (Song et al., 2002; Martinez et al., 2004; Dreyer & Radke, 2005). Supercritical-fluid extraction (Ali & Cole, 2002), pressurized liquid extraction (Wang et al., 1999; Lacorte et al., 2006; Liguori et al., 2006; Ackerman et al., 2008; Duedahl-Olesen & Ghorbani, 2008), microwave-assisted extraction (Navarro et al., 2006; Pena et al., 2006; Soclo et al., 2008), batch extraction enhanced by sonication (Jánska et al., 2006; Webster et al., 2007), matrix solid-phase dispersion (Pensado et al., 2005), and subcritical water extraction (Storelli & Marcotrigiano, 2001; Easton et al., 2002) have been developed as alternative techniques to replace classical extraction methods (Sanz-Landaluze et al., 2006; Ridgway et al., 2007). Supercritical fluid extraction is less frequently used, probably due to a strong dependence of optimal parameters setting on sample composition (fat and moisture), which is the cause of a rather low robustness of supercritical fluid extraction-based procedures (Jánska et al., 2006). Recently, the approach developed by Anastassiades et al. (2003) for pesticides extraction and named as quick, easy, cheap, effective, rugged, and safe (QuEChERS), was also evaluated to extract a selected group of 16 PAHs from homogenized fish samples (Ramalhosa et al., 2009). All these methods reduce extraction time and the volumes of solvent required, but some have the disadvantages of high investment and maintenance costs of the instruments (i.e., supercritical-fluid extraction, pressurized liquid extraction, and microwave-assisted extraction). Studies have shown that once optimized, these new extraction techniques are comparably efficient, with similar standard deviations (Ridgway et al., 2007; Ramalhosa et al., 2009). For evaluation of PAH in marine biota Soxhlet is, even nowadays, the principal extraction technique, especially for routine studies (Orbea et al., 2002; Oros & Ross, 2005; Tolosa et al., 2005).

Given the complexity of the matrices, after extraction more or less complicated clean up procedures need to be applied to provide extracts ready for the accurate analytical determination (Pena et al., 2006). Column chromatography (Wan et al., 2007; Cheung et al., 2007), solid phase extraction (SPE) (Duedahl-Olesen & Ghorbani, 2008; Malik et al., 2008; Siddiqi et al., 2009) and gel permeation chromatography (GPC) are the main sample purification techniques used for isolating PAHs from interfering matrix substances. Recently, especially the automatic GPC technique has been applied for cleaning up PAH sample extracts of edible marine species (Jánska et al., 2006; Llobet et al., 2006; Cheung et al., 2007; Duedahl-Olesen & Ghorbani, 2008; Beg et al., 2009).

Nowadays, the main analytical techniques sufficiently sensitive for determining PAH concentrations in foods are high-performance liquid chromatography (HPLC) coupled with fluorescence (FL) or UV absorbance detection (for non-fluorescent compounds) (Pena et al., 2006; Johnson et al., 2007; Perugini et al., 2007a, 2007b; Visciano et al., 2008; Ramalhosa et al., 2009) or gas chromatography (GC) with mass spectrometric detection (MS) (Varlet et al., 2007a, 2007b; Beg et al., 2009; Cho et al., 2009). These two separation–detection alternatives were chosen as US Environmental Protection Agency methods 8310 (EPA, 1986a) and 8100 (EPA, 1986b), respectively. GC-MS methods have become popular due to the selectivity of the MS-detector, the use of mass spectrum data for reliable confirmation of PAHs, and the possibility to use isotope labeled PAHs as internal standards. Single quadrupole MS is the most applied technique but the use of tandem mass spectrometry is increasing, since it gives more specific mass fragments (daughter ions) and hence improves specificity and sensitivity of the MS-methods (Varlet et al., 2007a, 2007b). Limit of detections and recoveries for PAHs are compound, food matrix and method dependent. The detection limits for PAHs typically range from 0.01 to 1 μg/kg. However, for some PAHs lower and higher values are determined (EFSA, 2007c, 2008a).

In what concerns sample preparation and according to the survey performed in the European Union during 2006 and 2007 (EFSA, 2007c), the most common methods referred by the involved laboratories were saponification in a shaking water bath at 60°C and liquid/liquid extraction. Concerning the analytical method applied, 4% of the participants indicated GC with a flame ionization detector (FID), 28% HPLC-FL, 26% HPLC-FL/UV and 43% GC-MS (EFSA, 2007c). Limits of detection reported for the 25 PAHs determined in the different food categories varied between 0.0002 and 1 μg/kg for the respective PAH except for cyclopenta(*cd*)pyrene with a maximum of 6 μg/kg (EFSA, 2007c).

Recently, a wide range of immunoassays and immunosensors for environmental analytes such as PAHs are being investigated, using various detection systems such as amperometric, capacitative, conductimetric, potentiometric, fluorimetric, radioactive and UV detection (Li et al., 2000; Fähnrich et al., 2002, 2003; Baggiani et al., 2007; Tudorache & Bala., 2007; Del Carlo et al., 2008; Palchetti & Mascini, 2008). Despite offering a number of advantages, such as low cost, ease of use, often portability, disposability and rapid analyte detection, they are normally restricted to aqueous solutions or solutions containing only small amounts of organic solvents. The antibodies and enzymes involved are frequently of limited stability and for PAHs they show strong cross-reactivities towards other PAH compound or structurally related molecules (Li et al., 2000; Karsten, 2002; Fähnrich et al., 2002, 2003; Baggiani et al., 2007; Tudorache & Bala., 2007; Del Carlo et al., 2008; Palchetti & Mascini, 2008).

Conclusion

Seafood is a nutrient-rich food that makes a positive contribution to a healthful diet. It is a good source of proteins, and relative to other protein foods, e.g., meat, poultry, and eggs, is generally lower in saturated fatty acids and higher in the omega-3 fatty acids (eicosapentaenoic acid and docosahexaenoic acid) as well as selenium (Nesheim & Yaktine, 2007). It is also a good source of calcium, phosphorus, iron, trace elements like copper, and a fair proportion of the B-vitamins (Nesheim & Yaktine, 2007). Dietary guidelines recommend that healthy adults eat at least two servings of fish (particularly fatty fish) per week (Kris-Etherton et al., 2002, 2003). There are large variations across countries and regions of the world in the amount of total fish supply for human consumption, reflecting different eating habits and traditions, availability of fish and other foods, prices, socio-economic levels, and seasons. Differences are also evident within countries, with consumption usually higher in coastal areas (FAO, 2009). *Per capita* fish consumption in higher-income countries is expected to continue growing, but at a slower pace than in recent decades. Rising incomes and the ensuing diversification of diets are leading to a shift towards significantly higher fish consumption in developing countries (FAO, 2009).

Beside attractive health benefits of fish, there were many reports on contamination of fish by environmental chemicals. Some PAHs are known genotoxic and carcinogenic compounds that are unavoidably present in some seafood products and cannot be completely avoided in the diet. They are natural and man-made chemical contaminants that result from environmental pollution and/or products of food processing. In order to provide risk managers and consumers with health advice, genotoxic and carcinogenic PAHs require the fullest possible risk assessment (EFSA, 2008b; Barlow & Schlatter, 2009). State of art of analytical methodologies based on extraction of the PAHs from the matrix, clean-up procedure, separation by gas chromatography or high performance liquid chromatography, followed by detection and quantification by mass spectrometry or fluorescence/ultraviolet detectors, respectively, allow to determine individual PAH in marine biota at concentrations of 0.01

μg/kg or less (Stołyhwo & Sikorski, 2005; EFSA, 2007c; EFSA, 2008). As scientific community has recognized that there is no identifiable threshold below which these compounds do not pose risk to humans and aiming to minimize PAHs harmful effects on public health, the European Union settled maximum levels for benzo(a)pyrene in foodstuffs containing fats and oils and foods where environmental pollution or smoking and drying processes might cause high levels of contamination, such as seafood. Further analyses of the relative proportions of genotoxic and carcinogenic PAHs in foods would be necessary to inform a future review of the suitability of maintaining benzo(a)pyrene as a marker.

Available information indicated that the contents of benzo(a)pyrene in several seafood categories are, on average and except for particular highly contaminated locations, not higher than the limits set by international or national regulations. For high-risk geographic areas, domestic or foreign government agencies should consider the option of mandatory labeling and the existing regulations to minimize chemical and biological contamination of the aquatic environment should be strengthened and enforced (Ahmed, 1991). In general terms, the highest PAH concentrations were found in bivalve mollusks and in crustaceans. Some of these species may contribute significantly to the intake of PAHs if such foods are a large part of the usual diet. The extent of PAHs bioaccumulation in seafood depends on such factors as geographic location, feeding patterns, solubility and lipophilicity of the compounds (related to the number of aromatic rings of PAHs), and their persistence in the environment. Moreover, species of fish that contribute to the human diet are generally predators of other fish and, in some cases, predators of predators. Consequently, PAHs may bioaccumulate along the food chain. Absorption of contaminants combined with certain lifestyles may result in a marked increase in the cancer risk related to these contaminants. For example, the ingestion of seafood contaminated with PAHs combined with the inhalation of cigarette smoke (Castro et al., 2009) gives the smoker a much higher risk of developing cancer than that predicted by an additive model for these two substances. Furthermore, using a body weight of 70 kg for contaminant intake estimations in adults necessarily underestimated the intakes and risks for children because they eat three to four times more food in proportion to their body size than do adults and therefore ingest larger amounts of chemical per unit of body mass (EPA 2003).

Balancing adequately the risks and benefits of seafood consumption is currently a nutritional/environmental health key issue. In order to minimize risks and PAHs impact on public health, continuous monitoring of their presence in food and in the environment is necessary. As it has already been stated by other authors (Domingo, 2007b), regional/national food and health administrations should be able to provide uniform and consistent advice to consumers on the most recommendable species. The main objective will be to maximize the intake of omega-3 fatty acids and minimize that of chemical pollutants, and inform about the most suitable frequency of consumption, and the most adequate meal size for each species.

References

Ackerman, LK; Schwindt, AR; Simonich, SLM; Koch, DC; Blett, TF; Schreck, CB; Kent, ML; Landers, DH. Atmospherically deposited PBDEs, pesticides, PCBs, and PAHs in Western US National Park fish: Concentrations and consumption guidelines. *Environmental Science and Technology*, 2008, 42, 2334-2341.

Ahmed, FE. *Seafood Safety*. Committee on Evaluation of the Safety of Fishery Products. Washington, DC: National Academy Press; 1991.

Al-Hassan, JM; Afzal, M; Rao, CVN; Fayad, S. Polycyclic aromatic hydrocarbons (PAHs) and aliphatic hydrocarbons (PAHs) in edible fish from the Arabian Gulf. *Bulletin of Environmental Contamination and Toxicology*, 2003, 70, 205-212.

Ali, MdY; Cole, RB. One-step SFE-plus-C-18 selective extraction of low-polarity compounds, with lipid removal, from smoked fish and bovine milk. *Analytical and Bioanalytical Chemistry*, 2002, 374, 923-931.

Al-Omair, A; Helaleh, MIH. Selected-ion storage GC-MS analysis of polycyclic aromatic hydrocarbons in palm dates and tuna fish. *Chromatographia*, 2004, 59, 715-719.

Alomirah, H; Al-Zenki, S; Husain, A; Ahmed, N; Al-Rashdan, A; Gevao, B; Sawaya, W. Dietary exposure to polycyclic aromatic hydrocarbons from commercially important seafood of the Arabian Gulf. Journal *of Food Agriculture and Environment*, 2009, 7, 9-15.

Al-Saleh, I; Al-Doush, I. Gas chromatography-mass spectrometric determination of polycyclic aromatic hydrocarbons in five species of fish from three sites in the Arabian Gulf. *International Journal of Environmental Health Research*, 2002, 12, 193-200.

Amodio-Cocchieri, R; Amoroso, S; Arnese, A; Cirillo, T; Montuori, P; Triassi, M. Pollution by mercury, arsenic, lead, chromium, cadmium and polycyclic aromatic hydrocarbons of fish and mussels from the Gulf of Naples, Italy. *Bulletin of Environmental Contamination and Toxicology*, 2003, 71, 551-560.

Anastassiades, M; Lehotay, SJ; Stajnbaher, D; Schenck, FJ. Fast and easy multiresidue method employing acetonitrile extraction/partitionng and "dispersive solid-phase extraction" for the determination of pesticide residues in produce. *Journal of AOAC International*, 2003, 86, 412-431.

Anyakora, C; Ogbeche, A; Palmer, P; Coker, H. Determination of polynuclear aromatic hydrocarbons in marine samples of Siokolo Fishing Settlement. *Journal of Chromatography A*, 2005, 1073, 323-330.

Baggiani, C; Anfossi, L; Baravalle, P; Giovannoli, C; Giraudi, G. Molecular recognition of polycyclic aromatic hydrocarbons by pyrene-imprinted microspheres. *Analytical Bioanalytical Chemistry*, 2007, 389, 413-422.

Baird, SJS; Bailey, EA; Vorhees, DJ. Evaluating human risk from exposure to alkylated PAHs in an aquatic system. *Human and Ecological Risk Assessment*, 2007, 13, 322-338.

Barlow, S; Renwick, AG; Kleiner, J; Bridges, JW; Busk, L; Dybing, E; Edler, L; Eisenbrand, G; Fink-Gremmels, J; Knaap, A; Kroes, R; Liem, D; Müller, DJG; Page, S; Rolland, V; Schlatter, J; Tritscher, A; Tueting, W; Würtzen, G. Risk assessment of substances that are both genotoxic and carcinogenic-report of an International Conference organized by EFSA and WHO with support of ILSI Europe. *Food Chemistry and Toxicology*, 2006, 44, 1636-1650.

Barlow, S; Schlatter, J. Risk assessment of carcinogens in food. *Toxicology and Applied Pharmacology*, 2009, doi:10.1016/j.taap.2009.11.004.

Baumard, P; Budzinski, H; Garrigues, P; Narbonne, JF; Burgeot, T; Michel, X; Bellocq, J. Polycyclic aromatic hydrocarbon (PAH) burden of mussels (*Mytilus sp.*) in different marine environments in relation with sediment PAH contamination and bioavailability. *Marine Environmental Research*, 1999, 47, 415-439.

Beg, MU; Gevao, B; Al-Jandal, N; Beg, KR; Butt, SA; Ali, LN; Al-Hussaini, M. Polycyclic aromatic hydrocarbons in three varieties of fish from Kuwait bay. *Polycyclic Aromatic Compounds*, 2009, 29, 75-89.

Binelli, A; Provini, A. Risk for human health of some POPs due to fish from Lake Iseo. *Ecotoxicology and Environmental Safety*, 2004, 58, 139-145.

Bordajandi, LR; Gomez, G; Abad, E; Rivera, J; Fernandez-Baston, MD; Blasco, J; Gonzalez, MJ. Survey of persistent organochlorine contaminants (PCBs, PCDD/Fs, and PAHs), heavy metals (Cu, Cd, Zn, Pb, and Hg), and arsenic in food samples from Huelva (Spain): Levels and health implications. *Journal of Agricultural and Food Chemistry*, 2004, 52, 992-1001.

Castro, D; Slezakova, K; Oliva-Teles, MT; Delerue-Matos, C; Alvim-Ferraz, MC; Morais, S; Pereira, MC. Analysis of polycyclic aromatic hydrocarbons in atmospheric particulate samples by microwave-assisted extraction and liquid chromatography. *Journal of Separation Science*, 2009, 32, 501-510.

Causeret, J. Fish as a source of mineral nutrition. In: Borgstrom, G, editor. *Fish as food*. New York: Academic Press; 1962; pp. 205-234.

Chen, BH; Lin, YS. Formation of polycyclic aromatic hydrocarbons during processing of duck meat. *Journal of Agricultural and Food Chemistry*, 1997, 45, 1394-1403.

Cheung, KC; Leung, HM; Kong, KY; Wong, MH. Residual levels of DDTs and PAHs in freshwater and marine fish from Hong Kong markets and their health risk assessment. *Chemosphere*, 2007, 66, 460-468.

Cho, J-Y; Son, JG; Park, B-J; Chung, B-Y. Distribution and pollution sources of polycyclic aromatic hydrocarbons (PAHs) in reclaimed tidelands and tidelands of the western sea coast of South Korea. *Environmental Monitoring Assessment*, 2009, 149, 385-393.

Chow, CK. Fatty acids in foods and their health implications, 3rd ed., CRC Press, New Boca Raton, USA 2008.

Commission Regulation (EC) No. 466/2001 of 8 March 2001 setting maximum levels for certain contaminants in food stuffs. *Official Journal of the European Union*, L 077.

Commission Regulation (EC) No. 2065/2003 of 10 November 2003 on smoke flavourings used or intented for use in or on foods. *Official Journal of the European Union*, L 309.

Commission Regulation (EC) No. 208/2005 of 4 February 2005 amending Commission Regulation (EC) No. 466/2001 as regards polycyclic aromatic hydrocarbons. *Official Journal of the European Union*, L 034.

Commission Regulation (EC) No. 1881/2006 of 19 December 2006 setting maximum levels for certain contaminants in food stuffs. *Official Journal of the European Union*, L 364.

Culp, SJ; Gaylor, DW; Sheldon, WG; Goldstein, LS; Beland, FA. A comparison of the tumours induced by coal tar and benzo[a]pyrene in a 2-year bioassay. *Carcinogenesis*, 1998, 19, 117-124.

da Silva, TF; Azevedo, DD; de Aquino, FR. Polycyclic aromatic hydrocarbons in fishes and sediments from the Guanabara Bay, Brazil. *Environmental Forensics*, 2007, 8, 257-264.

Deb, SC; Araki, T; Fukushima, T. Polycyclic aromatic hydrocarbons in fish organs. *Marine Pollution Bulletin*, 2000, 40, 882-885.

Del Carlo, M; Di Marcello, M; Perugini, M; Ponzielli, V; Sergi, M; Mascini, M; Compagnone, D. Electrochemical DNA biosensor for polycyclic aromatic hydrocarbon detection. *Microchimica Acta*, 2008, 163, 163-169.

Domingo, JL; Bocio, A; Falco, G; Llobet, JM. Benefits and risks of fish consumption Part I. A quantitative analysis of the intake of omega-3 fatty acids and chemical contaminants. *Toxicology*, 2007, 230, 219-226.

Domingo, JL. Health risks arising from the dietary intake of chemical contaminants: a case study of the consumption of edible marine species in Catalonia, NE Spain. Contributions to Science, 2007a, 3, 459-468.

Domingo, JL. Omega-3 fatty acids and the benefits of fish consumption: Is all that glitters gold? *Environment International*, 2007b, 33, 993-998.

DouAbul, AAZ; Heba, HMA; Fareed, KH. Polynuclear aromatic hydrocarbons (PAHs) in fish from the Red Sea coast of Yemen. *Hydrobiologia*, 1997, 352, 251-262.

Dreyer, A; Radke, M. Evaluation and optimization of extraction and clean-up methods for the analysis of polycyclic aromatic hydrocarbons in peat samples. *International Journal of Environmental Analytical Chemistry*, 2005, 85, 423-432.

Duedahl-Olesen, L; White, S; Binderup, ML. Polycyclic aromatic hydrocarbons (PAH) in Danish smoked fish and meat products. *Polycyclic Aromatic Compounds*, 2006, 26, 163-184.

Duedahl-Olesen, L; Ghorbani, F. Optimization of large volume injection for improved detection of polycyclic aromatic hydrocarbons (PAH) in mussels. *Polycyclic Aromatic Hydrocarbons*, 2008, 28, 282-301.

Duyar, HA; Erdem, ME; Samsun, S; Kalayci, F. The Effects of the Different Woods on Hot-Smoking Vacuum Packed Atlantic Bonito (Sarda sarda) Stored at 4 degrees C. *Journal of Animal and Veterinary Advances*, 2008, 7, 1117-1122.

Easton, MDL; Luszniak, D; Von der Geest, E. Preliminary examination of contaminant loadings in farmed salmon, wild salmon and commercial salmon feed. *Chemosphere*, 2002, 46, 1053-1074.

EFSA, 2005. Opinion of the Scientific Committee on a request from EFSA related to a harmonized approach for risk assessment of substances which are both genotoxic and carcinogenic. Adopted 18 October 2005. *The EFSA Journal*, 2005, 282, 1-31 Available from: http://www.efsa.europa.eu/EFSA/Scientific_Opinion/sc_op_ej282_gentox_en 3,0.pdf.

EFSA, 2007a. Opinion of the Scientific Panel on Contaminants in the Food Chain on a request from the Commission related to the potential increase of consumer health risk by a possible increase of the existing maximum levels for aflatoxins in almonds, hazelnuts and pistachios and derived products. Adopted 25 January 2007. *The EFSA Journal*, 2007, 446, 1-127 Available from: http://www.efsa.europa.eu/EFSA/efsa_locale 1178620753812_ 1178620761977.htm.

EFSA, 2007b. Opinion of the Scientific panel on contaminants in the food chain on a request from the European Commission on ethyl carbamate and hydrocyanic acid in food and beverages. Adopted 20 September 2007. *The EFSA Journal*, 2007, 551, 1-44 Available from: http://www.efsa.europa.eu/EFSA/efsa_locale-1178620753812_1178655060600. htm.

EFSA, 2007c. Findings of the EFSA data collection on polycyclic aromatic hydrocarbons in food. A report from the Unit of data Collection and Exposure on a Request from the European Commission. 2007. EFSA/DATEX/002. Available from: http://www. efsa.europa.eu/EFSA/Scientific_Document/datex_report_pah.pdf.

EFSA, 2008a. Scientific Opinion of the Panel on Contaminants in the Food Chain on a Request from the European Commission on Polycyclic Aromatic Hydrocarbons in Food. Adopted 9 June 2008. The EFSA Journal, 2008, 724, 1-114 Available from: http://www.efsa.europa.eu/EFSA/efsa_locale-1178620753812_1211902034842.htm.

EFSA, 2008b. Monitoring polycyclic aromatic hydrocarbons presence across the EU. *EFSA in focus- Food,* 2008; pp 10. ISSUE 01 - AUG. 2008 Available from: http://www.efsa.europa.eu/EFSA/efsa_locale-1178620753812_1178642214248.htm.

El Deeb, KZ; Said, TO; El Naggar; MH; Shreadah, MA. Distribution and sources of aliphatic and polycyclic aromatic hydrocarbons in surface sediments, fish and bivalves of Abu Qir Bay (Egyptian Mediterranean Sea). *Bulletin of Environmental Contamination and Toxicology*, 2007, 78, 373-379.

EPA, 1986. Guidelines for Carcinogen Risk Assessment. Federal Register 51(185), available at http://www.epa.gov/ncea/raf/car2sab/guidelines_1986.pdf.

EPA, 1986a. Polynuclear aromatic hydrocarbons, EPA method 8310.

EPA, 1986b. Polynuclear aromatic hydrocarbons, EPA method 8100.

EPA, 1995. The use of the benchmark dose approach in health risk assessment.

EPA/630/R-94/007. Risk Assessment Forum, Washington DC.

EPA, 1999. Guidelines for carcinogen risk assessment (review draft). NCEA-F-0644, July 1999. Risk Assessment Forum, United States Environmental Protection Agency, Washington DC. Available from: http://www.epa.gov/ncea/raf/cancer.htm.

EPA, 2003. Children's Environmental Exposures. United States Environmental Protection Agency, Office of Children's Health Protection. Washington, DC.

EPA, 2008. Benchmark Dose Software (BMDS) Version 2.0 (and subsequent updates). National Center for Environmental Assessment. U.S. Environmental Protection Agency. Available from: http://www.epa.gov/ncea/bmds.htm.

Fähnrich, KA; Pravda, M; Guilbault, GG. Immunochemical detection of polycyclic aromatic hydrocarbons (PAHs). *Analytical Letters*, 2002, 35, 1269-1300.

Fähnrich, KA; Pravda, M; Guilbault, GG. Disposable amperometric immunosensor for the detection of polycyclic aromatic hydrocarbons (PAHs) using screen-printed electrodes. *Biosensors and Bioelectronics*, 2003, 18, 73-82.

Falcó, G; Domingo, JL; Llobet, JM; Teixidó, A; Casas, C; Műller, L. Polycyclic aromatic hydrocarbons in foods: human exposure through the diet in Catalonia, Spain. *Journal of Food Protection*, 2003, 66, 2325-2331.

FAO, 2009. The State of World Fisheries and Aquaculture-2008. FAO Fisheries and Aquaculture Department. Food and Agriculture Organization of the United Nations. Rome.

Gagnon, F; Tremblay, T; Rouette, J; Cartier, JF. Chemical risks associated with consumption of shellfish harvested on the north shore of the St. Lawrence River's lower estuary. *Environmental Health Perspectives*, 2004, 112, 883-888.

Gomaa, EA; Gray, JJ; Rabie, S; Lopez-Bote, C; Booren, AM. Polycyclic aromatic hydrocarbons in smoked food products and commercial liquid smoke flavourings. *Food Additives and Contaminants*, 1993, 10, 503-521.

Hellou, J; Payne, JF; Upshall, C. Bioaccumulation of aromatic hydrocarbons from sediments: a dose-response study with flounder (*Pseudopleuronectes americanus*). *Archives of Environmental Contamination and Toxicology*, 1994, 27, 477-485.

Hellou, J; Mackay, D; Fowler, B. Bioconcentration of polycyclic aromatic compounds from sediments to muscle of finfish. *Environmental Science and Technology*, 1995, 29, 2555-2560.

Hyötyläinen, T. Critical evaluation of sample pretreatment techniques. *Analytical and Bioanalytical Chemistry*, 2009, 394, 743-758.

IARC, 1983. Polynuclear Aromatic Compounds, Part 1: Chemical, Environmental and Experimental Data. IARC Monographs on the Evaluation of Carcinogenic Risks to Humans 32. International Agency for Research on Cancer, Lyon.

IARC, 2002. Some Traditional Herbal Medicines, Some Mycotoxins, Naphthalene and Styrene. IARC Monographs on the Evaluation of Carcinogenic Risks to Humans 82. International Agency for Research on Cancer, Lyon.

IARC, 2008. Air Pollution, Part 1, Some Non-heterocyclic Polycyclic Aromatic Hydrocarbons and Some Related Industrial Exposures. IARC Monographs on the Evaluation of Carcinogenic Risks to Humans 92 - in preparation. International Agency for Research on Cancer, Lyon.

Iliadis, KN; Zotos, A; Taylor, AK; Petridis, D. Effect of pre-treatment and smoking process (cold and hot) on chemical, microbiological and sensory quality of mackerel (Scomber scombrus). *Journal of the Science of Food and Agriculture*, 2004, 84, 1545-1552.

IPCS, 1998. Selected Non-heterocyclic Polycyclic Aromatic Hydrocarbons. Environmental Health Criteria 202. International Programme on Chemical Safety, World Health Organization, Geneva.

Jánska, M; Tomaniova, M; Hajslova, J; Kocourek, V. Optimization of the procedure for the determination of polycyclic aromatic hydrocarbons and their derivatives in fish tissue: Estimation of measurements uncertainty. *Food Additives and Contaminants*, 2006, 23, 309-325.

Johnson, LL; Ylitalo, GM; Arkoosh, MR; Kagley, AN; Stafford, C; Bolton, JL; Buzitis, J; Anulacion, BF; Collier, TK. Contaminant exposure in outmigrant juvenile salmon from Pacific Northwest estuaries of the United States. *Environmental Monitoring and Assessment*, 2007, 124, 167-194.

Karacik, B; Okay, O.S; Henkelmann, B; Bernhöft, S; Schramm, K.-W. Polycyclic aromatic hydrocarbons and effects on marine organisms in the Istanbul Strait. *Environment International*, 2009, 35, 599-606.

Karsten, A. Development of Disposable Immunosensors for Polyaromatic Hydrocarbons (PAHs) and Development of a Novel Immunosensor System Based on Electrogenerated Chemiluminescence (ECL) Detection. 2002. Academic dissertation, Department of Chemistry, National University of Ireland Cork, Cork, Ireland.

Kong, KY; Cheung, KC; Wong, CKC; Wong, MH. The residual dynamic of polycyclic aromatic hydrocarbons and organochlorine pesticides in fishponds of the Pearl River delta, South China. *Water Research*, 2005, 39, 1831-1843.

Kris-Etherton PM; Harris WS; Appel LJ. AHA Nutrition Committee. Fish consumption, fish oil, omega-3 fatty acids, and cardiovascular disease. *Circulation*, 2002, 106, 2747-2757.

Kris-Etherton PM; Harris WS; Appel LJ. AHA Nutrition Committee. Omega-3 fatty acids and cardiovascular disease: new recommendations from the American Heart Association. *Arteriosclerosis Thrombosis and Vascular Biology*, 2003, 23, 151-152.

Lacorte, S; Raldua, D; Martinez, E; Navarro, A; Diez, S; Bayona, JM; Barcelo, D. Pilot survey of a broad range of priority pollutants in sediment and fish from the Ebro river basin (NE Spain). *Environmental Pollution*, 2006, 140, 471-482.

Lall, SP. Macro and trace elements in fish and shellfish. In: Ruiter, A, editor. *Fish and fishery products: Composition, nutritive properties and stability*. Wallingford: Cab International; 1995; pp. 187-213.

Law, RJ; Kelly, CA; Nicholson, MD. The QUASIMEME laboratory performance study of polycyclic aromatic hydrocarbons (PAHs): Assessment for the period 1996-1999. *Journal of Environmental Monitoring,* 2000, 2, 517-523.

Lech, JJ; Vodicnik, MJ. Biotransformation. In: Rand, GM, Petrocelli, SR editors. Fundamentals of Aquatic Toxicology: Methods and Applications. Hemisphere Publishing Corporation, New York, USA; 1985; 526-557.

Li, K; Woodward, LA; Karu, AE; Li, QX. Immunochemical detection of polycyclic aromatic hydrocarbons and 1-hydroxypyrene in water and sediment samples. *Analytica Chimica Acta*, 2000, 419, 1-8.

Liang, Y; Tse, MF; Young, L; Wong, MH. Distribution patterns of polycyclic aromatic hydrocarbons (PAHs) in the sediments and fish at Mai Po Marshes Nature Reserve, Hong Kong. *Water Research*, 2007, 41, 1303-1311.

Liguori, L; Heggstad, K; Hove, HT; Julshamn, K. An automated extraction approach for isolation of 24 polyaromatic hydrocarbons (PAHs) from various marine matrixes. *Analytica Chimica Acta*, 2006, 573, 181-188.

Llobet, JM; Falcó, G; Bocio, A; Domingo, JL. Exposure to Polycyclic Aromatic Hydrocarbons through Consumption of Edible Marine Species in Catalonia, Spain. *Journal of Food Protection*, 2006, 69, 2493-2499.

Malik, A; Ojha, P; Singh, KP. Distribution of polycyclic aromatic hydrocarbons in edible fish from Gomti River, India. Bulletin *of Environmental Contamination and Toxicology*, 2008, 80, 134-138.

Martinez, E; Gros, M; Lacorte, S; Barcelo, D. Simplified procedures for the analysis of polycyclic aromatic hydrocarbons in water, sediments and mussels. *Journal Chromatography A*, 2004, 1047, 181-188

McIntosh, AD; Moffat, CF; Packer, G; Webster, L. Polycyclic aromatic hydrocarbon (PAH) concentration and composition determined in farmed blue mussels (*Mytilus edulis*) in a sea loch pre- and post-closure of an aluminium smelter. *Journal of Environmental Monitoring*, 2004, 6, 209-218.

Meador, JP; Stein, JE; Reichert, WL; Varanasi, U. Bioaccumulation of polycyclic aromatic hydrocarbons by marine organisms. *Reviews of Environmental Contamination and Toxicology*, 1995, 143, 79-165.

Means, JC. Compound-specific gas chromatographic/mass spectrometric analysis of alkylated and parent polycyclic aromatic hydrocarbons in waters, sediments, and aquatic organisms. *Journal of AOAC International*, 1998, 81, 657-672.

Moret, S; Conte, L; Dean, D. Assessment of polycyclic aromatic hydrocarbon content of smoked fish by means of a fast HPLC/HPLC method. *Journal of Agricultural and Food Chemistry*, 1999, 47, 1367-1371.

Mostafa, GA. Monitoring of polycyclic aromatic hydrocarbons in seafoods from Lake Timsah. *International Journal of Environmental Health Research*, 2002, 12, 83-91.

Navarro, P; Cortazar, E; Bartolome, L; Deusto, M; Raposo, JC; Zuloaga, O; Arana, G; Etxebarria, N. Comparison of solid phase extraction, saponification and gel permeation chromatography for the clean-up of microwave-assisted biological extracts in the analysis of polycyclic aromatic hydrocarbons. *Journal of Chromatography A*, 2006, 1128, 10-16.

Nesheim, MC; Yaktine, AL. Consumption Patterns and Composition of Seafood. In: Nesheim, MC, Yaktine, AL editors. *Seafood Choices: Balancing Benefits and Risks*. Washington DC: National Academies Press; 2007; pp. 30-66.

Nisbet, ITK; LaGoy, PK. Toxic equivalency factors (TEFs) for polycyclic aromatic hydrocarbons (PAHs). *Regulatory Toxicology and Pharmacology*, 1992, 16, 290-300.

Oehlenschläger, J. Marine fish – A source for essential elements? In: Luten JB, Borresen T, Oehlenschläger, J editors. *Seafood from producer to consumer*. Amsterdam: Elsevier; 1997; pp. 641-652.

Orbea, A; Ortiz-Zarragoitia, M; Sole, M; Porte, C; Cajaraville, MP. Antioxidant enzymes and peroxisome proliferation in relation to contaminant body burdens of PAHs and PCBs in bivalve molluscs, crabs and fish from the Urdaibai and Plentzia estuaries (Bay of Biscay). *Aquatic Toxicology*, 2002, 58, 75-98.

Oros, DR; Ross, JRM. Polycyclic aromatic hydrocarbons in bivalves from the San Francisco estuary: Spatial distributions, temporal trends, and sources (1993-2001). *Marine Environmental Research*, 2005, 60:466-488

Oros, DR; Ross, JRM; Spies, RB; Mumley, T. Polycyclic aromatic hydrocarbon (PAH) contamination in San Francisco Bay: A 10-year retrospective of monitoring in an urbanized estuary. *Environmental Research*, 2007, 105, 101-118.

Palchetti, I; Mascini, M. Nucleic acid biosensors for environmental pollution monitoring. *The Analyst*, 2008, 133, 825-964.

Pena, T; Pensado, L; Casais, C; Mejuto, C; Phan-Tan-Luu, R; Cela, R. Optimization of a microwave-assisted extraction method for the analysis of polycyclic aromatic hydrocarbons from fish samples. *Journal of Chromatography A*, 2006, 1121, 163-169.

Pensado, L; Casais, C; Mejuto, C; Cela, R. Application of matrix solid-phase dispersion in the analysis of priority polycyclic aromatic hydrocarbons in fish samples. *Journal of Chromatography A*, 2005, 1077, 103-109.

Perelló, G; Marti-Cid, R; Castell, V; Llobet, JM; Domingo, JL. Concentrations of polybrominated diphenyl ethers, hexachlorobenzene and polycyclic aromatic hydrocarbons in various foodstuffs before and after cooking. *Food and Chemical Toxicology*, 2009, 47, 709-715.

Perugini, M; Visciano, P; Giammarino, A; Manera, M; Di Nardo, W; Amorena, M. Polycyclic aromatic hydrocarbons in marine organisms from the Adriatic Sea, Italy. *Chemosphere*, 2007a, 66, 1904-1910.

Perugini, M; Visciano, P; Manera, M; Turno, G; Lucisano, A; Amorena, M. Polycyclic aromatic hydrocarbons in marine organisms from the Gulf of Naples, Tyrrhenian Sea. *Journal of Agricultural and Food Chemistry*, 2007b, 55, 2049-2054.

Potrykus, J; Albalat, A; Pempkowiak, J; Porte, C. Content and pattern of organic pollutants (PAHs, PCBs and DDT) in blue mussels (*Mytilus trossulus*) from the southern Baltic Sea. *Oceanologia*, 2003, 45, 337-355.

Ramalhosa, MJ; Paíga, P; Morais, S; Delerue-Matos, C; Oliveira, MBPP. Analysis of polycyclic aromatic hydrocarbons in fish: evaluation of a quick, easy, cheap, effective, rugged, and safe extraction method. *Journal of Separation Science*, 2009, 32, 3529-3538.

Ridgway, K; Lalljie, SPD; Smith, RM. Sample preparation techniques for the determination of trace residues and contaminants in foods. *Journal of Chromatography A*, 2007, 1153, 36-53.

Roche, H; Buet, A; Ramade, F. Accumulation of lipophilic microcontaminants and biochemical responses in eels from the Camargue Biosphere Reserve. *Ecotoxicology*, 2002, 11, 155-164.

Romano, E; Ausili, A; Zharova, N; Magno, MC; Pavoni, B; Gabellini, M. Marine sediment contamination of an industrial site at Port of Bagnoli, Gulf of Naples, southern Italy. *Marine Pollution Bulletin*, 2004, 49, 487-495.

Said, TO; El Agroudy, NA. Assessment of PAHs in water and fish tissues from Great Bitter and El Temsah lakes, Suez Canal, as chemical markers of pollution sources. *Chemistry and Ecology*, 2006, 22, 159-173.

Said, TO. Determination of persistent organic pollutants in sediment and fish of the western coast of Alexandria, Egypt. *Chemistry and Ecology*, 2007, 23, 289-302.

Sanz-Landaluze, J; Bartolome, L; Zuloaga, O; González, L; Dietz, C; Cámara, C. Accelerated extraction for determination of polycyclic aromatic hydrocarbons in marine biota. *Analytical Bioanalytical Chemistry*, 2006, 384, 1331-1340.

Siddiqi, HA, Ansari, FA, Munshi, AB. Assessment of hydrocarbons concentration in marine fauna due to Tasman Spirit oil spill along the Clifton beach at Karachi coast. *Environmental Monitoring and Assessment*, 2009, 148, 139-148.

Sijm, DTHM; Wever, H; Opperhuizen, A. Influence of biotransformation on the accumulation of PCDDs from fly-ash in fish. *Chemosphere*, 1989, 19, 475-480.

Soclo, HH; Budzinski, H; Garrigues, Ph; Matsuzawa, S. Biota Accumulation of Polycyclic Aromatic Hydrocarbons in Benin Coastal Waters. *Polycyclic Aromatic Compounds*, 2008, 28, 112-127.

Song, YF; Jing, X; Fleishmann, S; Wilke, BM. Comparative study of extraction methods for the determination of PAHs from contaminated soils and sediments. *Chemosphere*, 2002, 48, 993-1001.

Srogi, K. Monitoring of environmental exposure to polycyclic aromatic hydrocarbons: a review. *Environmental Chemistry Letters*, 2007, 5, 169-195.

Stołyhwo, A; Sikorski, ZE. Polycyclic aromatic hydrocarbons in smoked fish - a critical review. *Food Chemistry*, 2005, 91, 303-311.

Storelli, MM; Marcotrigiano, GO. Polycyclic aromatic hydrocarbons in mussels (*Mytilus galloprovincialis*) from the Ionian Sea, Italy. *Journal of Food Protection*, 2001, 64, 405-409.

The Decision of the Government of Republic of Estonia, 2000. The list of allowed contaminantes in food and action of allowable concentration on food groups, 12 January, N°. 14, appendix 4 (in Estonian).

Tolosa I, Mora SJ, Fowler SW, Villeneuve J-P, Bartocci J, Cattini C. Aliphatic and aromatic hydrocarbons in marine biota and coastal sediments from the Gulf and the Gulf of Oman. *Marine Pollution Bulletin*, 2005, 50, 1619-1633.

Topping, G; Davies, JM; Mackie, PR; Moffat, CF. The Impact of an Oil Spill in Turbulent Water: The Braer. Ed. J. M. Davies and G. Topping, The Stationary Office, Edinburgh, 1997.

Tudorache, M; Bala, C. Biosensors based on screen-printing technology, and their applications in environmental and food analysis. *Analytical Bioanalytical Chemistry*, 2007, 388, 565-578.

van der Oost, R, Beyer, J, Vermeulen, NPE. Fish bioaccumulation and biomarkers in environmental risk assessment: a review. *Environmental Toxicology and Pharmacology*, 2003, 13, 57-149.

Varanasi, U. *Metabolism of Polycyclic Aromatic Hydrocarbons in the Aquatic Environment.* Boca Raton, FL, USA: CRC Press; 1989.

Varlet, V; Serot, T; Monteau, F; Le Bizec, B; Prost, C. Determination of PAH profiles by GC-MS/MS in salmon processed by four cold-smoking techniques. *Food Additives and Contaminants Part A*, 2007a, 24, 744-757.

Varlet, V; Serot, T; Knockaert, C; Cornet, J; Cardinal, M; Monteau, F; Le Bizec, B; Prost, C. Organoleptic characterization and PAH content of salmon (*Salmo salar*) fillets smoked according to four industrial smoking techniques. *Journal of the Science of Food and Agriculture*, 2007b, 87, 847-854.

Vermeulen, NPE., Donné-Op den Kelder, G., Commandeur, JNM., 1992. Formation of and protection against toxic reactive intermediates. In: Testa, B., Kyburz, E., Fuhrer, W., Giger, R. (Eds.), *Perspectives in Medicinal Chemistry*. Verlag Helvetica Chimica Acta, Basel, pp. 573-593.

Verweij, F; Booij, K; Satumalay, K; van der Molen, N; van der Oost, R. Assessment of bioavailable PAH, PCB and OCP concentrations in water, using semipermeable membrane devices (SPMDs), sediments and caged carp. *Chemosphere*, 2004, 54, 1675-1689.

Visciano, P; Perugini, M; Conte, F; Amorena, M. Polycyclic aromatic hydrocarbons in farmed rainbow trout (*Oncorhynchus mykiss*) processed by traditional flue gas smoking and by liquid smoke flavourings. Food *and Chemical Toxicology*, 2008, 46, 1409-1413.

Wan, Y; Jin, XH; Hu, JY; Jin, F. Trophic dilution of polycyclic aromatic hydrocarbons (PAHs) in a marine food web from Bohai Bay, North China. *Environmental Science and Technology*, 2007, 41, 3109-3114.

Wang, G; Lee, AS; Lewis, M; Kamath, B; Archer, RK. Accelerated solvent extraction and gas chromatography/mass spectrometry for determination of polycyclic aromatic hydrocarbons in smoked food samples. *Journal of Agricultural and Food Chemistry*, 1999, 47, 1062-1066.

Webster, L; Russell, M; Phillips, L; McIntosh, A; Walsham, P; Packer, G; Dalgarno, E; McKenzie, M; Moffat, C. Measurement of organic contaminants and biological effects in Scottish waters between 1999 and 2005. *Journal of Environmental Monitoring*, 2007, 9, 616-629.

WHO, 2006. Evaluation of Certain Food Contaminants. Sixty-fourth report of the Joint FAO/WHO Expert Committee on Food Additives. WHO Technical Report Series 930. World Health Organization, Geneva.

WHO, 2008. Principles and Methods for the Risk Assessment of Chemicals in Food. Chapter 7: Risk Characterisation. Draft document for comment. Available from: http://www.who.int/ipcs/food/update_project/en/index.html

Yurchenko, S; Molder, U. The determination of polycyclic aromatic hydrocarbons in smoked fish by gas chromatography mass spectrometry with positive-ion chemical ionization. *Journal of Food Composition and Analysis*, 2005, 18, 857-869.

In: Nutritional Insights and Food Safety
Editor: Jaroslava Švarc-Gajiæ

ISBN: 978-1-61122-130-5

Chapter VIII

Veterinary Drugs Residues

Slavica Vesković, Srdjan Stefanović and Saša Janković
Institute of Meat Hygiene and Technology; Kaćanskog 13; 11 000 Belgrade, Serbia

Abstract

The last several decades modern animal breeding and veterinary practice cannot be imagined without the use of veterinary drugs. Tremendous progress in chemical synthesis and pharmacological research has led to the production of a large number of pharmacologically active substances that are used as veterinary drugs in everyday veterinary practice. These substances are, besides being a part of good practices in animal husbandry and animal welfare legislation, responsible for preserving and/or improving animals' health and their productive characteristics. Therefore, one can say that one of the pillars of modern veterinary practice from both curative and preventive aspect is the utilization of veterinary drugs.

However, application of veterinary drugs during treatment or prevention of various diseases, inevitably leads to the presence of residual quantities of these substances in animal's body or products. Although extremely small (concentrations usually expressed in µg/kg), veterinary drugs residues in animal tissues and primary animal products, when ingested, can induce various pharmacological side effects in humans. In rare cases, these side effects are acute, i.e. clinically visible (e.g. allergic reactions to beta-lactam antibiotics). More often, accumulation of veterinary drugs residues due to their prolonged ingestion leads to large variety of harmful effects (depending on the class of compound, period of intake, concentration of drug, its metabolism and many other factors) that are not readily observed and can lead to serious detoriation of humans' health. As a consequence, the awareness of hazards associated with the usage of veterinary drugs has increased leading to the extensive research by both regulatory bodies and scientific community. Furthermore, legislation framework and analytical methodology are functionally integrated aiming the restriction of the utilization of veterinary drugs to the minimum. Accordingly, concentrations of veterinary drugs necessary to achieve the beneficial effects to health and productivity of animals are balanced to protect consumers as efficiently as possible from the risks associated with the intake of residues.

This chapter addresses the issue of veterinary drugs residues in food of animal origin. The authors provide a brief historical overview of analytical methods for detection and quantification of veterinary drugs residues, legislation basis for action in case of positive findings with special attention paid on EU legislative as well as Codex Alimentarius recommendations. Basic facts on sample selection, preparation and purification are also presented as well as the most suitable analytical techniques for unambiguous identification and accurate quantification of veterinary drugs residues. Finally, issues concerning future trends in legislation and analytical methodology are also given in this chapter.

Introduction

Veterinary drugs residues including their metabolites in meat and other foods of animal origin may cause adverse effects on consumers' health. The European Food Safety Authority has recently issued an opinion on the effects of hormones residues in meat and suggested that epidemiological data provided evidence for an association between some forms of hormone-dependent cancers and red meat consumption (EFSA, 2007). Other important effects due to the presence of some classes of antibacterial compounds (Figure 1) include the manifestations of allergic reactions or the selection of resistant bacteria that could be transferred to humans through the food chain (Butaye, et al. 2001). In addition, the consumption of trace levels of antimicrobial residues in foods from animal origin may have consequences on the indigenous human intestinal microflora, which constitutes an essential component of human physiology. This flora acts as a barrier against colonization of the gastrointestinal tract by pathogenic bacteria (Vollard & Clasener, 1994) and has an important role in food digestion. So, the ingestion of trace levels of antimicrobials in foods must take into account potentially harmful effects on human gut flora.

The analysis of residues of chemicals, including veterinary drugs in foods of animal origin, begun approximately five decades ago. One can say that in the Benelux (Belgium, The Netherlands and Luxemburg) the residue analysis started in the late 1960s or the early 1970s. The Benelux SP/Lab/h documents (Huis et al, 1978) illustrate the cooperation in residue analysis between several laboratories in The Netherlands and Belgium, producing the first traceable document dating from 1978. These scientific efforts at the time focused mainly on the development of analytical methods and were shortly joined by other European countries. Regulatory framework concerning the field of residues emerged as a consequence of the ability of analytical methodology to detect and quantify the presence of veterinary drugs in animal originating matrix. A close relation of these two areas (analytical and regulatory) has led to the establishment of first legislation setting zero tolerances for veterinary drugs residues. From today's point of view, this may seem both over-restrictive and unrealistic goal. However, in late seventies (Table 1), analytical techniques available at that time were not capable of detecting ppb concentrations of non-volatile compounds (almost all veterinary drugs) due to technical limitations in high performance liquid chromatography hardware. In the early 70s thin layer chromatography (TLC) was the method of choice for the qualitative detection of banned substances (thyreostats and some anabolics) due to specificity, the simplicity of chromatographic development in two dimensions and the possibility of reaching relatively low limits of detection for an acceptable budget (De Brabander et al., 2009). The only instrumental alternative with acceptable limits of detection, at that moment, gas gas chromatography with electron captures detection (GC-ECD).

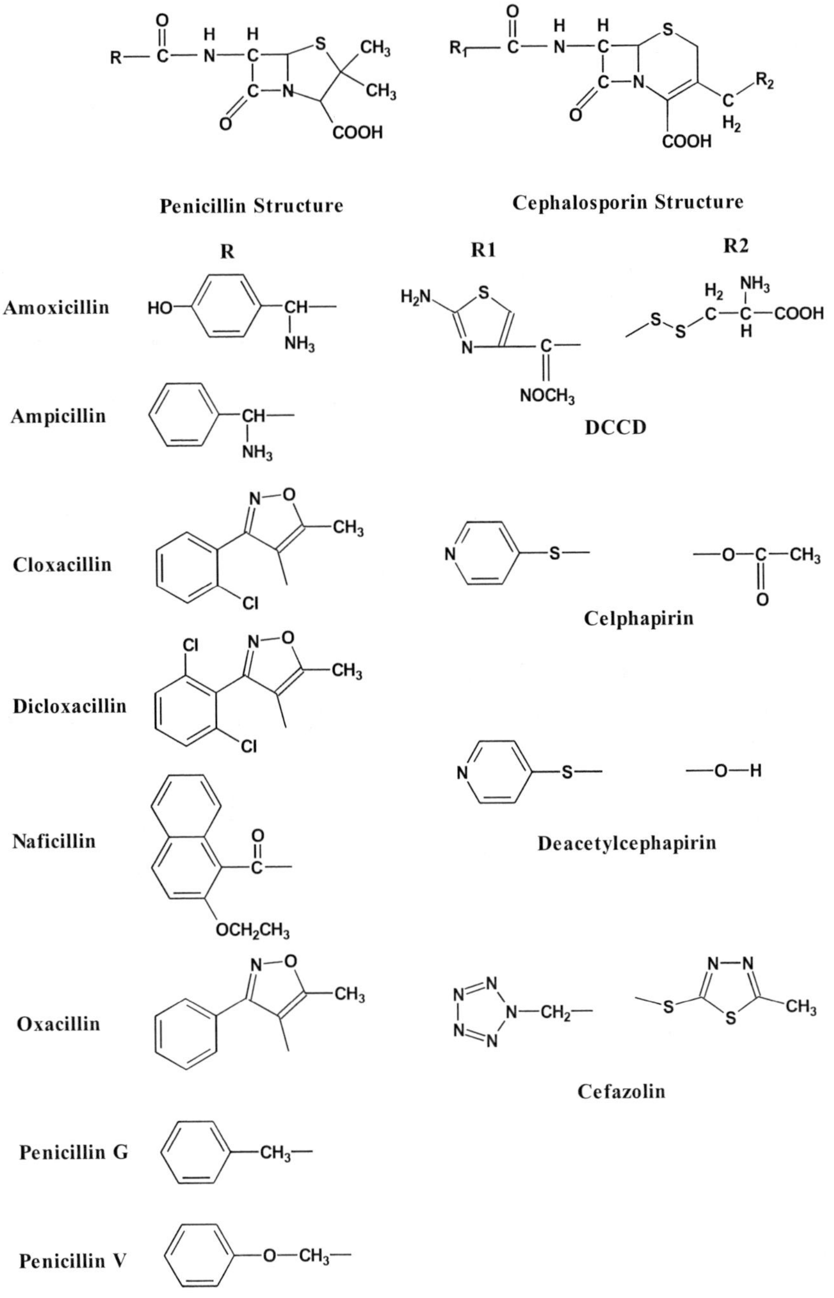

Figure 1. Chemical structure of some penicillin's and cephalosporins.

Electron capture detectors were at the time available and satisfied the need for sensitivity although they responded to the limited group of halogenated compounds implying the necessity for derivatization step with its (among the other limitations) inherent reproducibility difficulties. High-performance liquid chromatography with UV detection did not correspond to the specificity and limits of detection in many cases. More specific and much more sensitive fluorescence detectors were only introduced later. During the 90s more and more affordable gas chromatography–mass spectrometry (GC–MS) apparatus appeared on the market and the transition from TLC (and HPLC) to GC–MS methods was ongoing. From the late '90s on, LC–MS^n became the mandatory standard equipment in a residue laboratory. Although mass spectrometry was available *per se* much earlier, lack of appropriate interfaces between liquid chromatograph and mass spectrometer was the technical obstacle that prevented accurate identification of the veterinary drugs potentially present in foodstuffs. Having in mind these limitations it is clearer why, at the time, legislation couldn't be more specific in prescribing mandatory limits for veterinary drugs.

Table 1. Historical overview of the development of analytical methods for veterinary drugs residues

Year	1970s	1970-1980s	mid 1980s	1990-2000	2000-2010
Analytical technique	TLC GC-ECD	HPLC	GC-MS	GC-MS/MS LC-MS (TQD)	RapidRes HPLC (UPLC) ToF

A veterinary residue may be defined as a trace of a substances, present in a matrix (e.g. meat, urine, etc.) after some kind of administration (e.g. within the framework of veterinary practice or illegal use) to an animal. Normally this implies the concentration levels in the ppb (μg/kg) or ppt (ng/kg) range of the substances.

The prohibition of the use of growth-promoting agents such as, e.g., hormones and β-agonists is laid down in Council Directive 96/22/EC. Council Directive 96/23/EC includes the control of food-producing animals as well as their primary products like meat, milk, eggs and honey. This means that samples are taken from the living animal on the producing farms as well as from carcasses in the slaughterhouse. According to the Council Directive 96/23/EC, the substances may be divided into two major groups - A and B substances (Table 2). Group A involves the growth promoters abused in animal fattening and the "no maximum residue limit (MRL)" substances and may be subdivided into four major groups: anabolics or anabolic steroids, thyreostats, beta-agonists and substances belonging to the Annex IV. Group B encompasses the veterinary drugs or veterinary medicinal products (VMPs): antibacterial substances, other VMPs as anthelmintics, coccidiostats, carbamates and pyrethroids, sedatives, non-steroidal anti-inflammatory drugs (NSAIDs) and other pharmacologically active substances. The analytical requirements for both groups of substances are different.

Table 2. Groups of substances according to the Council Directive 96/23/EC

Group A		Group B	
A1	Stilbenes	B1	Antibacterial substances including silfonamides and quinolones
A2	Antithyroid agents	B2a	Antihelmintics
A3	Steroids, androgens, gestagens, estrogens	B2b	Anticoccidials including nitroimidazoles
A4	Resorcylic acid lactones	B2c	Carbamates and pyrethroides
A5	β-agonists	B2d	Sedatives
A6	Substances from Annex IV	B2e	Non-steroidal antiimflamatory drugs
		B2f	Other pharmacologically active substances

In the EU the use of veterinary drugs is regulated via Council Regulation 2377/90/EC. This regulation describes the procedure for the establishment of maximum residue limits (MRLs) for veterinary medicinal substances in foodstuffs of animal origin. Its Annexes present the following information:

- Annex I (Appendix I) includes the substances for which final MRLs have been established.
- Annex II includes the substances for which it is not considered necessary to establish MRL values in the light of public health protection. These substances can be used in food-producing species and for indicated animal species according to the conditions established.
- Annex III (Appendix II) includes the substances with provisional MRLs established for a defined period of time, when not all requirements for the establishment of an MRL have yet been fulfilled.
- Annex IV includes the substances for which no MRL can be established because residues of these substances, at whatever limits, in foodstuffs of animal origin constitute a hazard to the health of consumers. The administration of substances listed in this Annex is prohibited for food-producing animals.

Directive 96/23/EC also establishes National Monitoring Program for monitoring the residues. Control for Group A substances is more critical, i.e., has a higher priority, because of public-health concerns, thus relatively large numbers of samples have to be analyzed and more stringent criteria have to be used (Commission Decision 2002/657/EC). The Directive also lays down that samples collected for the National Monitoring Program have to be analyzed in accredited laboratories. Accordingly, an extensive network of analytical residue laboratories has been created for the purpose of residue inspections. This hierarchical system comprises, at the lowest level, so-called Routine and/or Field Laboratories, next some forty National Reference Laboratories (NRLs) and, at the top, four Community Reference Laboratories (CRLs). The four CRLs, which are located in Germany, France, Italy and The Netherlands, are hierarchically equal. However, each of them is responsible for a specific set of compounds.

The Annexes given in the Appendixes I and II present Comparative lists of EU and Codex Alimentarius MRLs (Council Directive 2377/90/EC, Anex I, III, consolidated version, updated 2009, Codex Alimentarius, updated at the 32nd session of the Codex Alimentarius Commission, July 2009).

In 2009, Council Regulation 2377/90/EC has been repealed by the Regulation (EC) No 470/2009 laying down Community procedures for the establishment of residue limits of pharmacologically active substances in foodstuffs of animal origin, repealing Council Regulation (EEC) No 2377/90 and amending Directive 2001/82/EC of the European Parliament and of the Council and Regulation (EC) No 726/2004 of the European Parliament and of the Council.

The keystone of this document is technical progress in analytical chemistry resulting in the ability to detect extremely low levels of veterinary medicinal products. The document also stresses the necessity to re-establish maximum residue limits in accordance with generally recognized principles of safety assessment and toxicological risks and environmental contamination, as well as the microbiological and pharmacological effects of residues. Furthermore, since the EU contributes, in the context of the Codex Alimentarius, to the development of international standards on maximum residue limits, the Community takes over those Codex Alimentarius maximum residue limits that it has supported in the relevant Codex Alimentarius Commission meetings without a further risk assessment. Consistency between international standards and Community legislation on residue limits in food is expected to be further enhanced.

For the purposes of ensuring food safety, the Regulation also lays down rules and procedures for establishing the maximum concentration of a residue of a pharmacologically active substance which may be permitted in food of animal origin (maximum residue limit). Similarly, the Regulation addresses the substances for which a maximum residue limit has not been laid down in accordance with this Regulation (reference point for action) for control reasons.

On contrary to EU requirements that are mandatory for both member states and third countries importing food of animal origin in the EU, Codex Alimentarius MRLs are not legally binding, however, large number of countries incorporates these values in their national legislative, thus providing the framework for national surveillance programs.

In the Council Directive 2377/90/EC, for banned (A) substances the emphasis lays on the identification of the substances in a large number of matrices (e.g. meat, urine, hair) in a concentration as low as possible (zero tolerance principle). In this case, at first qualitative multi-residue methods have to be developed and secondly, the methods for accurate quantification. For B substances having a MRL, methods for the quantitative determination of the substances in edible matrices only (e.g. meat, liver) have to be worked out. In most cases the MRLs of B substances are a magnitude 10–100 times higher than the recommended concentrations (minimum required performance levels; MRPLs) of the A substances.

Scientific community regularly publishes articles concerning analytical methods for the determination of veterinary drugs residues. Next to the traditional peer-reviewed journals, the proceedings of the two main Benelux conferences in the field: “Euroresidue” (six editions) and the international conference on hormone and veterinary drug residue analysis “the Ghent conference” (seven editions) are very important.

The analytical method and its performance must always be seen in the light of the interpretation of the analytical results. Food inspection services are interested mainly in yes or no answers: has this animal been treated illegally? Is the concentration of the residue higher than a certain value (MRL)? In fact all questions may be resumed to one major question: is the sample compliant or is the law violated? When the answer to that last question is YES, legal actions have to be taken. Therefore the analytical results must be accurate and “beyond any reasonable doubt”.

The Commission Decision 657/2002/EC establishes the performance criteria for analytical residue methods. In this revised version of earlier Commission Decisions the number of substances as well as the matrix spectrum have been enlarged. Briefly, hormonally active substances, thyreostats, β-agonists, pharmacologically active substances, e.g., anthelmintics, anticoccidiostats and sedatives, growth-promoting agents such as antibiotics and also contaminants such as pesticides and heavy metals, are now included. Relevant matrices now include honey, eggs, milk and aquacultural samples. In addition, the decision takes recent technical developments into account, with LC–MS taking the foremost position.

Next to the general performance requirements, e.g., detection level, selectivity and specificity, Decision 657/2002/EC defines additional requirements for confirmatory methods by introducing the concept of identification points (IPs) and defining criteria for ion intensities of mass spectra of the compounds. During confirmatory analysis a specific number of IPs has to be collected. For the confirmation of the identity of Group A substances – commonly referred to as unauthorized, illegal, banned or prohibited substances – a minimum of four IPs is required. For the confirmation of the identity of substances listed in Group B, a minimum of three IPs is required. More detailed explanation on this is to be found later in this chapter .

1. The Determination of Veterinary Drug Residues

1.1. Selection of Samples

The first selection that has to be made when setting up monitoring program regards the type of sample material. Ideally, a method of analysis for veterinary drug residues should be validated for the analysis of four tissues generally classed as "edible tissues", which are fat, liver, kidney and muscle. Specific dietary preferences may require validation of methods for other tissues, which are normally consumed in specific country or region. In addition, there may be a regulatory requirement to analyze urine or other body fluids for residues, particularly if live animal testing is part of a regulatory program. From a practical approach, the usual minimum requirement is that an analytical method should be validated for what is defined as "target tissue", which is the tissue from a treated animal in which the highest and most persistent concentrations of the drug residue are expected to be found. This would usually be the tissue collected for a national residues monitoring program. In addition, there is a requirement to test the "tissue in trade" when products are shipped between countries. This is most commonly muscle tissue, but may include other tissues. Knowledge of the metabolism and tissue distribution should ideally be gained for each drug residue before a final selection of appropriate tissues for validation is made.

Table 3. Suitable tissues and organs for the detection of veterinary drugs residues

Species/Primary product for method validation	Usual target tissue or matrix for method validation	
	Water-soluble	Fat-soluble
Ruminant (e.g. cattle, sheep, goat)	Liver or kidney, muscle	Fat, muscle
Non-ruminant (e.g. pig)	Liver or kidney, muscle	Fat, muscle
Poultry (e.g. chicken, turkey, duck)	Liver, muscle	Fat, or muscle with adhering skin in normal proportions
Fish	Muscle with adhering skin in normal proportions	Muscle with adhering skin in normal proportions
Shellfish/Crustacean	Muscle	Muscle
Milk (usually cows' milk)	Whole milk	Whole milk
Honey	Honey	Honey

It is also essential to assure that the method is validated for the appropriate marker residue, which may be either the parent compound, a metabolite or a representative compound. Table 3 provides data on selection of biological matrices appropriate for analysis of veterinary drugs residues depending on basic chemical properties of the analytes.For monitoring drugs having an MRL, animal tissues such as liver, kidney, muscle, milk or fat are selected. Since the drug concentrations in the consumable parts of an animal have to be below the MRL, these matrices are therefore of most interest and, because kidney and liver are the target organs for most veterinary drugs, the drug concentrations in these organs are higher than in, e.g., heart or lungs. One disadvantage of selecting animal organs or muscle is that they can be analyzed only after slaughtering.

1.2. Sample Preparation

The determination of trace contaminants in complex matrices, such as food, often requires extensive sample extraction and preparation regimes prior to instrumental analysis (Ridgway et al., 2007) The amount of the sample needed to be prepared depends on the sample matrix and the properties and level of analyte to be determined. The typical steps within sample preparation include sampling/homogenization, extraction, clean-up and concentration followed by the final analysis. Another step that can be included at several points is derivatization. More on derivatization step can be found later in this chapter.

Careful sampling techniques are required for foodstuffs in particular and any portion or aliquot taken for analysis must represent the original bulk sample. For food component analysis, smaller sample size can be used, but in trace analysis relatively large sample sizes are often required. Larger sample size results in the need for more efficient clean-up techniques and therefore possibly higher costs. However, in general, larger sample size taken for extraction provides more precise results (Horwitz et al, 1980).

The selective extraction of analytes is based on differences in their chemical and physical properties. These typically include molecular weight, charge, solubility (hydrophobicity), polarity, or differences in volatility.

Food samples cover a wide range of physical types from dry powders to biological matrices, such as meat, fats and liquids or solutions. Particle size of the samples can be an important parameter for reproducible results as the extent to which the matrix is broken up can influence the extraction rates and efficiency. The analyte is desorbed from the matrix and dissolved into a solvent or fluid. Extraction of an analyte is therefore influenced by solubility of the analyte, penetration of the solvent into the sample (mass transfer) and matrix effects (Mitra, 2003). Most of the extraction methods transfer multiple substances into an organic or aqueous solution, requiring additional clean-up and further concentration. The extract solutions can then be treated as a liquid samples. Liquid samples can be handled directly by solvent–solvent extraction methods or sorption methods.

As regards sample treatment, liquid extraction (LE) and liquid–solid extraction (LSE) were found to be very popular techniques, which were used in, respectively, 30 and 60% of all studies. Here, LE comprises conventional liquid–liquid extraction (LLE) as well as the liquid extraction of homogenized tissues such as liver, kidney and meat, referred to as liquid-phase extraction (LPE). LSE is almost always performed in the form of solid-phase extraction (SPE). The application of matrix solid-phase dispersion and immunoaffinity extraction is not often used. In many instances LE and LSE were used in combination. After the analyte isolation by means of LE has been completed, the extract is further purified, by using a suitable SPE procedure. The introduction of various types of co-polymeric sorbents has helped to make SPE a more robust extraction technique with a wider application range than the conventional silica-based sorbents. These SPE phases are used in multiresidue analytical methods where extraction of chemically different compounds is to be achieved. The most widely used polymeric sorbents are the (poly)styrene-divinylbenzene co-polymers. A polymeric sorbent frequently used for the extraction of drug residues from biological samples is Oasis-HLB. This is a hydrophilic-lipophilic balanced copolymer (HLB) of N-vinylpyrrolidone and divinylbenzenes. The hydrophilic N-vinylpyrrolidone increases the water wettability of the polymer, and the lipophilic divinylbenzene provides the reversed-phase retention necessary to retain analytes (Waters, 2009).

Other sample-preparation techniques used for the analysis of veterinary drugs are pressurized liquid extraction (PLE) also called "Accelerated solvent extraction" - ASE and ultrafiltration (UF). PLE, and also the closely related supercritical fluid extraction (SFE), have been shown to be very effective techniques for analyte isolation from fat-containing matrices (Carabias-Martinez et al, 2005). Here one should consider that, while optimization of a PLE procedure is fairly straightforward, optimization of SFE is often rather time-consuming because of the many parameters that are involved.

1.3. Screening and Confirmatory Analytical Methods

The controls within national monitoring programs are based on the screening of a large number of samples. Compliant samples are accepted while those suspected non-compliant samples have to be confirmed through other confirmatory methods that are described later. The basic requirements of screening methods are high throughput with low cost and ability to detect an analyte or class of analytes at the level of interest. They should be easy to use and handle. Possibility of automatization and reduced time to obtain the result, as well as good sensitivity and specificity are also required. Detection capability (CCβ) with an error probability (β)<5% is mandatory for all screening methods according to the Commission Decision 2002/657/EC. In case the residue has a maximum residue limit (MRL), the screening method must be capable to detect the residue below this limit. The screening methods must also avoid or reduce to a minimum the number of false negative results because they will be considered as compliant samples and will not be further analyzed. On the other hand, it must not give an excessive number of false non-compliant samples that will be later confirmed as compliant, due to the excessive cost and time involvement.

Analytical methods for veterinary drug residues in foods must be capable of reliably detecting the presence of a veterinary drug of interest or concern (screening methods), quantifying how much is present (quantitative methods), and providing unequivocal identification (confirmatory methods) of the drug. When an analytical method is used to determine whether the defined Maximum Residue Limit (MRL) for an approved veterinary drug has been exceeded, it is imperative that the test results are confirmed before regulatory action is taken. Regulatory action could include denying the product market access, destroying the product and/or the administration of financial penalties. In cases when the detected veterinary drug is not permitted, banned or prohibited from use in that commodity because no acceptable daily intake (ADI) and MRLs have been defined for toxicological reasons, detection of such drug at any concentration should be confirmed since this finding may automatically result in regulatory action.

Selecting a suitable method of residue analysis will, in many instances, depend on the problem at hand as well as on the final goal. When large sample series have to be monitored for a group of antibiotics, sample throughput will be an important criterion since speed is of the essence. In this situation a screening method is selected because high sample throughput and speed are the characteristics of such method. When, on the other hand, samples are suspected to contain an illegal growth-promoter, or banned antibacterial (e.g. chloramphenicol) (Figure 2), method selectivity will no doubt be the main criterion due to avoiding false non-compliant results. In this situation, a confirmatory method is of great significance because it provides full or complementary information enabling to confirm the identity of the substance.

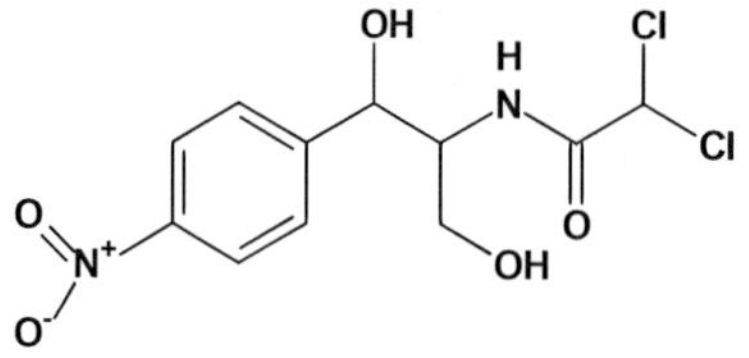

Chloramphenicol

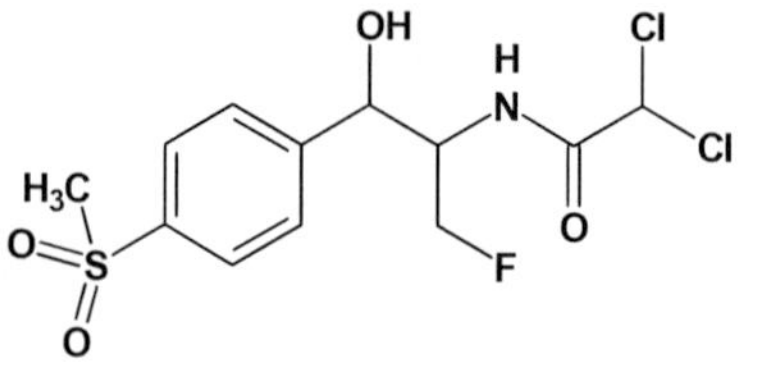

Florfenicol

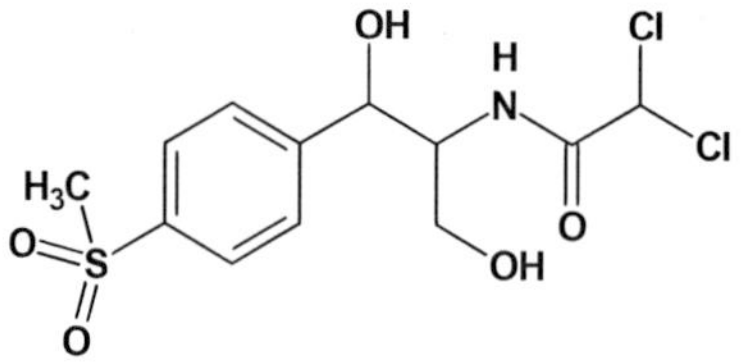

Thiamphenicol

Figure 2. Chemical structure of fenicols.

However, to increase efficiency and sample throughput, many laboratories are turning to the use of multi-residue analytical methods. Multi-residue analytical methods are methods, which can be used for the detection of multiple analytes of the same or different classes. These methods are most commonly used by laboratories for screening samples for the possible presence of veterinary drugs in samples but they can also be used for both quantitative and confirmatory analyses.

Proficiency testing (or other inter-laboratory testing procedures), where practicable, provides an important means for verifying the general accuracy of results generated by a method, and provides information on the between-laboratory variability of the results. However, proficiency testing generally does not address analyte stability or homogenity and extractability of analytes in the processed sample.

1.4. Suitability of Some Analytical Techniques Approved for Confirmatory Purposes by the EU Legislation

According to the Commission Decision 2002/657/EC1, total of eight confirmatory methods, under various conditions, are set for analysis of group B compounds (Annex I, 96/23/EC). Numerous methods of analysis were published in the past decade, employing several detection techniques. Besides the mass spectrometry (LC-MS), most often used detection methods in liquid chromatography are LC-Fl and LC-DAD. Both these methods are considered confirmatory according to the Commission Decision 2002/657/EC and further confirmation by LC-MS is not mandatory. Fluorescence (LC-Fl) is suitable confirmatory technique for molecules that exhibit native fluorescence and molecules that exhibit fluorescence after either transformation or derivatization. LC-Full Scan DAD (LC-DAD) is also suitable confirmatory technique under conditions stated in article 2.3.5.2 of the Decision.

However, in some cases, the data obtained by LC-FI and LC-DAD can be ambiguous. Therefore, it is necessary to employ other confirmatory techniques in order to obtain accurate results. One example of this can be found in the case of analysis of fluoroquinolone residues. The authors observed some limitations of LC-Fl and LC-DAD techniques that may question their suitability for confirmatory purposes (Stefanović et al., 2006). The instrumentation used during the experiment was as follows: Waters Alliance 2695 Separations Module, Waters 2475 Multi λ Fluorescence Detector, Waters 2996 PDA Detector (serial connection to Fl detector, on-line data acquisition from both instruments) and Micromass Quattro Micro MS Detector.

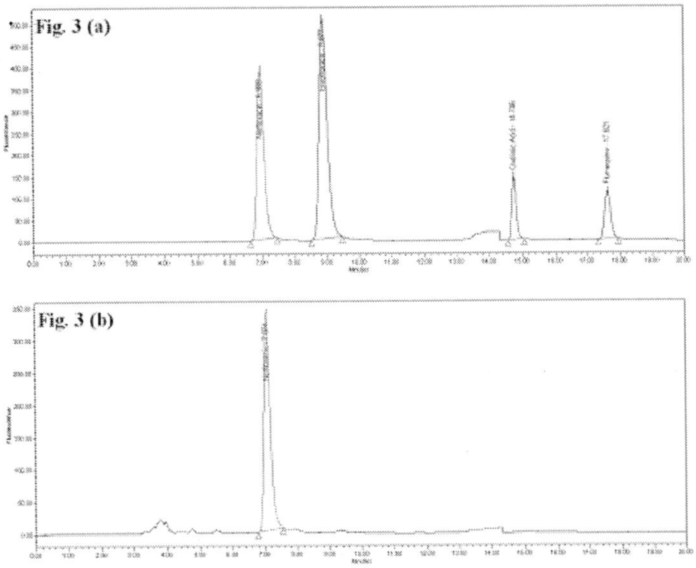

Figure 3. Chromatograms (LC-Fl) of quinolones standard solution (a) and suspect sample (bovine kidney) with norfloxacine peak at 7.071 minutes (b).

Figure 3 (a) shows the chromatograms obtained from the fluorescence system of standard solutions of quinolone antibacterals (a): norfloxacine, enrofloxacine, oxolinic acid and flumequine in concentration of 0.2 μg/ml. Figure 3 (b) shows the sample of bovine kidney with the peak corresponding to the retention time of norfloxacine. Relative difference in retention times of norfloxacin peak and suspect compound from the sample is 1.90%, which, considering the fluorescence technique as confirmative for B group of substances, can lead to the conclusion that the sample is non-compliant (providing that MRL is exceeded). However, since norfloxacine has no MRL set by the Council Regulation 2377/90/EC or Codex Alimentarius, the authors ran the suspect sample on diodearray and MS detectors in order to confirm the findings from the fluorescent detector.

Figure 4 shows the spectra recorded in the 190-400 nm range of norfloxacine standard (a) and suspect sample (b). As it is clearly seen there is no match between the spectra, regarding intensities, absorption maxima or general shape. Acquisition and processing system software confirmed mismatch between two spectra.

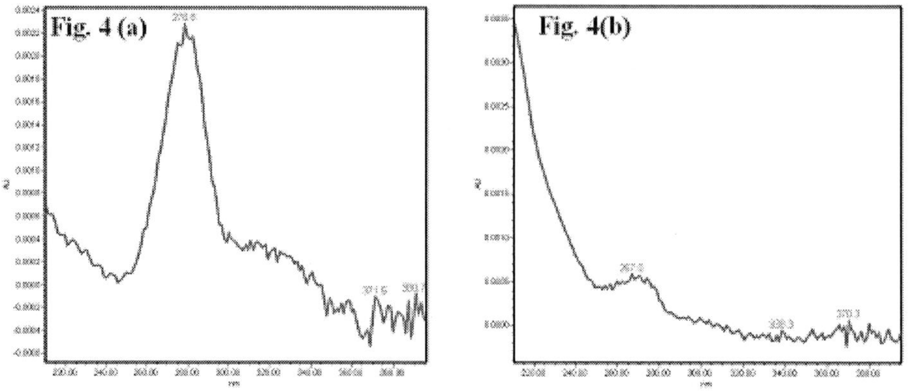

Figure 4. UV spectra (210-400 nm) of norfloxacine standard (a) and suspect sample (b).

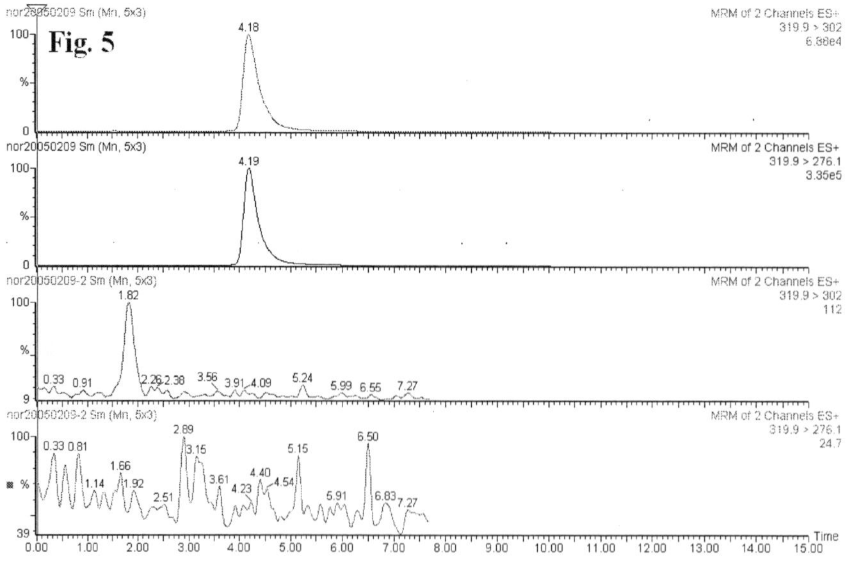

Figure 5. MS chromatogram of norfloxacine standard solution and suspect sample.

Figure 5 shows MS chromatogram of norfloxacine standard solution and suspect sample on both transitions (319.9>302, 319.9>276.1). The chromatogram shows that the norfloxacine is not present in the sample. This indicates that in this case study, fluorescent detection gave false non-compliant results, which raises an issue of its suitability for confirmatory purposes.

Although LC-DAD results, in most cases matched LC-MS/MS data, we observed some limitations of the technique concerning analytes with relatively low MRL (e.g. 50 µg/kg for flumequine in milk), i.e. low ng quantities of an analyte on column.

Figure 6 shows flumequine spectrum obtained from standard solution (a) and flumequine spectrum recorded in blank milk sample fortified at the level of 50 µg/kg (b). It can be observed that, although two spectra are visually similar, their absorption maxima do not match within the optical resolution of the detector (1.2 nm in the case of Waters 2996 instrument) which is the requirement of Commission Decision 2002/657/EC, article 2.3.5.2.). The disagreement of absorption maxima between spectra originates from low intensities of the detector response due to the low quantities of the analyte on column. Although these problems may be overcome by increasing sample weight or injection volume, this can result in other problems related to sample preparation and/or amount of impurities present in the sample extract. Therefore, in the cases where small amounts of some analytes are analyzed with LC-DAD technique, data obtained by spectrum scanning may be inconclusive which questions this technique's fitness for confirmatory purposes.

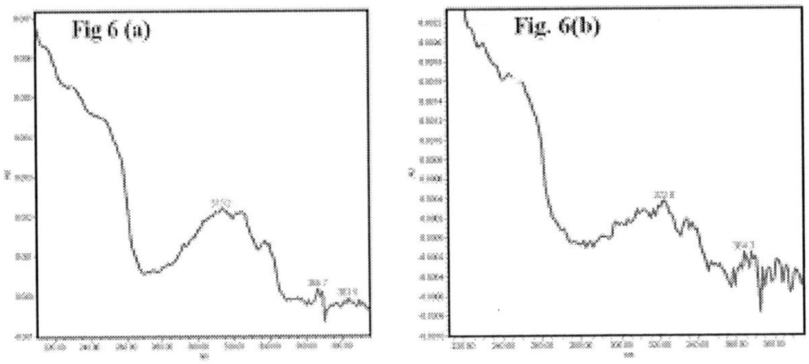

Figure 6. UV spectra of flumequine in standard solution (a) and fortified milk sample at the level of 50 µg/kg.

Similar results were reported in case studies on sodium salycilate in drinking water samples and proficiency test of emamectine in milk. Also, certain limitations of LC-DAD technique were observed in cases where low amounts of analyte are present resulting in mismatch of obtained and reference spectra thus yielding false compliant results.

1.5. Mass Spectrometry in Veterinary Drugs Residues Analysis

With the mass spectrometry emerging in the past decade as sensitive, relatively affordable and far more selective technique, it is safe to assume that future analytical techniques for veterinary drugs residues will be based solely on this method. Mass spectrometry was theoretically known to be the most accurate technique for confirming the presence of the compounds in the sample for a long time. However, the fact that the vast majority of veterinary drugs were non-volatile, polar compounds prevented its usage in analysis of veterinary drugs residues, since mass spectrometry, until the engineering breakthrough in coupling interfaces, was "reserved" for gas chromatography. The development of atmospheric pressure ionization (API) as a commercial interface technique, coupled to high-performance liquid chromatography and tandem mass spectrometry (LC–MS–MS) has opened a new chapter in qualitative and quantitative analysis of veterinary drug residues. API, which includes electrospray ionization (ESI) and atmospheric pressure chemical ionization (APCI), complements the classical GC–MS technology and enables the determination of compounds with high molecular masses and non-volatile substances without recourse to derivatization. This technique, based on triple quadrupole, ion trap, and recently time-of-flight technologies, has become accessible and affordable to residue control laboratories.

According to performance criteria and other requirements for mass spectrometric detection of substances listed in groups A and B of Annex I of Council Directive 96/23/EC, if full scan and single ion monitoring is performed, the relative intensities of the detected ions of the analytes in the matrix, expressed as a percentage of the intensity of the most intense ion or transition, must correspond to those of the standard solution.

In the case when mass fragments are measured using techniques other than full scan, a system of identification points shall be used to interpret the data. For the confirmation of substances listed in group A of Annex I, Council Directive 96/23EC (banned substances), a minimum of four identification points are mandatory. For the confirmation of substances listed in group B of Annex I of Council Directive 96/23/EC (substances with assigned MRLs), a minimum of three identification points are required. Table 4 shows the number of identification points that each of the basic mass spectrometric techniques can provide. Table 5 shows the examples for the calculation of identification points using LC/MS-MS.

Table 4. Number of identification points depending on identified mass fragments

MS technique	Number of identification points per ion
Low-res mass spectrometry (LR-MS)	1
Low-res mass spectrometry – precursor ion	1
Low-res mass spectrometry – transition products	1.5
High-res mass spectrometry (HR-MS)	2
High-res mass spectrometry – precursor ion	2
High-res mass spectrometry – transition products	2.5

Table 5. Number of identification points in different MS technique used in the confirmation of analyte

LC/MS techniques	Number of ions and transition products	Number of identification points scored (n)
LC/MS-MS	1 precursor ions + 2 daughters	4
LC/MS-MS	2 precursor ions + 1 daughter from each precursor	5
LC-MS/MS	1 precursor ion, 1 daughter, 2 granddaughters	5.5

In order to qualify for the confirmatory identification point, at least one ion ratio must be measured and the maximum of three separate techniques can be combined to achieve a minimum number of identification points. Commission Decision 2002/657/EC also provides maximum permitted tolerances for relative ion intensities depending on the used MS techniques (Table 6).

Table 6. Permitted tolerances for relative ion intensities established by the EU regulations

Relative intensity (% of the base peak)	EI-GC-MS[a]	CI-GC-MS[b], GC-MS^n, LC-MS, LC-MS^n (relative)
>50 %	± 10 %	± 20 %
>20 % to 50 %	± 15 %	± 25 %
>10 % to 50 %	± 20 %	± 30 %
≤ 10 %	± 50 %	± 50 %

[a]Electron ionization gas chromatography mass spectrometry.
[b]Chemical ionization gas chromatography mass spectrometry.

There is no fundamental chemometric basis for the number of IPs and the applied tolerances, but it is interesting to note that they do not differ too much from the criteria established by the Association of Official Racing Chemists (AORC), the US Food and Drug Administration (FDA), the International Olympic Committee (IOC) and the World Anti-Doping Agency (WADA) (Stolker et al., 2005). The main difference is that the EU is the only organization that allows the use of a combination of independent techniques to confirm the identity of a substance. Other regulatory bodies only allow the use of either GC–MS or LC–MS.

LC–MS–MS is an instrumental technique that has been established in statutory residue laboratories for a number of years. For MS–MS (Multiple reaction monitoring - MRM) investigations two types of mass spectrometers are predominant: triple quadrupole and ion trap mass spectrometer (or a hybrid of both of them - the combination of ion trap and a triple quadrupole system where the last quadrupole of the triple quadrupole mass spectrometer can serve as a linear ion trap, as well). The benefit of this hybrid system is the selective detection of multiple-charged ions over single charged ions that increase the signal/noise ratio, especially in case of the determination of proteins or peptides. For the analysis of banned compounds only two transitions are needed, provided the method meets other criteria, for example, maximum permitted tolerance for relative ion intensities.

Depending on the type of analysis (quantitative analysis for the substances with MRL, or confirmation of banned substances, where achieving the low limit of detection is necessary), quadrupole or ion trap instruments can be employed, although triple quadrupole instruments generally show higher sensitivity. Development of Time-of-Flight high resolution mass spectrometers coupled to ultra performance liquid chromatography which utilizes sub-2μm column particle size enabled the development of multiresidue methods for detection of about 100 compounds of veterinary drugs (Kaufmann et al, 2008).

Another advantage of LC–MS is that it enables the determination of compounds with high molecular weights as well as polar, non-volatile and thermolabile analytes without derivatization. Derivatization has been the only option for detection of substances using GC-

MS, if the substances were non-volatile, which is the case with most polar and hydrosoluble veterinary drugs. The drawbacks of this technique were rather tedious sample preparation process and generally poor reproducibility having in mind the stability of the derivatives and changes in the ambient parameters during derivatization step and waiting period for samples to be injected. Few are the examples of derivatization processes that still find its application in modern residues analysis. Derivatization of macrocyclic lactones for fluorescent detection with 1-methylimidazole and trifluoroacetic acid is perhaps one of the last remaining techniques where better sensitivity is obtained by fluorescent detection comparing to mass spectrometry.

For complex matrices, such as liver, kidney, muscle or urine, used to detect veterinary drugs, an appropriate sample preparation is necessary in order to avoid matrix effects (e.g. ion suppression) in the ionization processes during the mass spectrometric analysis. This is also a limiting factor in the light of the increasing trend in the development of multiresidue analytical methods. Chemical structure of veterinary drugs varies significantly inter or intra-class, which makes the efficient extraction of such compounds in single step very difficult, if not impossible to achieve.

The lack of volatility and chemical stability of most drugs essentially prevents the use of gas chromatography coupled to mass spectrometry (GC–MS) in the control of veterinary drug residues. The wide polarity range among various drugs also poses difficulties for extraction and clean-up. Furthermore, extraction is hindered by strong adsorption or even covalent bindings (e.g. nitro furans) to the matrix. The high concentration of proteins in animal-originating matrix complicates extraction and clean-up steps. Proteins can precipitate during clean-up steps and cause irreversible adsorption of some analytes. Last but not least, some veterinary drugs have to be determined and confirmed at rather low concentrations (e.g. 0.3 μg/kg for chloramphenicol) in order to meet legal requirements.

Most published veterinary drug residue methods focus on one class of compounds (e.g. sulfonamides, quinolones, macrolides, etc.). There are still only few papers describing approaches that cover several classes of veterinary drugs. Most published real multiresidue methods were designed for matrices like urine and milk, which can often be analyzed after a simple dilution step (Van Rhijn et al., 2006). Methods designed for the analysis of drugs in tissues, cover a significantly narrower range of drugs than the methods listed for urine or milk. Most of them are screening methods or can be considered semi-quantitative.

Matrix effects in quantitative LC–MS–MS analysis of biological fluids were demonstrated by several authors. Kebarle et al, 1993, reported that ESI responses of organic bases decreased with an increase in the concentrations of other organic bases. They concluded that not detected matrix components can reduce the ion intensity of the analytes and can lead to poor reproducibility and accuracy. After applying more selective extraction step the ion suppression was overcome.

Nelson et al. (2002) concluded that the elimination of the suppression peak should be made either through sample clean up or by simply modifying the chromatographic conditions. Gradient changes can be insufficient to solve the problem. A great change of the selectivity in HPLC can be obtained, for example, by change in the mobile phase chemistry (e.g. change the organic solvent). Furthermore, they suggested that the elimination of ion suppression problems is no different than dealing with other chromatographic interferences.

In summary, investigations of matrix effect, ion suppression and "cross-talk" effects should be a part of the validation of quantitative LC–MS–MS assays in residue analysis.

Quantification of a large range of analytes fundamentally different in structure and chemical properties is unlikely to be done by internal standards and even less by isotope-labeled analogs. One of the approaches that can be used is the calculation of recoveries and signal suppression for each individual compound by producing two fortified blanks - one before the extraction and another into the injection-ready final extract. This relative method is referred as "standard addition method".

The high sensitivity and selectivity requirements promoted the use of LC–MS–MS techniques. This will probably change with the recent introduction of high performance time of flight mass spectrometry (ToF), which provides selectivity and sensitivity somewhere between single stage and tandem mass spectrometry. This technique coupled with high-resolution chromatographic systems, produces full scan high-resolution data and theoretically permits the extraction of an unlimited number of analyte traces. Such an approach breaks classical limits imposed by LC–MS–MS and even permits the monitoring of drugs or metabolites where no reference material is available (Kaufmann et al, 2008).

However, the methods involving ToF mass spectrometry also have some limitations, which currently prevent the successful development of a reliable multiresidue method, one of them being linked to sample preparation and involving the limited extraction efficiency for highly polar and non-polar compounds due to the problems with the selection of appropriate extraction solvents. Poor sensitivity and strong signal suppression effects could be improved by extensive clean-up and concentration steps, which are aimed primarily at deproteinization, at the same time negligibly affecting analyte recovery. Losses of analytes by selective SPE clean-up step can be significantly reduced by employing a generic polymeric reversed phase material. From the other side, limitations inherent to LC-MS-MS such as dwell time considerations and time window problems related to synchronization of chromatographic separation and MS detection, were overcome by LC–ToF.

ToF mass spectrometry offers high degree of flexibility which cannot be provided by MS–MS technology. ToF does neither require the extremely time consuming set-up of transition retention time windows, nor is there any limitation regarding the number of analytes. Furthermore it allows the monitoring of new drugs or metabolites for which no reference substances are yet available. This "back-tracing" of unknown substance is possible because ToF mass spectrometers collect very large amount of data during full-scan meaning that the spectrum of unknown substance is permanently recorded by the acquisition system and can be used any time for the comparison with the standard of the same substance that became available after the analysis of the sample.

Conclusion

Wide use of veterinary drugs in modern animal breeding certainly improves both the animal health and productivity. Efficient prevention and therapy for animal diseases is not possible without utilization of these substances. However, application of veterinary drugs inevitably leads to the occurrence of their residues in animal tissues and primary animal products. The prevention of residues entering the food chain in quantities that can pose risk to consumers' health has been the common goal of both scientists and regulatory bodies in many countries.

With the evolution of technology during the past 40 years, it became possible to detect sub-ppb levels of veterinary drugs residues in biological matrices. Simultaneously with the developments in the field of engineering and information technologies, significant work was carried out in the field of toxicological research and risk-assessment methodology enabling, so far, the most effective way of managing human's health regarding veterinary drugs residues.

Structural, i.e. unequivocal identification of residues became possible with the introducetion of mass spectrometric techniques in residue laboratories. The instrumentation evolved tremendously in the past decade enabling even the back tracing of substances that, for whatever reason, are not available to the control laboratories at the time of the analysis.

Regulatory aspect of the veterinary drugs residues is following the analytical progress laying out more stringent criteria for compliance of animal originating food and prescribing even lower detection limits for banned substances. The European Union entered the process of central registration of all pharmacologically active substances that are present on the market and instructed EFSA to re-evaluate the existing MRLs of these substances. The possibility to adopt Codex Alimentarius MRLs that are established at the relevant Codex Alimentarius meetings is also a step forward to the harmonization of regulatory criteria at the global level.

All this implies that current and future trends in veterinary drugs residues analysis and legislation are leading to the establishing of the globally effective and balanced system for maximal protection of consumer's health and at the same time providing the unrestricted and free food trade.

References

A. A. M. Stolker, U. A. Th. Brinkman, Analytical strategies for residue analysis of veterinary drugs and growth-promoting agents in food-producing animals – a review, *Journal of Chromatography A*, 2005, 1067, 15-53.

Anton Kaufmann, Patrick Butcher, Kathryn Maden, Mirjam Widmer Quantitative multiresidue method for about 100 veterinary drugs in different meat matrices by sub 2-μm particulate high-performance liquid chromatography coupled to time of flight mass spectrometry, *Journal of Chromatography A*, 2008, 1194, 66-79.

Butaye, P., L.A. Devriese, and F. Haesebrouck. 2001 Differences in antibiotic resistance patterns of *Enterococcus faecalis* and *Enterococcus faecium* strains isolated from pet and farm animals. *Antimicroial Agents Chemotheraphy*, 45, 1347-1378.

Codex Alimentarius Commission, Maximum residue limits for veterinary drugs in food, Official Codex Alimentarius website http://www.codexalimentarius.net/mrls/vetdrugs/jsp/vetd_q-e.jsp.

Commission Decision 2002/657/EC *Off. Journal of the European Community*, 2002 L. 221.

Comparative list of EU and Codex Alimentarius MRLs (Council Directive 2377/90/EC, Anex I, III, consolidated version, updated 2009, Codex Alimentarius Commission, Updated as at the 32nd session of the Codex Alimentarius Commission, July 2009).

Council Directive 1996/22/EC, *Off. Journal of the European Community*, 1996 L125.

Council Directive 1996/23/EC, *Off. Journal of the European Community*, 1996 L125.

Council Regulation 2377/90/EC *Off. Journal of the European Community*, 1997 L125.

De Brabander HF, Noppe H, Verheyden K, Vanden Bussche J, Wille K, Okerman L, Vanhaecke L, Reybroeck W, Ooghe S, Croubels S. Residue analysis: Future trends from a historical perspective, *Journal of Chromatography A*. 2009, 1216(46),7964-76

J. Van Rhijn, C. Bourgeon, J. Lasaroms, E. Oosterik, D. McMillan, *Proceedings of the 15th International Symposium on Hormone and Veterinary Drug Residues* Antwerp, 2006.

L.G. Huis in't Veld, Doc. Benelux Econom, Union SP/Lab/h, 78, 1.

N. S. Wilson, M. D. Nelson, J. W. Dolan, L. R. Snyder, R. G. Wolcott, P. W. Carr Column selectivity in reversed-phase liquid chromatography: I. A general quantitative relationship. *Journal of Chromatography A*, 961, 2, 2002, 171-193.

Opinion of the Scientific Panel on contaminants in the food chain (CONTAM) related to hormone residues in bovine meat and meat products .http://www.efsa.europa.eu/EFSA/efsa_locale-1178620753812_1178622336805.htm

R. Carabias-Martinez, E. Rodriguez-Gonzalo, P. Revilla-Ruiz, J. Hernandez-Mendez, Pressurized liquid extraction in the analysis of food and biological samples. *Journal of Chromatography A* 1089, 2005, 1.

Regulation (EC) No 470/2009 of the European Parliament and of the Council, laying down Community procedures for the establishment of residue limits of pharmacologically active substances in foodstuffs of animal origin, repealing Council Regulation (EEC) No 2377/90 and amending Directive 2001/82/EC of the European Parliament and of the Council and Regulation (EC) No 726/2004 of the European Parliament and of the Council, *Off. Journal of the European Community*, 2009, L 152/11.

Ridgway K, Lalljie SP, Smith RM. Sample preparation techniques for the determination of trace residues and contaminants in foods, *Journal of Chromatography A*. 2007 15, 1153(1-2), 36-53.

S. Mitra (Ed.), Sample Preparation Techniques in Analytical Chemistry, *Wiley-Interscience*, New Jersey, 2003.

S. Stefanovic, Tatjana Radicevic, Aurelija Spiric, Valentina Batas, S. Jankovic, and R. Petronijevic, Comparison of three confirmatory methods in residue analysis of (fluoro)quinolone antibacterials, *Annual meeting of the NRLs, Fougeres,* France, 2006.

Tang L, Kebarle P. Dependence of ion intensity in electrospray mass spectrometry on the concentration of the analytes in the electrosprayed solution. *Anal. Chem.* 1993; 65:3654–68.

Tina Zuidema et al., "Can fluorescence be considered as a sufficiently conclusive confirmatory method for B-group substances", poster presented at 5th International Symposium on hormone and veterinary drug residue analysis, Antwerp, Belgium, May 16-19 2006.

VOLLARD, E.J. and CLASENER, H.A.L., 1994. Colonization resistance. Antimicrobial *Agents and Chemotherapy,* 38 (3), 409-414.

W. Horwitz, L. R. Kamps, K. W. Boyer, *J. Assoc. Off. Anal. Chem.* 63, 1980, 1344.

Waters Inc official website http://www.waters.com/waters/nav.htm?locale=en_usandcid=513209.

In: Nutritional Insights and Food Safety
Editor: Jaroslava Švarc-Gajiæ
ISBN: 978-1-61122-130-5

Chapter IX

Food Color Additives

***Slavica Grujić*[1] *and Radoslav Grujić*[2]**
[1]University of Banja Luka, Faculty of Technology, Bulevar vojvode Petra Bojovića 1A, 78000 Banja Luka, Republika Srpska
[2]Department Food Science and Food Technology, University of East Sarajevo, Faculty of Technology, Vuka Karadžića 30, 71123 Istočno Sarajevo, Republika Srpska

Abstract

Numerous social, technical and economic factors have influenced the food industry over the last 20 or so years. Over this time the food market has changed rapidly with a much larger proportion of food being `processed before sale and ready prepared to meet the needs of new consumers such as working mothers, single parent families and the increasing number of older people in household. Accordingly, visually appealing foods that taste good and meet the consumers' demands on quality and price became the challenge to the food industry.

Consumers buy and consume food products for a number of reasons most of which relate predominantly to the characteristics of products. Some of the quality determinants refer to physical characteristics of products, such as taste, texture and shelf life. These factors can be measured in an objective manner. Other quality characteristics of food products can be determined by sensory perception, like the appearance and the smell of a food, and the feeling that the products produce in consumers. Colorants are added to many foods to make them appear healthier and more appealing, reinforcing the fact that color plays an important role in consumer choice. What is important is that the colors that are applied are safe, and that colors should not be used to mask unhealthy products

In order to produce food with good properties which is safe for consumer's health the food indutry uses food additives. The subject area of food additives is complex and includes both natural and synthetic substances, covering wide range of chemical entities. In general, consumers support the use of food additives in food production providing that they do not become hazards to human health. Different food color materials, including those defined as artificial, natural and nature identical are in use in manufacturing the food products. Developments of new and improved colors have aim to be in line with current consumer interests for incorporation of more natural products into food. There is however constant ongoing developments directed to improve the stability and handling properties of colors, new processing methods and to a much lesser extent (mainly restricted by legislative controls) development of totally new pigments. This chapter analyzes the positive and negative aspects of food additives in food production and elaborates their benefits and risks.

Introduction

Ever since, natural colors from spices and herbs, berries and vegetables have been a part of human's everyday diet. They have been consumed for generations, helped to identify food and evaluate its palatability. Color mainly defines the aesthetic value of food, predetermines consumers' expectations of flavor and taste and modulates appetite (Stintzing & Carle, 2004). Therefore, color is a major issue for the food industry and the manufacturers. However, owing to processing and storage of foods color may be altered through the action of light, temperature, oxygen, metal ions and endogenous enzymes. In addition, the color of fruits and vegetables vary during seasons, having an impact on the consistency of food products. Consequently, there is a technological need for coloring food in order to restore its initial appearance, compensate the fluctuation of the quality of raw materials and batch to batch variations. The application of food additives is further reinforced to meet consumers' expectations, protect photolabile vitamins and aromas and finally color the food for reasons of visual appeal (Stintzing & Carle, 2004). While synthetic pigments are increasingly rejected by the consumers and supposed to being unwholesome, the acceptance of natural or nature-derived alternatives is promoted by their psychological comprehension of being healthy. Natural sources used for coloring foods do not only carry chromophores like chlorophylls (kiwi, spinach, stinging nettle), carotenoids (carrot, pumpkin), anthocyanins (aronia, cherry, elderberry, grape, purple sweet potato, red cabbage, red radish) and betalains (red beet), but also contain other non-volatile and volatile ingredients which may bring about positive or negative qualities to the target food commodity. Coloring foodstuffs are labeled as ''coloring fruit- and plant extracts'' on the ingredient list. A good hygienic status, high color stability and purity together with a faint flavor and taste are the primary prerequisites for a promising coloring food sources.

Downham and Collins (2000) made a review of the importance of food colors through history. The addition of colorants to foods is thought to have occurred in Egyptian cities, where candy makers around 1500 BC added natural extracts and wine to improve the products appearance. Up to the middle of the 19th century ingredients, such as the spice saffron, were added for decorative effect to certain foodstuffs. Following the industrial revolution both the food industry and `processed food' developed rapidly. In 1856 the first synthetic color was developed by Sir William Henry Perkin and, by the turn of the century, unmonitored color additives had spread through the USA and Europe in all sorts of popular foods, including ketchup, mustard, jellies, and wine. Sellers at the time offered more than 80 artificial coloring agents to food manufacturers, some even intended for dyeing textiles, not foods. Many color additives were never tested for toxicity or other adverse effects. As the 1900s began, the bulk of chemically synthesized colors were derived from aniline, a petroleum product that is toxic. Originally, these were dubbed `coal-tar' colors because the starting materials were obtained from bituminous coal (Downham & Collins, 2000). Even though colors from plant, animal and mineral sources, which had been used in earlier times, remained in use early in this century, manufacturers had strong economic incentives to phase them out. Chemically synthesized colors were simply easier to produce, less expensive, and superior in coloring properties. Only tiny amounts were needed. They blended easily and didn't impart unwanted flavors to foods. But, as their use grew, so did their safety concerns. This lead to numerous regulations throughout the world, which, for example, in the USA reduced the permitted list of synthetic colors to seven from 700 been used! However `adulteration' continued for many years and this, together with more recent adverse press comments on food colors and health, has continued to contribute to the consumers concerns about color addition to the foodstuffs.

Consumer pressure, sociological changes, and technological advances improving the food processing industry have increased the overall color market. The most significant growth has been marked for naturally derived colors owing to the improvements in their stability and the intention of food industries to meet the consumers perception that the `natural is the best'. Future growth is expected to be greatest for naturally derived colors.

Nowadays, food products development is a continuous process that is of great concern to all companies active in this field. As a consequence of changing consumer needs, tomorrow's consumer may not want the products that were in great demand yesterday. These changing needs are apparent in, for instance, the increasing number of people who suffer from obesities and the increase of the ageing population (Linnemann et al., 2006). Moreover, the development of new food products serves as a competitive tool for food companies and as such it represents a mean to strengthen their position in the market. On a global scale, food product development is needed to provide growing populations with sufficient food of desired quality and also as a mean to increase the sustainability of food supply systems. This article gives an overview of factors that are relevant for successful food product development and presents methods for structured ways to develop new foods.

1. Definition of Food Quality

The contamination of food by chemical hazards is a worldwide public health concern and is a leading cause of international trade problems. Contamination may occur through environmental pollution of the air, water and soil, or through the intentional use of various chemicals, such as food additives or contaminants resulting from food manufacturing and processing. Chemicals can be a significant source of foodborne illness, although effects are often difficult to link with a particular food. Chemical contaminants in food include natural toxicants and environmental contaminants. Food additives and nutrients such as vitamins and essential minerals, pesticide and veterinary drug residues, are used to increase or improve the food supply, but assurance must first be obtained that all such uses are safe. Chemical contamination of food can affect health after a single exposure or, more often, after a longterm exposure; however, the health consequences of exposure to chemicals in food are often inadequately understood. While assessments of the risks associated with the exposure to pesticides, veterinary drugs and food additives are usually supported by extensive information; fewer data are available on the toxicology of other contaminants in food. New findings related to the potential of the chemicals to affect the immune, endocrine and developing nervous systems should continue to be incorporated into hazard characterizations of chemicals in food (WHO, 2002).

Food standards at national and international levels are defined based on a Codex of an internationally agreed framework for risk analysis. WHO has a long history of providing assessments of chemical risks in food to Codex and to Member States. The Joint FAO/WHO Expert Committee on Food Additives (JECFA) and the Joint FAO/WHO Meeting on Pesticide Residues (JMPR) are recognized as being at the forefront of scientific knowledge in assessing the risks of chemicals in food. In addition to more traditional tasks, JECFA and JMPR must also deal with issues such as cumulative exposure to low concentrations of chemicals, fetal neurotoxicity and the special risks in vulnerable subpopulations. WHO also reviewes the procedures used by the expert bodies to ensure consistency and transparency, and to avoid conflict of interests.

In utilitarian terms, quality can be defined as ''fitness for use'' or, more appropriately for foodstuffs, ''fitness for consumption'', which leads to what the experts in ISO standards call ''customer'' or ''consumer'' satisfaction. Thus, quality can be described as the requirements necessary to satisfy the needs and expectations of the consumer (Peri, 2006). Food quality could be defined as a set of consumer requirements for safety, authenticity and conformity of a product.

The most important are nutritional and sensory food quality characteristics, which correlate to the biological quality, and represent the core of food value. Safety, nutritive and sensory requirements have important role in integrated quality of the food product and consumer choices (Peri, 2006). Nutritional requirements are obviously extremely important because the main purpose of eating is to satisfy nutritional needs. Regular consumption of specific food may have beneficial effects on health and strengthen the body's defenses against a number of chronic diseases. Sensory requirements interlace the products quality characteristics and consumers' expectations (Linnemann et al., 2006; Peri, 2006). During the consumption of certain food brain transforms sensations into perceptions. Sensory perceptions are further related to other brain functions such as memory, culture, values, emotions, etc. Knowledge or memory of food sensory characteristics is compared to our sensory reactions to the product.

Additives are used to enhance the quality or stability of a food or to improve its sensory properties, provided that this does not change the nature of the food and does not deceive the consumer. This joint sensory and psychological perception of quality is one of the most important areas for the development of food sciences.

2. Food Colorants

According to the CODEX General standard for food additives (CODEX STAN 192-1995) definition of *food additive* means any substance not normally consumed as a food by itself and not normally used as a typical ingredient of the food, whether or not it has nutritive value. The intentional addition of that substance to food is for a technological (including organoleptic) purpose in the manufacture, processing, preparation, treatment, packing, packaging, transport or holding of such food results, or may be reasonably expected to result (directly or indirectly), in it or its byproducts becoming a component of or otherwise affecting the characteristics of such foods. The term does not include contaminants or substances added to food for maintaining or improving nutritional qualities.

In terms of color adding as additive, labeling the terms `natural color' and `food color' are not permitted as they may indicate that the color occurs naturally, when it doesn't. There are numerous options available: `artificial color'; `artificial color added'; and `color added'. When using naturally derived colors, a preferred option to indicate it on label is `colored with x' or `x (color)' naming the color source. If the name of the specific color is not included the label declaration must then say `artificially colored or `artificial color added'. The European Union has authorized use of colorants as food additives, naturally derived or inorganic pigments found in nature, synthetic pigments synthesized to match the naturally occurring counterparts. Each one has assigned an `E number' (Grujić, 2005). Having regard to Council Directive 89/107/EEC on the approximation of the laws of the Member States concerning food additives authorized for use in foodstuffs intended for human consumption, EU Directive 94/36/EC harmonized all previous individual country legislation and details these colors and Commission Directive 2008/128/EC is laying down specific purity criteria concerning colours for use in foodstuffs in EU. This was in response to the development of a single market for the free movement of goods, consumer demand for health and safety and the prevention of food adulteration.

Over the last 10-15 years within many countries there has been a distinct move towards the use of natural and nature identical colors. This was a response to consumer and major retailer pressure to develop more natural products and to limit the inclusion of synthetic colors. Furthermore such approach has been enforced by legislation. Nevertheless the food market is very diverse and the constant need for cost effective, readily available foods and a major increase in the number of people eating in restaurants (where ingredients used are not declared) means artificial colors will continue to be used in substantial quantities (Downham & Collins, 2000).

In the USA, certified (i.e. synthetic) colors have historically been used, mainly because of achievable shades, the low cost and the good stability. Synthetic colors are also highly concentrated and they are widely available. However, there is a growing move towards natural products and growth in the `natural color' market is predicted, especially owing to the fact that only seven synthetic colors are approved.

2.1. Natural Colors

A large number of vegetables harbor shining colors. These colors are conferred by the pigments contained in the plants cells. On the basis of their chemical structures, natural pigments can be classed into four families, i.e. tetrapyrroles (e.g. chlorophyll), carotenoids, polyphenolic compounds (e.g. anthocyanins), and alkaloids (e.g. betalains). Natural pigments are also found in animal tissues and, eventually in transformed food products as additives. Although animal tissues contain plant pigments, such as carotenoids, these tissues are usually not able to synthesize them but the pigments are introduced from food. Natural pigments have an important impact on the commercial value of foods, because the colors establish the first contact with the consumer. In addition, plant pigments may have an influence on the health of the consumers. Pigments are labile: they can be easily altered and destroyed.

Natural colors are spread widely throughout the nature in fruits, vegetables, seeds and roots. In our daily diets we consume large quantities of many pigments, especially anthocyanins, chlorophylls and carotenoids. Nature is thought to produce about 100 million tonnes *per annum* of carotenoids, of which more than 600 structures have been identified. Compared to this, our intake from naturally colored processed food is fairly insignificant.

Pigments from nature vary widely in their physical and chemical properties. Many are sensitive to oxidation, pH change and light and their inherent solubility varies widely. There are currently 13 permitted naturally derived colors within the EU and 26 colors exempt from certification in the USA. Natural colors are considered much less stable, more difficult to use and more expensive than the synthetic colors they aimed to replace. Furthermore it is thought that the color shades achievable with natural pigments are less vibrant and appealing. Prior to any FDA petitioning and EU approval for use in food, new natural pigment sources require safety assessment, which is costly and time consuming.

Since their wider commercialization around 25 years ago significant developments have occurred in the production and use of natural colors. The growth in the use of natural colors comes from increasing consumer pressure for `natural' products and from general distrust in food industry, based on unsubstantiated health scares related to additives in general, but especially related to perceived association with many azo dyes such as tartrazine (Downham & Collins, 2000). Suppliers of natural colors are focused on the development of the currently permitted pigments in three main areas: formulation technology, processing technology; and alternative sources of pigments. These approaches have proved to be very successful and have contributed to the increase in the usage of natural colors throughout the food and drink industry. At present food manufacturers can produce most color shades in a natural form providing the vibrancy and stability.

Annatto extract is a yellow-orange natural food color, which is obtained from the outer coatings of the seeds of the Annatto tree (*Bixa orellana* L.), a small tree which grows in Central and South America (Oka et al., 2007). It has been used as a food colorant by peoples in Latin America for many centuries. Although the plant species originated in northern South America, it is now widely cultivated in tropical areas for commercial production (Hagiwara et al., 2003). Annatto extract containing carotenoids, is employed in the food industry as an important colorant, mainly in dairy products such as cheese and butter. The main components of this natural pigment are bixin and norbixin. It has been reported that annatto extract does not exert any genotoxicity, subacute and chronic toxicity, reproductive toxicity or carcinogenicity.

Anthocyanins. The colored phenolic compounds present in many red fruits such as grapes, blueberries, cherries and cranberries are thought to play a significant role in preventing or delaying the onset of many diseases (Downham & Collins, 2000). The plants pigments include anthocyanins, phenolic acids, flavanols, tannins and resveratrol. Much research has focused on these phytochemicals which are present in in black grape skins and consequently red wine, linking the red wine intake to a reduced incidence of heart disease and cancers. The compounds present in red wine are known to be powerful antioxidants and have been identified as having a wide range of biochemical and pharmacological effects including anticarcinogenic, anti-inflammatory and antimicrobial, and preventing both the LDL (low density lipoprotein) oxidation and the subsequent onset of cardiovascular disease.

Currently there is a tendency in developing of food ingredients based on natural anthocyanins for inclusion into functional food products. Anthocyanins play important roles both in plant physiology, visual attraction, but also in food mainly defining its esthetic value. Physiological effects that the pigments exert in plants are supposedly similar to those shown in humans following ingestion of colored food. Therefore, anthocyanins in fresh and also processed fruit and vegetables serve two functions: They improve the overall appearance, but also contribute to consumers' health and well-being (Stintzing & Carle, 2004). In addition to their immediate function ameliorating the visual quality, colored foodstuffs such as juice, their respective concentrates but also fruit and vegetable powders incorporating anthocyanins, may improve the nutritional value of the target food. These potential nutraceutical properties are even more important at a time, when human diet is increasingly based on processed foods.

Anthocyanins are derivatives of 2-phenylbenzopyrylium salts. In fruit juices and as purified food coloring materials in foodstuffs, they interact readily with other naturally occurring materials, such as flavonols. Such interactions depend on intermolecular association through, for instance, hydrogen bonds, and may therefore affect anthocyanin stability. The reactions are usually accompanied with decolorization. The rate of anthocyanin degradation depends on pH, temperature, oxygen partial pressure, metal ions, ascorbate concentration, and other components. In most food processing operations, the anthocyanins are relatively stable, especially when low pH conditions are maintained.

Naturally present ascorbic acid can be problematic for the stability of anthocyane colors. In the presence of iron or copper ions and oxygen, the oxidation of ascorbic acid to dehydroascorbic acid is accompanied by the formation of hydrogen peroxide, which in turn can oxidize anthocyanins, a reaction implicated in the loss of color. The exact mechanism, however, is not clear. Under anaerobic conditions, anthocyanins and ascorbic acid may react via condensation-type mechanisms. The products of these interactions, some of which are complex polymers, have not been well characterized.

Red cabbage color is an anthocyanins red dye obtained by extracting the red leafs of the *Brassica oleracea* with water and hydrolyzing under weak acidic conditions. The red color of the dye is derived from derivatives of cyanidin acylglucoside (Oka et al., 2007). This color shows a red-purple color under acidic conditions, is highly heat- and light-resistant, especially at pH lower than 3.0. By exploiting these properties, it is widely used for coloring of juices, candies, jelly, chewing gums, fruit wines etc.

Betalains are the red and yellow plant pigments obtained from members of the order Centrospermae, the most food-significant of these being the beetroot (*Beta vulgaris* L.). The betalains are divided into two groups, the betacyanins which are purplish-red in color and the less common yellow-colored betaxanthins. The betacyanins comprise about 90% of beetroot betalains. Betacyanins differ from other naturally occurring water-soluble plant pigments, especially anthocyanins, in that their color is hardly affected by pH changes in the range normally encountered in foodstuffs. Betacyanins are fairly stable under food-processing conditions, although heating in the presence of air at neutral pH causes breakdown to brown compounds.

From a technological point of view, anthocyanins and betalains complement each other for their use to color the food from yellow, orange to red and purple. While the first gradually lose their tinctorial power from pH 2 to 3, the latter are chemically stable from pH 3 to 7. Red and purple shades can be achieved both by anthocyanins and betacyanins, whereas orange and yellow hues are mainly obtained with betalain mixtures and betaxanthins, respectively.

Caramel colors form a significant segment of the overall color market (around 11%), principally owing to their use in cola beverage drinks (Downham & Collins, 2000). They are produced by the controlled heating of carbohydrates, such as sucrose, glucose and fructose. Four classes of caramels are commercially produced for specific applications. They differ in the catalyst used to promote the caramelization process. The market for caramel colors is thought to be reasonably static, with annual increases at around 2-3% *per annum*. The growth in caramel use is expected to occur through market development and in line with the predicted growth in `brown' food products such as toffee flavored products, colas and ready meals.

Caramel food colors are chemically heterogeneous hence their chemistry is complex and constitutes a large subject area. For this reason, this important group of food additives and Maillard-type reactions are described just where other additives are involved too (Scotter & Castle, 2004). Where appropriate, the importance of interactions of food additives with other components of food (i.e. nutrients and non-nutrients) is discussed, as well as certain aspects of toxicology.

The *carotenoids* include the carotenes, which are hydrocarbons, and the xanthophylls, which are oxygen-containing analogues. Carotenoids are widespread in nature with more than 600 been identified. The health benefits of carotenoids lie in two main areas: antioxidant activity by protecting cells against oxidative damage, which is thought to lead to degenerative diseases such as atherosclerosis, cancer, arthritis and macular degeneration and pro-vitamin A activity. β-carotene and α-carotene have an pro-vitamin A activity and as such can be converted within the intestinal mucosa to vitamin A. Carotene color formulations can therefore be used to contribute to any vitamin A claim that is made, as well as providing the coloring effect.

Much scientific research has been completed on the health benefits of carotenoids. A great deal of research has focused on β-carotene alone, but there is now increasing evidence that the carotenoids work synergistically and therefore an intake of mixed carotenoids is more beneficial, as this is how carotenoids would be taken from food sources, such as carrots. Mixed carotenoids from the fruit of the palm oil tree have a very similar composition to the carotenoids in the carrot.

Based on extensive epidemiological observations, fruits and vegetables that are a rich source of carotenoids are thought to provide health benefits by decreasing the risk of various diseases, particularly certain cancers and eye diseases. The carotenoids that have been most studied in this regard are β-carotene, lycopene, lutein and zeaxanthin. In part, the beneficial effects of carotenoids are thought to be due to their role as antioxidants. β-carotene may add the benefits to the food due to its ability to be converted to vitamin A. Additionally, lutein and zeaxanthin may be protective in eye diseases because they absorb blue light that enters the eye and could damage it (Krinsky & Johnson, 2005).

Food sources of carotenoides include a variety of fruits and vegetables, although the primary sources of lycopene are tomato and tomato products. Additionally, egg yolk is a highly bioavailable source of lutein and zeaxanthin. These carotenoids are available in supplement form. However, intervention trials with large doses of β-carotene have demonstrated adverse effects on the incidence of lung cancer in smokers and workers exposed to asbestos. Until the efficacy and safety of supplements containing these nutrients are examined, diets high in fruits and vegetables are advised.

Naturally occurring carotenoid pigments, such as astaxanthin and canthaxanthin, may be applied in animal feed so that the resulting food products are appealing to the consumer. Whilst arguably, these pigments may be seen to be of cosmetic value, astaxanthin and canthaxanthin are both known to exert benefits on animal health and welfare (Baker & Günther, 2004). Evidence suggests that carry-over of these pigments into the human food chain could also be beneficial to human health.

Carotenoids are amongst the most widely distributed pigments in biological systems. Carotenoid pigments found in nature are safe for coloring food and have health benefits for people (Baker & Günther, 2004). β-carotene is routinely used in soft drinks, cheeses and butter or margarines. The pigment is well regarded as being safe, and indeed positive health effects are also ascribed to this carotenoid due to a provitamine A role. In wild salmon, the carotenoid pigment 'astaxanthin' provides a majority of the color. Canthaxanthin, a carotenoid pigment abundant in plants, microbes, crustacea and birds, can also impart color to salmon and trout. In these applications, the carotenoid is not referred to as a colorant (or a dye), but rather a pigment, as the animal itself selectively retains the pigment because it is biologically programmed to do so.

The tomato color is carotenoid coloring obtained by extraction from the fruit of *Lycopersicon esculentum* Mill. and contains several components. The main component is lycopene. This color is yellow-red and highly heat- and light-resistant, but readily oxidized. This color is used for coloring tomato processed foods, processed marine products, jelly, and candies.

The orange color is carotenoid coloring obtained from the fruit or rind of *Citrus sinensis* Osbeck and contains several components. The main component is a fatty acid ester of ß-cryptoxanthin. This color is yellow–orange and is used for the coloring of citrus fruit beverages, confectionery, and sherbet.

Within the context of food additives, carotenoids may exist in the free state, in solutions in the lipid phase, or associated with proteins or polysaccharides. They can also exist as esters and glycosides. In food, the main causes of carotenoid degradation are various oxidative reactions.

Carotenoids act as very effective scavengers in the photosensitized oxidation of unsaturated fatty acids, where chlorophylls may act as sensitizers. The oxidative stability of carotenoids is improved by the addition of antioxidants, such as BHA, BHT, tocopherol and ascorbyl palmitate. The addition of ascorbic acid is reported to improve the color stability.

Carminic acid from cochineal is a pale yellow quinone compound which complexes readily with aluminium (as in cochineal carmines), tin and other metals to give brilliant red pigments. A red pigment is obtained from the insect Coccus cactus that lives on various cactus plants. The insect is native to tropical South and Central America and produces the pigment as a deterrent against other insects (Oka et al., 2007). This color is used for the coloring of candies and jelly. The cochineal complexes are relatively stable under food processing conditions. Carminic acid has close structural and chromogenic properties to the highly toxic anthracycline antitumour drug doxorubicin and is reported to redox cycle to produce free radicals (Gutteridge & Quinlan 1986; Scotter & Castle, 2004). These radicals, in the presence of trace amounts of iron salts, readily damage cell membrane lipids and degrade the carbohydrate deoxyribose. Damage to cell membrane lipids appears to involve mainly organic oxygen radicals, such as alkoxy and peroxy radicals, whereas that to deoxyribose implicates the hydroxyl radical formed in a fentontype reaction. α-tocopherol, the phenolic antioxidants BHA and butylated hydroxytoluene (BHT), the hydroxyl radical scavengers mannitol, benzoate, and thiourea, and iron chelators, such as EDTA, were all reported to prevent such damage. The product of the reaction between carmine and hot ammonia solution has been reported to be the acid-stable 4-amino analogue, which is permitted for food use in the USA (Sugimoto et al., 2002, Scotter & Castle, 2004).

Carthamus yellow is flavonoid yellow dye obtained by extracting the flower of the *Carthamus tinctorius* Linne with water. The yellow color of the dye is mainly derived from the flavonoids, saffronin A and saffronin B. This color shows a yellow color under acidic conditions and a reddish yellow color under basic conditions, and is highly heat- and light-resistant. By exploiting these properties it is widely used for the coloring of juices, candies, jelly, chewing gums, fruit wines, chocolate, etc. (Oka et all , 2007).

Chlorophyll has been shown to have wound healing, antigenotoxic and antimutagenic properties. It has also been cited as a deodorizer to reduce body odor and bad breath. Chlorophyll degradation during food processing can proceed as an acid-, base- or enzyme-catalyzed reaction. Weak acids liberate the magnesium bound in porphyrin ring to form pheophytins by substitution with hydrogen. This results in a color change from green to dull brown. Magnesium may be replaced by copper (as in copper chlorophyll additives, i.e. chemically modified chlorophylls) and by tin and zinc. Alkaline salts may also be produced, but these are very unstable. Chlorophylls may also undergo photo-oxidation accompanied by the loss of desirable color. Lipoprotein-bound chlorophylls are somewhat protected against acids, but can be affected by cooking and processing. In alkaline media, the decomposition of chlorophylls is very rapid and they are not stable against the action of free-radicals, e.g. during lipoxygenase-catalysed oxidation of lipids, probably due to the effect of hydroperoxides (Scotter & Castle, 2004). Even though chlorophylls have received far less interest than carotenoids, they appear to have appreciable potential against environmental and dietary mutagens.

Curcumin is the collective term given to the yellow colored compounds obtained from rhizomes of *Curcuma domestica*. Historically turmeric, the source of the curcumin pigment, has been used in medical treatments for its anti-inflammatory and antiseptic properties, as well as a spice. Curcumin is a potent antioxidant and protects the cellular components against oxidative damage. It has been found to inhibit the initiation, promotion and progression of cancers, enhance the activities of specific enzymes responsible for digestion, act as an antibacterial agent and promote liver detoxification. There are even reports of its anti-HIV properties (Downham & Collins, 2000).

Curcumin is relatively stable to heat processing except in alkaline medium, where it degrades. The compound is sensitive to light, which limits its applications in food. Curcumin gives a lemon-yellow color with a distinct green shade in solution. Cations tend to induce a more orange-brown shade and SO_2 reduces the color intensity.

Gardenia yellow extracted from gardenia fruit (*Gardenia jasminoides* Ellis) is a yellow natural food additive and is widely used for coloring foods. It is known that the yellow color is derived from a water soluble pigment including crocin and crocetin as major components (Oka et al., 2007).

Lac dye is quinone coloring, a natural food additive extracted from a stick lac, which is a secretion of the insect Coccus laccae (*Laccifer lacca* Kerr) and is widely used for coloring food. It is known that the red color is derived from a water-soluble pigment including laccaic acids A, B, C, and E (Oka et al., 2007).

Lutein. The xanthophyll pigment lutein has been recognized as an antioxidant. It is one of the two carotenoids found in the macular region of the eye and evidence suggests that lutein may protect against age related macular degeneration, a leading cause of blindness in people over the age of 65. Lutein based supplements are widely available in the USA based on this evidence. A diet rich in lutein is also thought to decrease the incidence of cataracts. There is also increasing evidence that lutein has anticancer properties.

Lycopene, the natural pigment found in tomatoes may help in reducing the risk of several cancers such as prostrate and cervical cancer. Studies have indicated that lycopene may be more efficiently absorbed from processed tomato products such as ketchup and sauces than from raw tomatoes.

Paprika color is carotenoid coloring obtained by extraction of the fruits of red peppers (*Capsicum annuum*). The pigment contains capsanthin and its esters, such as lauric acid, myristic acid, and palmitic acid, in large amounts as its color components (Oka et al., 2007). Commercially available paprika colors are known to have different compositions of these color components depending on the material the paprika color is extracted from, making the determination of paprika color based on the analysis of the color components impossible.

Turmeric Oleoresin is a yellow pigment obtained by extracting the tubers of *Curcuma longa* Linn, with volatile solvents and subsequent concentration to remove the solvent. The main component is curcumin. This color is used for the coloring of pickle and curry powder (Oka et al., 2007).

Within the EU numerical ADIs have been allocated only for the natural coloring materials annatto, carmines, carotenes and the copper complexes of chlorophyll. Annatto is permitted for use in a restricted range of foodstuffs, whereas the carmines and carotenes can be used in food in restricted concentration. The copper complexes of chlorophylls may be used according to the *quantum satis*.

Pigment analysis constitutes a real analytical challenge because pigments are often part of complex structures and/or mixtures. Therefore, addressing these issues is never straightforward. To take up this challenge, it is necessary to have at disposal a diversified number of analytical procedures, able to rapidly and precisely quantify the different pigments and their degradation products present in the samples. The development of powerful analytical methods is also of prime importance in the control of quality. In this contribution, Schoefs (2004) briefly reviewed the methods for pigment extraction and separation describing the ways of pigment identification and quantification.

2.2. Nature Identical Colors

'Nature identical' colors have been developed to match their counterparts in nature. The most common pigments that are synthesized are carotenoids consisting of conjugated hydrocarbons, and as such they are prone to oxidative attack and a subsequent loss of color. Color formulations have been developed with antioxidant systems, such as tocopherol and ascorbyl palmitate, to reduce this effect (Downham & Collins, 2000).

'Nature identical' β-carotene has a large portion of the colorant market. Its principal use is in yellow fats (margarines, low fat spreads etc.), soft drinks, confectionery and bakery products (Downham & Collins, 2000, Grujić & Grujić, 2009). For most food and drink applications the challenge to suppliers is to provide oil and water dispersible forms, especially for the yellow fat and soft drink producers. This could be achieved by using methods such as emulsification and pigment suspension as follows:

- Emulsion formulations consist of very fine β-carotene oil droplets dispersed throughout an aqueous phase. These can be spray dried to give water dispersible powders.
- Oil dispersible suspensions are made using micronization to form nano sized β-carotene crystals suspended in vegetable oil. Dispersing this suspension through a protective colloid/polymer matrix, which coats and stabilizes the pigment, makes water dispersible beadlet forms. This suspension is then spray dried to form high strength powders.

By using these methods water and oil dispersible nature identical colors with pigment contents from 1% to 10% have been developed. The shade achieved is dependent on the formulation and processing used and varies from golden yellow to a red/orange shade.

2.3. Synthetic Colors

Food colors are used for maintenance and improvement of color appearance in foods. Synthetic colors are added to foods to replace the loss of natural colors during processing, to reduce batch-to-batch variations and to produce products with consumer appeal where no natural color exists. In recent years, natural food colors have been increasingly used for the consumer preference (Tripathi et al., 2007). However, they are relatively unstable and their costs are higher than synthetic food colors. Therefore, synthetic food colors are still used instead of natural colors in many foods such as drinks, candies, and sweets. The list of permitted synthetic food colors vary from country to country. Some people are sensitive to particular food colors, so the colors in the food products must be the same as those on their labels. Thus, determination of synthetic food colors is required to ensure the food safety.

The synthetic food dyes amaranth, sunset yellow FCF, indigo carmine and synthetic azo dyes are often used in foods processed at higher temperatures, especially sugar-based confectionery commodities. Their interaction with other food additives has been reviewed (Scotter & Castle, 2004). It was found that many factors can and do contribute to colorant stability, such as excessive heat, light, pH, redox systems, other food ingredients and reactions with proteins, reducing ions and reducing sugars. The majority of color additives are unstable in combination with oxidizing and reducing agents. Since color depends on the existence of a conjugated unsaturated system within the dye molecule, any substance which modifies this system (e.g. oxidizing or reducing agents, sugars, acids, and salts) will affect the color. All dyes, those with an azo group in particular, will exhibit accelerated fading under both acid and alkaline conditions in the presence of metals, including zinc, tin, aluminium, iron and copper, especially at higher temperatures. This is mostly due to the reducing effects of the liberated hydrogen. Dyes will often react with the metals in food cans. Yoshioka and Ichihashi (2008) published results of the determination of forty synthetic food colors determined in drinks and candies by reversed-phase high-performance liquid chromatography with photodiode array detection, and described an analytical method.

Currently seven permitted synthetic pigments are used in the USA. Before 1906 the USA `adulterated' foods were common and used more than 700 colorants, many of which were highly toxic. Within the EU 17 synthetic pigments are permitted (Downham & Collins, 2000). These are all in the form of water soluble dyes. Lake pigments and dispersions are also permitted six of which are used in the USA. The lake of erythrosine is not permitted because of concerns over its iodine content.

Water soluble dyes were originally produced as fine powders. The suppliers of water soluble dyes have addressed the problem of dusting and clumping by making granules, pre-weighed sachets and gels.

Lake pigments are insoluble compounds precipitated onto an `aluminium hydrate substrate' and are produced as extremely fine powders. The dye content and the particle size determine the color shade of the powder. Lakes are primarily used when (Downham & Collins, 2000):

- there is insufficient solvent to dissolve the dyes (for example in fat based applications);
- when color migration is a problem;
- when an ultra fine powder is required (for example in powdered desserts and soups to color the dry mix);
- in confectionery for colored panned sugar coatings, providing less drying time and a more even coating than water soluble pigments.

Lakes tend to be more stable to light and other chemicals than their parent dyes, but are usually unsuitable in strongly acidic products as the color-aluminium bond is broken down, resulting in delaking and color change/precipitation problems. Liquid dispersions are also made of lake pigments for the ease of handling and customer preference.

Although cited as having excellent stability, soluble dyes do lose color in certain food manufacturing circumstances. The most common problems with soluble dyes are:

- decolorization by ascorbic acid (vitamin C);
- loss of color resulting from microbial attack (often used as an indicator for `off' foodstuffs);
- precipitation/color loss resulting from the presence of metal ions;
- reactions with proteins at high temperatures causing color fade.

These problems are difficult to overcome without chemical modifications to the pigments, which is not permitted. Color suppliers offer technical support to recommend the most suitable dye for the application and advice on the stage of color addition as well as on other ingredients such as sequestrants and antioxidants that can be added to reduce color loss.

2.4. Determination of Food Colorants

The establishment of appropriate methods for the analysis of natural colorings is necessary in order to rapidly evaluate food quality and safety. Natural colorings derived from natural materials have a wide variety and are frequently used in foods in Japan. Natural carotenoids, quinods, flavonoids, and anthocyane colorings, as well as many synthetic dyes are used in various foods, so in terms of food safety, the establishment of accurate and rapid analytical methods for their determination is important. Synthetic colors are generally analyzed by thin-layer chromatography, as method which allows a fast analysis and the simultaneous analysis of many samples (Oka et al., 2007). Recommended rapid analytical methods for identification of natural colorings in foods such as annatto extract, orange color, gardenia yellow, paprika color, tomato color, marigold color, β-carotene, turmeric oleoresin (carotenoid colorings), lac color, cochineal color (quinoid colorings), carthamus yellow (flavonoid coloring), and red cabbage color (anthocyanin coloring) have been proposed.

3. Additive–Food Interactions

It is well established that food additives and to a lesser extent their degradation products can interact with one another and with food constituents to form an array of new products. In some instances, such products have been identified, whereas, in others they are poorly characterized or remain of unknown structure. The consequences of such interactions are the main consideration in food safety implications being of particular concern. From the information and data in the key references and other important articles relating to additive–additive and additive–food component interactions, it is clear that the bulk of the research effort in this area has targeted a few classes of food additives, such as synthetic food coloring materials. The consequences of these interactions are not fully understood yet. The availability of this information in the literature has been summarized as review paper by Scotter and Castle (2004). The effects of pH, temperature, light, reactive species, oxygen, and other parameters on the reactivity of these food additives have been discussed. Other important aspects that have been addressed include the formation of toxic reaction products and mutagenic compounds, protective effects and inhibition, kinetics and mechanisms, and where appropriate, the likelihood and significance of additive reactions in food and model systems. The amount of available information on the interactions of certain additives, which may have the potential for interaction is sparse, the same as for safety (toxicity) testing of food additives based on a quantitative structure–activity relationship (QSAR) approach.

Additive–food interactions are more problematic than additive–additive interactions because the knowledge of the detailed chemical composition of food is still surprisingly limited, beyond the major food constituents and trace nutritional components. Scotter and Castle (2004) state that in order to define the 'whole food' safety is not enough to take into account only the toxic factors present in a food. There are also possible interactions with other beneficial chemicals, present as food constituents, such as nutrients, protective factors and the substances that modify toxicity. This approach does not attempt to provide a complete chemical description of foods, but it could be used to assess the balance between beneficial and detrimental effects of natural food constituents, individually and in combination. Such an approach may be useful in assessing the additive and synergistic combination of effects of all food additives that may be present in any given foodstuff. The identification and quantification of degradation products may also be important in discussing the potential toxicity of food additives, as these products may react further with other food components including other additives, to form undesirable compounds.

4. Additives - Additives Interaction

Very important area with respect to food colors is the simultaneous use of multiple ingredients constituting a food color (Downham & Collins, 2000). Additives are usually used in a color formulation to fulfill a technological need, together with the carriers or diluents to impart functionality such as water/oil dispersibility, to improve stability or for the enhancement of shelf life. The stability of a specific pigment is dictated by its chemical structure and the medium to which it is exposed. Chemical modification to enhance performance/stability is not acceptable, consequently the route to improved performance of colorants is via the use of process and/or formulation technologies. In order to improve the performance of food colorants it is permitted to use the carrier/diluent according to the miscellaneous additives directive, to use food ingredients (e.g. sugar, oil), whose use is not restricted by additive regulations, or to use a processing aid having an impact on the color formulation, but no technological function in the final foodstuff.

Scotter and Castle (2004) published critical reviews of the key literature on some food additive–additive chemical interactions and food additive–food component interactions, published over the last 30 years. The review includes the chemistry (reactivity), functionality, stability, use and reactions with other specific food additives for five main classes of synthetic food coloring materials. Where appropriate, the importance of interactions of food additives with other components of food (i.e. nutrients and non-nutrients) has been assessed and certain aspects of toxicology included. A practical outcome of the review includes a set of recommendations for future research in studied area.

5. The Safety of Food Colorants

Food is a heterogeneous mixture of chemicals, both natural and man-made; hence, the science of food and food chemistry is complex. The subject area of food additives is similarly complex and includes both natural and synthetic substances, covering a wide range of chemical entities. The industry of food additives is growing rapidly. Consumers have created demands for processed foods and usually one or more additives are needed to meet their demands. Furthermore low-calorie foods require substitutes for (principally) fats and sugars. To meet regulatory compliance, not only each additive must demonstrate technological need, but it is also subjected to extensive toxicity testing before approval and addition to the list of additives (Scotter & Castle, 2004). These tests are oriented towards establishing a level of exposure, i.e. the acceptable daily intake (ADI), which is associated with the acceptable risk. Whilst being important for the appearance, nutritional value, taste, and safety of food, food additives may have different implications *in vivo* (Grujić, 2005; Grujić et al., 2009).

Food safety and the protection of consumer's interests is of increasing concern to general public, non-governmental organizations, professional associations, international trading partners and trade organizations. It is necessary to ensure that consumer confidence and the confidence of trading partners is secured through the open and transparent development of food law and through public authorities taking the appropriate steps to inform the public where there are reasonable grounds to suspect that a food may present a risk to health.

The Joint Food and Agriculture Organization of the United Nations (FAO/WHO) Food Standards Programme were established in 1963. The Joint FAO/WHO Codex Alimentarius Commission (Codex) was its principal organ. The objective of Codex is to develop standards for food, protecting the health of the consumers and ensuring fair practices in the food trade. Codex has elaborated many international standards on food safety, and Member States have often used these in national legislation. Recent international agreements managed by the World Trade Organization (WTO) have put even further emphasis on the importance of Codex standards. Under WTO, health and safety requirements must be justifiable on the grounds of protecting public health and must be based on a sound, scientific risk assessment.

The Joint FAO/WHO Expert Committee on Food Additives (JECFA) has been meeting since 1956 to evaluate the safety of food additives, contaminants, naturally occurring toxicants and residues of veterinary drugs in food. JECFA has evaluated more than 1500 food additives, approximately 40 contaminants and naturally occurring toxicants, and residues of approximately 90 veterinary drugs. Currently, the Committee develops principles for the safety assessment of chemicals in food that are consistent with risk assessment and take account the recent developments in toxicology and other relevant sciences.

Concerns related to food additives have focused mainly on adverse reactions to certain additives such as the artificial food coloring tartrazine or the sulfite group of preservatives. The chemical interactions between food additives permitted for use in the European Union (EU) are the main considerations given in this review. The term 'interaction' may be interpreted differently, depending on the particular scientific point of view. In toxicological terms, for instance, interaction may be used as a general term to describe an altered outcome arising from the presence of two compounds and could be antagonistic, additive or synergistic.

5.1. Examination of Food Additives Intake

The first step toward defining the permitted use of food additives are the toxicological studies conducted by the Joint Expert Committee on Food Additives (JECFA), the establishment of an Acceptable Daily Intake (ADI), and the elaboration of identity and purity criteria. In the second step responsible governmental agencies or the Codex commodity committees, propose the permitted use of an additive in different foodstuffs to the Codex Committee on Food Additives and Contaminants (CCFAC).

Different approaches exist to estimate the probable daily intake, some of them being very expensive and time consuming. Some countries have therefore difficulties in initiating studies on the intake of food additives. For this reason, CCFAC requested the Working Group on Intake of Food Additives and Contaminants to prepare guidelines for simple evaluation of food additive intake (Codex Alimentarius, 1989).

The Acceptable Daily Intake (ADI) is estimated by JECFA and represents the amount of a food additive, expressed on a body weight basis, that can be ingested daily over a lifetime without appreciable health risk (standard man - 60 Kg) (WHO Environmental Health Criteria document No. 70, Principles for the Safety Assessment of food Additives and Contaminants in Food, Geneva, 1987). The ADI is expressed in milligrams of the additive per kilogram of body weight (Codex Alimentarius, 1989). A body weight of 60 kg is usually taken to represent the average weight of the population. However, in some countries, and especially in the developing ones, a 50 kg body weight would better represent the average body weight of the population.

The Theoretical Maximum Daily Intake (TMDI) of food additive is calculated by multiplying the average per capita daily food consumption for each foodstuff and the legal maximum level for specific additive established by Codex standards or by national regulations. The values obtained for different food are summarized to calculate the TMDI. The TMDI gives only a rough indication of the dietary intake of substance since it does not take into consideration the food habits of special population groups, and it assumes that:

- all foods in which the additive is permitted contain that additive;
- the additive is always present at the maximum permitted level;
- the foods in question containing the additive are consumed by people each day of their lives at the average per capita level;
- the additive does not undergo a decrease in level as a result of cooking or processing techniques;
- all foods permitted to contain the additive are ingested and nothing is discarded.

The Estimated Daily Intake (EDI) of a food additive is the amount of an additive ingested by the average consumer based on a) the actual use of the additive by industry, b) according to Good Manufacturing Practice (GMP), or c) an approximation as close as possible to the actual use level. There is a wide variety of procedures for calculating intakes that closely approach actual intakes.

Maximum Use Level of an additive is the highest concentration of the additive determined to be functionally effective in a food or food category and agreed to be safe by the Codex Alimentarius Commission. It is generally expressed as mg additive/kg of food. The maximum use level will not usually correspond to the optimum, recommended, or typical level of use. Under GMP, the optimum, recommended, or typical use level will differ for each application of an additive and are dependent on the intended technical effects and the specific food in which the additive will be used, taking into account the type of raw material, food processing and post-manufacture storage, transport and handling by distributors, retailers, and consumers.

5.1.1. The Estimation of Acceptable Daily Intake

Before discussing different approaches used in estimating food additive intake, the methods of establishing an ADI need to be reviewed (Codex Alimentarius, 1989). Groups of experimental animals (e.g. rats) are given daily diets containing different levels of the additive under examination. For example, levels of the additives in the diet could be: 0.1%, 1%, 2%, 5%. If a toxic effect is found at the 2% level and a "no toxic effect" at 1% level, the

1% level (expressed in mg/kg body weight) will be the "no-observed-effect level", and it is from this level that the extrapolation to humans is done. In this case, the no-observed-effect level lies between the 1% and 2% levels, and if no toxicological evaluations are done at intermediary levels (1.25%, 1.50%, 1.75%) the choice of the 1% level as the no-observed-effect level introduces a first safety factor.

The extrapolation from the no-observed-effect level to an ADI is often done by using a safety factor of 100 (10 x 10) which assumes that humans are 10 times more sensitive than experimental animals and that there is a 10-fold variation in sensitivity within the human population. This safety factor of 100 is based on the experience and common sense of toxicologists.

Estimations of the intake may be sequentially calculated starting with the simplest TMDI and proceeding to more refined EDI if necessary. When precise data on consumption of foodstuff exist, they should be used. When such precise data do not exist, approximations can be adequate to support a safe use. A hypothetical figure based on extreme theoretical cases such as the TMDI can give adequate assurance of safety if such figure is lower than the ADI (Codex Alimentarius, 1989; Grujić, 2005). However, if the ADI is exceeded using this approach, the actual intake must be approximated before decision making. The TMDI, for example, can be improved by taking into account intake of special population groups.

An example of estimation of acceptable daily intake can be given for annatto extract (norbixin), a natural food color extracted from the Bixa orellana L. Subchronic oral toxicity study was conducted in groups of 10 male and 10 female Sprague–Dawley rats that were fed with annatto extract at dietary levels of 0%, 0.1%, 0.3% and 0.9% for 13 weeks (Hagiwara et al., 2003). At the level of 0.1% there were no treatment-related adverse effects on body weight, food and water consumption, ophthalmology and hematology data. Thus, the No-Observed-Adverse-Effect-Level (NOAEL) was judged to be a dietary level of 0.1% (69 mg/kg body weight/day for males, 76 mg/kg body weight/day for females) of annatto extract (norbixin) under the present experimental conditions.

Lima et al. (2003) published the results on the evaluation of the mutagenicity and antimutagenicity of annatto. The micronucleus test was performed in bone marrow cells from Swiss male mice treated with one of the three concentrations of annatto (1330, 5330 and 10,670 ppm), incorporated into the diet. The animals were fed with the diets for 7 days and sacrificed 24 h after the last treatment. For the evaluation of the antimutagenic potential of annatto, at day 7, the animals received an intraperitoneal injection of cyclophosphamide (50 mg/kg body weight). Under the concentrations tested annatto did not present mutagenic or antimutagenic activities on the mice bone marrow cells. However, an increased frequency of micronucleated cells was observed when the highest concentration (10,670 ppm) was administered simultaneously with cyclophosphamide. In conclusion, the data indicate that annatto color, for the conditions used, is neither mutagenic nor an inhibitor of induced mutations, although it should be used carefully since high doses may increase the effect of a mutagen.

Purple corn color (Maize morado color, PCC), is extracted from the cobs and kernel of *Zea mays* Linne, and it has been consumed in Peru by Incan. In Japan, it is widely used in beverages, jellies, and candies since 1970s. The number of toxicological studies of anthocyanins have been limited, and the acceptable daily intake (ADI) was earlier determined as 0–2.5 mg/kg/day based on a short-term toxicity study of grape-skin extract only.

A subchronic oral toxicity study of purple corn color (PCC) was performed with groups of 10 male and 10 female F344 rats fed the agent at dietary levels of 0%, 0.5%, 1.5% and 5.0% for 90 days (Nabae et al., 2008). No mortalities occurred during the treatment period. No treatment-related changes in the body weight, food and water consumption, ophthalmology, hematology, organ weight data and histopathology were observed. Regarding general conditions and gross pathology, staining of fur and black feces were noted in rats of the 1.5% and 5.0% diet groups. Moreover, brown urine and black material in the stomach, small and large intestine were evident in rats receiving 5.0%. These changes were considered due to the anthocyanin content. On clinical chemistry analysis, total cholesterol, phospholipid and triglyceride were significantly lowered in both sexes of the 5.0% group, but these were not considered to be toxicologically significant. Thus, the No-observed-adverse-effect-level (NOAEL) was judged to be 5.0% in diet for both sexes (male: 3542 mg/kg/day, female: 3849 mg/kg/day) for PCC under the present experimental conditions.

When examining existing food consumption data, the possible variation in food habits within groups of population should not be forgotten. Some groups within the population will show patterns of food consumption that are significantly different from those of the population as a whole and include, for example, ethnic and cultural minority groups within a community; people using some additives at home (glutamates, intense sweeteners); heavy eaters and drinkers; and the sick (e.g. diabetics). In some countries, incomplete regulations for the use of food additives can make the problem even more complicated, especially when the majority of processed food is imported.

In deciding for which additives an evaluation of intake would have first to be done, a priority list defined in CODEX Guidelines CAC/GL 03-1989 (Codex Alimentarius, 1989) can be used:

1. additives authorized at high level in highly consumed foodstuffs,
2. additives authorized in highly consumed foodstuffs,
3. additives having received a low ADI (0-5 mg/kg of body weight)

A low priority can be given to additives which have a non specified ADI when they are used as additives according to good manufacturing practice. Great importance for food safety evaluation via the acceptable daily intake (ADI) or provisional tolerable weekly intake (PTWI) is given for chemicals that produce adverse effects and that are thought to show a threshold in their dose–response relationships (WHO, 2006). For the compounds that are both genotoxic and carcinogenic no-observed-effect level (NOEL) represents the limit of detection in that bioassay, rather than an estimate of a possible threshold. For compounds that are genotoxic and carcinogenic NOEL can not be used as a base for establishing health-based guidance values. For compounds that are both genotoxic and carcinogenic, it is adviced that intakes should be reduced to as low as reasonably achievable (ALARA). Such advice is of limited value, because it does not take into account either human exposure or carcinogenic potency, and has not allowed risk managers to prioritize different contaminants or to target risk management actions. In addition, ever-increasing analytical sensitivity means that the number of chemicals with both genotoxic and carcinogenic potential detected in food will increase.

The threshold of toxicological concern (TTC) is a pragmatic risk assessment tool that is based on the principle of establishing a human exposure threshold for all chemicals, below which there is a very low probability of an appreciable risk to human health. The concept that there are levels of exposure that do not cause adverse effects is inherent in setting acceptable daily intakes (ADIs) for chemicals with known toxicological profiles. The TTC principle extends this concept by proposing that a *de minims* value can be identified for many chemicals, in the absence of a full toxicity database, based on their chemical structures and the known toxicity of chemicals, which share similar structural characteristics (Kroes & Kozianowski, 2002).

The establishment and application of widely accepted TTC values would benefit consumers, industry and regulators. By avoiding unnecessary toxicity testing and safety evaluations when human intakes are below such threshold, application of the TTC approach would focus limited resources of time, cost, animal use and expertise on the testing and evaluation of substances with the greatest potential to pose risks to human health. An Expert Group of the European branch of the International Life Sciences Institute (ILSI Europe) has examined the TTC principle for its wider applicability in food safety evaluation (Kroes et al., 2004). The Expert Group examined metabolism and accumulation, structural alerts, endocrine disrupting chemicals and specific endpoints, such as neurotoxicity, teratogenicity, developmental toxicity, allergenicity and immunotoxicity, and determined whether such properties or endpoints had to be taken into consideration specifically in a step-wise approach. The Expert Group concluded that the TTC principle can be applied for low concentrations of chemicals in food that lack toxicity data, provided that there is a sound intake estimate.

5.2. Risk Assessment and Safety Menagement

The health status of a population can be evaluated applying the risk assessment for a product or product group to which a risk is associated. The control of hazards potentially associated with foods typically involves the application of control measures in the food chain, from primary production, through processing, to consumption. Validation of these control measures acquires increased importance. It is through the validation process that one demonstrates that the selected control measures are actually capable on a consistent basis of achieving the intended level of hazard control. Governmental risk management may choose to implement specific risk management measures (standards, microbiological criteria, hygiene code, labeling, education, etc.).

A risk assessment can give an absolute or a relative indication of the health status. This is applicable on the food products originating from one country or for the imported ones. The food industry and competent authorities are not only responsible for producing safe food but also for demonstrating in a transparent manner how food safety has been planned. This is done through the development of HACCP studies. HACCP plans as part of the food safety assurance system represents a straightforward and logical system of the control based on the prevention of problems.

Risk assessment is a science-based investigation consisting of four steps: hazard identification, exposure assessment, hazard characterization and risk characterization. Hazard identification identifies the issues of concern and provides the focus of the risk assessment. The exposure assessment generates estimates of the likelihood and magnitude of exposure to the hazard, setting the stage for the next two steps of the assessment, hazard characterization and risk characterization, in which the exposure outputs are translated into a measure of risk (Aruoma, 2006).

Risk assessment for specific food additive represents the evaluation of the substance potential to share common sites and mechanisms of action or common pathways of elimination with essential body molecules. All food additives approved for use in the EU are allocated with numerical ADIs based on reports by Food and Agricultural Organization (FAO)–World Health Organization (WHO) Joint Expert Committee for Food Additives (JECFA). Approved additives demonstrated insignificant health concern (Scotter & Castle, 2004; Grujić & Blesić, 2007).

For food additives and veterinary drug residues, JECFA normally establishes ADIs on the basis of available toxicological data and other information. The identity and purity of food additives is strictly specified and ensures that the commercial product is of appropriate quality and can be manufactured consistently, representing an equivalent to the material that was subjected to the toxicological testing.

For contaminants and naturally occurring toxicants, levels corresponding to 'tolerable' intakes such as the provisional maximum tolerable daily intake (PMTDI) or the provisional tolerable weekly intake (PTWI) are normally established when there is an identifiable no-observed-effect level. When a no-observed-effect level cannot be identified, the Committee gives the recommendation depending on the circumstances and the available data.

For veterinary drug residues, maximum residue limits (MRLs) in target animal tissues, milk and eggs, are developed taking into account Good Practice in the use of Veterinary Drugs. The application of these MRLs assures that when the drug is used properly, the intake of residues from animal products is unlikely to exceed the ADI.

In addition to the review of information's submitted by sponsors and national governments, JECFA experts are expected to conduct extensive literature searches on the substances for consideration. JECFA also develops general principles and methods for the risk assessment of chemicals in food. To keep abreast in the variety of scientific disciplines necessary to conduct up-to-date risk assessments, continuous review and update of the evaluation processes are necessary. Moreover, JECFA plays an important role in the international harmonization of risk assessments of chemicals in food.

Measures adopted by legislation governing food and feed should generally be based on risk analysis except when not appropriate. The risk assessments should be undertaken in an independent, objective and transparent manner, on the basis of the available scientific information and data. It is recognized that scientific risk assessment alone cannot, in some cases, provide all the information on which a risk management decision should be based, and that other factors relevant to the matter should legitimately be taken into account.

The landscape of food safety management in Europe has undergone recent changes as a result of the European Community's policy towards strengthening public confidence in food safety. The large number of food safety problems experienced in the last decade in Europe and elsewhere has brought to light the vulnerability of modern food production systems. As a part of management policy, the European Community has implemented its regulation (EC) No 178/2002, better known as the "General Food Law". This law describes, among others, the establishment of the European Food Safety Authority (EFSA), which has become the independent European agency for risk assessment of all categories of potential food hazards. General Food Law clearly describes the food safety framework in the Europe Union including the role and responsibilities of the different parties involved. It is anticipated that this new law will ensure the improvement in the safety of the food supply and will contribute to the restoration of a public trust.

Public trust in regulatory institutions responsible for the governance of food safety has declined due to public distrust in how such risks have been handled and managed (Grujić & Blesić, 2007; Marvin et al., 2009). The process of decision-making consists of the major components: risk assessment, risk management and risk communication. Risk is defined as the likelihood that, under particular conditions of exposure, an intrinsic hazard will represent a threat to human health. Hence, risk is a function of hazard and exposure where hazard is defined as the potential of an agent or situation to cause an adverse health effect(s)/event(s).

It is apparent that food safety risks can be reduced if food safety hazards are recognized in an early stage and if necessary information is exchanged between parties engaged in maintaining food safety. Many information's and monitoring systems on food safety (Marvin et al., 2009) have been put in place at international level (such as Rapid Alert System on Food and Feed (RASFF) in Europe; WHO-INFOSAN) and at national levels (national monitoring and survey programmes) and demonstrated their usefulness in the control of food safety risks.

The Rapid Alert System for Food and Feed (RASFF) hosted by the statistical service of the European Commission demands that national food control authorities of the European Union (EU) member states are obliged to notify any measures regarding to food safety, such as recalls of food and feed products and arrestment of imported consignments not complying with food legislations. The introduction of RASFF has further formalized a procedure of centralized reporting that existed before RASFF. Two types of notifications to RASFF are discerned:

- ''Alert'' notifications of findings/measures that may have implications for other members of the RASFF system, such as other EU member states.
- ''Information'' notifications, where members report findings or measures that may not necessarily have implications for other members, since the pertinent products have not reached their markets.

The study made by Kleter and coworkers (2009) explored the utility of notifications filed through RASFF to identify emerging trends in food safety issues. RASFF information and alert notifications published in the four-year period of July 2003–June 2007 were assigned to categories of products and hazards. For chronological trend analysis, a basic time unit of three months was chosen. Data within each hazard category were analyzed for chronological trends, relationships between products and hazard categories, regions of origin, and countries filing the notifications. Conspicuous trends that were observed included a rise in the incidence of food contact substances, as well as of chemical substances migrating from utensils and fraud related issues. Temporary increases were noted in the incidences of the unauthorized dye Para Red, genetically modified organisms, the pesticide isophenfos-methyl, and herring worm *Anisakis simplex*. National and European authorities have signaled these conspicuous trends and have taken measures. For a holistic approach towards early identification of emerging hazards, it is recommended to add complementary data to RASFF data, including safety assessments, risk management measures, background data on hazards and surveillance patterns.

6. Legislation on Food Coloring Additives

An essential aspect of the market is the free movement of safe and wholesome food. The market also protects the social and economic interests supporting the health and well-being of citizens. The free movement of food and feed can be achieved only if food and feed safety requirements do not differ significantly between countries.

There are important differences in concepts and principles between the food regulations in different parts of the world. Therefore it is important to adopt measures for governing food on a global scale, and to assure the free movement of food. Accordingly, it is necessary to harmonize the legal concepts, principles and procedures and to adapt the relevant legislation as a common basis for measures governing food and feed market.

According to regulation (EC) No 178/2002, the term 'food' (or 'foodstuff') is denoted as any substance or product, whether processed, partially processed or unprocessed, intended to be, or reasonably expected to be ingested by humans. 'Food' includes drink, chewing gum and any substance, including water, intentionally incorporated into the food during its manufacture, preparation or treatment.

According to the Regulation (EC) No 178/2002, term 'food' does not include:

- feed;
- live animals unless they are prepared for placing on the market for human consumption;
- plants prior to harvesting;
- medicinal products;
- cosmetics;
- tobacco and tobacco products;
- narcotic or psychotropic substances within the meaning of the United Nations Single Convention on Narcotic Drugs, 1961, and the United Nations Convention on Psychotropic Substances, 1971;
- residues and contaminants.

Use of colors as additives in food is defined by the European Parliament and Council Directive 94/36/EC on colors for use in foodstuffs and amending directive. The colors listed in the directive are included on the basis of the general criteria set down in Annex II of the Directive 89/107/EEC. As with all other additives used in food, colors may only be used if they perform a useful purpose, are safe and do not mislead the consumer. The Colors Directive 94/36/EC state that color may be used to:

- reinforce colors already present in food
- restore the original appearance of food whose color has been affected by processing, storage, etc.
- make food visually appealing and give color to otherwise colorless food

Colors add or restore color in a food. They are not substances that are normally consumed as foods by themselves or used as characteristic ingredients of foods. There is general agreement that basic and unprocessed food should not be colored. This Regulation is not intended to catch products such as fruit juices (for example, elderberry juice added to yoghurt) or tomato concentrates. These would be regarded as ingredients, to be labeled as such, even when added principally for coloring purposes.

In European Union, quality, safety and conditions of use of food additives are given by the Directive 89/107/EEC (Grujić 2005; Grujić & Blesić, 2007). It is applicable to food additives, the various categories of which are given in Annex I of the Directive, and which are used or intended to be used as ingredients during the manufacture or preparation of a foodstuff. The compounds the Directive refers to are present in the final product, in native or altered form.

The Directive denotes the 'food additive' as any substance not normally consumed as a food and not normally used as a characteristic ingredient of food independently on its nutritive value. The intentional addition of food additives to food during manufacturing, processing, preparation, treatment, packaging, transport or storage of such food results, or may be reasonably expected to result, in direct or indirect incorporation of the compound or its by-product as a component of such foods.

The Directive 89/107/EEC does not apply to:

- processing aids;
- substances used in the protection of plants and plant products in conformity with Community rules relating to plant health;
- flavorings for use in foodstuffs, falling within the scope of Council Directive 88/388/EEC;
- substances added to foodstuffs as nutrients (for example minerals, trace elements or vitamins).

The categories of food additives are: Colors, Preservatives, Anti-oxidants, Emulsifiers, Emulsifying salts, Thickeners, Gelling agents, Stabilizers, Flavor enhancers, Acids, Acidity regulators, Anti-caking agents, Modified starch, Sweeteners, Raising agents, Anti-foaming agents, Glazing agents, Flour treatment agents, Firming a gents, Humectants, Sequestrants, Enzymes, Bulking agents, Propellent gases and packaging gases. The inclusion of food additives in one of the categories of the Annex I is performed on the basis of the principal function of the food additive. However, the allocation of the additive to a particular category does not exclude the possibility of the additive being authorized for several functions.

Food additives can be approved only in case of reasonable technological need and if the purpose cannot be achieved by other means which are economically and technologically practicable. Additives must not present hazard to the health of consumers at the level of their proposed use, and must not mislead the consumer.

The use of food additives may be considered only where there is evidence that the proposed use of the additive demonstrates the advantages or benefit to the consumer. The additives can be approved for use aiming the preservation of the nutritional quality of the food. The intentional reduction in the nutritional quality of food is justified only if the food does not constitute a significant item in a normal diet or where the additive is necessary for the production of foods for groups of consumers having special dietary needs.

If the primary function of a substance added to food is anything other than a color, whether or not it has a secondary coloring effect, then it is not caught by the definition of color. The topic of `coloring foodstuffs' or ingredients that have a secondary coloring effect, can always be guaranteed to generate a debate and strong opinions, mainly with regard to definition and labeling. As it only relates to natural colors, in practice, there are two extremes (Downham & Collins, 2000):

- Use of a `coloring foodstuff' that happens to be highly colored, and which has not been selectively extracted to enrich the color.
- Selectively extracted color substances derived from `coloring foodstuff', which is a permitted color additive.

In order to protect human health the safety of additives, enzymes and flavourings used in foodstuffs must be assessed before they are placed on the market. So, Regulation (EC) No 1331/2008 was adapted to complete the regulatory framework concerning the authorization of the substances by laying down the various stages of the procedure, the deadlines for those stages, the role of the parties involved and the principles that apply. This Regulation lays down a common procedure for the assessment and authorization of food additives, food enzymes, food flavourings and source materials of food flavourings and of food ingredients with flavoring properties, used or intended for use in the foodstuffs. The Regulation contributes to the free movement of food within the Community and to a high level of protection of human health, as well as to a high level of consumer protection, including the protection of consumer interests. The common procedure includes updating the lists of authorized substances in the Community pursuant to Regulation (EC) No 1333/2008 [on food additives], Regulation (EC) No 1332/2008 [on food enzymes] and Regulation (EC) No 1334/2008 [on flavourings and certain food ingredients with flavoring properties for use in and on foods].

In the USA the use of food colors is governed by the Code of Federal Regulations (2010). This is divided into 50 titles and title 21 is assigned to the Food and Drug Administration. Parts 70/82 list color additives. These are divided into two categories:

1. Certified color additives FD and C colors. These are synthetically produced organic molecules that have had their purity checked by the FDA. There are seven of these which are water soluble dyes and six insoluble lakes.
2. Colorants exempt from certification. These are derived to those of animal, vegetable, mineral origin or are synthetic duplicates of naturally existing colors. As such they contain complex mixtures of numerous components. There are 26 of these. From a regulatory point of view there is no such thing as a `natural color'. Although, it is generally accepted that colorants exempt from certification are usually naturally derived.

Specific conditions for the use of the food additives may include the foodstuff to which it can be added, the conditions under which it may be added and the maximum permitted levels of use. Most food additives may only be used in limited quantities in certain foodstuffs. For certain food additives, no maximum levels are specified. However, they must be used in accordance with good manufacturing practice, at a dose level no higher than necessary to achieve the intended purpose and its use should not mislead the consumer. This is commonly referred to as the *'quantum satis'* principle.

Labeling of food additives sold to the manufacturers or directly to the consumer is regulated by the Directive 89/107/EC. The information's related to the additive must be conspicuous, clearly legible and indelible marked on packaging and must include:

- for food additives sold singly or mixed with each other, the name and its EEC number must be denoted. In the absence of such provisions, a description of the additive that is sufficiently precise to enable the distinction from additives with which it could be confused, in descending order of the proportion by weight in the total mast be available. When other substances, materials or food ingredients to facilitate storage, sale, standardization, dilution or dissolution of a food additive or food additives are incorporated in the additives, the name of the additive in accordance with the first indent and an indication of each component in descending order of the proportion by weight in the total must be given.
- either the statement 'for use in food', or the statement 'restricted use in food', or a more specific reference to its intended use, must be given;
- if necessary, the special conditions of storage and use must be contained.

Other information that must be included encompasses:

- directions for use, if the omission thereof would preclude appropriate use of the additive;
- a mark identifying the batch or lot;
- the name or business name and address of the manufacturer or packager, or of a seller established within the Community;
- an indication of the percentage of any component which is subject to a quantitative limitation in a food or adequate compositional information to enable the purchaser to comply with any Community provisions, or in their absence national provisions, applying to the food. Where the same quantitative limitation applies to a group of components used singly or in combination, the combined percentage may be given as a single figure;
- the net quantity;
- any other information.

Food additives must at all times comply with the approved criteria of purity. Approval for food additives must (Directive 89/107/EEC):

- specify the foodstuffs to which these additives may be added and the conditions under which they may be added;
- be limited to the lowest level of use necessary to achieve the desired effect;
- take into account any acceptable daily intake, or equivalent assessment, established for the food additive and the probable daily intake of it from all sources. Where the food additive is to be used in foods eaten by special groups of consumers, account

should be taken of the possible daily intake of the food additive by consumers in those groups.

In addition to the general criteria for food additives, the Directive 89/107/EEC recommends that the detailed provisions on categories of food additives are included in separate Directives. Three technical Directives have addressed the use of the Sweeteners (94/35/EC), Colors (94/36/EC) and all other additives (95/2/EC) (the so called 'miscellaneous additives'), outlining the foods in which they can be used and their maximum levels of use.

7. Future Outlook in the Use of Food Colors

In constantly changing food market it is important to identify the future outlook for colors with respect to legislation, innovations in formulation and processing technology (Downham & Collins, 2000). Developments in color formulation over the last years have focused on augmenting the stability of natural and nature identical pigments, as they have much variation in their natural stability and solubility (Downham & Collins, 2000). Improvements in synthetic colors have focused around process developments. Additives used in natural color formulations can have a major effect on the colors' stability, ease of use and color shade. Additives can also affect the application characteristics. Formulation developments have focused on improvement in four main areas. For the convenience of color use, it is important to make water dispersible forms of oil soluble pigments by forming a dispersion of oil solubilized pigments throughout an aqueous disperse phase by using emulsifiers, antioxidants and stabilizers. Color stability to oxidation could be enhanced, for example, via the synergistic use of antioxidants such as tocopherol and ascorbyl palmitate. Improved acid stability and clarity of food colors makes their applications in soft drinks, jellies and conserves easier. Producers, scientific workers and food technologist engaged in new food product development must work on replacement of consumer `unfriendly' (often allergenic) ingredients.

The fundamental principle in safety assessment of food colorants is to ensure that consumer safety is not compromised. This applies to all additives and is a consideration that is taken without preference over one type of color or another. Future developments in this field should include prompt response of the industry to changes in the regulations with respect to safety issues. For the additives whose assessment was performed a long time ago a reassessment may be deemed appropriate. There is expected to be an extra impetus in this area as all additives are due for an intake assessment, which will identify certain candidates for closer scrutiny (Downham & Collins, 2000).

The aim of color manufacturers, whether synthetic, nature identical or naturally derived, is to constantly support the correct selection and application of colors. Time pressures and ingredient rationalization often mean that the most suitable color is not used. Such approach carries a manufacturing risk and can cause lack of consumer appeal and the failure of potential new products. Color suppliers will continue to mirror the flavor industry by offering bespoke formulations and pre blends along with a comprehensive technical advice and sample service.

7.1. Colors as Functional Food Ingredients

There is growing evidence that many food components perform additional beneficial functions in the body. Our instinctive preference for eating naturally occurring colored foods (fruits and vegetables) is thought to be natures' way of providing our diet with certain phytochemicals along with micronutrients and vitamins. Natural antioxidants are now thought to possibly prevent the increasing incidence of many diseases such as cancers and heart disease, thus these diseases have been linked to a lack of fruit and vegetables in the diet (Downham & Collins, 2000). Although most people know that they are recommended to eat 5 portions of fruit and vegetables every day, less than 10% of the population achieve this target.

Although many advances in the developments of food colors have been made over the last 25 years, particularly in terms of harmonized legislation and advances in processing and formulation technologies, there is still a room for future developments. The physicochemical principles that have evolved in plants to enhance and modify color should be considered in the future by plant breeders, horticulturists, food technologists and dieticians for selection, growing, processing, utilization of the respective color sources as well as the nutritional benefits offered by the ingested compounds (Stintzing & Carle, 2004). The overall color market is forecast to grow in line with technological and sociological changes that will lead to an overall increase in processed foodstuffs. It is thought that the natural color market will grow on a global scale at a greater rate than synthetic colors owing to a continued consumer pressure to `go natural'.

Developments in artificial colors will continue to focus on customized blends and technical support as well as further improved handling properties. Significant developments in natural colors have occurred over the last 10 years and this is likely to continue in the area of stabilizing the currently permitted range of pigments by the development of their formulations and processing technologies, as well as the continued searches for `untapped' sources of permitted pigments. Developments are only likely to cease when colors such as a heat and acid stable natural red color are developed or alternatively a stable non pH dependant natural blue shade! The growing market of functional food ingredients is likely to see natural pigments used for their health rather than their coloring properties. This is a very exiting area `waiting to happen', which should be realized in the future.

Undoubtedly at some time in the future the colors directive will be subject to amendment, but this seems a distant prospect at present. Currently a proposal for food additives developed from new source materials, such as genetically modified crops, is already under discussion by the Scientific Committee on Food. It seems eminently sensible that new source materials or new production processes, such as the fermentative source of β-carotene, will happen in the future.

7.2. Novel Pigment Sources

Many novel pigment sources have been identified as potential new sources of natural colors. As example, Downham and Collins (2000) write about some food colorants currently used in certain countries, but unfortunately approval in EU and/or US would involve lengthy and expensive safety testing, which prohibits their commercialization today.

Monascus is a heat stable red and yellow colorant derived from the fermentation of rice by the fungus *Monascus purpureus* and *Monascus anka*. It is one of the most commonly used natural colors in Japan and the Orient for applications such as meat and fish products. It is not permitted within the EU or the USA owing to concerns over potentially toxic coumarin compounds produced during the fermentation process.

Spirulina sp. contains the pigment *phycocyanin* which gives it a blue shade. The highest stability of the pigment is at pH 5-7. Phycocyanin is not permitted as a colorant source within the EU or the USA. The FDA has classified *Spirulina* sp. as cyanobacteria and considers it a food, not a vegetable, and as such it does not conform to the regulation 21CFR 73.260 on `Vegetable Juice'. It is, however, used in Japan. The application areas of phycocyanin are limited to non acidic foodstuffs such as chewing gum and dairy products.

Other sources of pigments include blue gardenia, the traditional orange carrot and purple corn, however the stability, price and legislation limit their application.

7.3. Process of Pigments Microencapsulation

The process of pigments microencapsulation encompasses both formulation and process technology. There have been some developments within this area for both the nature identical and natural colors. Complete microencapsulation aims to totally entrap the pigment particles in a protective network, which isolates and stabilizes the pigment from the common factors that can cause color loss or change such as oxidation or acidic conditions. The release mechanism is often more limiting for colors in comparison to other ingredients, such as flavors. It is the visual appearance of the food at the point of purchase, or prior to consumption, which really matters. Release in the mouth or during food processing may not always be appropriate. The protection provided by encapsulation depends on the encapsulating matrix, efficiency of coating and the point in time when the pigment is released. The inner core material may be released upon addition of water, heating or fracturing (Downham & Collins, 2000). If the pigment is designed not to be released, the encapsulating material must be transparent to light and the microencapsules ought to be very small.

A range of encapsulating materials is suitable for colors such as carbohydrates, gums, phospholipids and proteins. Consideration has to be given to the sources of these materials. For marketing success they must not be derived from genetically modified organisms and must be nut oil free, as well as kosher and suitable for vegetarians. Encapsulating methods available include spray drying, spray coating and spinning disc technology. Microencapsulation is an area of great potential in the protection of synthetic, nature identical and natural pigments. Continued advances in ingredient and processing technologies should see a vast array of stabilized colors in the future.

References

Aruoma O.I. The impact of food regulation on the food supply chain. *Toxicology*, 2006, 221, 119–127.

Baker R. and Günther C. The role of carotenoids in consumer choice and the likely benefits from their inclusion into products for human consumption. *Trends in Food Science and Technology*, 2004, 15, 484–488.

Codex Alimentarius . Guidelines for simple evaluation of food additive intake, CAC/GL 03-1989.

Downham A.; Collins P. Coloring our foods in the last and next millennium. *International Journal of Food Science and Technology*, 2000, 35, 5-22.

Grujić R., Grujić S., Basic of Food Technology and Food Storage, Pan-Europien University Banja Luka, 2009 (in Serbian).

Grujić R., Grujić S., Đurašinović P., Pavlović P. Workers responsibility in food businesses during implementation of food safety system, Applied Innovations and Technologies, 2010a, Vol 1, No 1 143-48.

Grujić R., Grujić S., Đurašinović P., Pavlović P. Satisfaction of the employed in food businesses and success of food safety management system implementation, *Perspectives of Innovations, Economics and Business*, 2010b. Vol 5, 38-41.

Grujić S. Food Additives (Prehrambeni aditivi funkcionalna svojstva i primjena), Faculty of Technology, Banja Luka, 2005 (in Serbian).

Grujić S; Blesic M. Food Regulations; Faculty of Technology Banja Luka, 2007 (in Serbian).

Grujić S.; Grujić R.; Savanović D.; Odžaković B.; Dejanović M. Uticaj odabranih aditiva na poboljšanje kvaliteta i stabilnosti boje fino usitnjenih barenih kobasica od pilećeg mesa, *Tehnologija mesa*, 2009, vol. 50, br. 3-4, pp. 232-237.

Hagiwara A; Imai N; Ichihara T; Sano M; Tamano S; Aoki H; Yasuhara K; Koda T; Nakamura M; Shirai T. A thirteen-week oral toxicity study of annatto extract (norbixin), a natural food color extracted from the seed coat of annatto (*Bixa orellana* L.), in Sprague–Dawley rats. *Food and Chemical Toxicology*, 2003, 41, 1157–1164.

Kleter G.A; Prandini A; Filippi L; Marvin H.J.P. Identification of potentially emerging food safety issues by analysis of reports published by the European Community's Rapid Alert System for Food and Feed (RASFF) during a four-year period. *Food and Chemical Toxicology*, 2009, 47, 932–950.

Krinsky N. I; Johnson E. J. Carotenoid actions and their relation to health and disease. *Molecular Aspects of Medicine*. 2005, 26, 459–516.

Kroes R; Renwick A.G; Cheeseman M; Kleiner J; Mangelsdorf I; Piersma A; Schilter B; Schlatter J; Schothorst F; Vos J.G., Würtzen G. Structure-based thresholds of toxicological concern (TTC): guidance for application to substances present at low levels in the diet. *Food and Chemical Toxicology*, 2004, 42, 65–83.

Kroes R; Kozianowski G. Threshold of toxicological concern (TTC) in food safety assessment. *Toxicology Letters*, 2002, 127, 43–46.

Lima R.O.A.; Azevedb L.; Ribeiro L.R; Salvadori D.M.F. Study on the mutagenicity and antimutagenicity of a natural food color (annatto) in mouse bone marrow cells. *Food and Chemical Toxicology*, 2003, 41, 189–192.

Linnemann, A.R; Benner, M; Verkerk, R; van Boekel, M.A.J.S. Consumer-driven food product development. *Trends in Food Science and Technology,* 2006, 17, 184–190.

Marvin H.J.P; Kleter G.A; Prandini A; Dekkers S; Bolton D.J. Early identification systems for emerging foodborne hazards. *Food and Chemical Toxicology*, 2009, 47, 915–926.

Nabae K; Hayashi S; Kawabe M; Ichihara T; Hagiwara A; Tamano S; Tsushima Y; Uchida K; Koda T; Nakamura M; Ogawa K; Shirai T. A 90-day oral toxicity study of purple corn color, a natural food colorant, in F344 rats. *Food and Chemical Toxicology*, 2008, 46, 774–780.

Oka H; Ozeki N; Hayashi T; Itakura Y. Analysis of Natural Colorings in Foods by Thin Layer Chromatography. *Journal of Liquid Chromatography and Related Technologies*, 2007, 30, 2021–2036.

Peri C.. The universe of food quality. *Food Quality and Preference*, 2006, 17, 3–8.

Schoefs B. Determination of pigments in vegetables. *Journal of Chromatography* A, 2004, 1054, 217–226.

Scotter M.J; Castle L. Chemical interactions between additives in foodstuffs: a review . *Food Additives and Contaminants*, 2004, 21, No. 2, pp. 93–124.

Stintzing FC; Reinhold C. Functional properties of anthocyanins and betalains in plants, food, and in human nutrition. *Trends in Food Science and Technology*, 2004, 15, 19 –38.

Tripathi M; Khanna S; Das M. Surveillance on use of synthetic colors in eatables vis a vis Prevention of Food Adulteration Act of India. *Food Control*, 2007, 18, 211–219.

World Health Organization. WHO global strategy for food safety: safer food for better health. Food Safety Department World Health Organization, Geneva, Switzerland, 2002, http://www.who.int/fsf.

WHO, Evaluation of certain food contaminants, S*ixty-fourth report of the Joint FAO/WHO Expert Committee on Food Additives,* Technical Report Series 930, World Health Organization, Geneva, *2006.*

Yoshioka N; Ichihashi K. Determination of 40 synthetic food colors in drinks and candies by high-performance liquid chromatography using a short column with photodiode array detection. *Talanta*, 2008, 74, 1408 –1413.

Food Law Used in Chapter

Codex Alimentarius. Guidelines for the validation of food safety control measures, CAC/GL 69 – 2008.

Codex Alimentarius. Codex general standard for food additives, C*odex Stan 192-1995, Rev.* 2009.

Code of Federal Regulations (2010), Color additives, http://ecfr.gpoaccess.gov/cgi/t/text/text-idx?c=ecfrandtpl=/ecfrbrowse/Title21/21cfr70_main_02.tpl.

Commission Directive 2008/128/EC laying down specific purity criteria concerning colours for use in foodstuffs, OJ L 6, 10.1.2009. p. 20.

Council Directive 89/107/EEC on the approximation of the laws of the Member States concerning food additives authorised for use in foodstuffs intended for human consumption, OJ L40, p27., Amended by: European Parliament and Council Directive 94/34/EC of 30 June 1994 L 237, p1.

EU Parlament. Regulation (EC) No 1331/2008 of the European Parliament and of the Council of 16 December 2008 establishing a common authorisation procedure for food additives, food enzymes and food flavourings OJ L354, p1. http://eur-lex.europa.eu/ LexUriServ/ LexUriServ.do?uri=CELEX:32008R1331.

EU Parlament. Regulation (EC) No 1332/2008 of the European Parliament and of the Council of 16 December 2008 on food enzymes (OJ L354, p7) and amending Council Directive

83/417/EEC, Council Regulation (EC) No 1493/1999, Directive 2000/13/EC, Council Directive 2001/112/EC and Regulation (EC) No 258/97. http://eur-lex.europa.eu/ LexUriServ/LexUriServ.do?uri=CELEX:32008R1332

EU Parlament. Regulation (EC) No 1333/2008 (OJ L354, p16) of the European Parliament and of the Council of 16 December 2008 on food additives http://eur-lex.europa.eu/LexUriServ/LexUriServ.do?uri=CELEX:32008R1333.

EU Parlament. Regulation (EC) No 1334/2008 (OJ L354, p34) of the European Parliament and of the Council of 16 December 2008 on flavourings and certain food ingredients with flavouring properties for use in and on foods and amending Council Regulation (EEC) No 1601/91, Regulations (EC) No 2232/96 and (EC) No 110/2008 and Directive 2000/13/EC http://eur-lex.europa.eu/LexUriServ/LexUriServ.do?uri=CELEX: 32008R 1334.

EU Parlament. European Parlament and Council Directive 94/35/EC on sweetener for use in foodstuffs, OJ No. 237, p. 3, amended by Directive 96/83/EC, No. 48, p. 16.

EU Parlament. European Parlament and Council Directive 94/36/EC on colors for use in foodstuffs, OJ No. 237, p. 13.

EU Parlament. Regulation (EC) No 178/2002 of the European Parliament and of the Council laying down the general principles and requirements of food law, establishing the European Food Safety Authority and laying down procedures in matters of food safety. OJ L 31, 1.02.2002 p.1.

World Health Organization. WHO global strategy for food safety: safer food for better health. Food Safety Department World Health Organization, Geneva, Switzerland, 2002, http://www.who.int/fsf.

WHO, Evaluation of certain food contaminants, *Sixty-fourth report of the Joint FAO/WHO Expert Committee on Food Additives,* Technical Report Series 930, World Health Organization, Geneva, 2006.

WHO, Evaluation of certain food contaminants, *Sixty-fourth report of the Joint FAO/WHO Expert Committee on Food Additives,* Technical Report Series 956, World Health Organization, Geneva, 2010.

In: Nutritional Insights and Food Safety
Editor: Jaroslava Švarc-Gajiæ

ISBN: 978-1-61122-130-5

Chapter X

Nitrosamines in Food: Formation, Occurrence and Analytic

Przemysław Andrzejewski[1,]*and Anastasia Nikolaou[2,] **
*Adam Mickiewicz University, Faculty of Chemistry, Poznan, Poland
**University of the Aegean, Department of Marine Sciences, Faculty of the Environment, University Hill, 81100 Mytilene, Greece

Abstract

Nitrosamines, mainly N-nitrosodimetylamine (NDMA), N-nitrosomethylethylamine (NMEA) and N-nitrosodiethylamine (NDEA) are mutagenic compounds and are suspected to be carcinogenic in humans. American Environmental Protection Agency (US EPA) classified them into group B2 – i.e. the compounds which are probably carcinogenic to humans. US EPA detected these compounds in potable water at levels of 7 ng/l (N-nitrosodimethylamine - NDMA), 20 ng/l (N-nitrosomethylethylamine - NMEA) and 2 ng/l (N-nitrosodiethylamine - NDEA).

Rocket fuel, namely the incomplete oxidation of present hydrazines, polymers, plasticizers, batteries and other industrial products are identified as the main anthropogenic sources of nitrosamines. On the other hand, microbial transformation of N-precursors within feedlots is the main natural source of nitrosamines. Nitrosamines are widespread in the environment. Their appearance has been confirmed in drinking water, groundwater (mainly that supplied by recharged water) and tobacco smoke. Furthermore many foodstuffs such as beer, meat, cheese and pickles, contain measurable quantities of these compounds and they are also probably produced in the course of human digestive activity.

This chapter presents an extensive review of international literature concerning the current state of the art on nitrosamines, particularly N-nitrosodimethylamine, and their occurrence in solid food and beverages. Authors focused their attention on nitrosamines characteristics, their occurrence in solid food and beverages (including water), mechanisms of their formation, on the influence of food processing on nitrosamines formation and nitrosamines analysis in solid food and beverages. Since Lijinski in 1999

[1]e-mail: pandrz@amu.edu.pl.
[2]e-mail: nnikol@aegean.gr

presented very interesting and comprehensive review concerning occurrence of nitrosamines in food, authors of this chapter discussed mainly the results published after 1999.

Introduction

Nitrosamines are group of compounds with the general molecular structure shown in Figure 1 with R_1 and R_2 representing hydrogen, aliphatic or aromatic group.

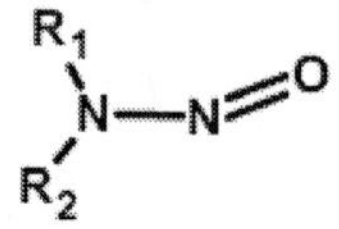

Figure 1. A general molecular structure of nitrosamines.

An abundance of possible functionalities which can occurs in nitrosamine structure produces significant number of different nitrosamines. Nitrosamines as a group of chemicals have been known for over 100 years but they have not been studied extensively. However, in 1956 John Barnes and Peter Magee reported that N-nitrosodimethylamine has a carcinogenic effect in rats. The discovery resulted in an increased interest in this group of compounds. It was found out that 90% of 300 identified nitrosamine compounds have shown to be carcinogenic (Domański, 2003). US EPA, however, put only eight of known nitrosamines on the list of compounds possible harmful to humans. These nitrosamines, which belong to sub-group of secondary nitrosamines, are listed below in Table 1 and their structures are shown in Figure 2.

Table 1. Nitrosamines on the US EPA list of compounds possible harmful for human (US EPA, 2010)

	Nitrosamine	CASRN[a]	Estimate of Carcinogenic Risk from Oral Exposure	
			Slope[b] (per mg/kg-day)	Nitrosamine concentration in water associated with the risk of 10^{-5} (ng/l)
1	N-Nitrosodimethylamine (B2)	62-75-9	51	7
2	N-Nitroso-N-methylethylamine (B2)	10595-95-6	22	20
3	N-Nitrosodiethylamine (B2)	55-18-5	150	2
4	N-Nitrosopyrrolidine (B2)	930-55-2	2.1	200
5	N-Nitrosodi-N-propylamine (B2)	621-64-7	7	50
6	N-Nitroso-di-n-butylamine (B2)	924-16-3	5.4	60
7	N-Nitrosodiethanolamine (B2)	1116-54-7	2.8	100
8	N-Nitrosodiphenylamine (B2)	86-30-6	0.0049	70 000

[a]CASRN - The Chemical Abstracts Service Registration Numbers;
[b]Carcinogenicity Assessment for Lifetime Exposure, oral administration.

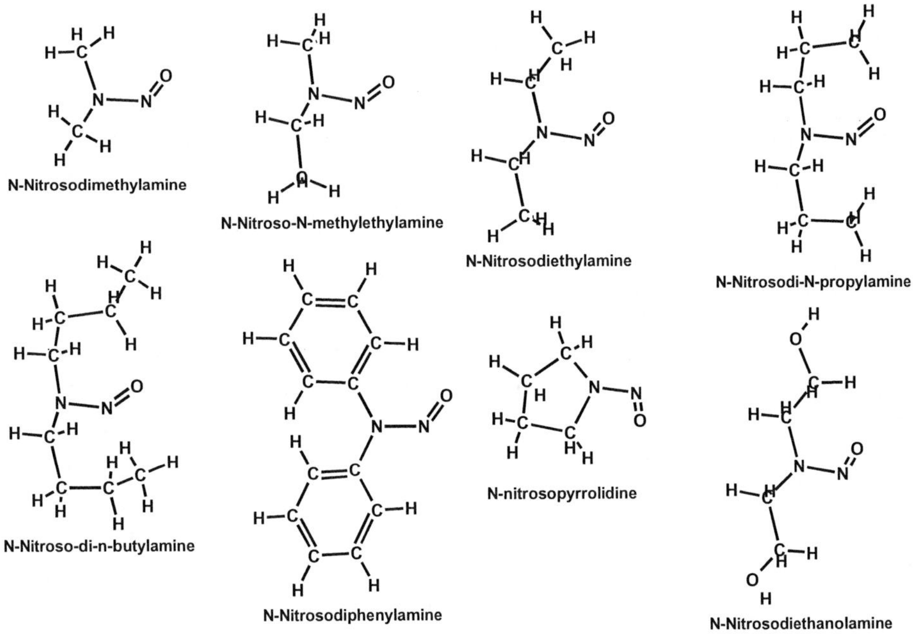

Figure 2. Structures of nitrosamines from the US EPA list of compounds possible harmful to humans.

All nitrosamines listed above belong to the group B2 classified by US EPA, i.e. probable human carcinogens, based on sufficient evidence of their carcinogenicity in animals. Moreover, three of them, i.e. N-Nitrosodimethylamine (NDMA), N-Nitroso-N-methylethylamine (NMEA) and N-Nitrosodiethylamine (NDEA), seems to be the most dangerous to humans on the basis of their lowest concentrations in water associated with risk of 10^{-5} and their highest slope factors in carcinogenity assessment (Table 1). According to US EPA data nitrosamines, particularly NDMA, cause tumors, at multiple sites including lung, liver, and kidney, in both rodents (Wistar rats and Balb/C mice) and nonrodent mammals exposed by various routes. Other experiments on mice indicated that NDMA, regardless of the manner of absorption, causes cancer of liver, lung and kidney in adult mice and cancer of liver and lung in the young specimens fed with milk from mothers exposed to NDMA. Experiments on other animal species, including hamsters, guinea pigs, rabbits, ducks, different type of fish, frogs or newts, also demonstrated the carcinogenic character of NDMA (US EPA, 2010). Also the International Agency for Research on Cancer has classified some of the more commonly encountered nitrosamines, N-Nitrosodimethylamine (NDMA) and N-nitrosodiethylamine (NDEA), as probable carcinogens and N-nitrosodibutylamine, N-nitrosopiperidine and N-nitrosopyrrolidine (NPYR) as possible carcinogens.

N-nitrosodimethylamine, the most recognized member of nitrosamines group, is a yellow, volatile and oily liquid, which is characterized by a low viscosity. It is highly soluble in water, alcohols, ethers and other organic solvents as well as in fat. This compound is sensitive to light, especially ultraviolet light and it undergoes fast photolytic degradation. NDMA is a flammable compound. The molecular weight of NDMA is 78.08 g mol^{-1} and partition coefficient octanol/water ($\log K_{o/w}$) is -0.57 (ChemFinder, 2007).

Incomplete oxidation of hydrazines present in rocket fuel (Gunnison et al, 2000), polymers, plasticizers, batteries and other industrial products are recognized as the main anthropogenic sources of nitrosamines (Richardson, 2003). On the other hand, microbial transformation of N-precursors within feedlots is the main natural source of nitrosamines within the environment (Gunnison et al, 2000). Nitrosamines are widespread in the environment and they have been detected in drinking water (Jobb et al. 1995), groundwater (mainly that supplied by recharged water) (Mitch et al., 2002) and tobacco smoke (Gunnison et al, 2000), as well as in foodstuffs like beer, meat, cheese and pickles.

Nitrosamines, particularly NDMA, can be introduced into food mainly via poor quality ingredients, spices or food preparing technology. Moreover, water used in food processing can be the source of nitrosamines or its precursors. In 2001 Najm and Trussell suggested that NDMA appears to be a by-product of the chloramination of water and wastewater, with the level of NDMA formed directly related to the chloramine dose (Najm & Trussell, 2001). Choi and Valentine (Choi & Valentine, 2002) and Mitch and Sedlak (Mitch & Sedlak, 2002) in 2002 reported that N-nitrosodimethylamine is formed during the disinfection of water and sewage with chloramines or chlorine (in presence of ammonia). Until that nitrosamines were linked only with food products of deteriorating quality. It was believed that their presence resulted only from biochemical process taking place in oxygen-free conditions, in the presence of a particular strain of bacteria. The presence of nitrosamines in water was explained by the wastewater migration to drinking water intakes bringing indirectly the new potential source of nitrosamines in food and beverages as well.

This chapter presents an extensive review of international literature concerning the current state of the art on nitrosamines, particularly N-nitrosodimethylamine, and their occurrence in solid food and beverages. Authors focused their attention on nitrosamines characteristics, their occurrence in solid food and beverages (including water), mechanisms of their formation, on the influence of food processing on nitrosamines formation and nitrosamines analysis in solid food and beverages. Since Lijinski in 1999 presented very interesting and comprehensive review concerning occurrence of nitrosamines in food, authors of this chapter discussed mainly the results published after 1999.

1. Nitrosamines in Solid Food and Beverages

1.1. Nitrosamines in Solid Food

1.1.1. Meat and Fish

Besides wild fruits and vegetables, meat of killed animals and fish were the first, food of primitive human beings. In the course of time human race started to preserve the meat and fish in order to prevent its deterioration and as a consequence improvement of meat and fish quality and taste followed. Meat preservation, for example, with nitrites protects it against very danger anaerobic bacteria *Clostridium botulinum*, which produces compound lethal for human known as botulin. On the other hand the addition of some ingredients to meat and its processing as well as improper storage, may result in the formation of compounds, like NDMA, dangerous to consumers. To present NDMA and other nitrosamines were found in many kinds of solid food including meat and fish. It is obvious that both presence as well as the amount of nitrosamines in meat and fish strongly depend on the method of processing, processing temperatures and time, residual and added nitrite concentrations, concentrations of nitrosamines precursors, presence of nitrosation catalysts and inhibitors, and storage conditions (Yurchenko & Molder, 2006).

The first reports about the presence of nitrosamines (particularly NDMA and NDEA) in bacon and other cured meats date in early 1960s. The results of these analysis were, however not very accurate nor specific (Lijinski, 1999). An implementation of new analytical techniques including new detectors like TEA (Thermal Energy Analyzer) or MS (Mass spectrometer) allowed to increase the credibility of results in nitrosamines analysis.

1.1.1.1. Fish

Between 1988 and 1996 Mitacek et al. systematically collected and tested over 1800 samples of fresh and preserved food. All the food items identified by anthropological studies to be consumed frequently in four major regions of Thailand were analyzed for volatile nitrosamines using gas chromatography combined with a thermal energy analyzer. The six kinds of fermented fish contained NDMA ranging from 3.7 to 7.95 µg/kg, and in five kinds of fish N-nitrosopyrrolidine (NPYR) was found at levels from 5.6 to 18.1 µg/kg, and in four kinds of fermented fish N-nitrosopiperidine (NPIP) at levels from 1.8 to 8.7 µg/kg. Relatively high levels of N-nitrosodimethylamine (NDMA), N-nitrosopiperidine (NPIP) and N-nitrosopyrrolidine (NPYR) were detected in fermented fish ('Pla-salid''). NDMA was also detected at levels ranging from trace amounts to 66.5 µg/kg in several salted and dried fish samples. Two dishes `Larb-pla' and ``Pla-siu'' (salted and dried fish) contained NDMA at levels of 7.2 and 6.5 µg/kg respectively, but without detectable levels of NPYR and NPIP (Mitacek et al., 1999).

Yurchenko and Molder, during the period 2001-2005 investigated the presence and concentration of five nitrosamines, notably N-nitrosodimethylamine, N-nitrosodiethylamine, N-nitrosodibutylamine, N-nitrosopiperidine, and N-nitrosopyrrolidine, in 294 various samples of fish. They divided fish samples to eight groups according to their processing, i.e. fresh fish (50 samples), cold smoked fish (35 samples), hot smoked fish (135 samples), fried fish (20 samples), salted fish (34 samples), pickled fish (10 samples), salted/dried fish (10 samples) and fractions of smoked sprats in oil (13 samples). Applying two-steps solid-phase extraction prior to GC-MS (with positive-ion chemical ionization) Yurchenko and Molder found NDMA in all groups of samples except in fresh fish. The mean concentrations of NDMA ranged from 0.52 µg/kg (cold-smoke salmon) to 1.99 µg/kg (sprats in tomato sauce into group of fried fish). In samples of fresh fish the presence of other nitrosamines was not detected. The mean concentrations of sum of five nitrosamines ranged from 1.70 µg/kg (cold-smoke salmon) to 9.62 µg/kg (sprats in tomato sauce in group of fried fish). In 117 of 294 samples of various fish products the concentration of NDMA exceeded 1 µg/kg. The level of five nitrosamines in cold-smoked fish was lower than the level in hot-smoked and fried fish samples. In 8 of 294 samples of various fish products the concentration of the sum of NDMA and NDEA exceeded the tolerance limit of 3 µg /kg. The highest levels of nitrosamines were found in samples of fried and pickled fish. Relatively high level was found in hot-smoked fish, in sprats in oil, in salted- and in salted/dried fish. On the opposite, low levels of nitrosamines were detected in cold-smoked fish. Yurchenko and Molder attributed the formation of significant amounts of volatile nitrosamines in the fish to the interaction of nitrites and amines from the fish. Moreover, higher temperature of food processing (hot-smoking and particularly frying) resulted in higher concentrations of nitrosamines in comparison to low temperature processes such as cold-smoking. The concentrations of nitrosamines in fish prepared without thermal treatment (pickled and salted fish) were comparable to nitrosamines concentrations in hot-fried fish. Authors explained this phenomenon as the result of nitrate (and probably nitrite) presence in the crude salt used for pickling and salting of the fish (Yurchenko & Molder, 2006).

1.1.1.2. Meat

Mitacek et al., between 1988 and 1996, also investigated the presence of nitrosamines in some meat dishes consumed in Thailand. The pork meat, specially the `Nam' (fermented sausage) and the `Nam-moo-som" (fermented pork) contained NDMA and NPYR at levels of 1.6 µg/kg - 3.4 µg/kg and 2.1 µg/kg - 2.9 µg/kg, respectively (Mitacek et al., 1999).

Yurchenko and Molder, during years 2001-2005, also investigated the presence and concentrations of five nitrosamines i.e. N-nitrosodimethylamine, N-nitrosodiethylamine, N-nitrosodibutylamine, N-nitrosopiperidine, and N-nitrosopyrrolidine in 386 various samples of meat. They divided meat samples to six groups according to their processing, i.e. raw meat, smoked meat, grilled meat, fried meat, canned meat and picked meat. Applying the same analytical tools i.e. two-steps solid-phase extraction prior to GC-MS (with positive-ion chemical ionization), Yurchenko and Molder found NDMA in more than 88% of samples, NDEA in 27%, NPYR in 90%, NPIP in 65%, and NDBA in 33% at the mean levels of 0.85, 0.36, 4.14, 0.98, and 0.37 µg/kg, respectively. In 189 of 386 samples of various meat products, the concentration of NDMA exceeded 1 µg/kg. NDMA was found in all groups of samples except in raw meat. The mean concentrations of NDMA ranged from 0.16 µg/kg (frankfurters in group of smoked meat) to 4.93 µg/kg (pork fat with paprika in group of fried meat). In all samples of raw meat the presence of other nitrosamines was not detected. The mean concentrations of the sum of five nitrosamines ranged from 0.64 µg/kg (frankfurters in group of smoked meat) to 32.46 µg/kg (pork fat with paprika in group of fried meat). The concentrations of nitrosamines in meat prepared without thermal treatment (pickled and canned meat) were similar to average values of nitrosamines concentrations obtained for smoked, grilled and fried meat. Authors explained this phenomenon as the result of addition of salt both to pickled and canned meat (Yurchenko and Molder, 2007).

Andrade et al., examined the presence and concentrations of four nitrosamines i.e. N-nitrosodimethylamine (NDMA), N-nitrosodiethylamine (NDEA), N-nitrosopiperidine (NPIP) and N-nitrosopyrrolidine (NPYR) in two samples of hot-dog sausages. Applying head-space solid-phase micro-extraction technique prior to GC-TEA analysis Andrade et al. found NDMA in these two samples in concentration of 43.5±6.5 µg/kg and 15.0±2.2 µg/kg (Andrade et al., 2005).

NDMA and NDEA presence in various types of meat as well as the influence of meat treatment on concentration of both nitrosamines was also investigated by Rywotycki. He examined 15 sorts of meat of a different origin (young sows, sows, hogs, boars, heifers, cows, bullock, bulls, claves, mares, geldings, ewes, wethers, rams and goat) and compared NDMA and NDEA concentrations in raw samples of these meat with amines concentrations in these meats after baking, salting, baking/salting or adding sodium ascorbate. Applying GC-MS (with ion-trap detector) Rywotycki found NDMA and NDEA in all analyzed samples including raw meat. The experiment revealed the greatest nitrosamine concentrations in pork and beef and the lowest in veal and goat meat. The mean concentrations of NDMA in raw meat ranged from 2.34 μg/kg (goat meat) to 12.00 μg/kg (bull meat). The mean concentrations of NDEA in raw meat ranged from 2.19 μg/kg (goat meat) to 12.68 μg/kg (boars meat) (Rywotycki, 2007). Results obtained by Rywotycki (Rywotycki, 2007) seem to be higher than results obtained by (Yurchenko & Molder, 2007).

1.1.2. Other Solid Food and Food Ingredients

In the period between 1988 and 1996 Mitacek et al., have also extensively investigated the presence of nitrosamines in some vegetables consumed in Thailand. NDMA and NPYR were frequently detected in several vegetables, particularly fermented beans ("Tau-chiau") at levels ranging between 1 and 95.1 μg/kg and 0÷146 μg/kg, respectively (Mitacek et al.,1999).

Beresford et al. in their review focused on cheese microbiology, mentioned that the presence of nitrite in cheese may results in nitrosamines formation during it manufacturing. Nitrite can react with aromatic amino acids to form nitrosamines. On the other hand, cheese has definitely higher pH then optimal for nitrosation process, and therefore this fact slows down the reaction leading to the formation of nitrosamines (Beresford et al., 2001). Kyriakidis et al. examined the concentrations of nitrite and nitrate in 140 samples of Greek cheeses produced from sheep's milk. Although nitrite accumulation in cheese is temporary as it is soon transformed to other reduction products, its presence in cheese may lead to the formation of nitrosamines. On the other hand, it has been reported that no relationship appears to exist between nitrosamine content and either the initial or the residual nitrate in the cheese and that nitrosamines have also been found in cheese to which no nitrate was added (Kyriakidis et al, 1997).

Yurchenko and Molder, during years 2001-2005, investigated the presence and concentrations of five nitrosamines i.e. N-nitrosodimethylamine, N-nitrosodiethylamine, N-nitrosodibutylamine, N-nitrosopiperidine, and N-nitrosopyrrolidine in 77 samples of vegetable oils (olive oil, rape oil, refined and not refined sunflower oil, soybean oil, corn oil and peanut oil). Applying the same analytical tool i.e. two-steps solid-phase extraction prior to GC-MS (with positive-ion chemical ionization) Yurchenko and Molder found NDMA and NDEA in all types of oils. The mean concentrations of NDMA and NDEA ranged from 0.24 μg/kg and 0.18 μg/kg respectively (soybean oil) to 0.71 μg/kg and 0.47 μg/kg, respectively (not refined sunflower oil). In all samples of oils the presence of other nitrosamines was not detected, however it is worth noting that NDMA and NDEA are considered to be the most dangerous ones for humans (Yurchenko & Molder, 2006).

1.2. Nitrosamines in Beverages

1.2.1. Beer

Beer is, at present, the most consumed alcoholic beverage in the world, and is the most popular drink after water and tea. The history of beer production is also impressive. Beer was made first in Mesopotamia between 3500 and 2900 BC (according to other sources in ancient Egypt). This beverage is made from malted cereals, hops, yeasts, water and other ingredients (Nelson, 2005). The NDMA was probably co-occurring in this beverage from the beginning of beer production, however the presence of this compound in beer first was reported in 1977 by Sen et al (Sen et al. 1980).

The investigation of Sen et al. was focused on the presence of NDMA and other nitrosamines in selected types of food and beverages including beer. They detected about 1.5 μg/kg of N-nitrosodimethylamine (NDMA) in 21 of 22 samples of beers and ales (Sen et al. 1980a). Later on Sen et al. examined the origin of beers from 30 countries and five continents: Africa, North, Middle and South America, Asia, Australia and New Zealand and Europe. The mean values of NDMA concentrations in investigated beers, in principle, did not exceed 1 ppb in most samples and ranged from below LOD to 2.1 ppb, except in beer from Mexico. Sen et al. observed in this beer an extremely high (up to 9.1 ppb) concentration of NDMA (Sen et al. 1996). The concentration of NDMA higher than FDA limit (5 μg/L) was also notified by Perez et al. (Perez et al., 2008) in one of the samples of Mexican beer. After Sen et al. have published their first report concerning NDMA presence in beers, considerable amount of papers dealing with this problem have been published. Results presented in some of it are described below.

Spiegelhalder et al., using GC-CD (gad chromatography with chemiluminescence detector) technique, analyzed 158 samples of commercially available draft, bottled and canned beers of different types for contamination with volatile nitrosamines. 111 (70%) of these samples were found to contain N-nitrosodimethylamine, in mean concentration of 2.7 ppb (μg/kg) with maximum levels reaching 68 ppb (dark or smoky beer 'Rauchbier'). Other hazardous nitrosamine N-nitrosodiethylamine, was detectable in only two samples at 0.5 and 3.0 ppb levels (Spiegelhalder et al., 1979).

In 1994 Izquierdo-Polido et al. investigated the presence of NDMA in 21 beers originating from Spanish breweries (Special Lager, Extra and non-alcoholic). Applying solid phase extraction prior to GC- TEA (thermal energy analysis detector) analysis, they found NDMA in 52% of Spanish beers at or above the method detection level (0.05 μg/kg). The mean level for all samples was 0.11 μg/kg and ranged from not detected to 0.55 μg/kg (Izquierdo-Polido et al., 1996).

During their impressive studies Yurchenko and Molder, between 2003 and 2004, analyzed 158 Estonian beers originating from six Estonian breweries (Saku, Tartu, Viru, Parnu, Saaremaa and Nigula) and 106 imported beers originating from Czech, Ukraine, Denmark, England, Russia, Ireland, Finland, Germany, Netherland, Austria and Spain, on NDMA presence. Applying two-steps solid phase extraction prior to GC-MS analysis with positive chemical ionization, they found NDMA in Estonian beers at level ranging from <0.15 to 1.31 μg/l with an average of 0.20 μg/l. In 106 imported beers they found close NDMA levels ranging from <0.15 to 1.1 μg/l with an average of 0.21 μg/l. The highest NDMA concentrations they found in domestic beers, in Estonian porter (0.57 ppb, the average of 12 samples) and Estonian dark beer (0.48 ppb, the average of 15 samples). Moreover they discovered several regularities concerning the influence of alcohol percentage in beer, type of beer and storage conditions. The highest concentration of NDMA was observed in alcohol-free beers and weak beers (<0.5%) contained higher concentrations of N-nitrosodimethylamine than strong beers (>0.5%). Also NDMA concentrations in dark beers were higher than in light beers with the same percent of alcohol. Moreover, temperature of beer storage had significantly impact on the NDMA concentration. The beers were stored at 4, 20, 25 and 30°C in the dark and usually analyzed after two weeks. No detectable changes were found in bottles stored at temperature of 4°C, but a loss of NDMA was observed in samples kept at 20, 25 and 30°C. Yurchenko and Molder also put together the results of earlier investigations on NDMA occurrence in beers conducted between 1991 and 1994 by

Sen et al. and compared them with own ones. Results obtained by these two groups of researches for beers originating from the same countries were similar and generally did not exceed 1 ppb (Yurchenko & Molder, 2005).

According to the evaluation of the daily intake of NDMA for average beer consumer, for approximate daily beer consumption of 0.5 l and an average NDMA concentration in beer of 0.3 μg/l i.e. 300 ng/l, daily intake of NDMA is calculated to be 150 ng. According to US EPA recommendations daily oral intake associated with health risk of 10^{-5} should not exceed 14 ng (2 liters of water containing 7 ng/l a day) (USEPA, 2010). The relation between alcohol content and nitrosamines influence was established by Anderson et al. who demonstrated the influence of ethanol presence on NDMA metabolism. Experiments made be Anderson et al. and conducted with rodents and primates, demonstrated the increased exposure of posthepatic organs to nitrosamines when given in combination with ethanol, followed by enhancement of DNA adduct formation and, at least in rodents, of tumor development (Anderson et al., 1995).

Eleven years ago, in 1999, Lijinski, based on reports concerning nitrosamines occurrence in beer, especially data published by Spiegelhalder et al., (Spiegelhalder et al., 1979) stated, that contamination of food with nitrosamines was considered a more serious matter in beer than in other foods contaminated with carcinogens, especially in Germany, so the problem was solved with some haste (Lijinski, 1999). On the other hand, Sen et al. noticed significant decrease in NDMA concentration both in Canadian and imported beers, based on results obtained in 1978-1980 and 1991-1994, resulting from improvement in malt-drying technologies. In 162 of Canadian beers analyzed during 1982-1996, the average NDMA level was found to be 0.098 ppb (range, <0.1-0.6 ppb) as compared to average levels of 1.4 and 0.7 ppb detected in two earlier (1978 and 1980, respectively) surveys. In the two surveys of imported beers carried out during 1991-1992 and 1994, the respective averages were 0.71 ppb (106 samples; range, <0.1-9.1 ppb) and 0.15 ppb (36 samples; range, <0.1-3.2 ppb). According to their calculations the daily intake of NDMA via beer by an average Canadian in 1996 was about one-fifteenth of that estimated in 1978-1980 (Sen et al, 1996).

1.2.2. Water

Water is, definitely, the oldest and probably the most popular beverage all over the world. Drinking water is, at present, available from three sources: raw water from local wells (mainly in rural areas, in the case of lack of water-supply system), as treated tap water originating from water network system and as bottled water (mineral or table water).

Water from local wells can be contaminated with both inorganic and organic impurities including NDMA. Presence of NDMA in wells is connected to infiltration of N-nitrosodimethylamine containing raw waters and to discharge waters or wastewaters to groundwater aquifer. Mitch et al. reported NDMA presence in drinking water wells polluted by rocket engine testing facilities in Sacramento County, CA, that used unsymmetrical dimethylhydrazine (UDMH)-based rocket fuel. NDMA concentration of up to 400 000 ng/l on site and 200 000 ng/l off site, forced local authorities to close downgradient drinking water wells. Other causes of pollution of drinking water wells by NDMA have also been recognized. Mitch et al. reported the pollution of drinking water wells by NDMA by means of recharging of aquifer with discharge waters. For example, in 2000, two drinking water production wells suspended operations due to the presence of NDMA resulting from the recharge water from the advanced wastewater treatment system of the Orange County Water District's Water Factory 21 (Mitch et al., 2003). As it turned out, NDMA concentration during chlorination of secondary wastewater effluent exceeded 100 ng/L (Najm & Trussell, 2001). California Department of Health Services conducted a survey of 32 water treatment plants for NDMA presence. The survey confirmed a presence of NDMA in some raw waters (Charrois et al, 2007). Year after, Zhao et al. also found NDMA in some influent waters (Zhao et al., 2008).

NDMA were also found in tap water from municipal water treatment plants. One of the first studies on nitrosamines occurrence was focused on NDMA presence in US and Canadian drinking water treatment plants and was carried out by Barrett et al. between years 2001 and 2002. Samples of raw waters, effluents and from distribution systems of 21 water treatment plants were analyzed for nitrosamine presence. There was almost no NDMA in raw waters found. The effluents were divided into two kinds: chlorinated and chloraminated. Slightly higher concentrations of NDMA were found in chloraminated waters (10 ng/l) comparing to chlorinated ones: 9 ng/l (Barrett et al, 2003). Charrois et al. have surveyed 179 Ontario water treatment plants for nitrosamine presence. The study concerned influent, effluent and distribution water samples and altogether more than 3000 samples have been analyzed. Except for NDMA, also nanogram quantities of N-nitrosomorpholine and N-nitrosopyrrolidine have been detected in some waters. Moreover 20 samples from Alberta public drinking water distribution systems were analyzed and NDMA up to 100 ng/l in one of the samples was found. The sample was taken from the distribution system located at the furthest distance from the water treatment utility. Another sample taken from the middle of the same distribution system had the NDMA concentration of 66 ng/l (Charrois et al. 2007).

Based on their studies in 2001Najm and Trussell suggested that NDMA appears to be a by-product of the chloramination of water and wastewater, with the level of NDMA formed directly related to the chloramine dose. According to results obtained by authors NDMA, however, did not form on contact with free chlorine or ozone (Najm & Trussell, 2001). In 2002 Choi and Valentine (2002) and Mitch and Sedlak (2002) reported that N-nitrosodimethylamine is formed during the chloramination of water or sewage containing dimethylamine. Moreover, the concentration of NDMA was closely related to the ratio of chlorine, ammonia ions and dimethylamine. Furthermore, the concentration of NDMA increased with the reaction time and the concentration of monochloramine. It should be emphasized that the maximum concentration of NDMA is formed at a neutral pH of 7 - 8. Andrzejewski et al. showed that NDMA is produced in water containing dimethylamine (DMA) and disinfected with chlorine dioxide (Andrzejewski et al., 2005), ozone (Andrzejewski et al., 2008), hydrogen peroxide (Andrzejewski & Nawrocki, 2007) and permanganate (Andrzejewski et al., 2009). Although the use of ozone and chlorine dioxide in the treatment of water containing DMA also leads to formation of essential, from technological point of view, amounts of NDMA, chloramination is commonly blamed for NDMA formation during water treatment. These results ultimately explain the reasons of NDMA presence in finished drinking waters, even if nitrosamines were absent in raw waters.

Problems linked to NDMA presence as well as to other potentially hazardous substances in water are definitely more serious than the problem related to the occurrence of these compounds in other beverages. Water is used not only as beverage, but also for body washing and recreation. During shower, taking bath or swimming, humans are exposed to water impurities via alimentary canal (accidental ingestion), respiratory system (volatile water impurities) and skin. Walse and Mitch (Walse & Mitch, 2008) and Jurado-Sanchez et al.

(Jurado-Sanchez et al., 2010) reported the presence of nitrosamines (including NDMA) in chlorinated waters of swimming pools.

The reports concerning the presence of NDMA or other nitrosamines in bottled waters have not been available to authors.

1.2.3. Other Beverages

As much as the data on nitrosamine content in beer and water were extensive, no published data concerning nitrosamine content in wine have been found, probably due to principal differences in technological processes in the production of these beverages (i.e. lack of high temperature processes in wine production). The informations concerning the presence of nitrosamines in tea were also impossible to attain. On the other hand Choi et al. reported the possible health impact of some species of tea extracts on consumers exposed to nitrite and secondary amines in their diet. The formation of carcinogenic nitrosamines under simulated gastric conditions was studied during the incubation of amine rich food and nitrate, and its possible inhibition by adding kumquat, sweet orange, strawberry, garlic, kale juices, Maesil (*Prunus mume*) and green tea extracts. The strawberry, kale juices, Maesil and green tea extracts turned out to be equally effective in reducing the formation of N-nitrosodimethylamine (NDMA) (Choi et al., 2002).

2. Mechanism of Nitrosamines Formation

The 'classic' nitrosamine formation pathway assumes that these compounds are formed during direct nitrosation of secondary amines by nitrous acid at low pH (about 3.0-3.5), in which NO^+ plays a particular role. Tertiary amines do not react with nitrite (Figure 3, reaction #3).

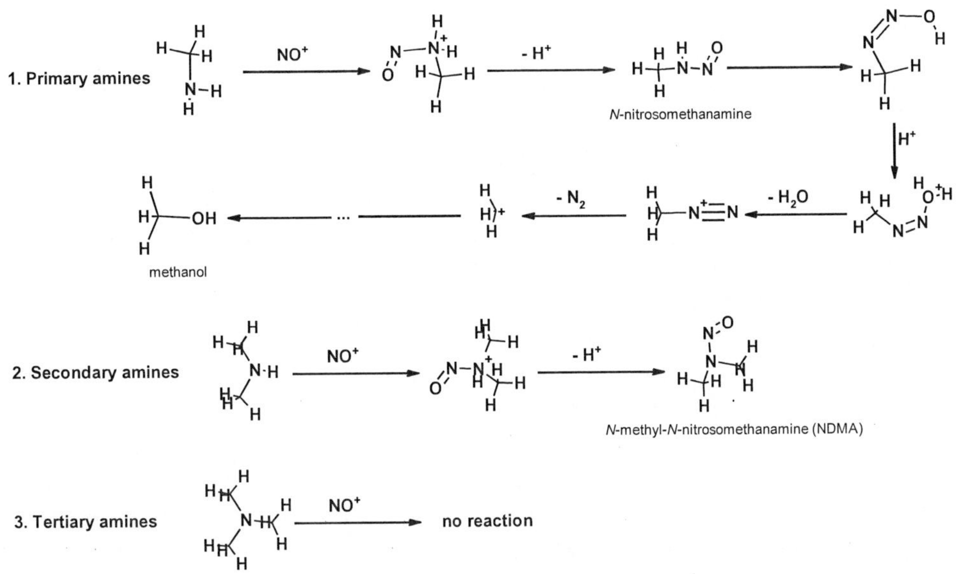

Figure3. The 'classic' nitrosation pathway of primary (methylamine), secondary (dimethylamine) and tertiary amines (trimethylamine).

In the case of primary amines the reaction leads to the formation of several unstable compounds like diazo- base or diazonium cation (Figure 3, reaction #1) and nitrosamine is only intermediate product of the reaction. Finally, the appropriate alcohol can be formed as stable product of this reaction. Only the reaction with secondary amines results in the formation of the corresponding nitrosamines (Figure 3, reaction #2) (Wunsch et al., 1979).

Based on above presented scheme, only secondary amines can be considered as final precursors of nitrosamines. Thus, other compounds, i.e. structures containing dialkylamino groups should be considered as primary nitrosamines precursors, which during preliminary reactions release dialkylamino groups. These groups subsequently undergo nitrosation to form nitrosamines.

Mechanism of the formation of NDMA and other nitrosamines in solid food likes meat and fish is linked to the reaction of direct nitrosation of secondary (or tertiary) amines with nitrite or nitrogen oxides. Fresh food (meat and fish) are sources of nitrosamine precursors (secondary or tertiary amines) and nitrosation agent, originating from added ingredients, is formed during food treatment subsequently reacting with nitrosamines precursors. Tozawa and Kawabata proposed two pathways for N-nitrosothiazolidine (NT) formation during fish meal manufacturing. Both cysteamine and thiazolidine were found to be precursors of NT. The cysteamine content decreased during boiling and drying of the fish; but that of thiazolidine increased during boiling. They showed that N-nitrosothiazolidine 4-carboxylic acid (NTCA) was formed in sardine meal after treatment with nitrogen dioxide gas, and the rate of formation of NT from NTCA added to sardine meal was as high as 10% when the meal was heated at 160°C for 60 min. According to authors N-nitrosothiazolidine is formed according to two pathways: (1) cysteamine→thiazolidine→NT; and (2) cysteine→ (thiazolidine 4-carboxylic acid) →NTCA→NT (Tozawa & Kawabata, 1991). Rywotycki stresses the role of autotrophic and numerous heterotrophic organisms participating in biochemical and chemical processes of nitrosamine formation, which are also active in biochemical processes of nitrification and de-nitrification together with numerous bacteria. He quoted the results of experiments which demonstrated that some strains of enterococcus and Clostridium bacteria have the ability to synthesize nitrosodimethylamine (NDMA), while some Proteus are capable of nitrosodimethylamine production. The role of bacteria in nitrosamine formation consists in nitrate reduction to nitrite, protein degradation to secondary amines, production of an enzymes catalyzing nitrosating reactions and formation of a suitable reaction environment by acidification (Rywotycki, 2007). On the other hand, Yurchenko and Molder evaluated the influence of baking temperature on the content of volatile nitrosamines in samples of oil and fish. In all experiments concentration of nitrosamines increased with temperature increasing. Processing temperature of 200°C seemed to be the critical value. The concentrations of nitrosamines below this value increased insignificantly, but above 200°C significant increase in nitrosamine concentration was observed. (Yurchenko & Molder, 2007).

The mechanism of nitrosamines formation during cheese production was investigated by Klein et al. They explained the process by the activity of several strains of micromycetes in the course of cheese ripening. Selected strains of micromycetes commonly used as fermentation agents in cheese industry or contamination during cheese making were responsible for the formation of nitrosamines in 60% of the cases. The concentrations observed were similar to those found by other authors with other identified microorganisms. The results obtained in experiments on experimental camembert type cheese, made from milk containing nitrates and cultured with a strain of *Penicillium camemberti*, showed that the amount of nitrosodimethylamine formed in this cheese increases from 5 to 20 ppb during ripening (Klein et al., 1980).

The NDMA formation in beer is mainly attributed to one of the steps of malting process: drying, which can be conducted both in extremely high temperatures, such as in direct-fire drying (from 1500 to 1800°C) or lower with hot air (below 100°C). During this process nitrogen oxides are formed and their amount strongly depends on the processing temperatures. Higher temperatures result in higher nitrogen oxides formation. Nitrogen oxides react, during this step, with certain alkaloids to form NDMA. Thus, higher temperatures of drying process lead to formation of significantly higher amounts of NDMA (Yurchenko & Molder, 2005). The mechanism of NDMA formation in beer (from gramine), proposed by Rubenchik, denies however above presented exceptional role of secondary amines in the NDMA formation. According to him gramine, even though is tertiary amine, undergoes nitrosation to form NDMA (Yurchenko & Molder, 2005). This mechanism of NDMA formation from gramine is shown in Figure 4.

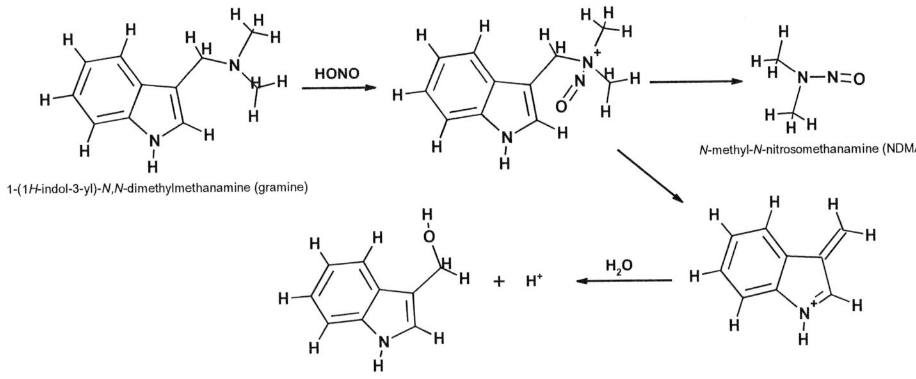

Figure4. Mechanism of NDMA formation from gramine, proposed by Rubenchik.

The mechanism proposed by Rubenchik, however does not correspond completely to conditions of nitrosation during beer brewing. Rubenchik defines HONO (nitrous acid) as nitrosation agent. In 1978 Powell and Adams presented the mechanism of N_2O_4 formation - strong nitrosation agent, during direct reaction of two molecules of NO_2 in gaseous phase (Powell & Adams, 1978):

$$NO_{2(g)} + NO_{2(g)} \leftrightarrow N_2O_{4(g)}$$

Understanding the mechanism of NDMA (and other nitrosamines) formation is strictly connected to the problem of nitrosamines (particularly NDMA) precursors. Dimethylamine and other secondary dialkylamines are, no doubt, some of them. Yurchenko and Molder pointed out that two alkaloids (hordenine and gramine), formed in malt roots during germination, may act as amine precursors in nitrosation during beer manufacturing (Yurchenko & Molder, 2005). The main components necessary for understanding the mechanism of NDMA formation as the result of nitrosation of dialkylamino group-containing compound during beer brewing seems to be explained:

- hot spots in brewing process i.e. direct-fire drying step of the malting process is responsible for NDMA formation

- the main precursors in raw material are certain group of alkaloids containing dialkylaminogrups (including hordenine and gramine), which can be considered, from point of view of amine structure, as tertiary amines
- the source of nitrosation agent i.e. nitrogen oxides in hot flue gases originate from coal burning

On oppose to NDMA formation during beer brewing which was explained, the problem of mechanism of NDMA formation is still discussed. As stated in chapter 1, in 2002, Mitch and Sedlak (Mitch & Sedlak, 2002) and Choi and Valentine (Choi & Valentine, 2002) reported that NDMA is formed during the chloramines disinfection of water or in wastewater treatment plant effluents containing dimethylamine (DMA). The mechanism proposed by Choi and Valentine (Choi & Valentine, 2002) and Mitch and Sedlak (Mitch & Sedlak, 2002) is based on chloramination leading to the formation of 1,1-dimethylhydrazine, known as unsymmetrical dimethylhydrazine (UDMH). Furthermore, 1,1-dimethylhydrazine undergoes oxidation to yield many different by-products, including NDMA. The proposed mechanism was subsequently modified by Schreiber and Mitch. The authors emphasized the role of dichloroamine and dissolved oxygen in NDMA formation due to the reaction of chloramination of DMA (Schreiber & Mitch, 2006). In 2003, Choi and Valentine proposed other model of mechanism of NDMA formation during reaction of dimethylamine with chlorine. According to the proposed mechanism, HOCl reacts with nitrite present in water to form very reactive nitrosating intermediate i.e. dinitrogen tetroxide (N2O4), which subsequently reacts with dimethylamie to form NDMA. Nevertheless, the paper states that in chloraminated water NDMA is formed mainly by the reaction of HOCl with ammonia and subsequent formation of UDMH (Choi & Valentine, 2003).

Schreiber and Mitch made an attempt to clarify doubts concerning mechanism of NDMA formation during DMA chloramination. They investigated the mechanism of this reaction under conditions which occurred during chlorination near the breakpoint. The authors proposed two independent paths of NDMA formation: a relatively slow reaction of dichloramine with NDMA precursors in the presence of oxygen at molar ratio $Cl_2/NH_3 \leq 1,5$; and the fast reaction of reactive breakpoint chlorination intermediates which are involved in the direct nitrosation of DMA. The authors postulated, depending on pH, the formation of peroxynitrous acid (O=N-O-OH; p*K*a=6.8) or peroxynitrite ion ($O{=}N{-}O{-}O^-$), which subsequently releases $*NO_2$ and OH* or $^*NO$ and O_2^{*-} radicals, respectively. The peroxynitrous acid-derived HO* could react with DMA to form an amine radical and then be nitrosated by nitric oxide (*NO), a one-electron transfer oxidation product of NO^- to form NDMA. Alternatively, peroxynitrite-derived $^*NO$ radical could react with DMA to form NDMA. The authors also pointed out the crucial role of dissolved oxygen in the peroxynitrous acid or peroxynitrite ion formation. However, they observed no differences in NDMA formation in the presence or absence of dissolved O_2 during breakpoint chlorination (Schreiber & Mitch, 2007). The above presented NDMA formation pathway via peroxynitrous acid or peroxynitrite ion could explain the mechanisms of other oxidants reactions with DMA as well, because peroxynitrite can be formed also as a result of hydrogen peroxide reaction with nitrite (Uppu & Pryor, 1996).

As reported above, Andrzejewski et al. demonstrated the possibility of NDMA formation in water containing dimethylamine (DMA) disinfected with chlorine dioxide (Andrzejewski et al., 2005), ozone (Andrzejewski et al., 2008), hydrogen peroxide (Andrzejewski &

Nawrocki, 2007) and permanganate (Andrzejewski et al., 2009). Provided that the reactions with chlorine dioxide, ozone, hydrogen peroxide and permanganate take place in the absence of ammonium ions, the mechanism of NDMA formation must be different from the one proposed by Choi and Valentine (Choi & Valentine, 2002) and Mitch and Sedlak (Mitch & Sedlak, 2002).

On the basis of the nitrosamine formation pathway, proposed by Keefer and Roller (Keefer & Roller, 1973) and Andrzejewski et al. (Andrzejewski et al., 2008), assuming that NDMA, which is the product of strong non-chlorine oxidants reaction with DMA, is formed as a result of a multi-step reaction. In the first stage, part of DMA is oxidized and formaldehyde, formic acid, nitrite and nitrate are formed. Subsequently, nitrite reacts with the remaining part of DMA to form NDMA. Andrzejewski and Nawrocki also applied labeled nitrite ^{15}N in order to explain the mechanism of NDMA formation during permanganate/ferrate reactions with aqueous solution of DMA. The presence of ^{15}N nuclide (added as $^{15}NO_2^-$ ion to reaction mixture) in the NDMA molecule, in the higher than normal abundance, clearly showed that nitrite is the source of nitroso group in the NDMA molecule. Thus the mechanism of nitrosation of DMA is responsible for NDMA formation during these reactions (Andrzejewski & Nawrocki, 2010).

Formation of NDMA upon ozonation of DMA was confirmed by Yang et al. They proposed other mechanism of NDMA formation based on the generation of hydroxylamine as a by-product of DMA oxidation. According to Yang et al.'s hypothesis, formation of nitrosamines proceeds through UDMH formation and then oxidation of this hydrazine (Yang et al. 2009).

The list of possible NDMA precursors in water is relatively long and contains dimethylamine (Mitch & Sedlak, 2002; Choi &Valentine, 2002), still incompletely defined dissolved organic nitrogen as a part of natural organic matter (Chen & Valentine, 2006; Gerecke & Sedlak, 2003), other amines (tertiary- or quaternary-) (Lee et al., 2007; Kemper et al., 2010), cationic flocculants (Wilczak at al., 2004) or anion exchange resins used for ion-exchange in water treatment (Najm & Trussell, 2001; Kimoto et al., 1980; Kemper et al., 2009). According to Lee et al. tertiary amines should be consider the precursors of the final precursor i.e. DMA (Lee et al., 2007).

The mechanism of nitrosamines formation in food and beverages is still matter of discussion, particularly in case of water. Chemical reactions of nitrosation seem to be responsible for nitrosamines formation in beers or high temperature processed meats and fish. The strong nitrosation agent i.e. N_2O_2, formed as the result of direct reaction of two molecules of NO_2 in gaseous phase, may play crucial role in the nitrosation reaction, during the production of these types of food and beers. On the other hand, microorganisms and bacteria play crucial or important role during nitrosamines formation in cheese or canned, pickled and salted meat and fish. Precursors of nitrosamines are also still topic of discussion. Dialkylamines seem to be the final precursors of nitrosamines in water, i.e. these compounds undergo reaction, which directly leads to nitrosamine formation. On the other hand, dialkylamine containing tertiary amines serve as kind of potential precursors releasing dialkylamine groups during reactions preceding final reaction of nitrosamine formation. Mechanism of nitrosamines formation in food, reported by part of above cited authors, includes possible direct nitrosation of dialkylamine containing tertiary amines precursors and subsequent release of formed nitrosamine.

3. The Influence of Food Processing on Nitrosamines Formation

Results of investigations presented in this review and also in previous ones clearly show that nitrosamines, particularly NDMA, were detected in processed meat, fish, vegetables, oils as well as in beverages like beer. The EU has set the maximum level of sodium nitrite in processed meat to 150 mg/kg to limit nitrosamine formation but, in practice, about 120 mg/kg is usually added.

In a recent study, Drabik-Markiewicz et al. (2010) performed a research on the effects of food processing on nitrosamine formation. In particular, they used fresh minced pork that was injected with brine containing sodium chloride and pentasodium triphosphate then spiked with sodium nitrite and one of the three free amino acids proline, hydroxyproline and pyrrolidine. The prepared food was cooked for 30 minutes at different temperatures to mimic industrial process: 85, 120 and 120-220°C for pasteurization, sterilization and baking/roasting, respectively. N-nitrosodipropylamine was used as an internal standard on cooked samples, which were then basified before vacuum distillation and extraction with dichloromethane. The dried extracts were analyzed by GC with a thermal energy analyzer as detector. The analytes were separated on a packed column. Under these conditions, all nitrosamines were baseline-separated and the detection and quantitation limits were 0.125 and 0.375 μg/ml, respectively.

For cooked ham fortified with all three amino acids, only NDMA and NPYR were detected at levels up to 0.751 and 2.472 μg/ml, respectively.

The presence of proline and pyrrolidine clearly increased the number of detections of NPYR from 12% to 35% and 88%, respectively, although hydroxyproline had no detectable effect. Pyrrolidine concentrations had a greater effect than nitrite concentrations. The highest NPYR level was observed after heating to 220°C or following the addition of 480 mg/kg of nitrite, well above EU legislative levels. In blank samples containing nitrite but no added amino acid, NDMA was detected more frequently than NPYR. NDMA formation was principally due to the addition of nitrite and, to a lesser extent, elevated temperatures, and was limited when nitrite was added within the legal limits. Hydroxyproline and pyrrolidine increased NDMA levels to maximum levels of 0.654 and 0.751 μg/ml, respectively.

This study has extended current knowledge on the effects of free amino acids on nitrosamine formation in cooked meat. Overall, higher nitrite levels and higher temperatures produced higher yields of NDMA and NPYR, the nitrite effect generally being the greater. However, nitrosamine formation was low for legal nitrite levels. Free amino acids increased the levels of nitrosamines, particularly pyrrolidine and proline for NPYR and, less markedly, hydroxyproline and pyrrolidine for NDMA (Drabik-Markiewicz et al., 2010).

Chen et al. (1991) investigated the effects of microwave heating on the formation of nitrosamines in bacon. Bacon was cooked in a teflon-coated frying pan and in transparent and susceptor packages in a 700 W microwave oven. Bacon slices were prepared to three "degrees of doneness": "undercooked", "overcooked" and "similar" to standard pan frying (3 minutes on each side at 340°F) by controlling the time in the microwave oven. Final bacon temperatures of 167°C (330°F) and 143°C (290°F) were observed for samples cooked to the same "degree of doneness" as fried bacon in the susceptor (2.5 minutes) and transparent (3 minutes) packages, respectively. Compared to frying, lower concentrations of N-nitrosopyrrolidine (NPYR) and N-nitrosodimethylamine (NDMA) were present in bacon cooked either in the transparent or susceptor packages. Greater concentrations of NPYR were found in bacon cooked on susceptors in comparison to cooking in a transparent package. Formation of NPYR in pan-fried bacon was correlated with the concentration of nitrite in the raw product.

Huang et al. (1981) investigated nitrosamines formation in uncooked, steamed and fried samples of salted fish, by gas chromatography with detection by chemiluminescence and some were also analyzed by combined gas chromatography and high-resolution mass spectrometry. N-Nitrosodimethylamine (NDMA) was detected in all of the samples that were analyzed, whether cooked or uncooked. It was also detected in the aqueous phases derived from the steamed samples, and in the oil from frying in two out of three batches. In one of these the NDMA level was the highest encountered in the present study. N-Nitrosodiethylamine (NDEA), on the other hand, was detected in more batches of the steamed fish than of the uncooked or fried fish. It was not detected in the oil used for frying. In half of the steamed batches NDEA was detected only in the aqueous phases and in one batch it was detected only in the steamed fish. N-Nitrosodi-n-propylamine (NDPA) was detected in both the steamed and fried samples and N-nitrosodi-n-butylamine (NDBA) in only the fried samples. Neither was detected in the uncooked samples. N-Nitrosomorpholine (NMOR) occurred in the uncooked samples. Salted fish heads are sometimes used by southern Chinese to prepare soup. NDMA and NDEA occurred in both uncooked fish heads and in the soups prepared from them. The results confirm that certain nitrosamines are formed from precursors during cooking.

Lintasa et al. (1990) analyzed aqueous extracts of uncooked and cooked samples of squid and shrimp, characterized by their high amine content, exposed to nitrite. The samples were cooked following traditional Italian recipes: stewing, grilling and deep-frying for squid; boiling, grilling and deep-frying for shrimp. Incubation of the aqueous extracts with nitrite in acidic medium yielded appreciable amounts of N-nitrosodimethylamine. Ascorbic acid and α-tocopherol were effective in preventing nitrosation of seafood amines only in the presence of molar excesses of these vitamins.

Lee et al (2003) analyzed NDMA in seven dried seafood products, either uncooked or cooked. The cooking methods used were a briquette fire, a gas range, an electric oven, a microwave oven, a steam cooker and an electric coil cooker. The contents of NDMA ranged from 1.0 to 46.9 μg/kg in uncooked products. When these samples were cooked, regardless of the cooking method, the content of NDMA tended to increase, ranging from 1.1 to 630.5 μg/kg. In general, indirect heating such as a steam cooker and a microwave oven, as compared with direct heating such as a gas range and a briquette fire, caused less increase in NDMA during cooking.

Fiddler et al. (1992) conducted studies to determine the feasibility of using Alaska pollock mince as a partial substitute for red meats in the formulation of frankfurters. Their research included the effects of fish form (unwashed and washed mince and surimi), percentage substitution (15 and 50) and five different methods of cooking the fish-meat franks on their N-nitrosodimethylamine (NDMA) content. The amount of formed NDMA depended on the method of cooking. Broiling and frying generated the highest levels. Microwave and boiling generated the lowest levels of NDMA, which were equivalent to the level in uncooked franks. Broiling was observed to increase the amount of dimethyl-and trimethylamine formed.

Key et al. (2007) determined the NDMA content in fish, in raw fish and after baking in pre-heated and not pre-heated ovens and after grilling using electrical and natural gas heated domestic cookers. In many cases there was an increase in NDMA levels in natural gas heated cookers but the increase was not so significant in comparison to variations observed in levels in raw fish obtained on different occasions. There was no significant increase in NDMA levels with electric cookers.

Gough et al. (2006) examined over 500 samples of foodstuffs, including meat, fish and dairy products, vegetables, fruit and soups for the presence of volatile nitrosamines. Cooked complete meals were studied in order to assess the possibility of interactions of the constituents which could result in nitrosamine formation. The extracts of foods were subjected to gas chromatography and the presence of nitrosamines confirmed using on-line high resolution mass spectrometry. The most frequently occurring nitrosamines were N-nitrosodimethylamine and N-nitrosopyrrolidine which were present in many cooked bacon samples. N-nitrosodimethylamine also occurred in some other meat products, but other nitrosamines were rarely found. N-nitrosodimethylamine also occurred in fish and cheese, but neither this nitrosamine nor any other was found above the detection limit of 1 μg/kg in any of the other foods.

Yurchenko and Molder (2006) investigated the formation of nitrosamines in samples of fish, and in samples of oil during 2001–2005. Increased levels of nitrosamines were observed after baking and frying. The concentration of nitrosamines in the fish after baking in pre-heated electrical oven was found to depend on the cooking temperature. There was significant increase in nitrosamines levels in the fish and in the oil after baking with electrical oven at temperature around 150°C. In most cases NDMA concentration in gas-frying sample was higher than that in the electric oven-baking fish. They also investigated the influence of cooking time on nitrosamines formation. The concentration of nitrosamines increased rapidly in first 20 min and then remained stabile.

The same researchers performed another investigation in meat (2007), where they determined the level of five nitrosamines in raw, fried, grilled, smoked, pickled, and canned meat products. The authors also performed experiments with nitrite addition to the samples, and from the results, it may be concluded that meat curing with sodium nitrite increases remarkably the level of nitrosamines. The process of frying causes increased sensitivity of all amines to nitrosation about 10 times compared to raw mutton samples. The dependence of concentration of nitrosamines produced in fried mutton with added sodium nitrite was roughly linear in selected range of concentrations. Most sensitive for sodium nitrite addition was NPYR (about 0.16 μg pro 1 mg $NaNO_2$). Lower concentrations of other nitrosamines were formed. The concentration increase pro 1 mg added $NaNO_2$ was about 0.020 μg for NDMA, 0.014 μg for NPIP, 0.005 μg for NDEA and NDBA, respectively. Increased levels of nitrosamines were observed after baking and frying indicating the formation of these compounds during preparing. Particularly important is the role of fat in baked mutton. It appears that about 73% of nitrosamines are concentrated in fat of baked mutton. Thereby, at baking temperatures lower than 200°C about 90% of NDMA is concentrated in fat whereas NPYR abundance in fat reaches 30% by these temperatures. At 250°C baking temperature, the abundance of NDMA in fat is 73% and NPYR 64%, respectively. Nitrosamines in gas frying samples of mutton were formed at higher levels than in the electricoven and in microwave oven-baking mutton. The formation of nitrosamines increased with time and temperature of frying. The increase was rapid in range from 40 to 100°C and then stabilized. Hence, the formation of nitrosamines takes place at temperatures below 100°C.

In pork fried in a frying pan with olive oil by using natural gas, after frying for 30 min per side, nitrosamines were found in 5 of 5 samples of pork. The total yield of nitrosamines from the fat of pork was much greater than that from either the lean or even whole rasher. In fried pork with paprika, the concentration of nitrosamines in fat exceeded the concentration in lean 6 times (among them NDMA 8 times, NDEA 2.5 times, NPYR 6.7 times, NPIP 3.2 times, and NDBA 1.9 times). In fried pork without paprika, the concentration of nitrosamines in fat exceeded the concentration in lean 5.4 times. Therefore, the effect of paprika in meat did not prevail in the formation of nitrosamines in frying process (Yurchenko & Molder, 2006, 2007).

4. Nitrosamines Determination in Solid Food and Beverages

The determination of nitrosamines in water at ultra-trace levels is an analytical challenge due to their specific properties such as low molecular weight, high polarity and high water solubility. Analytical problems in their determination by mass spectrometry related to interfering compounds are very common, as the molecular weight of NDMA 74.08 g/mol is close to many daughter ions from other common water contaminants. Therefore, traditional Gas Chromatography-Mass spectrometry (GC-MS) analytical methods cannot differentiate between these small differences in mass weight between interfering compounds and NDMA, especially in trace concentration levels, resulting often in false positives for NDMA. The proposed solution to this problem is the application of high resolution MS (HRMS) analysis, the technique capable of distinguishing these compounds.

NDMA was first reported as a new disinfection by-product (DBP) in drinking water in Canada by Graham et al (1995). Since then, many researchers worldwide tried to develop and optimize analytical methods for the determination of NDMA and other nitrosamines in water samples. Thereafter, modifications of these methods have been developed, to enable their analysis also in beverages and in food, as their occurrence in these matrices has been well documented, as discussed in the previous section. Solid phase extraction, liquid-liquid extraction and solid phase microextraction have been used for the extraction of nitrosamine from the samples, while GC-MS and more recently GC-HRMS have been applied for separation and quantification of the analytes. In 2000s the USEPA nitrosamines determination method #521 and method developed by Charrois et al. established new standard in nitrosamines identification in water by applying chemical positive ionization mass spectrometric detector (MSD-CI) with methanol/acetonitrile (Method 521, EPA Document # EPA/600/R-05/054) or ammonia (Charrois et al., 2007). Table 2 summarizes selected analytical methods developed during the last years for the analytical determination of nitrosamines in food and beverages.

Table 2. Selected analytical methods developed for the determination of nitrosamines in food and beverages

Sample matrix	Analytical Instrumentation	Sample Preparation	Reference
Sausages	Micellar Electrokinetic Chromatography	SPE	Filho et al., 2002
Model food protein matrix systems (meat, fish)	GC-MS	SPME-DED	Ventanas & Ruiz, 2006
Fish	GC-CI-MS	Two-step SPE	Yurchenko & Mölder, 2006
Meat	GC-CI-MS	Two step SPE	Yurchenko & Mölder, 2007
Whisky	GC-MS	LLE	Goff and Fine, 1979
Beer	HPLC-fluorescence	Microwave-assisted Dansylation	Cárdenes et al., 2001
Beer	GC-CI-MS	Two-step SPE	Yurchenko & Mölder, 2005

To obtain best results in terms of accuracy, isotope dilution GC-MS is mostly used by applying either high resolution GC-MS with chemical ionization (CI) or electron impact (EI), or low resolution GC/MS with selected ion monitoring (SIM), using deuterated NDMA (NDMA-d6) as an internal standard. Detection limits down to 2 ppt level and recoveries between 60-120% have been reported (references cited in Table 1).

Analytical methods to detect volatile N-nitrosamines in beer have also been reported by Fine (1983), Spiegelhalder et al. (1983), Tateo and Roundbehler (1983), Song and Fu (1988), Osterdahl (1988), Frommberger (1989), Kubacki et al. (1989), Scanlan et al. (1980), Sen et al. (1996) and Tricker and Preussmann (1991a, 1991b). Thermal Energy Analyzer has been used as a selective detector for NDMA, enabling LODs ranging from 0.05 to 0.3 μg/l (Leppanen & Ronkainen, 1982; Kubacki et al., 1989; Scanlan et al., 1980; Song & Fu, 1988; Frommberger, 1989; Andrzejewski et al., 1981). With GC-HRMS, LODs of 0.1 – 0.5 μg/l were achieved (Sen et al., 1980; Goff & Fine, 1979; Yin et al., 1982).

Regarding the extraction methods, SPE remains the predominant method used, with two-step SPE as a good alternative for enhancement of the sensitivity of the method (Yurchenko & Mölder, 2005). SPME has found limited application to date, with the Direct Extraction Device (DED) having recently been used with promising results (Ventanas & Ruiz, 2006). Other sample preparation methods that have been applied for both beverage and food samples include vacuum distillation and steam distillation (Andrzejewski et al., 1981; Scanlan et al., 1980; Sen et al., 1982; Spiegelhalder et al., 1979), mineral oil distillation of solid samples (Tricker & Preussmann, 1991a,1991b), direct extraction with dichloromethane, celite column extraction method (Hotchkiss et al., 1981; Sen et al., 1980, 1996) and solid-phase extraction with Extrelut sorbent (Osterdahl, 1988; Raoul, et al., 1997; Tateo & Roundbehler, 1983).

More recently, Yurchenko and Mölder (2005) developed and applied a positive-ion chemical ionization GC-MS method for the determination of N-nitrosodimethylamine in Estonian beer. For cleaning of the sample the two-step solid-phase extraction with Extrelut and Florisil sorbents were used. NDMA was separated by GC-MS (SIM mode) and detected by positive-ion chemical ionization using ammonia as reagent gas. The recovery of the method was 70-80% and the limit of detection for NDMA was 0.15 ppb. The reproducibility of results (at the 2.5 ppb level), was satisfactory with relative standard deviations (RSD) of 1–13%. The recovery of NDMA was 74% with standard deviation of 0.22 % and relative standard deviation of 9.1% in a spiked beer sample.

Different analytical methods have been developed for the determination of nitrosamines in fish, using thermal energy analyzer, by Howard et al. (1970), Pensabene et al. (1990), Sen et al. (1985) and Zou et al. (1994). GC-HRMS was used by Huang et al. (1981), GC-positive-ion chemical ionization-MS by Fish et al. (1976), Fong et al., (1984), Gadbois et al., (1975) and Prest and Hermann (1999). Similar methods have been applied for the determination of nitrosamines in meat, with thermal energy analyzer been used by Fiddler et al. (1971), Zhukova et al. (1999), a Coulson electrolytic conductivity detector by Mottram et al. (1977), a fluorometric method by Pokrovskii et al. (1978), micellar electrokinetic chromatography (Filho et al., 2003), and GC-HRMS by Stephany et al. (1978).

Yurchenko and Mölder (2006, 2007) developed an analytical method for the analysis of nitrosamines in fish (2006) and in meat (2007). The samples were prepared by a two step SPE with Extrelut and Florisil sorbents. GC-positive-ion chemical ionization MS (SIM mode) was used, with pulsed splitless injection, and with ammonia as reagent gas. For both methods, the limit of detection was 0.10 μg/kg, respectively, with about 85% recovery.

Overall, a significant effort have been made by many researchers to develop and optimize sensitive and accurate analytical methods for the determination of nitrosamines in various kinds of food, cooked and preserved meat and fish, as well as beverages, mainly beer. GC-MS methods have gained much interest, while the sample preparation methods have been enhanced by additional steps for better results. The challenge is to achieve as low detection limits as possible for these compounds in the difficult matrices of food and beverages. There is a need for their determination in other matrices as well (tea, coffee, other beverages and other kinds of food), as, to the author's knowledge, no data on their occurrence in such matrices, is yet available.

Conclusion

Nitrosamines, particularly NDMA, are present in most often consumed food and beverages like meat, fish or beer, despite both the stric regulations on maximum nitrite amount in processed food and the improvement in food and beverages processing technologies. On the other hand significant decrease of nitrosamines concentration is noticed, particularly in beers.

Analytical methods of nitrosamines determination in food and beverages, including water, have been significantly developed during last ten years. The most popular method of analyte enrichment i.e. the liquid-liquid extraction was successfully replaced by more efficient and lower reagents consuming methods of solid-phase extraction (SPE) or solid-phase micro-extraction (SPME). The Thermal Energy Analysis (TEA) detector, so widely used in 1980s and in the first years of 1990s was replaced by electron impact ionization low resolution mass spectrometric detector (MS) and recently by positive chemical ionization high resolution mass spectrometric detector (MS-CI). The application of spectrometric detector increased the credibility of the identification of nitrosamines in very complicated food and beverages matrixes in low nanogram levels.

The nitrosamines formation mechanism, particularly mechanism of nitrosamines formation in water, is still discussed, but fortunately this is mainly challenge for scientist, but not for food and beverages consumers.

References

Andrade R., Reyes F.G.R., Rath S. (2005) Analytical, Nutritional and Clinical Methods: A method for the determination of volatile N-nitrosamines in food by HS-SPME-GC-TEA. *Food Chemistry*, 91, 173–179.

Anderson L.M., Chhabra S.K., Nerurkar P.V., Souliotis V.L., Kyrtopoulos S.A. (1995) Alcohol related cancer risk: A toxico-kinetic hypothesis. *Alcohol*, 12, 97-104.

Andrzejewski D., Havery D. C., Fazio, T. (1981) Determination and confirmation of N-nitrosodimethylamine in beer. *Journal of the Association Official Analytical Chemists*, 64, 1457–1461.

Andrzejewski P., Kasprzyk-Hordern B., Nawrocki J. (2008) N-nitrosodimethylamine (NDMA) formation during ozonation of dimethylamine-containing waters. *Water Research*, 42, 863-870.

Andrzejewski P., Kasprzyk-Hordern B., Nawrocki J. (2005). The hazard of N-nitrosodimethylamine (NDMA) formation during water disinfection with strong oxidants. *Desalination*, 176, 37-45.

Andrzejewski P., Nawrocki J. (2007) N-nitrosodimethylamine formation during treatment with strong oxidants of dimethylamine containing water. *Water Science and Technology*, 56, 125–131.

Andrzejewski P., Nawrocki J. (2009) N-nitrosodimethylamine (NDMA) as a product of potassium permanganate reaction with aqueous solutions of dimethylamine (DMA). *Water Research*, 43, 1219-1228.

Andrzejewski P., Nawrocki J. (2010). Mechanism of NDMA formation during ferrate or permanganate reactions with aqueous solutions of dimethylamine (DMA). *Desalination and Water Treatment*, in press.

Barrett S., Hwang C., Guo Y., Andrews S.A., Valentine R.: Occurrence of NDMA in drinking water: A North American survey, 2001-2002. In: Proceedings of AWWA Annual Confenece, Anaheim, Ca, 15-19 June 2003. AWWA, Denver, CO.

Beresford T.P., Fitzsimons N.A., Brennan N.L., Cogan T.M. (2001) Recent advances in cheese microbiology. *International Dairy Journal*, 11, 259–274.

Cárdenes L., Ayala J.H., González V., Afonso A.M. (2001) Fast microwave-assisted dansylation of N-nitrosamines: Analysis by high-performance liquid chromatography with fluorescence detection. *Journal of Chromatography A*, 946, 133-140.

Charrois J.W.A, Boyd J.M, Froese K.L., Hrudey S.E. (2007) Occurrence of *N*-nitrosamines in Alberta public drinking-water distribution systems. *Journal of Environmental Engineering and Science* 6, 103–114.

ChemFinder (2007) ChemFinder.com.

Chen Z., Valentine R.L. (2006) Modeling the Formation of N-Nitrosodimethylamine from the Reaction of Natural Organic Matter (NOM) with Monochloramine. *Environmental Science and Technology*, 40, 7290-7297.

Choi S.Y., Chung M.J., Sung N.J. (2002) Volatile N-nitrosamine inhibition after intake Korean green tea and Maesil (Prunus mume SIEB. et ZACC.) extracts with an amine-rich diet in subjects ingesting nitrate *Food and Chemical Toxicology* 40, 949–957.

Domański W. (2003) Bezpieczeństwo pracy 4, 23-27 (in Polish).

oi J., Valentinmański W. (2003) Bezpieczeństwo pracy 4, 23-27 (in Polish).

Fiddler W., Doerr R. C., Ertel J.R., Wasserman, A.E. (1971) Gas–liquid chromatographic determination of N-nitrosodimethylamine in ham. *Journal of the Association Official Analytical Chemists*, 54, 1160–1163.

Filho P.J.S., Rios A., Valcárcel M., Zanin K.D., Caramão E.B. (2003) Determination of nitrosamines in preserved sausages by solid-phase extraction–micellar electrokinetic chromatography. *Journal of Chromatography A*, 985, 503-512.

Fine D.H. (1983). Determination of volatile Nitrosamines in beer and other alcoholic beverages using a cellulose extraction cartridge. In: *Environmental carcinogens selected methods of analysis,* Vol. 6, pp. 462.

Fish R.H., Holmstead R.L., Gaffield, W. (1976) Chemical ionization mass spectrometry of N-nitrosamines. *Tetrahedron*, 32, 2689–2692.

Fong Y., Ding J., Liu S. (1984) Chemical ionization mass spectrometry of nitrosamines. *Talanta*, 31, 619–620.

Frommberger R. (1989) N-nitrosodimethylamine in German beer. *Food and Chemical Toxicology*, 27, 27–30.

Gadbois D.F., Ravesi E.M., Lundstrom R.C., Maney R.S. (1975) N-nitrosodimethylamine in cold-smoked Sablefish. *Journal of Agricultural and Food Chemistry*, 23, 665–668

Gerecke A.C., Sedlak D.L. (2003) Precursors of N-Nitrosodimethylamine in Natural Waters; *Environmental Science and Technology*, 37, 1331-1336.

Goff U., Fine D.H. (1979) Analysis of volatile N-nitrosamines in alcoholic beverages. *Food Cosmetical Toxicology*, 17, 569–573.

Graham, J. (1995) Factors affecting the formation of NDMA formation during drinking water treatment. Proceedings Water Quality Technology Conference New Orleans, LA p 757-772.

Gunnison D, Zappi M.E., Teeter C., Pennington J., Bajpai R. (2000) Attenuation mechanisms of N-nitrosodimethylamine at operating intercept and treat groundwater remediation system, *Journal of Hazardous Materials*, B73, 179-197.

Hotchkiss J.H., Vecchio A.J. (1985). Nitrosamines in fried-out bacon fat and its use as a cooking oil. *Food Technology*, 39, 67–73.

Howard, J.W., Fazio T., Watts J.O. (1970) Extraction and gas chromatographic determination of N-nitrosodimethylamine in smoked fish. *Journal of the Association of Official Analytical Chemists*, 53, 269–274.

Huang D.P., Ho J.H., Webb K.S., Wood B.J., Gough T.A. (1981) Volatile nitrosamines in salt processed fish before and after cooking. *Food and Cosmetics Toxicology*, 19, 167–171.

Izquierdo-Polido M., Barbour J. F., Scanlan R.A. (1996) N-nitrosodimethylamine in Spanish beers. *Food and Chemical Toxicology*. 34, 297-299.

Jobb D.B., Hunsinger R.B., Meresz O., Taguchi V.Y., Proc. Am. Water Works Assoc. Water Qual. Technol. Conf. Denver, CO, USA, 1995;103.

Jurado-Sánchez B., Ballesteros E., Gallego M. (2010) Screening of N-nitrosamines in tap and swimming pool waters using fast gas chromatography. *Journal of Separation Science*, 33, 610-616.

Keefer L.K., Roller P.P. (1973) N-nitrosation by nitrite ion in neutral and basic medium. *Science*, 181, 1245-1247.

Kimoto W. I., Dooley C. J., Carre J., and Fiddler, W. (1980) Role of strong ion exchange resins in nitrosamine formation in water. *Water Research*, 14, 869-876.

Kemper J., Walse S.S., Mitch W.A. (2010) Quaternary Amines As Nitrosamine Precursors: A Role for Consumer Products? *Environmental Science and Technology*, in press.

Kemper J., Westerhoff P., Dotson A., Mitch W.A. (2009) Nitrosamine, Dimethylnitramine, and Chloropicrin Formation during Strong Base Anion-Exchange Treatment. *Environmental Science and Technology*, 43, 466–472.

Klein D., Keshavarz A., Lafont P., Hardy J., Derby G. (1980) Formation of nitrosamines in cheese products. *Annales de la nutrition et de l"alimentation* 34, 1077-1088.

Kubacki S.J., Havery D.C., Fazio T. (1989) Volatile N-nitrosamines in beer. *Food Additives and Contaminants*, 6, 29–34.

Kyriakidis N.B. , Tarantili-Georgiou K. and Tsani-Batzaka E. (1997) Nitrate and Nitrite Content of Greek Cheeses. *Journal of Food Composition and Analysis.* 10, 343–349.

Lee C., Schmidt C., Yoon J., von Gunten U.(2007) Oxidation of N-Nitrosodimethylamine (NDMA) precursors with ozone and chlorine dioxide: Kinetics and effect on NDMA formation potential. *Environmental Science and Technology*, 41, 2056-206.3

Leppanen O., Ronkainen P. (1982) A sensitive method for the determination of nitrosamines in alcoholic beverages. *Chromatographia*, 16, 219–223.

Lijinsky W. N-nitroso compounds in the diet. *Mutation Research* 443, 129–138.

Method 521: Determination of nitrosamines in drinking water by solid phase extraction and capillary column gas chromatography with large volume injection and chemical ionization tandem mass spectrometry (MS/MS), Ver.1.0, *EPA Document # EPA/600/R-05/054.*

Mitacek E. J., Brunnemann K. D., Suttajit M., Martin N., Limsila T., Ohshima H. and Caplan L. S. (1999) Exposure to N-Nitroso Compounds in a Population of High Liver Cancer Regions in Thailand: Volatile Nitrosamine (VNA) Levels in Thai Food. *Food and Chemical Toxicology,* 37, 297-305.

Mitch W.A., Sharp J.O, Trussell R.R., Valentine R.L. Alvarez-Cohen L., Sedlak D.L. (2003) N-nitrosodimethylamine (NDMA) as drinking water contaminant. *Review, Environment Eng. Sci.* 20, 389-404.

Mitch W.A., Sedlak D.L. (2002) Formation of N-nitrosodimethylamine (NDMA) from dimethylamine during chlorination. *Environmental Science and Technology*, 36, 588-595.

Mottram D.S., Patterson R.L., Edwards R.A., Gough T.A. (1977) The preferential formation of volatile N-nitrosamines in the fat of fried bacon. *Journal of the Science of Food and Agriculture*, 28, 1025–1029.

Najm I., Trussell R.R., (2001). NDMA formation in water and wastewater. *Journal of American Water Works Association.* 93, 92–98.

Nelson M. The Barbarian's Beverage: A History of Beer in Ancient Europe. Abingdon, Oxon: Routledge, 2005.

Osterdahl B.G. (1988) Volatile nitrosamines in foods on the Swedish market and estimation of their daily intake. *Food Additives and Contaminants*, 5, 587–595.

Pensabene J.W., Fiddler W., Phillips, J.G. (1990) Gas chromatographic chemiluminescence method for determination of volatile N-nitrosamines in minced fish-meat and surimi-meat frankfurters: collaborative study. *Journal of the Association of Official Analytical Chemists*, 73, 947–952.

Perez D.M., Alatorre G.G., Alvarez E.B., Silva E.E., Alvarado J.F.J. (2008) Solid-phase microextraction of N-nitrosodimethylamine in Beer. *Food Chemistry*, 107, 1348–1352.

Pokrovskii A.A., Kostiukovskii Ya.L., Melamed, D.B., Medvedev, F.A. (1978). Determination of the N-nitrosamine content in meat and meat products. *Voprosy Pitaniya*, 2, 65–72 (in Russian).

Powell D.R., Adams Jr. E.T. (1978) Self-association of gases. 1. Theory. Application to the nitrogen dioxide-dinitrogen tetraoxide system. *Journal of Physical Chemistry*, 82, 1947-1952.

Prest H.P., Hermann R.E. (1999) An approach to the determination of N nitrosodimethylamine at part-per-quadrillion levels using positive chemical ionization and large-volume injection. Hewlett–Packard Company, Application Note 23, 5968-5747E. Available from <www.hp.com/go/chemsupplies>.

Raoul S., Gremaud E., Biaudet H., Tureski R. (1997) Rapid solid-phase extraction method for the detection of volatile nitrosoamines in food. *Journal of Agricultural and Food Chemistry*, 45, 4706–4713.

Richardson S.D. (2003) Disinfection by-products and other emerging contaminants in drinking water. *Trends in Analytical Chemistry*, 22, 666-684.

Rywotycki R. (2007) The effect of baking of various kinds of raw meat from different animal species and meat with functional additives on nitrosamine contamination level. *Food Chemistry*, 101, 540–548.

Scanlan R.A., Barbour J.F., Hotchkiss J.H. (1980) N-nitrosodimethylamine in beer. *Food and Chemical Toxicology*, 18, 27–29.

Schreiber M., Mitch W.A. (2006) Nitrosamine Formation Pathway Revisited: The importance of chloramine speciation and dissolved oxygen. *Environmental Science and Technology*, 40, 6007-6014.

Schreiber M., Mitch W.A. (2007) Enhanced Nitrogenous Disinfection By-Product Formation near the Breakpoint: Implications for Nitrification Control. *Environmental Science and Technology*, 41, 7039-7046.

Sen, N. P., Seaman, S., and McPherson, M. (1980). Nitrosamines In alcoholic beverages. *Journal of Food Safety*, 2, 13–18.

Sen, N. P., Seaman, S. W., Begeson, C., and Brousseau, R. (1996). Trends in the levels of N-nitrosodimethylamine in Canadian and imported beers. *Journal of Agricultural and Food Chemistry*, 44(6), 1498–1501.

Song P.J., Fu J.F. (1988) N-nitrosamines in Chinese foods. *Food and Chemical Toxicology*, 26, 205–208.

Spiegelhalder, B., Eisenbrand, G., and Preussmann, R. (1979). Contamination of beer with trace quantities of N-nitrosodimethylamine. *Food and Cosmetics Toxicology*, 17, 29–31.

Spiegelhalder B., Eisenbrand G., Preussmann R. (1983). Volatile N-nitrosamines in beer and other beverages by direct extraction using a Kieselguhr column. In: *Environmental carcinogens selected methods of analysis*, Vol. 6, pp. 135–142. Lyon: International Agency for Research on Cancer, Sci. Publ.

Stephany R.W., Freudenthal J., Schuller P.L. (1978) *Meat and meat products – mass spectrometric determination of volatile N-nitrosamines*, pp. 151–161. Science Publications 18. International Agency of Research on Cancer.

Tateo F., Roundbehler D.P. (1983) Use of thermal energy analyzer in the analysis of nitrosamines – volatile nitrosamines in samples of Italian beers. *Mitteilungen aus dem Gebiete der Lebensmitteluntersuchung*, 74, 110–120.

Tozawa H., Kawabata T. (1991) Volatile N-nitrosamines in fish meal, with special reference to the mechanism of formation of N-nitrosothiazolidine, *IARC Scientific Publications* (105), 214-218.

Tricker A.R., Preussmann R. (1991a) Carcinogenic N-nitrosamines in the diet: occurrence, formation, mechanisms and carcinogenic potential. *Mutation Research*, 259, 277–289.

Tricker, A.R., Preussmann R. (1991b). Volatile and non-volatile nitrosamines in beer. *Journal of Cancer Research and Clinical Oncology*, 117, 130–132.

USEPA (2010). www.epa.gov/iris/subst/index.html.

Uppu, - Uppu, R.M., Pryor W.A. (1996) Synthesis of peroxynitrite in a two-phase system using isoamyl nitrite and hydrogen peroxide *Analytical Biochemistry* 236 242-249.

Ventanas S., Martín D., Estévez M., Ruiz J. (2006) Analysis of volatile nitrosamines from a model system using SPME–DED at different temperatures and times of extraction, *Food Chemistry*, 99, 842-850.

Walse S.S., Mitch W.A. (2008) Nitrosamine carcinogens also swim in chlorinated pools. *Environmental Science and Technology*, 42, 1032-1037.

Wilczak, A. Assadi-Rad, H.H. Lai, L.L. Hoover, J.F. Smith, R. Berger, F. Rodigari, J.W. Beland, L.J. Lazzelle, E.G. Kinicannon, H. Baker, C.T. Heaney, Formation of NDMA in chloraminated water coagulated with DADMAC cationic polymer, *J. Am. Water Works Assoc.* 95 (2003) 94–106.

Wunsch, K-H. Miethchen R., Ehlers D. *Organische Chemie Grundkurs*, 1979, PWN.

Yang L., Chen Z., Shen J., Xu Z., Liang H., Tian J., Ben Y., Zhai X., Shi W., Li G. (2009) Reinvestigation of the Nitrosamine-Formation Mechanism during Ozonation. *Environmental Science and Technology*, 43, 5481–5487.

Yin F., Ding J.H., Liu S. (1982) N-nitrosodimethylamine in domestic beer in China. *Food Chemical Toxicology*, 20, 213–214.

Yurchenko S., Molder U. (2005) Analytical, Nutritional and Clinical Methods: N-nitrosodimethylamine analysis in Estonian beer using positive-ion chemical ionization with gas chromatography mass spectrometry. *Food Chemistry,* 89, 455–463.

Yurchenko S., Molder U. (2006) Analytical, Nutritional and Clinical Methods: Volatile N-Nitrosamines in various fish products. *Food Chemistry,* 96, 325–333.

Yurchenko S., Molder U. (2007) Analytical, Nutritional and Clinical Methods: The occurrence of volatile N-nitrosamines in Estonian meat products. *Food Chemistry,* 100, 1713-1721.

Zhao Y.–Y., Boyd J. M ., Woodbeck M., Andrews R. C ., Qin F., Hrudey S. E ., Li X.–F. (2008) Formation of N-Nitrosamines from Eleven Disinfection Treatments of Seven Different Surface Waters. *Environmental Science and Technology*, 42, 4857–4862.

Zhukova G.F., Torskaia M.S., Rodin V.I., Khotimchenko S.A. (1999) N-nitrosamines and nitrites in meat and meat products. *Voprosy Pitanija*, 68, 32–34 (in Russian).

Zou X.N., Lu S.H., Liu B. (1994) Volatile N-nitrosamines and their precursors in Chinese salted fish – a possible etiological factor for NPC in China. *International Journal of Cancer*, 59, 155–158.

In: Nutritional Insights and Food Safety
Editor: Jaroslava Švarc-Gajiæ

ISBN: 978-1-61122-130-5

Chapter XI

Toxigenic Fungi and Mycotoxins

***Bulent Kabak*[1] *and Alan D. W. Dobson*[2]**

[1]Hitit University, Faculty of Engineering, Department of Food Engineering, Corum, Turkey

[2]Microbiology Department and Environmental Research Institute, University College Cork, National University of Ireland, Cork, Ireland

Abstract

The contamination of food and feed with mycotoxins is a significant source of food-borne illnesses. Mycotoxins are toxic secondary metabolites produced by certain fungi belonging predominantly to the *Aspergillus*, *Penicillium* and *Fusarium* genera, which can cause a variety of adverse effects to both humans and animals, ranging from allergic responses to death. While *Aspergillus* and *Penicillium* strains are generally found as contaminants in food during drying and storage, *Fusarium* spp. are typically field contaminants and their production of mycotoxins is limited to a few plant products, and is mainly associated with cereal crops. The most important *Aspergillus* mycotoxins, which frequently occur at biologically significant concentrations in various food commodities, are aflatoxins, ochratoxin A (OTA), citrinin, cyclopiazonic acid, penicillic acid and sterigmatocystin. Some of these mycotoxins (OTA, citrinin, cyclopiazonic acid, penicillic acid) can also be produced by *Penicillium* species. Other potent *Penicillium* mycotoxins which have to date been poorly studied include patulin, roquefortine C, rubratoxins and PR toxin. The main mycotoxins produced by *Fusarium* species and which are present in cereal grains include trichothecenes (T-2 toxin, HT-2 toxin, deoxynivalenol, nivalenol), fumonisins, zearalenone and moniliformin. *Fusarium* species are also destructive plant pathogens and are responsible for diseases in crops such as ear rot which can result in significant losses in both crop yield and quality. This paper will focus on an update of our current knowledge on the mycotoxigenic fungi (*Aspergillus*, *Penicillium*, *Fusarium*) which are most commonly found as food contaminants and on the mycotoxins they produce. The review will focus on the toxicity, the sources in foods and the associated human health risks.

Introduction

Toxigenic fungi are ubiquitous in nature, and occur regularly in worldwide food supplies due to mould infestation of susceptible agricultural products, such as cereal grains, nuts and fruits. Depending on the host crop and the fungal species, toxigenic fungi may cause plant diseases, such as *Aspergillus* fruit rot on grapes, blue mould rot of apple caused by *Penicillium expansum*, as well as *Fusarium* head blight (FHB), maize ear rot and seedling diseases (Murphy et al., 2006).

Mycotoxins have become increasingly important worldwide in the context of food safety. They occur in agricultural products mainly as a result of the activity of three genera: *Aspergillus*, *Penicillium* and *Fusarium* (Pitt et al., 2000). Fungi from the genera *Fusarium* are mainly active in the field, while both *Aspergillus* and *Penicillium* species are considered as mostly storage fungi. Up until know, approximately 400 secondary metabolites with toxigenic potential produced by more than 100 moulds, have been reported, with the Food and Agriculture Organisation (FAO) estimating that as much as 25% of the world's agricultural commodities are contaminated with mycotoxins, leading to significant economic losses.

Mycotoxins have been associated with severe toxic effects to vertebrates, from allergic responses to cancer and death, depending on a number of factors including intake levels, duration of exposure, toxin species, mechanisms of action, metabolism and defense mechanisms. The mycotoxins of most significance from both a public health and agronomic perspective include the aflatoxins, ochratoxin A (OTA), trichothecenes, fumonisins and zearalenone (ZEA) (Kabak et al., 2006).

1. Aspergillus Mycotoxins

The fungal genus *Aspergillus* was established in 1729, and represents a large family of fungi that are adapted to a wide range of environmental conditions (Wilson et al., 2002). Although *Aspergillus* species are distributed worldwide, these fungi are more common in the warmer, subtropical and tropical areas in comparison with more temperate environments. They are usually considered to be saprophytes that can grow on a large number of substrates. Their growth at high temperatures and low water activity (a_w) allows their involvement in the colonization of a variety of crops, sometimes with limited parasitism especially under favourable conditions (CAST, 2003). Within this genus, some of the Aspergilli can cause decay and deterioration in stored products and may cause disease in plants and various animals, including humans. Some species of *Aspergillus* including *A. candidus*, *A. clavatus*, *A. flavus*, *A. fumigatus*, *A. niger*, *A. nomius*, A. *ochraceus*, *A. parasiticus*, *A. restricus*, *A. tamarii*, *A. terreus*, *A. versicolor*, *Emericella nidulans* and *Eurotium amstelodami* have the ability to colonize agricultural crops of economic importance and produce highly toxic and carcinogenic mycotoxins (Frisvad & Samson, 1991). The most important groups of mycotoxins produced by *Aspergillus* species are aflatoxins, ochratoxins, citrinin, cyclopiazonic acid (CPA), sterigmatocystin (STC) and penicillic acid. Some of these mycotoxins can also be produced by *Penicillium* species.

1.1. Aflatoxins

Aflatoxins are produced primarily by two species of toxigenic Aspergilli, *A. flavus* and *A. parasiticus*. Since the discovery of aflatoxins, *A. flavus* has become the most widely reported foodborne fungus, reflecting its economic and medical importance and ease of recognition, as well as its universal occurrence. *A. parasiticus* is apparently less widely distributed, but the extent of its occurrence may be obscured by the tendency for both *A. flavus* and *A. parasiticus* to be reported only as *A. flavus*. *A. nomius* is also known to produce this toxin, but it is not of practical importance (Pitt, 2000). While *A. parasiticus* is well adapted to a soil environment, *A. flavus* is more adapted to the aerial parts of plants (leaves, flowers) (EFSA, 2004a).

According to morphological, genetic and physiological criteria, *A. flavus* can be divided into two morphotypes, S strain (sclerotia of < 400 μm in diameter) and L strain (sclerotia of $>$ 400 μm in diameter) (Cotty, 1994). S-strain isolates generally produce much more aflatoxin than L-strain isolates (Cotty, 1994), with many L-strain isolates producing no aflatoxins ("atoxigenic"). All members of *A. flavus* produce only B-aflatoxins most likely as a result of a 0.8-1.5-kb deletion in the aflatoxin gene cluster (Ehrlich et al., 2004), while *A. parasiticus* and *A. nomius*, produce both B-and G-aflatoxins (Ehrlich et al., 2003).

Fungal contamination and subsequently aflatoxin formation can occur in commodities in the field, at harvest, during post-harvest and in storage. The rate and degree of contamination are dependent on temperature, humidity and on soil and storage conditions (Boutrif, 1998). Both *A. flavus* and *A. parasiticus* can grow over a wide range of temperatures (10 to 43°C), with an optimum in the 32-33°C range (ICMSF 1996a), with aflatoxins being produced between 12-40°C (Koehler et al., 1985). Although both species grow over the pH range of just above 2.0 to $\geq$10 at 25°C, aflatoxin production for *A. parasiticus* has been reported at between pH 3.0 and 8.0, with an optimum near pH 6. The optimum a_w for growth is 0.99 with a minimum value of 0.80-0.83. Aflatoxins are produced at a_w values ranging from 0.95 to 0.99, with a minimum a_w value of 0.82 being reported for *A. flavus* (ICMSF, 1996a).

A number of nutritional factors are known to affect both mould growth and aflatoxin biosynthesis, including various carbohydrate and nutritional sources, lipoperoxides, trace metals (Mn, Fe, Zn, K, Cu, Mg, Mo) and phosphates in the growth medium (Luchese & Harrigan, 1993). How these different factors act to regulate aflatoxin biosynthesis is still as yet poor understood. Many of the effects may in fact however be exerted indirectly through interference with primary metabolism (Sweeney & Dobson, 1998).

Aflatoxins are extensively documented as a global contaminants of a wide variety of commodities including cottonseed, peanuts, tree nuts (pistachios, almonds, pecans, walnuts, brazil nuts), spices, dried fruits (figs, raisins) and a range of cereals (especially maize) (EFSA, 2004a). Even though contamination is generally considered to be a problem in tropical and subtropical regions of Africa, Asia and Latin America; aflatoxins have also been reported in temperate countries of Europe and North America (Boutrif, 1998).

These mycotoxins occur in several chemical forms; with approximately 19 different toxic derivatives of aflatoxins have been reported. The four main naturally produced aflatoxins are known as B_1, B_2, G_1 and G_2 (Figure 1). "B" and "G" refer to the blue and green fluorescent colours produced by these compounds under UV light on thin-layer chromatography plates, while the subscript numbers 1 and 2 indicate major and minor compounds respectively. Following ingestion, AFB_1 is metabolized in the liver through the cytochrome P450 enzyme system to various metabolites, including the endo- and exo-epoxides of AFB_1, the hydroxyl-metabolites AFM_1, AFM_2 and AFM_4, and aflatoxins P_1 and Q_1, as well as conjugated metabolites (McLean & Dutton, 1995). The carcinogenicity of AFB_1 arises from its interaction with the DNA-guanine moiety to produce to the aflatoxin-N7-guanine adduct, whereas the acute toxicity of AFB_1 is believed to stem from interaction between the dihydrodiol and protein amino groups to produce Schiff base adducts (Pitt et al., 2000).

AFM_1, the 4-hydroxy metabolite of AFB_1, is the predominant metabolite of AFB_1 in milk. When lactating animals such as cows, goats and humans are fed with feedstuffs contaminated with AFB_1, this metabolite can be transferred to milk as AFM_1 in the range of 0.3-6.3% (Choudhary et al., 1998). In addition to AFM_1 other aflatoxin metabolites are excreted with milk, including AFM_2 (the analogous metabolite of AFB_2) and AFM_4, another hydroxyl metabolite of AFB_1. Both AFM_2 and M_4, occur in milk at much lower concentrations compared to AFM_1 and thus are considered less significant from a public health perspective (EFSA, 2004a).

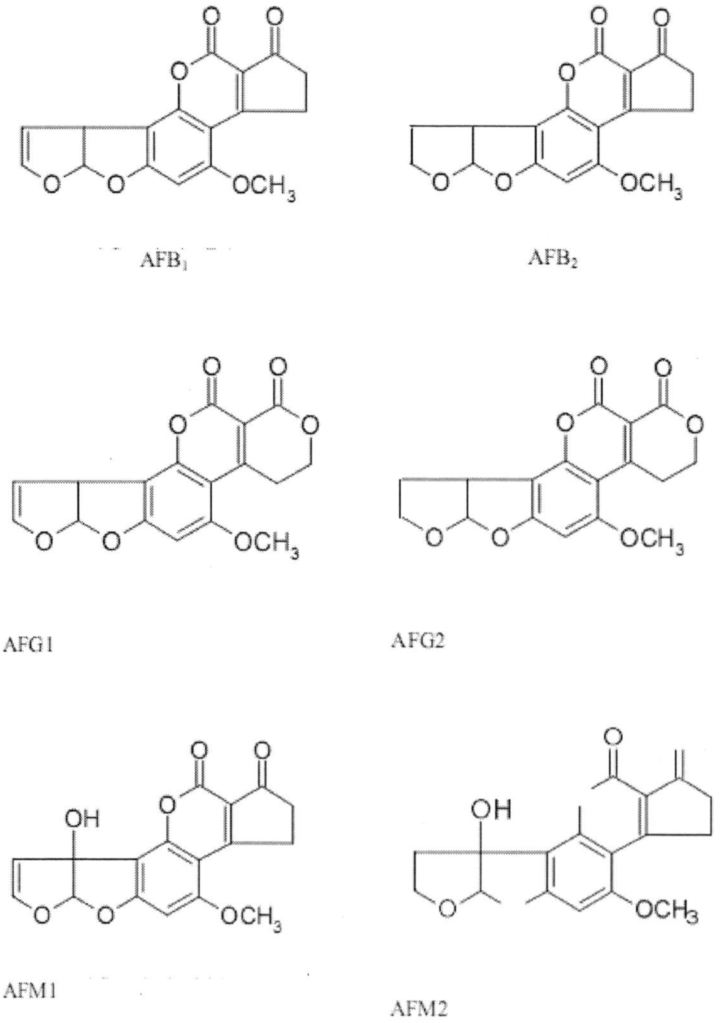

Figure 1. Structure of aflatoxins.

Aflatoxins are also both acutely and chronically toxic to various animal species, including humans, causing acute liver damage, liver cirrhosis, tumour induction and teratogenesis (Pitt, 2000). The aflatoxins were first discovered in 1959/1960 as a result of deaths of thousands of turkeys in the UK and this was referred to as "turkey x disease". Further investigation revealed that these outbreaks were associated with groundnut meal infected with *A. flavus* which was contaminated by a compound which fluoresced blue, under ultraviolet light (Moss, 2002). Since then aflatoxins have been the focus of intensive research all over the world.

Exposure to aflatoxins at high levels can lead to acute human aflatoxicosis leading to jaundice, edema, gastrointerstinal hemorrhage, and ultimately, death (Shephard, 2008a). There have been a number of reported outbreaks of acute toxicity resulting from aflatoxin ingestion in humans. One of the most serious outbreak of aflatoxicosis occurred in the region of western India in 1974, leading to 397 recognized cases and 106 deaths. The outbreak was traced to the consumption of maize heavily contaminated with aflatoxin ranged between 6.25 and 15.6 mg kg^{-1}. Daily consumption of toxin by some of the patients was calculated to be 2-6 mg of aflatoxin for several weeks (Krisnamachari et al., 1975). Other documented fatal human aflatoxicosis outbreaks have been reported in Kenya in 1981: 20 cases and 12 reported deaths (Ngindu et al., 1982); Malaysia in 1988: 13 deaths (Lye et al., 1995); and Ngieria in 2004: more than 100 deaths (Afla-guard, 2005). One of the largest outbreak of aflatoxicosis happened in the eastern and central districts of Kenya in 2004 where 317 people were ill and 215 died, following the consumption of contaminated maize (up to 8 mg kg^{-1} aflatoxin) (CDC (Center for Disease Control and Prevention, 2004). More recently, a similar outbreak in the eastern districts of Kenya during 2005 resulted in 75 cases, with 32 deaths (Shephard, 2008b).

Two human diseases, namely Kwashiorkor and Reye's syndrome may be associated with the ingestion of aflatoxin-contaminated food. Kwashiorkor, a disease of children in Northern Africa, is usually attributed to nutritional deficiencies, but may also be related to aflatoxin intake (Hendrickse et al., 1982). Similarly, Reye's syndrome, which is characterized by acute encephalopathy and fatty degeneration of the viscera has been linked to aflatoxin ingestion with the mycotoxin being detected in the organs of affected children in Thailand, Australia and New Zealand (Becroft & Webster, 1972).

Apart from these effects aflatoxins have been directly linked to hepatacellular carcinoma, impaired growth and to immune suppression. Epidemiological studies have shown a good correlation between aflatoxin intake and human liver cancer in African countries and in Thailand (Pitt, 2000). It is also clear that hepatitis B virus infection and aflatoxin ingestion interact synergistically in the epidemiology of human liver cancer (Moss, 2002). Earlier studies in the United States reported contradictory results, with studies involving individuals that had been exposed to appreciable levels of aflatoxin; indicating that aflatoxins were unlikely to contribute significantly to the incidence of liver cancer in the US (Stoloff, 1983). In 1999, however, the International Agency for Research on Cancer (IARC) evaluated aflatoxins as follows: "There is sufficient evidence in humans for the carcinogenicity of AFB_1 and naturally occurring mixtures of aflatoxins (Group 1)" and "AFM_1 is possible carcinogenic to humans (Group 2B), based on inadequate evidence for carcinogenicity in humans and sufficient evidence in animals" (IARC, 1993).

The maximum permissible level of aflatoxins in food materials has been regulated in many countries. The legal limits vary from one country to another, depending on the degree of economic and social development. The guidance levels for aflatoxins in human foods proposed by the European Union are shown in Table 1.

Table 1. European Union regulations for aflatoxins (European Commission, 2006)

Foodstuffs	Maximum levels ($\mu g\ kg^{-1}$)		
	AFB_1	Sum of AFs B_1, B_2, G_1 and G_2	AFM_1
Groundnuts to be subjected to sorting, or other physical treatment, before human consumption or use as ingredient in foodstuffs	8.0	15.0	-
Nuts to be subjected to sorting, or other physical treatment, before human consumption or use as an ingredient in foodstuffs	5.0	10.0	-
Groundnuts and nuts and processed products thereof, intended for direct human consumption or use as an ingredient in foodstuffs	2.0	4.0	-
Dried fruit to be subjected to sorting, or other physical treatment, before human consumption or use as an ingredient in foodstuffs	5.0	10.0	-
Dried fruit and processed products thereof, intended for direct human consumption or as an ingredient in foodstuffs	2.0	4.0	-
All cereals and all products derived from cereals, including processed cereal products	2.0	4.0	-
Maize to be subjected to sorting or other physical treatment before human consumption or use as an ingredient in foodstuffs	5.0	10.0	-
Species, including chillies, chilli powder, cayenne, paprika, white and black pepper, nutmeg, ginger and turmeric	5.0	10.0	-
Raw milk, heat-treated milk and milk for the manufacture of milk-based products	-	-	0.050
Processed cereal-based foods and baby foods for infants and young children	0.10	-	-
Infant formulae and follow-on formulae, including infant milk and follow-on milk	-	-	0.025
Dietary foods for special medical purposes intended specially for infants	0.10	-	0.025

1.2. Ochratoxins

Ochratoxin A (OTA) is the major mycotoxin in this group and it has received increasing recent interest within the scientific community, because of the hazard it poses to human health. OTA is a chlorinated isocoumarin derivative linked through an amine bond to L-beta-phenylalanine and is classified as a pentaketide (Figure 2) (Walker, 1999).

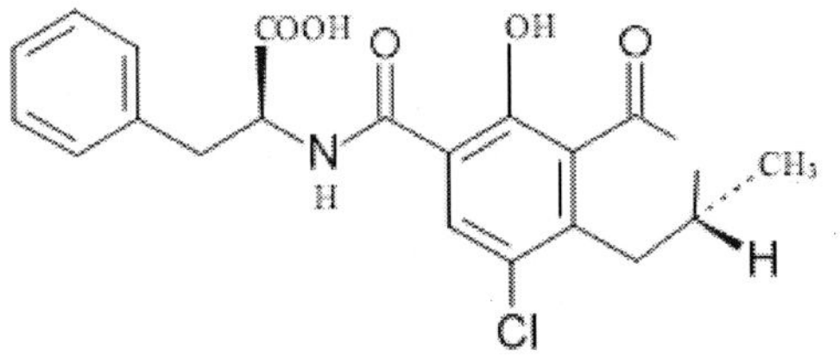

Figure 2. Structure of ochratoxin A.

It is produced by a single *Penicillium* species, *P. verrucosum*, by several *Aspergillus* species, *A. ochraceus* and Aspergilli of the section *Nigri*, especially *A. carbonarius* (EFSA, 2006). These three groups of species differ not only in their ecological niches, but also in the commodities affected and in the frequency of occurrence in different geographical regions. While *P. verrucosum* is the main producer in cereals and cereal products of OTA in cooler regions of Northern Europe (Olsen et al., 2003) and Canada (JECFA, 2001), *A. ochraceus* grows at moderate temperatures and can infect a wide range of stored commodities including coffee beans, cocoa, cereals and edible nuts (EFSA, 2006). However, there is little evidence of serious contamination of cereals by *A. ochraceus* and closely related species. *A. carbonarius* grows at high temperatures and is associated with maturing fruits, especially grapes. Because of its black spores, it is highly resistant to sunlight, and survives sun-drying. It is the source of OTA in grapes, wine and vine fruits (JECFA (Joint FAO/WHO Expert Committee on Food Additives, 2001). This species is now considered to be a major source of OTA in tropical and subtropical foods (Pitt et al., 2000).

The minimum moisture content for growth of *P. verrucosum* in cereals is 16-17%, with OTA being produced at approximately 1% higher (Codex Alimentarius Commission, 2002). *P. verrucosum* grows from 0 to 31°C, with an optimum at 20°C (ICMSF, 1996b). It is a xerophile, capable of growth at an a_w of 0.80 (Pitt & Hocking, 1997). OTA can be produced by this species over the entire temperature range, but not below an a_w of 0.86 (ICMSF, 1996b).

There is less information on OTA production by *Aspergillus* species in warmer climates, e.g., whether the infection and toxin production starts in the field on the growing plant (Codex Alimentarius Commission, 2002). *A. ochraceus* is a mesophile capable of growing at temperature between 8 and 37°C, with the optimum at 24-31°C. Its growth has been described at a minimum a_w level of 0.77-0.80, but toxin production does not occur below about 0.83 a_w (ICMSF, 1996a). *A. carbonarius* grows between 10-40°C, but little is known about factors affecting toxin production (Pitt et al., 2000).

Invasion with toxigenic species of *Aspergillus* and *Penicillium* has been reported throughout the world and subsequently OTA can be found as a natural contaminant in cereals (wheat, maize, oat, millet, rye, barley and rice), pulses, wine, grape juice, beer, coffee beans, cocoa, dried wine fruits as well as spices and nuts. Large differences in OTA levels have been reported, ranging from 0.066 to 8.8 ng g^{-1} in cereals, 0.001 to 2.34 ng ml^{-1} in beer (Kabak, 2009) and from 0.002 to 7.63 ng ml^{-1} in wine (Var & Kabak, 2007). In the European diet, cereals such as barley, wheat, maize, oats and their by-products are considered the major source of OTA intake, corresponding to 50%, followed by wine (approximately 13%), coffee (aprox. 12%) and spices (aprox. 8%), others (6%) beer (5%), cocoa (4%), dried fruits (3%) and meat (1%). As for the contribution from the wide category of 'others', fruit juice provide the most relevant contributors (European Commission, 2002b). OTA has been also detected in human blood, breast milk and animal derived products such as pork products (European Commission, 2002a). Levels reported range from 0.1 to 10 ng ml^{-1} (with an exceptional maximum of 160 ng ml^{-1}) in human blood in a wide range of European countries (European Commission, 2002b).

OTA is a well-known nephrotoxic agent and has been associated with fatal human kidney disease, referred to as Balkan Endemic Nephropathy (BEN) and with an increased incidence of tumours of the upper urinary effect (JECFA, 2001). The toxin has also been reported to have a number of toxic effects when tested in various experimental animals including: carcinogenic, teratogenic, immunotoxic, genotoxic and possibly neurotoxic effects (European Commission, 2002a). The toxin was evaluated by The Scientific Committee on Food, who proposed that exposure should be limited to below 5 ng kg^{-1} b.w. day^{-1} (SCF, 1998). In 2001, The Joint FAO/WHO Expert Committee on Food Additives (JECFA) set a provisional tolerable weekly intake (PTWI) of 100 ng kg^{-1} body weight (b.w.), corresponding to approximately 14 ng kg^{-1} b.w. per day (JECFA, 2001). However, the Panel on Contaminants in the Food Chain (CONTAM) of The European Food Safety Authority (EFSA) recently derived a tolerable weekly intake (TWI) of 120 ng kg^{-1} b.w. for OTA. Recent analyses of the dietary exposure of adult European consumers to OTA revealed that at present the weekly exposure ranges from 15 to 60 ng OTA per kg b.w. per week, including high consumers of foods containing OTA. This rate of exposure is below the TWI value of 120 ng kg^{-1} b.w. as derived by the Panel (EFSA, 2006). OTA was also classified by the IARC as a group 2B (possible human carcinogen) agent in 1993, based on sufficient evidence for carcinogenicity in animal studies and inadequate evidence in humans (IARC, 1993). The European Union has also set maximum levels for the presence of this mycotoxin in foodstuffs (Table 2).

Table 2. European Union regulations for OTA (European Commission, 2006)

Foodstuffs	Maximum levels ($\mu g\ kg^{-1}$)
Unprocessed cereals	5.0
All products derived from unprocessed cereals, including processed cereal products and cereal intended for direct human consumption	3.0
Dried vine fruits (currants, raisins and sultanas)	10.0
Roasted coffee beans and ground roasted coffee, excluding soluble coffee	5.0
Soluble coffee (instant coffee)	10.0
Wine (including sparkling wine, excluding liqueur wine and wine with an alcoholic strength of not less than 15% vol)	2.0
Aromatised wine, aromatised wine-based drinks and aromatised wine-product cocktails	2.0
Grape juice, concentrated grape juice as reconstituted, grape nectar, grape must and concentrated grape must as reconstituted, intended for direct human consumption	2.0
Processed cereal-based foods and baby foods for infants and young children	0.50
Dietary foods for special medical purposes intended specifically for infants	0.50

1.3. Cyclopiazonic Acid

Cyclopiazonic acid, a toxic indole tetramic acid, was firstly isolated from *Penicillium cyclopium* Westling (Holzapfel, 1968). Subsequently, it has been discovered to be produced by several *Penicillium* species, including *P. commune* and *P. camamberti* (Pitt et al., 1986), as well as by various Aspergilli such as *A. flavus* (Luk et al., 1977), *A. versicolor* (Ohmono et al., 1973) and *A. tamarii* (Dorner, 1983). The discovery that *A. flavus* isolates are capable of producing CPA has caused increased concern over the potentially harmful effects of this toxin (Norred et al., 1988). This compound can be found as a natural contaminant in feeds (Balachandran & Parthasarathy, 1996; Martins & Martins, 1999; Oliveira et al., 2008), maize (Hayashi & Yoshizawa, 2005; Lee & Hagler, 1991; Urano et al., 1992; Widiastuti et al., 1988), peanuts (Lansden & Davidson, 1983; Mphande et al., 2004; Pinto et al., 2001; Urano et al., 1992) and other foods. CPA has also been detected in edible tissues in poultry, and in milk, cheese and eggs (Chang et al., 2009). The co-occurrence of CPA with aflatoxins has been reported in peanuts (Mphande et al., 2004; Pinto et al., 2001) and maize (Urano et al., 1992).

CPA is an optically active colourless crystalline with the empirical formula $C_{20}H_{20}N_2O_3$ and a molecular weight of 33.39 (Figure 3). It has a melting point of 245°C (EMANa).

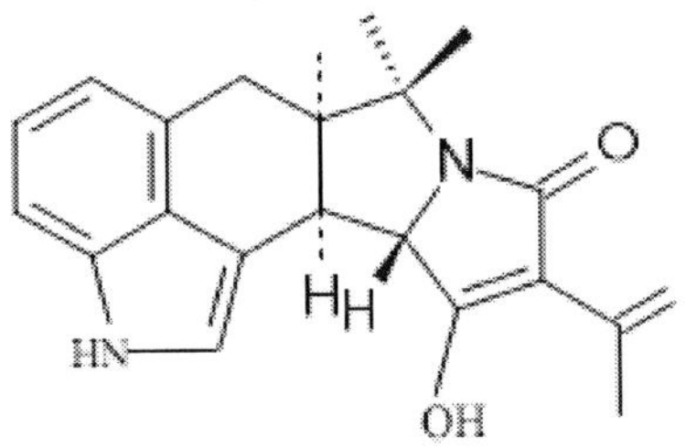

Figure 3. Structure of cyclopiazonic acid.

CPA is a specific inhibitor of calcium-dependent ATPase in the sarcoplasmic reticulum, where by altering Ca^{2+} levels, it results in increased muscle contraction (Rileyet al., 1992). It has been shown that high concentrations of CPA result in toxicity in various animals including rats, chicken, mice, rabbits, pigs and dogs (Burdock & Flamm, 2000). In rats, where CPA has an oral LD_{50} value of 36 mg kg^{-1} in males and 63 mg kg^{-1} in females, it has been reported to produce degenerative changes and necrosis in the liver, spleen, exocrine and endocrine pancreas, kidney, salivary glands, myocardium, and skeletal muscle. Intraperitoneal injection of CPA in male rats produced a 50% lethal dose of 2.3 mg kg^{-1}, causing lesions of the liver, kidney, pancreas, spleen and heart (Purchase, 1971). Surprisingly, among the large mammals, pigs appear to be quite sensitive to CPA with a no-observed-adverse-effect-level (NOAEL) of approximately 1 mg kg^{-1} (Lomax et al., 1984). As previously mentioned CPA can also co-occur with other mycotoxins, especially aflatoxins; and this may lead to a higher risk of adverse health effects than the intake of CPA alone. For instance, it has been reported that CPA at 50 mg kg^{-1} interacted synergistically with aflatoxin at 3.5 mg kg^{-1} in feed and adversely affected the growth of treated birds (Smith et al., 1992). CPA is also suspected to cause symptoms of "kodua poisoning" in humans, a non-lethal illness characterized by fatigue, tremors, slurring of speech and nausea after consumption of mouldy millet seeds in some parts of India (Rao & Husain, 1985).

1.4. Sterigmatocystin

Sterigmatocystin (STC) is a toxic metabolite structurally and biologically closely related to aflatoxins, and consists of a xanthone nucleus attached to a bifuran structure (Figure 4). STC crystallises from aqueous acetone solution in the form of pale yellow needles and is readily soluble in methanol, ethanol, acetonitrile, benzene and chloroform. It reacts with hot ethanolic KOH and is methylated by methyl sulphate and methyl iodide. Methanol or ethanol in acid produces dihydroethoxysterigmatocystin. Its melting point is 246°C, with an empirical formula of $C_{18}H_{12}O_6$, and a molecular weight of 324.3. The maximum absorptions in UV visible spectrum of STC in benzene were located at 245 and 325 nm (Veršilovskis & De Saeger, 2010).

Sterigmatocystin is produced by many *Aspergillus* species, primarily *A. versicolor* and *A. nidulans*. Other fungi including *Bipolaris* spp., *Chaetomium* spp., and *Emiricella* spp. are also known to produce this mycotoxin (Veršilovskis & De Saeger, 2010). *A. versicolor*, the main STC producer, is a xerophile which has been reported to grow at an a_w of 0.76 (ICMSF, 1996a). STC have been found (although quite infrequently) in cereals (Scott et al., 1972; Veršilovskis et al., 2008a), including wheat, buckwheat, maize, barley, oat, rye, as well as in bread (Veršilovskis & Mikelsone, 2008), beer (Veršilovskis et al., 2008b), spices (El-Kady et al., 1995) and cheese (El-Sayed et al., 1996; Northolt et al., 1980; Veršilovskis et al., 2009).

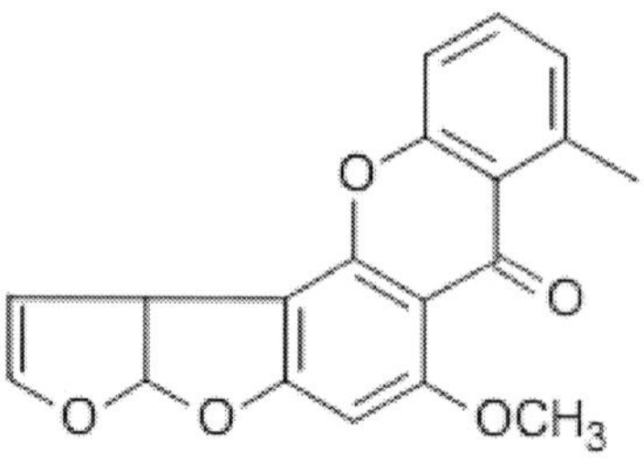

Figure 4. Structure of sterigmatocystin.

The acute toxicity, carcinogenicity, mutagenicity and cytotoxicity of STC have been reviewed extensively by Terao (1983). STC is an intermediate in the biosynthesis of aflatoxins, however, its acute and chronic toxicity is considerable lower than that of AFB_1. STC is associated with acute clinical symptoms of bloody diarrhea, with subsequent loss of milk production and death in some cases in dairy cattle fed with feed containing *A. versicolor* and high levels of STC (7.75 mg kg^{-1}) (Vesonder & Horn, 1985). The oral LD_{50} of STC in mice exceeds 800 mg kg^{-1}. The 10-day oral LD_{50} in Wistar rats is 166 mg kg^{-1} in males, 120 mg kg^{-1} in females, and 60 to 65 mg kg^{-1} for intraperitoneal administration in males. The intraperitoneal 10-day LD_{50} of STC for vervet monkeys is 32 mg kg^{-1}. It has been reported that STC is 125 times less toxic than AFB_1 when tested in ducks (Lillehoj & Ciegler, 1968).

Chronic symptoms of STC include induction of hepatocellular carcinomas in rats, pulmonary tumors in mice, renal lesions and alterations in the liver and kidneys of African green monkeys. It has been suggested that STC is about one tenth as potent carcinogen as AFB_1. STC has been shown to have genotoxic and toxicopathological effects in the fish *Oreochromis niloticus* where the effects on the tissues were manifested by different histopathological lesions in different organs including hyperplastic proliferation of branchial epithelium, necrobiotic changes in hepatic tissue and destruction of components of the spleen (Mahrous et al., 2006).

STC has been shown to be mutagenic in the *Salmonella typhimurium* test, the *Rec* assay, and the *Bacillus subtilis* assay (Wang & Groopman, 1999). It is obvious that the mutagenicities of AFB_1 and STC are far more potent than the other mycotoxins which contain the 2, 3 double bond in the bisdihydrofuran ring (Terao, 1983). The mechanism of STC mutagenicity is linked to its covalent binding to DNA after metabolic activation and its conversion to STC-N^7-Guanine adduct after hydrolysis (Essigmann et al., 1979). A cytotoxic effect of STC has been demonstrated in vervet monkeys, where like other myctoxins that contain an unsaturated 2, 3 bond in the bisdihydrofuran ring; it markedly affected nucleoli, inhibitory incorporation of ^{3}H-thymidine and ^{3}H-uridine and reduction in mitosis (Englebrecht & Altenkirk, 1972).

2. Penicillium Mycotoxins

Penicillium is a large genus, with 150 recognized species of which 50 or more are of common occurrence (Pitt, 1997). Like Aspergilli, *Penicillium* species are most commonly storage contaminants than field contaminants. While *Aspergillus* species are more common in warm climates, *Penicillium* and *Fusarium* species are more commonly found in cooler climates. Some *Penicillium* species are among the most common and destructive agents of postharvest diseases, affecting most kinds of fruits and vegetables. Several species also cause decay of grains and legumes during harvest, storage or transit. In addition to the losses caused by the rotting of fruits and vegetables, as well as by the deterioration of grains and legumes, some Penicillia are known to produce several mycotoxins (Logrieco et al., 2003), with almost 100 *Penicillium* species being reported as toxin producers. The major mycotoxins produced by *Penicillium* species include ochratoxins, patulin, citrinin, penicillic acid and CPA. Other mycotoxins include citreoviridin, penitrem A, PR toxin, roquefortine C among others.

2.1. Patulin

Patulin (4-hydroxy-4H-furo[3, 2c]pyran-2(6H)-one), a water-soluble lactone (Figure 5); was first isolated as an antibiotic during the 1940s from *P. patulum* (*P. urticae*, *P. griseofulvum*). Patulin ($C_7H_6O_4$) is a colourless, crystalline compound with a molecular weight of 154 daltons and a melting point of 111°C. It is soluble in water and polar organic solvents such as ethanol, acetone, ethyl acetate, ethyl ether and chloroform but insoluble in benzene and petroleum ether (Trucksess & Tang, 1999). Patulin is generally stable in acidic solutions at pH 2 or below. It is, however, unstable in alkali and is slowly decomposed in distilled water and methanol at ambient temperatures (Deshpande, 2002).

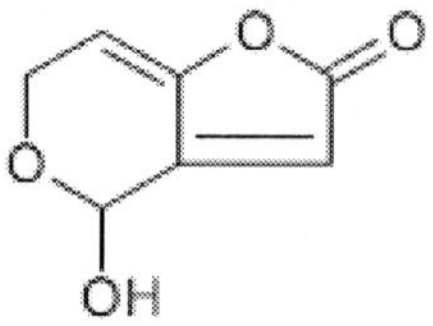

Figure 5. Structure of patulin.

Early studies showed that patulin inhibited more than 75 bacterial species including gram-positive and gram-negative bacteria. Later, clinical trials undertaken during the 1940s revealed that patulin was useful in the treatment of dermatomycosis (Ciegler et al., 1971; Moake et al., 2005). However, during the 1950s and 1960s, it became apparent that, in addition to its antibacterial, antiviral and antiprotozoal activity, patulin was toxic to both plants and animals, precluding its clinical use as an antibiotic. During the 1960s, patulin was subsequently reclassified as a mycotoxin (Bennet & Klich, 2003).

Patulin is produced by certain species of *Penicillium*, including *P. expansum* (*P. leucopus*), *P. patulum*, *P. claviforme*; by some Aspergilli (*A. clavatus*, *A. terreus*) and by *Byssochlamys fulva* and *B. nivea* (Jay, 1992). Among these *P. expansum*, commonly known as the blue mould which causes soft rot of apples, pears, cherries and other fruits, is the major producer of patulin in nature. *P. expansum* is a psychrophile which grows quite strongly at 0°C, but which can also grow at -2°C to -3°C. The optimal temperature for the growth of this mould is 25°C, and a maximum of 35°C. It has a minimum a_w of 0.82-0.83 for germination (Sweeney & Dobson, 1998), and a minimum a_w of 0.94 for patulin biosynthesis (Northolt & Bullerman, 1982). It has been reported that the minimum a_w for patulin production by *P. patulum* is 0.95 (Northolt et al., 1978). Similarly, the minimum a_w values for patulin production by *B. nivea* in apple juice are 0.978, 0.968, and 0.959 at 21°C, 30°C and 37°C, respectively (Roland & Beuchat, 1984).

Patulin has been found as a contaminant in many moldy fruits, vegetables, as well as cereals and other foods and feeds, however, the major sources of contamination are apples and apple based products (Table 3).

Patulin has been claimed to have a number of acute, chronic and toxic effects on health at a cellular level. These acute toxic effects include agitation, convulsions, edema, ulceration, hyperemia, epithelial cell degeneration, nausea, intestinal inflammation, vomiting and other gastrointestinal and kidney damage (Moake et al., 2005). The LD_{50} of patulin in various test animals by oral, subcutaneous, intraperitoneal and intravenous have been reported as 25 to 46, 10 to 33, 5 to 15 and 15 to 25 mg kg^{-1} b.w., respectively (McKinley & Carlton, 1991). Cellular level effects of patulin include inhibition of protein synthesis (Arafat & Musa, 1995), plasma membrane disruption (Mahfoud et al., 2002), disruption of transcripton and translation (Arafat et al., 1985) and inhibition of DNA synthesis (Cooray et al., 1982).

Patulin has been shown to be immunotoxic, neurotoxic and teratogenic in experimental animals, however there is no clear evidence that patulin is carcinogenic. JECFA established a provisional maximum tolerable daily intake (PMTDI) for patulin of 0.4 μg kg^{-1} b.w. day^{-1}, based on NOAEL of 43 mg kg^{-1} b.w. day^{-1} in long-term toxicological studies and the use of a 100-fold safety factor (WHO, 1995). The Scientific Commission of the European Community have regulated a maximum allowable level of 50 μg kg^{-1} for fruit juices, reconstituted concentrated fruit juices, fruit nectars, spirit drinks, cider and other fermented drinks derived from apples or containing juices; 25 μg kg^{-1} for solid apple products, including apple compote, apple puree intended for direct human consumption; and 10 μg kg^{-1} for apple juice and solid apple products, including apple compote and apple puree, for infants and young children, and baby foods other than processed cereal-based foods for infants and young children (European Commission, 2006).

Table 3. Worldwide occurrence of patulin in apple and fruit products

Natural source	Country	n	Positive (%)	Range (μg L^{-1})	Method	Reference
Fruit juices	UK	38	10 (26)	5-56	HPLC	(Mortimer et al., 1985)
Apple cider	USA	5	5 (100)	244-3990	TLC	(Wheeler et al., 1987)
Fruit products	Australia	328	72 (22)	51-1130	HPLC	(Burda, 1992)
Apple juice	Spain	18	15 (83)	2-34	HPLC	(Rovira et al., 1993)
Apple juice	Spain	100	82 (82)	0.5-170	HPLC	(Prieta et al., 1994)
Apple	Spain	12	-	-	HPLC	(Prieta et al., 1994)
Apple juice	Turkey	21	20 (95)	<20 - >50	HPLC	(Gökmen & Acar, 1996)
Apple juice	Brazil	73	15 (21)	6.4-77	HPLC	(Machinski & Midio, 1996)
Apple juice	Turkey	215	215 (100)	7-376	HPLC	(Gökmen & Acar, 1996)
Fruits/fruit juices	Brazil	111	1 (1)	17	HPLC	(De Sylos et al., 1999)
Apple juices	UK	300	58 (19)	>15-171	HPLC	(Ministry of Agriculture, Fisheries and Foods, 1999)
Apple products	South Africa	60	16 (27)	5-45	HPLC	(Leggott & Shephard, 2001)
Fruit products	Sweden	100	5 (5)	2-50	HPLC	(Thuvand et al., 2001)
Apple juice	Turkey	45	27 (60)	19-733	HPLC	(Saito et al., 1971)
Apple products	Italy	40	11 (28)	6-74	HPLC	(Ritieni et al., 2003)
Apple juice	Belgium	43	27 (62)	2.5-39	HPLC	(Tangni et al., 2003)
Apple cider	Belgium	7	2 (29)	2.8-6.1	HPLC	(Tangni et al., 2003)
Apple juice	Japan	76	15 (20)	1.4-45.6	LC-MS	(Ito et al., 2004)
Apple juice/concentrate	Iran	65	47 (72)	>15-285	TLC	(Cheragh et al., 2005)
Apple products	The Netherlands	63	1 (2)	25<	HPLC	(Boonzaaijer et al., 2005)
Fruit products	Italy	100	26 (26)	>0.5-53	HPLC	(Piemont et al., 2005)
Organic fruit products	Italy	69	31 (45)	>0.5-69	HPLC	(Piemont et al., 2005)
Apple-based products	Spain	53	14 (26)	1.5-51	HPLC	(González-Osnaya et al., 2007)
Apple-based drinks	Brazil	134	4 (3)	3-7	HPLC	(Iha &, Sabino, 2008)
Apple juice	Iran	58	54 (93)	10.5-121	HPLC	(Karimi et al., 2008)
Apple juice	Turkey	23	23 (100)	2.6-36.8	HPLC	(Moukas et al., 2008)
Apple juice	China	14	14 (100)	3.8-16.2	HPLC	(Moukas et al., 2008)
Apple juice	Greece	29	29 (100)	0.9-11.8	HPLC	(Moukas et al., 2008)
Apple juice	India	50	12 (24)	21-1839	HPLC	(Saxena et al., 2008)
Apricot juices	Italy	27	7 (26)	>1.7-32.4	HPLC	(Spadaro et al., 2008)
Pear juices	Italy	39	25 (64)	>1.7-33.4	HPLC	(Spadaro et al., 2008)
Peach juices	Italy	30	2 (7)	>1.7-5	HPLC	(Spadaro et al., 2008)
Mixed juices	Italy	29	9 (26)	>1.7-25.4	HPLC	(Spadaro et al., 2008)
Apple juice	Spain	100	66 (66)	0.7-119	MEKC	(Murillo-Arbizu et al., 2009)
Apple juice	Iran	150	150 (100)	6-106	HPLC	(Jalali et al., 2010)

HPLC: High performance liquid chromatography.
TLC: Thin layer chromatography.
LC-MS: Liquid chromatography-Mass spectrometry.
MEKC: Micellar electrokinetic chromatography.

2.2. Citrinin

Citrinin was first isolated as an experimental antibiotic from a culture of *P. citrinum* in 1931 (Hetherington & Raistrick, 1931) and was later associated with "yellow rice toxicosis" in Japan (Saito et al., 1971). It can also be produced by many species of *Penicillium* and several species of *Aspergillus*. Other citrinin-producing Penicillia include *P. expansum*, *P. viridicatum*, *P. fellutanum*, *P. lividum*, *P. implicatum*, *P. jeneni*, *P. citreoviride*, *P. steckni*, *P. velutinum*, *P. canescens*, *P. notatum*, *P. palitans*, and *P. caliviforme* (Deshpande, 2002). Among these, *P. citrinum*, *P. viridicatum* and *P. expansum* are known as postharvest pathogens of fruits and vegetables (Barkai-Golan, 2008). The Aspergilli which have been reported to this mycotoxin include *A. terreus*, *A. carneus* and *A. niveus*. More recently, citrinin has been isolated from fermentation cultures of *Monascus ruber* and *M. purpureus*, industrial species of fungi used to produce red pigments (Blanc et al., 1995; Liu et al., 2005a).

Citrinin has been found as a contaminant in feeds (Abdelhamid, 1990; Kononenko & Burkin, 2008; Scudamore et al., 1997) and cereal grains (Nguyen et al., 2007; Scott et al., 1972; Vrabcheva et al., 2000), including rice, wheat, oats, rye, maize, barley, and breakfast cereals (Molinié et al., 2005) and fruits (Aziz et al., 2002). It has also been detected in naturally fermented sausages from Italy (Anderson, 1995), *Monascus* fermentation products (Li et al., 2005) and traditional fermented maize products (Kpodo et al., 1996). Citrin has also been found together with OTA in cereals (Meister, 2003; Vrabcheva et al., 2000), as well as with patulin in fruits (Martins et al., 2002). Moreover, Bailly et al. (2002) showed that *P. citrinum* can produce citrinin at levels of up to 600 mg kg^{-1} in goat's cheeses.

Citrinin, (3R-*trans*)-4,6-dihydro-8-hydroxy-3,4,5-trimethyl-6-oxo-3H-2-benzo-pyran-7-carboxylic acid (Figure 6), crystallizes as lemon coloured needles, melting at 172°C. This compound is sparingly soluble in water but soluble in dilute sodium hydroxide, sodium carbonate or sodium acetate, in methanol, acetonitrile, ethanol, and in most other organic solvents (Deshpande, 2002).

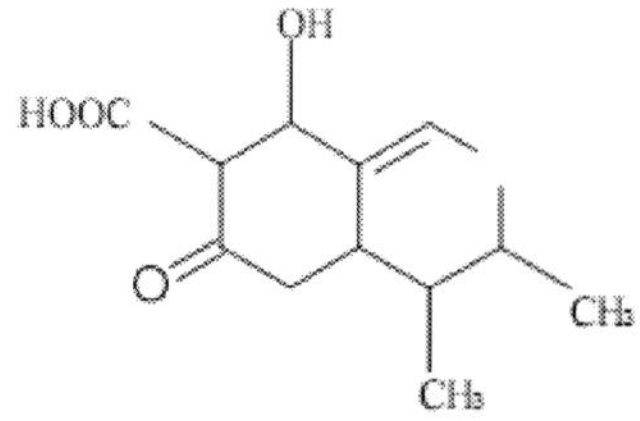

Figure 6. Structure of citrinin.

Like OTA, citrinin is a potent nephrotoxin in livestock, mice, rats, rabbits, dogs, pigs and poultry causing swelling and eventual necrosis of the kidneys and also affecting liver function to a lesser extent (Lawley et al., 2008). The nephropathy is characterized by degeneration of the tubules, with subsequent cortical fibrosis along with functional impairment of tubular activity (Deshpande, 2002). Its LD_{50} values have been reported to be 50 mg kg^{-1} for oral administration in rats, 35 to 38 mg kg^{-1} b.w. (intraperitoneally) in mice, 57 mg kg^{-1} b.w. in ducks, 95 mg kg^{-1} b.w. in chickens and 134 mg kg^{-1} b.w. in rabbits (Bennet & Klich, 2003; Deshpande, 2002). Citrinin is also embryodical, fetotoxic, and teratogenic at relatively high doses (Flajs & Peraica, 2009). However, there is limited evidence of the carcinogenicity of citrinin in experimental animals. In humans, citrinin in combination with OTA has been implicated as a putative cause of BEN, a chronic renal disease.

2.3. Penicillic Acid

Penicillic acid ($C_8H_{10}O_4$) is a toxic antibiotic produced by various *Penicillium* species including *P. cyclopium*, *P. martensii*, *P. palitans*, *P. canescens* and by some Aspergilli (*A. sclerotium*, for example) (Ciegler & Kurtzman, 1970; Kang et al., 2007; Keromnes & Thouvenot, 1985). It has been reported to be present infrequently in maize, beans, and other food crops as well as in Swiss cheese (Jay, 1992).

It has a molecular weight of 170.16 and crystallizes as anhydrous needles from pentane, hexane, or benzene with a melting point of 83-84.8°C. It is moderately soluble (2%) in cold water and in cold benzene; highly soluble in hot water, alcohol, ether, and chloroform, and insoluble in pentane-hexane (Ciegler et al., 1971).

Penicillic acid is cytotoxic to plant and animal cell lines and is moderately genotoxic to microorganisms (Logrieco et al., 2003). This metabolite has been reported to inhibit the growth of maize root by 50% at 500 $\mu g\ kg^{-1}$ (Khachatourians, 1990). It has been shown to be toxic to rat alveolar macrophages *in vitro* suggesting the possibility of a respiratory hazard to agricultural workers exposed to contaminated grain (Sorenson & Simpson, 1986). Its LD_{50} in mice by oral, intravenous, and subcutaneous routes was found to be 600, 250, and 110 $mg\ kg^{-1}$, respectively. The mechanism of toxicity of penicillic acid has been reported to involve the inhibition of sulfhydryl group-containing enzymes (Deshpande, 2002).

3. Fusarium Mycotoxins

Fusarium species are generally considered as field fungi, infecting growing plants in the field, although they can cause some problems in stored grains. The species are distributed worldwide and are important plant pathogens, as well as opportunistic colonisers of plants and agricultural commodities, or as saprophytes on debris and cellulosic plant materials. Several *Fusarium* species cause a range of plant diseases, including vascular wilt, root and stem rot, seedling blight; cereal ear rot and fruit rot (Logrieco et al., 2003). The *Fusarium* species mainly found associated with Fusarium head blight (FHB) in wheat and other small-grain cereals throughout Europe are *F. graminearum*, *F. avenaceum* and *F. culmorum*. Other species which are less frequently encountered, but also toxigenic include *F. poae*, *F. cerealis*, *F. equiseti*, *F. sporotrichioides* and to a lesser extent, *F. acuminatum*, *F. subglutinans*, *F. solani*, *F. oxysporum*, *F. verticillioides*, *F. semitectum* and *F. proliferatum* (Bottalico & Perrone, 2002). Infection of maize kernels, causing an ear rot, is associated mainly with *F. graminearum* and *F. moniliforme*. Apart from pathogenic activity, some *Fusarium* species can synthesise several mycotoxins. The Fusaria are probably the most prevalent toxin-producing fungi in northern temperate regions and are commonly found on cereals grown in the temperate regions of America, Europe and Asia (SCF, 2001). The most important *Fusarium* mycotoxins are trichothecenes (T-2 toxin, HT-2 toxin, deoxynivalenol and nivalenol), fumonisins, zearalenone (ZEA) and moniliformin (MON).

3.1. Trichothecenes

Trichothecenes are a very large family of naturally occurring sesquiterpenoid metabolites produced by a number of fungal genera including *Fusarium*, *Stachybotrys*, *Myrothecium*, *Trichoderma*, *Cephalosporium*, *Verticimonosporium* and others (Bennet & Klich, 2003; Ciegler, 1978). Although the number of trichothecenes runs into hundreds, only a few of them have been shown to be agriculturally important (Figure 7). Among Fusaria, *F. poae*, *F. sporotrichioides*, *F. moniliforme*, *F. culmorum* and *F. graminearum* are the most common trichothecene producers.

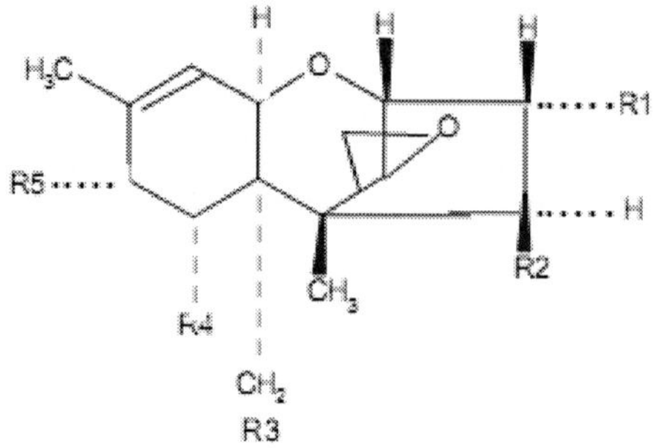

	R_1	R_2	R_3	R_4	R_5
T-2 toxin	OH	OAc	OAc	H	$OCOCH_2CH(CH_3)_2$
HT-2 toxin	OH	OH	OAc	H	$OCOCH_2CH(CH_3)_2$
Deoxynivalenol	OH	H	OH	OH	O
Nivalenol	OH	OH	OH	OH	O

Figure 7. Structure of some trichothecenes.

All trichothecenes contain an olefinic bond at 9, 10 and an epoxide group at C-12, 13, characterized as 12, 13-epoxytrichothecene (Ciegler, 1978). In the early stages of trichothecene research, Ueno and co-workers (1973) classified these toxins into two subclasses: type A having a functional group other than a ketone at C-8 position; with the type B having a carbonyl function at C-8. Later, two groups were added to this classification: type C containing a second epoxy group at C-7, C-8, C-9 or C-10, and type D containing a macrocyclic ring between C-4 and C-5 with two ester linkages (Ciegler, 1978; Smith et al., 1994). The most common type A trichothecenes are T-2 toxin, HT-2 toxin, neosolaniol, monoacetoxyscirpenol and diacetoxyscirpenol which are produced mainly by *F. sporotrichioides* and *F. poae*, while common type B trichothecenes include deoxynivalenol (DON), and its 3-acetyl and 15-acetyl derivatives (3-AcDON and 15-AcDON, respectively), nivalenol (NIV) and fusarenon-X produced principally by *F. graminearum* and *F. culmorum* (Placinta et al., 1999). The type C trichothecenes include crotocin and crotocol (Ciegler, 1978), while macrocyclic trichothences (type D) include satratoxins, verrucarins and roridins and are produced by members of the genus *Myrothecium* and *Stachybotrys* (Ciegler, 1978; Sudakin, 2003).

Trichothecenes mainly occur in cereal grains such as wheat, barley, maize, oats, rice, soya beans and in derived products such as breakfast cereals, bread and beer (Table 4). They are seldom detected in other food commodities such as sorghum, potatoes, bananas, mustard seed, groundnuts, mangoes and sunflower seed.

Table 4. Worldwide contamination of cereals and cereal-based foodstuffs with trichothecenes

Natural source	Country	n	Positive (%)	Range ($\mu g\ kg^{-1}$)	TRc	Method	Reference
Wheat	USA	483	193 (40)	<500-18000	DON	ELISA	(Trucksess et al., 1995)
Barley	USA	147	84 (57)	<500-26000	DON	ELISA	(Trucksess et al., 1995)
Maize	Indonesia	16	2 (13)	21-32	DON	HPLC	(Ali et al., 1998)
Maize	Indonesia	16	2 (13)	49-169	NIV	HPLC	(Ali et al., 1998)
Cereals	Norway	449	139 (31)	>20-1440	DON	GC-MS	(Langesth & Rundberget, 1999)
Cereals	Norway	449	22 (5)	>20-211	NIV	GC-MS	(Langesth & Rundberget, 1999)
Cereals	Norway	449	58 (13)	>20-380	T-2	GC-MS	(Langesth & Rundberget, 1999)
Cereals	Norway	449	148 (33)	>20-880	HT-2	GC-MS	(Langesth & Rundberget, 1999)
Maize meal and cornflakes	Argentina	38	-	-	DON	HPLC	(Solovey et al., 1999)
Cereals	Finland	68	54 (79)	5-111	DON	GC-MS	(Eskola et al., 2001)
Cereals	Finland	68	3 (4)	10-20	NIV	GC-MS	(Eskola et al., 2001)
Cereals	Finland	68	-	-	T-2	GC-MS	(Eskola et al., 2001)
Cereals	Finland	68	2 (3)	10-20	HT-2	GC-MS	(Eskola et al., 2001)
Wheat-based breakfast cereals	Portugal	88	64 (73)	103-6040	DON	HPLC	(Martins & Martins, 2001)
Cereals/pulses products	Turkey	50	13 (26)	450-1900	T-2	HPLC	(Omurtag and Yazıcıoğlu, 2001)
Wheat flour	Germany	60	59 (98)	15-1379	DON	GC-MS	(Schollonberger et al., 2002)
Wheat flour	Germany	60	7 (12)	25-40	NIV	GC-MS	(Schollonberger et al., 2002)
Wheat flour	Germany	60	1 (2)	4	T-2	GC-MS	(Schollonberger et al., 2002)
Wheat flour	Germany	60	4 (7)	12	HT-2	GC-MS	(Schollonberger et al., 2002)
Infant cereal foods	Canada	237	150 (63)	>20-980	DON	GC-MS	(Lombaert et al., Neil, R., 2003)
Infant cereal foods	Canada	237	-	-	HT-2	GC-MS	(Lombaert et al., Neil, R., 2003)
Infant cereal foods	Canada	237	-	-	NIV	GC-MS	(Lombaert et al., Neil, R., 2003)
Wheat/rye flours	Denmark	190	149 (78)	>10-2591	DON	GC-ECD	(Rasmussen et al., 2003)
Wheat/rye flours	Denmark	189	66 (35)	10-189	NIV	GC-ECD	(Rasmussen et al., 2003)
Wheat/rye flours	Denmark	63	23 (37)	10-193	T-2	GC-ECD	(Rasmussen et al., 2003)
Wheat/rye flours	Denmark	62	17 (27)	10-70	HT-2	GC-ECD	(Rasmussen et al., 2003)

Table 4. (Continued)

Natural source	Country	n	Positive (%)	Range ($\mu g\ kg^{-1}$)	TRc	Method	Reference
Beer	Kenya	75	75 (100)	1.6-6.4	DON	ELISA	(Mbugua & Gathumbi, 2004)
Cereals	Russia	5652	2166 (69)	100-8600	DON	TLC/HPLC	(Tutelyan, 2004)
Maize	Italy	46	20 (43)	5-3430	DON	LC-MS/MS	(Cavailere et al., 2005)
Maize	Italy	46	12 (26)	6-3500	3AcDON+15AcDON	LC-MS/MS	(Cavailere et al., 2005)
Maize	Italy	46	7 (15)	12-2440	NIV	LC-MS/MS	(Cavailere et al., 2005)
Rice	Korea	88	3 (3)	105-159	DON	LC-MS	(Park et al., 2005
Rice	Korea	88	5 (6)	182-462	NIV	LC-MS	(Park et al., 2005
Bread	Germany	101	93 (92)	15-690	DON	GC-MS	(Schollonberger et al., 2005a)
Bread	Germany	101	5 (5)	25-64	NIV	GC-MS	(Schollonberger et al., 2005a)
Bread	Germany	101	2 (2)	12	HT-2	GC-MS	(Schollonberger et al., 2005a)
Bread	Germany	101	1 (1)	4	T-2	GC-MS	(Schollonberger et al., 2005a)
Cereal-based foods	Germany	84	48 (57)	8-389	DON	GC-MS	(Schollonberger et al., 2005b)
Cereal-based foods	Germany	84	8 (10)	21-65	NIV	GC-MS	(Schollonberger et al., 2005b)
Cereal-based foods	Germany	84	10 (12)	6-12	T-2	GC-MS	(Schollonberger et al., 2005b)
Cereal-based foods	Germany	84	31 (37)	5-33	HT-2	GC-MS	(Schollonberger et al., 2005b)
Cereals	Ethiopia	84	41 (49)	40-2340	DON	HPLC	(Ayalew et al., 2006)
Cereals	Ethiopia	84	4 (5)	40-490	NIV	HPLC	(Ayalew et al., 2006)
Cereals	Lithuania	447	403 (90)	n.r.-987	DON	ELISA	(Mankevičiene et al., 2006)
Cereals	Lithuania	175	116 (66)	n.r.-319	T-2	ELISA	(Mankevičiene et al., 2006)
Wheat/wheat products	South Africa	210	51 (24)	10-8000	DON	TLC	(Mashinini and, Dutton, 2006)
Maize-based products	Brazil	78	1 (1)	767	T-2	GC-MS	(Milane et al., 2006)
Maize-based products	Brazil	78	1 (1)	555	HT-2	GC-MS	(Milane et al., 2006)
Maize-based products	Brazil	78	1 (1)	167	DON	GC-MS	(Milane et al., 2006)
Maize-based products	Brazil	78	1 (1)	166	NIV	GC-MS	(Milane et al., 2006)
Maize	Nigeria	180	40 (22)	226-745	DON	LC-MS	(Adejumo et al., 2007)
Maize	Nigeria	180	31 (17)	1-72	3AcDON	LC-MS	(Adejumo et al., 2007)
Maize	Nigeria	180	17 (9)	1-51	DAS	LC-MS	(Adejumo et al., 2007)
Maize	Nigeria	180	-	-	NIV	LC-MS	(Adejumo et al., 2007)

Natural source	Country	n	Positive (%)	Range (μg kg^{-1})	TRc	Method	Reference
Maize	Nigeria	180	-	-	T-2	LC-MS	(Adejumo et al., 2007)
Maize	Argentina	23	4 (17)	>12-834	DON	GC-ECD	(Broggi et al., 2007)
Cereals	Poland	24	19 (79)	1-1800	DON	HPLC	(Krysińska-Traczyk et al., 2007)
Cereals	Poland	15	19 (63)	4-5020	NIV	HPLC	(Krysińska-Traczyk et al., 2007)
Maize-based foods	Spain	175	47 (27)	26-132	DON	GC-ECD	(Castillo et al., 2008)
Maize-based foods	Spain	175	7 (4)	51-107	NIV	GC-ECD	(Castillo et al., 2008)
Cereals	Serbia	139	52 (37)	40-2460	DON	LC	(Jajić et al., 2008)
Maize-based products	Portugal	105	-	-	DON	TLC	(Martin et al., 2008b)
Maize/maize products	Germany	29	23 (80)	2-106	T-2+HT-2	HPLC	(Meister, 2008)
Oats/oat products	Germany	65	65 (100)	3-174	T-2+HT-2	HPLC	(Meister, 2008)
Wheat	UK/Ireland	1624	1396 (86)	>10-20333	DON	GC-MS	(Edwards, 2009)
Wheat	UK/ Ireland	1624	1088 (67)	>10-439	NIV	GC-MS	(Edwards, 2009)
Wheat	UK/Ireland	1624	260 (16)	>10-52	T-2	GC-MS	(Edwards, 2009)
Wheat	UK/Ireland	1624	503 (31)	>10-193	HT-2	GC-MS	(Edwards, 2009)
Foodstuffs	Jordan	51	2 (4)	250-950	DON	ELISA	(Salem & Ahmad, 2010)
Foodstuffs	Jordan	61	-	-	T-2	ELISA	(Salem & Ahmad, 2010)

TRc: Trichothecenes.
n.r.: not reported.
DON: Deoxynivalenol.
NIV: Nivalenol.
3Ac-DON: 3-Acetyldeoxynivalenol.
15Ac-DON: 15-Acetyldeoxynivalenol.
DAS: Diacetoxyscirpenol.
ELISA: Enzyme-linked immonosorbent assay.
HPLC: High performance liquid chromatography.
GC-MS: Gas chromatography-mass spectrometry.
GC-ECD: Gas chromatography-electron capture detection.
TLC: Thin layer chromatography.
LC-MS/MS: Liquid chromatograhphy-tandem mass spectrometry.
LC-MS: Liquid chromatography-mass spectrometry.
LC: Liquid chromatography.

The toxic potency of trichothecenes varies markedly depending on the structure. In general, type A trichothecenes tend to be more toxic than type B with decreasing order of toxicity from isovaleryl > hydrogen > hydroxyl relate to the substituent at the C-8 position (Rotter et al., 1993). An outbreak of trichothecene (such as DON, NIV, acetyldeoxynivalenol, T-2 toxin) "poisoning" in humans was reported from Kashmir Valley, India in 1987 and was associated with the consumption of bread made from moulds (such as *Fusarium* sp., *Aspergillus* sp.)-damaged wheat. Typical symptoms were abdominal pain, inflammation of the throat, diarrhoea, blood in stools, vomiting and allergic reaction (Bhat et al., 1989). Another human mycotoxicosis associated with eating bread made from scab-infested wheat, barley or other grains infected with *F. graminearum* has been reported in Japan, where it is known as "akabi-byo", red mould disease or scabby grain intoxication. Symptoms of this illness include anorexia, nausea, vomiting, headache, abdominal pain, diarrhea, chills, giddiness and convulsions. No published reports are available on any *Fusarium* toxins present in specific samples of scabby grain implicated in the outbreaks of fusariotoxicosis, however, NIV and DON are known to occur naturally in cereal grains in Japan (Bullerman, 1997).

3.1.1. T-2 Toxin and HT-2 Toxin

T-2 toxin and HT-2 toxin are type A trichothecenes, which are characterized by a functional group other than a carbonyl at C-8. These toxins are produced by certain *Fusarium* species, especially *F. sporotrichioides* (*F. tricinctum*), *F. poae*, *F. equiseti* and *F. acuminatum* (JECFA, 2001). The major producer of T-2 toxin and HT-2 toxin is *F. sporotrichioides*, a saprophyte, which is found in the temperate to colder regions of the world, including Russia, northern Europe, Canada, northern United States, and Japan. It grows from -2 to 35°C, with an optimum between 22.5 and 27.5°C. The minimum a_w for the growth of *F. sporotrichioides* is 0.88, whereas the maximum limit is reported as > 0.99 (Bullerman, 1997; FAO, 2001). The optimum temperature for T-2 production by *F. sporotrichioides* on maize grits is 15°C (Burmeister, 1971). Another producer, *F. poae* is most commonly found in temperate regions of Russia, Europe, Canada, and the northern United States, as well as in warmer regions, such as Australia, India, Iraq and South Africa. *F. poae* has an optimum growth range of between 22 to 27°C, but it can grow at temperatures as low as 2 to 3°C (Bullerman, 1997). The optimum temperature for the production of T-2 toxin by *F. acuminatum* is relatively low (8-14°C), with yields being much lower or negligible at temperatures of 25°C and above (Rabie et al., 1986).

T-2 and HT-2 toxins often occur together in grains such as maize, wheat, barley, oats and rye as wells as in some cereal-based products including malt, beer and bread (SCF, (2001). Among type A trichothecens, T-2 and HT-2 toxins were found to be two most frequent contaminants of cereal grains from EU Member States (European Commission, 2003).

T-2 toxin is only distinguished from HT-2 toxin by an acetyl group in the C-4 position (Eriksen & Pettersson, 2004). T-2 toxin (fusariotoxin T2) is defined as 12,13-epoxytrichothec-9-ene-3,4,8,15-tetraol 4,15-diacetate 8-(3-methylbutanoate), with an empirical formula of $C_{24}H_{34}O_9$ and a molecular weight of 466.58. HT-2 toxin is the 12,13-epoxytrichothec-9-α,4-β,8-α,15-tetraol 15 acetate 8-isovalerate. Its empirical formula is $C_{22}H_{32}O_8$, with a molecular weight of 424.54. T-2 toxin is readily metabolized by mammalian gut microflora to HT-2 toxin which is a major metabolite in the gut and therefore, a common risk assessment for T-2 toxin and HT-2 toxin appears reasonable (SCF, 2001). T-2 toxin and its metabolites, primarily HT-2 toxin may be found in trace amounts in animal products. The metabolites can transmitted into the milk of lactating animals and can represent about 0.2% of the administered dose (Yoshizawa et al., 1981).

T-2 toxin can inhibit DNA, RNA and protein synthesis both *in vitro* and *in vivo* (Shinozuka et al., 2001; Thompson & Wannamacher, 1990; Ueno et al., 1995). This compound also induces apoptosis both *in vitro* (at 10 ng ml^{-1} levels in HL-60 human promyelotic leukemia cells and at 0.2 g ml^{-1} in mouse thymocytes) (Shinozuka et al., 2001;

Ueno et al., 1995) and *in vivo* (at 10 mg kg^{-1} b.w. in intestinal crypt epithelial cells, and thymic and splenic lymphocytes in mice) (Li et al., 1997; Shinozuka et al., 1997) in various organs. Moreover, T-2 toxin can inhibit the mitochondrial electron transport system, with succinic dehyrogenase as the site of action (Khachatourians, 1990).

T-2 toxin, the most acute trichothecene, is about 10 times more toxic than DON (Ueno et al., 1973). Acute effects of T-2 toxin occur after oral exposure to 0.06-10 mg kg^{-1} b.w. in various species. The effects include non-specific symptoms like weight loss or poor weight gain, feed refusal or reduced feed intake, dermatitis, vomiting, diarrhea, hemorrhages and necrosis of the epithelium of stomach and intestine, bone marrow, spleen, testis and ovary (SCF, 2001). The LD_{50} values of T-2 toxin in adult male mice for oral, intraperitoneal, subcutaneous and intravenous administration are 10.5, 5.2, 2.1, and 4.2 mg kg^{-1} b.w., respectively (Ueno, 1984). Little data is available on the toxicity of HT-2 toxin alone. The few comparative *in vitro* and *in vivo* data available on T-2 and HT-2 toxins indicate that they induce adverse effects with similar potencies (JECFA, 2001). For a 6-week-old male mice, the intraperitoneal LD_{50} of HT-2 toxin is 9 mg kg^{-1} b.w. (Ueno et al., 1973).

Like DON and other trichothecenes, T-2 toxin can cause both stimulation and suppression of the immune system, depending on the doses and duration of exposure (JECFA, 2001). T-2 toxin has also been shown to be dermatotoxic (Rafai et al., 2000) and embryotoxic (Blakley et al., 1987).

T-2 toxin has been tested for carcinogenicity in mice and in trout by oral administration in the diet in rats by intragastric administration. In mice, it increased the incidences of pulmonary and hepatic adenomas in males, while it showed a weak carcinogenic effect in rats (Li, 1988). The IARC (1993) concluded that no data were available on the carcinogenicity to humans of toxins derived from *F. sporotrichioides* and there is limited evidence in experimental animals for the carcinogenicity of T-2 toxin. The overall conclusion was that toxins derived from *F. sporotrichioides* are not classifiable as to their carcinogenicity to humans (Group 3).

T-2 and HT-2 toxins have been associated with alimentary toxic aleukia (ATA) in humans. During World War II, a very severe human disease occurred in the former Soviet Union, particularly in the population in Orenburg. The disease, known as ATA is believed to be related to ingestion of over-wintered grains infected with *F. poae* and *F. sporotrichioides* that were milled into flour and made into bread (Bullerman, 1997). The most severe outbreak of the disease was in 1944, but outbreaks have also been reported in 1952, 1953, and 1955 particularly in people consuming over-wintered wheat (SCF, 2001). The first stage is characterized by symptoms that appear a short time after ingestion of the toxic grain. Clinical symptoms include vomiting, abdominal pain, and diarrhea followed by leukopenia, bleeding from the nose and throat, depletion of the bone marrow and fever. Necrotic lesions in the mouth, gums and mucosa may occur and the disease may be highly fatal, with up to 60% mortality. During the second stage, leukopenia, hemorrhagic diathesis, granulopenia, bone marrow aplasia and sepsis may occur (Bullerman, 1997; SCF, 2001).

In an outbreak of toxicosis in China, 97 out of 165 persons fell ill who had consumed rice infected with *F. heteresporum* and *F. graminearum*. The level of T-2 toxin in these mould rice was up to 420 μg kg^{-1}. The symptoms were nausea, dizziness, vomiting, chills, abdominal distension, abdominal pain, thoracic stuffiness and diarrhea (Wang et al., 1993).

The total intake of T-2 and HT-2 toxins, in combination, in Europe has been estimated to be 16.3 ng kg^{-1} b.w. per day. JECFA proposed a PMTDI of 60 ng kg^{-1} b.w. per day for T-2 and HT-2 toxins, alone or in combination, using a safety factor of 500 (JECFA, 2001). A temporary TDI (t-TDI) of 0.06 μg kg^{-1} b.w. for the sum of T-2 and HT-2 toxins was set by the SCF of the European Commission (SCF, 2001). No regulations exist for T-2 and HT-2 toxins but the EU plans to introduce regulatory limits for these mycotoxins in cereals and cereal based products.

3.1.2. Deoxynivalenol

Deoxynivalenol (DON) also known as vomitoxin belongs to the type B trichothecenes and is produced principally by *F. graminearum* (teleomorph *Gibberella zeae*) and *F. culmorum*. Both species are important plant pathogens, causing FHB in wheat and *Gibberella* ear rot in maize (JECFA, 2001). A direct relationship between the occurrence of FHB and contamination of wheat with DON has been established.

The distribution of the two species appears to be related to climatic conditions. *F. graminearum* predominates in the warmer, humid areas of the world such as the USA whilst *F. culmorum* has been shown to be one of the predominant *Fusarium* spp. in the cooler areas such as northern, central and western Europe and Canada (Wagacha et al., 2007). *F. graminearum* has an optimum growth temperature of between 24 to 26°C and grows down to about 0.88 a_w. Maximum production of DON has been reported to be at 30°C, while only small amounts of DON are produced at 15 and 20°C on maize by *F. graminearum* (Vesonder et al., 1982). The optimum pH for *F. graminearum* is 7.2 at 25°C, with minimum values of 2.4 at 30°C and 3.0 both at 25 and 37°C, being reported (Wheeler et al., 1991). *F. culmorum*, a psychrotrophic strain, is capable of growth at 0°C, with an optimum of between 20 and 25°C. *F. culmorum* grows optimally at 0.98 a_w and minimally at 0.90 a_w both at 15 and 25°C, while production of DON occurs over a much narrower range (0.995-0.96 a_w). The optimum a_w for DON production by *F. culmorum* is 0.97 and 0.99 at 15 and 25°C, respectively (Hope et al., 2005). It has also been reported that the optimum temperatures for DON, NIV and 3-AcDON production by both *F. graminearum* and *F. culmorum* are 28, 20 and 15°C, respectively (Llorens et al., 2004).

Deoxynivalenol has been found as a natural contaminant in various cereal crops such as wheat, buckwheat, maize, barley, oats, rye, rice, sorghum and triticale. It has also been detected in processed cereal products including malt, beer, bread and breakfast cereals etc. In contaminated cereals, 3-AcDON and 15-AcDON can occur in significant amounts (10-20%), concomitantly with DON (SCF, 1999). The transfer of DON from animal feed to meat and other animal products appears to be extremely small.

DON (12, 13-epoxy-3, 4,15-trihydroxytrichotec-9-en-8-one) has a molecular weight of 296.32 with the empirical formula of $C_{15}H_{20}O_6$ and a melting point of 131-135°C. DON contains one primary and two secondary hydroxyl groups and is soluble in water and polar solvents such as methanol and acetonitrile. Unlike many of the other trichothecenes the molecule contains a conjugated carbonyl system that results in some UV absorbance which can assist in its detection by thin layer chromatography (TLC) and high performance liquid chromatography (HPLC) (EMANb).

DON may have adverse health effects after acute, short-term, or long-term administration. The main overt effect at low dietary concentrations appears to be a reduction in food consumption (anorexia), while higher doses induce vomiting (emesis) (Rotter et al., 1996). In $B6C3F_1$ female mice, the LD_{50} values for DON are 78 mg kg^{-1} b.w. (oral) and 49 mg kg^{-1} b.w. (intraperitoneal), whereas oral and intraperitioneal LD_{50} values for 15-AcDON have been reported to be 34 and 113 mg kg^{-1} b.w., respectively. Acute doses of both DON (60-1000 mg kg^{-1}) and 15-AcDON (40-160 mg kg^{-1}) result in a variety of toxic effects ranging from necrosis of the gastrointestinal tract, bone marrow, lymphoid tissues, and focal lesions in kidney and cardiac tissue. The kidney of the mice appears to be 5 to 10 times more sensitive to 15-AcDON than DON, whereas the heart is more sensitive to DON than 15-AcDON (Forsell et al., 1987). 3-AcDON causes a dose-related depressed feed consumption in mice within the first seven days and reduced body weight until day 14 when fed at a level up to 10 mg kg^{-1} (Kasali et al., 1985).

Subchronic oral exposure in various species such as mice, rat and pigs may lead to reduced feed intake, reduced weight gain, and changes in some blood parameters including serum immunoglobulins (SCF, 1999). The IARC (1993) concluded that there is inadequate evidence in experimental animals to link DON with carcinogenicity. The overall conclusion was that the carcinogenicity was not classifiable.

DON has not been found to be teratogenic (Khera et al., 1984) and mutagenic, but does inhibit protein and DNA/RNA synthesis (Rogers & Héroux-Metcalf, 1983). DON shows immunosuppressive or immunostimulatory effect, depending upon the dose and duration of exposure (Rotter et al., 1996). JECFA have established a PMTDI of 1 μg kg^{-1} b.w. on the basis of the NOAEL of 100 μg kg^{-1} per day in mice and concluded that intake at this level would not result in effects of DON on the immune system, growth, or reproduction (JECFA, 2001).

As previously stated outbreaks of toxicosis associated with consumption of mould-contaminated wheat and maize and related to the presence of *F. graminearum* have been reported in Japan (red mould disease), India (DON toxicosis), and China (fusariotoxicosis). The epidemiological data in all three cases point toward DON-contaminated grain products as the causative factor (Rotter et al., 1996). In a large-scale human toxicosis caused by infected wheat in India in 1988, about 50 000 people were affected. Symptoms in humans included abdominal pain or a feeling of fullness in the abdomen, dizziness, headache, throat irritation, nausea, vomiting, diarrhea and blood in the stool. However, the exposure was not limited to DON but included also other *Fusarium* toxins (SCF, 1999).

The total intake of DON has been estimated to range from 0.77 μg kg^{-1} b.w. day^{-1} in the African diet to 2.4 μg kg^{-1} b.w. day^{-1} in the Middle Eastern diet. The major source of intake in three of the five regional diets (Middle Eastern, Latin American and European) was wheat (64-88% of the total intake), whereas the sources in the other two regional diets were more varied (wheat and rice in the far East and wheat, rice and maize in Africa) (JECFA, 2001).

The Scientific Commission of the European Community have introduced a maximum allowable level of 1750 μg kg^{-1} for unprocessed durum wheat, oats and maize; 1250 μg kg^{-1} for unprocessed cereals other than durum wheat, oats and maize; 750 μg kg^{-1} for pasta (dry) and cereals intended for direct human consumption, cereal flour, bran as end product marketed for direct human consumption and germ; 500 μg kg^{-1} for bread, pastries, biscuits, cereal snacks and breakfast cereals; and 200 μg kg^{-1} for processed cereal-based foods and baby foods for infants and young children (European Commission, 2006).

3.1.3. Nivalenol

Nivalenol (NIV) is produced mainly by *F. cerealis* (*F. crookwellence*) and *F. poae* and to a lesser extent by *F. culmorum* and *F. graminearum*. As with other trichothecenes, NIV can be found in various cereal crops such as maize, oats, wheat, barley and rye, and their derived products (SCF, 2000c). It may also co-exist with both its mono-acetylated derivative (fusarenon-X) and di-acetylated derivative (4,15-AcNIV), together with DON and ZEA in grains.

NIV belongs to the type B chemical class of non-macrocyclic trichothecenes. Its chemical structure can be defined as trichotec-9-en-8-one,12, 13-epoxy-3,4,7,15-tetahydroxy-(3α,4β,7α), with an empirical formula of $C_{15}H_{20}O_7$ and a molecular weight of 312.35 (SCF, 2000c). Its melting point is 138-140°C.

Like the other trichothecenes, NIV is a potent inhibitor of protein synthesis. It has been reported to be more toxic than DON. The LD_{50} values of NIV in 6-week-old male ddY mice by oral, intraperitoneal, subcutaneous and intravenous routes were found to be 38.9, 7.4, 7.2 and 7.3 mg kg^{-1} b.w., respectively. Most cases of death in mice were observed within 3 days, regardless of the routes of administration, and a marked congestion and hemorrhage in the intestines was observed (Ryu et al., 1988). Clinical symptoms in mice following NIV administration included sedation, diarrhea and congestion of both the lungs and the digestive tract (Kawasaki et al., 1990). A significant erythropenia and slight leukopenia have been reported in female mice given 30 mg NIV kg^{-1} diet for 24 days, but no marked changes were observed in other hematological parameters, feed consumption, body weight gain, or weights of liver, spleen, and thymus (Ryu et al., 1987). In addition, NIV is known to induce apoptosis in the lymphoid tissues of mice (Poapolathep et al., 2002).

NIV targets endocrine organs, especially the anterior pituitary in both sexes and the female reproductive organs, and the hematopietic and immune organs in rats following 90 days dietary exposure. Based on the hematological data, the NOAEL of NIV has been determined to be less than 6.25 μg kg^{-1} (0.4 μg kg^{-1} b.w. day^{-1} for both males and females) (Takahashi et al., 2008).

The major toxic manifestations observed in the C57BL/6CrSlc SPF female mice after chronic dietary exposure to NIV was reduced body weight gain, reduced feed efficiency, increased relative organ weights, and severe leukopenia. Both after 6 months and 1 year of treatment, absolute weights of liver, kidney and thymus were dose dependently decreased (statistically significant at 30 mg NIV kg^{-1}), while relative weights of these organs plus spleen were dose-dependently increased (statistically significant at 12 and 30 mg NIV kg^{-1}). However, no histopathological changes were observed in liver, thymus, spleen, kidneys, stomach, adrenal glands, ovaries, sternum, bone marrow, lymph node, brain and small intestines (Ryu et al., 1988).

With regard to carcinogenicity, Hsia et al. (2004) reported that food in high risk areas of esophagus cancer in two provinces of China contained higher levels of NIV, associated with DON. The authors also revealed papillomas and carcinomas in 23/49 (47%) of Balb/C mice exposed to NIV following 60 weeks exposure. In another study, carcinogenicity was not detected in a study female mice (C57BL/6CrSlc SPF mice) that were administered NIV at dietary concentrations up to 30 mg kg^{-1} for 2 years (Ohtsubo et al., 1989). The IARC have noted that there is inadequate evidence in experimental animals to classify NIV as a carcinogen and that toxins derived from *F. graminearum*, *F. culmorum* and *F. crookwellense* are not classifiable as to their carcinogenicity to humans (Group 3) (IARC, 1993).

The main daily intake of NIV in Nordic countries has been estimated to come from cereals and has been shown to be 0.05-0.09 μg kg^{-1} b.w. The SCF set t-TDI of 0.7 μg kg^{-1} b.w day-1 for NIV, using a large safety factor of 1000 due to the lowest-observed-adverse-efectlevel (LOAEL) and a limited database (SCF, 2001). While no regulations current exist for NIV, but given the relatively higher toxicity of NIV when as compared to DON; it appears likely than it may receive more attention from a regular perspective in the near future.

3.2. Fumonisins

The fumonisins are a group of recently (1988) discovered mycotoxins which are produced primarily by *F. verticillioides* (formerly *F. moniliforme*, telemorph = *Gibberella fujikuroi*) and *F. proliferatum*, fungi that commonly contaminate maize. These species cause *Fusarium* kernel rot of maize, an important disease in hot climates. As *F. verticillioides* and *F. proliferatum* grow over a wide range of temperature but only at relatively high water activities (above about 0.9), fumonisins are formed in maize only before harvest or during the early stage of drying (JECFA, 2001). Other fumonisin producing species are *F. napiforme*, *F. anthophilum*, *F. dlamini* and *F. nygamai* (Musser & Plattner, 1997; Nelson et al., 1992). Other than Fusaria, fumonisins can also be produced by certain strains of *Alternaria alternata* (Chen et al., 1992; Mirocha et al., 1996).

Fusarium moniliforme has an optimum growth range of between 25 to 30°C (Le Bars et al., 1994; Marin et al., 1995), a maximum of 32 to 37°C and a reported minimum of 2.5 to 5°C (FAO, 2001). It has a minimum a_w of 0.87 for growth and has been reported to produce very little toxin at an a_w of 0.925 at both 25 and 30°C, with a maximum at 0.968. *F. proliferatum*, the other major producer of fumonisins has a similar growth profile to *F. moniliforme*. Intermediate a_w levels (0.92-0.97) are particularly critical in partially dried maize where growth and fumonisin production by *F. proliferatum* and *F. moniliforme* can easily occur (Marin et al., 1995).

In addition to maize, various foodstuffs, such as sorghum, asparagus, rice and mung beans are reported to be infrequently contaminated with fumonisins. Surveillance has also shown that the toxin may be present in many finished products, including beer, bread, breakfast cereals, chilli pickles, corn flakes, curry paste, maize muffin, maize pops cereals, maize starch, maize-based infant cereals, noodles, spices and tandori (Arranz et al., 2004). Worldwide contamination of food and feed materials with fumonisins are shown in Table 5.

Fumonisins are characterized by a 19-20 carbon amino-polyhydroxyalkyl chain which is diesterified with propane-1,2,3-tricarboxylic acid (Bezuidenhout et al., 1988). The first fumonisins identified were fumonisin B_1 (FB_1) and fumonisin B_2 (FB_2) from cultures of *F. moniliforme* MRC 826, an isolate from South African maize (Gelderblom et al., 1988). The 28 fumonisin analogs that have been characterized since 1988 can be separated into four main groups identified as the fumonisin A, B, C, and P series. The fumonisin B analogs, comprising toxicology important FB_1, FB_2 and FB_3 (Figure 8), are the most abundant naturally occurring fumonisins, with FB_1 predominating and usually being found at the highest levels (Rheeder et al., 2002).

In contrast to most of the other mycotoxins, the fumonisins do not have cyclic structures. Their structures are based on a long hydroxylated hydrocarbon chain containing methyl and amino groups, which contribute to their water-solubility. FB_1 has an empirical formula of $C_{34}H_{59}NO_{15}$ with a molecular weight of 721.838, and a melting point of 103-105°C (Scott, 1993). FB_1 is the causative agent in the incidence of neurotoxic syndrome equine leukoencephalomalacia (LEM) (Marasas et al., 1988). LEM which is also known as "crazy horse disease" is characterized by liquefactive necrotic lesions in the white matter of the cerebral hemispheres of horses and other equine species. Marked neurotoxicity is evident, with aimless walking and loss of muscle control followed by death; which usually occurs about 2 weeks after toxin ingestion (Pitt, 2000). FB_1 also causes pulmonary edema syndrome and hydrothorax in pigs (Harrison et al., 1990; Ross et al., 1990) and it is also hepatotoxic and carcinogenic in rats (Gelderblom et al., 1988; Gelderblom et al., 1991; Gelderblom et al., 1996).

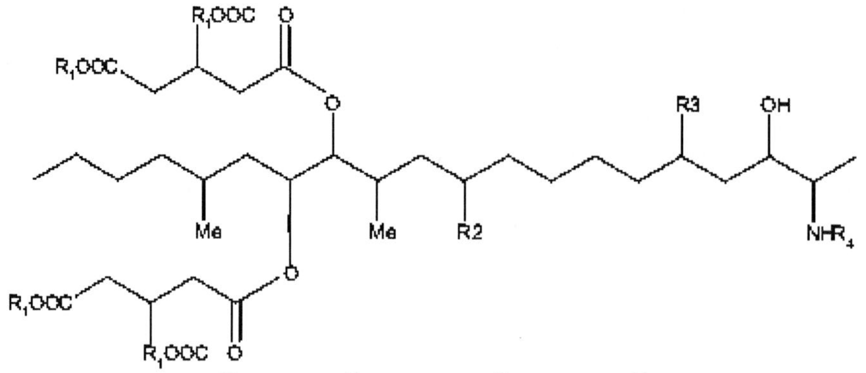

	R_1	R_2	R_3	R_4
Fumonisin B_1	H	OH	OH	H
Fumonisin B_2	H	H	OH	H
Fumonisin B_3	H	OH	H	H

Figure 8. Structure of some fumonisins.

FB_1 is not genotoxic and mutagenic (Gelderblom & Snyman, 1991). There is some *in vitro* evidence for developmental toxicity, but except for chicken no teratogenic effects have been reported in either *in vitro* or *in vivo* studies (SCF, 2000b). Other toxic effects of FB_1 such as neurotoxic (Ledoux et al., 1992) and immunotoxic (Stockmann-Juvala, 2007; Tryphonas et al., 1997) have also been reported.

Table 5. Worldwide contamination of foods and feeds with fumonisins

Natural source	Country	n	Positive (%)	Range ($\mu g\ kg^{-1}$)	Toxin	Method	Reference
Maize-based food/feed	Switzerland	120	44 (37)	55-790	FB_1	HPLC	(Pittet et al., 1992)
Maize-based food/feed	Switzerland	120	15 (13)	50-160	FB_2	HPLC	(Pittet et al., 1992)
Maize	Argentina	17	17 (100)	1585-9990	Fs	HPLC	(Sydenham et al., 1993)
Maize-based products	Spain	50	8 (16)	>25-200	FB_1	HPLC	(Sanchis et al., 1994)
Maize-based foodstuffs	Germany	19	16 (84)	12-1300	FB_1	ELISA	(Uslebe et al., 1994)
Cereals/animal feedstuffs	South Africa	80	66 (85)	200-11000	FB_1	HPLC	(Dutton & Kinsey, 1995)
Maize	India	35	26 (74)	10-5000	FB_1	HPLC	(Shetty and Bhat, 1997)
Sorghum	India	44	2 (5)	150-510	FB_1	HPLC	(Shetty and Bhat,

Natural source	Country	n	Positive (%)	Range (µg kg^{-1})	Toxin	Method	Reference
							1997)
Feeds	India	14	14 (100)	20-260	FB_1	HPLC	(Shetty and Bhat, 1997)
Maize-based foodstuffs	Taiwan	15 3	52 (34)	73-2395	FB_1	HPLC	(Tseng & Liu, 1997)
Maize-based foodstuffs	Taiwan	15 3	32 (21)	120-715	FB_2	HPLC	(Tseng & Liu, 1997)
Maize-based foods/ cereals	UK	29 1	76 (26)	10-2124	Fs	HPLC	(Patel et al., 1997)
Maize	Indonesia	16	16 (100)	51-2440	FB_1	HPLC	(Ali et al., 1998)
Maize	Indonesia	16	8 (50)	<50-376	FB_2	HPLC	(Ali et al., 1998)
Maize	Indonesia	16	4 (25)	57-222	FB_3	HPLC	(Ali et al., 1998)
Maize-based foods	The Netherlands	78	28 (36)	8-1430	FB_1	HPLC	(De Nijs et al., 1998b)
Maize	The Netherlands	62	61 (98)	30-3350	FB_1	HPLC	(De Nijs et al., 1998a)
Beer	Spain	32	14 (44)	5-86	FB_1	ELISA	(Torres et al., 1998)
Maize-based feeds/ cereals	Spain	17 1	136 (80)	200-23600	FB_1	HPLC	(Castellá et al., 1999)
Maize-based feeds/ cereals	Spain	17 1	25 (15)	200-5900	FB_2	HPLC	(Castellá et al., 1999)
Beer	USA	29	25 (86)	0.3-12.7	Fs	HPLC	(Hlywka and Bullerman, 1999)
Maize meal/cornflakes	Argentina	38	36 (95)	2-4964	FB_1+ FB_2+ FB_3	HPLC	(Solovey et al., 1999)
Maize	Taiwan	11 0	49 (45)	109-1148	FB_1	HPLC	(Tseng and Liu, 1999)
Maize	Taiwan	11 0	2 (2)	222-255	FB_2	HPLC	(Tseng and Liu, 1999)
Maize	Venezuela	37	31 (84)	25-15050	FB_1	HPLC	(Medina-Martínez and Martínez, 2000)
Maize	USA	10 0	71 (71)	43-1642	FB_1	HPLC	(Munimbazi and Bullerman, 2000)
Maize-based products	USA	34	22 (65)	28-2679	FB_1	HPLC	(Munimbazi and Bullerman, 2000)
Maize-based products	USA	34	10 (29)	30-797	FB_2	HPLC	(Munimbazi and Bullerman, 2000)
Maize	Iran	19	19 (100)	10-3980	FB_1	HPLC	(Shephard et al., 2000)
Maize	Iran	19	13 (68)	50-1175	FB_2	HPLC	(Shephard et al., 2000)
Maize	Iran	19	13 (68)	50-960	FB_3	HPLC	(Shephard et al., 2000)
Black tea/medical plants	Portugal	87	55 (66)	80-280	FB_1	HPLC	(Martins et al., 2001a)
Black tea/medical plants	Portugal	87	-	-	FB_2	HPLC	(Martins et al., 2001a)
Maize/maize-based products	Turkey	82	21 (26)	250-2660	FB_1	HPLC	(Omurtag, 2001)
Maize/maize-based products	Turkey	82	1 (1)	550	FB_2	HPLC	(Omurtag, 2001)
Maize-based foods	Denmark	70	26 (37)	1-1000	FB_1	HPLC	(Petersen and Thorup,2001)

Table 5. (Continued)

Natural source	Country	n	Positive (%)	Range ($\mu g\ kg^{-1}$)	Toxin	Method	Reference
Maize-based foods	Denmark	70	15 (21)	4-250	FB_2	HPLC	(Petersen and Thorup,2001)
Cornflakes/maize -based cereals	Italy	18	17 (94)	22-1092	FB_1	HPLC	(Solfrizzo et al., 2001)
Cornflakes/maize -based cereals	Italy	18	17 (94)	7-235	FB_2	HPLC	(Solfrizzo et al., 2001)
Maize/maize products	Argentina	18	8 (44)	603-1888	Fs	HPLC	(Torres et al., 2001)
Maize-based foodstuffs	Spain	228	52 (23)	16-938	FB_1	HPLC	(Velluti et al., 2001).
Maize-based feeds	Spain	58	50 (86)	89-8757	FB_1	HPLC	(Velluti et al., 2001)
Maize	Brazil	57	52 (91)	90-17690	FB_1	HPLC	(Almeida et al., , 2002)
Maize	Brazil	57	33 (58)	50-5240	FB_2	HPLC	(Almeida et al., , 2002)
Maize-based foods	Korea	76	38 (50)	13-1210	FB_1	ELISA	(Kim et al., 2002)
Maize-based foods/feeds	Indonesia	105	78 (74)	10-3307	Fs	ELISA	(Nuryono et al., 2002)
Barley and maize foods	Korea	127	11 (9)	15-122	FB_1	ELISA	(Park et al., 2002)
Food samples	Italy	202	51 (25)	10-2870	FB_1	LC/MS	(Cirillo et al., 2003)
Food samples	Italy	202	70 (29)	10-790	FB_2	LC/MS	(Cirillo et al., 2003)
Infant cereal foods	Canada	142	42 (30)	>10-130	Fs	HPLC	(Lombaert et al., 2003)
Beer	Kenya	75	54 (72)	>0.2-0.8	FB_1	ELISA	(Mbugua & Gathumbi, 2004)
Maize silage	USA	89	86 (97)	21-1824	FB_1	HPLC	(Kim et al., 2004)
Maize silage	USA	89	64 (72)	21-276	FB_2	HPLC	(Kim et al., 2004)
Maize silage	USA	89	51 (57)	10-161	FB_3	HPLC	(Kim et al., 2004)
Maize-based foodstuffs	Brazil	82	76 (93)	145-16455	Fs	HPLC	(Scaff & Scussel, 2004)
Maize-based infant foods	Brazil	196	117 (60)	60-5825	FB_1	HPLC	(De Castro et al., 2004)
Maize-based infant foods	Brazil	196	106 (54)	28-1687	FB_1	HPLC	(De Castro et al., 2004)
Maize-based infant foods	Brazil	196	106 (54)	16-549	FB_1	HPLC	(De Castro et al., 2004)
Maize	Croatia	49	49 (100)	142-1378	FB_1	HPLC	(Domijan et al., 2005)
Maize	Croatia	49	3 (6)	68-3084	FB_2	HPLC	(Domijan et al., 2005)
Maize/ maize products	Taiwan	76	11 (15)	50-160	Fs	HPLC	(Liu et al., 2005c)
Asparagus	China	30	24 (80)	47-714	FB_1+ FB_2	HPLC	(Liu et al., 2005b)
Breakfast cereals	France	32	30 (94)	1-1110	FB_1	HPLC	(Molinié et al., 2005)
Cornflakes	Belgium	205	135 (66)	20-464	FB_1	LC/MS-MS	(Paepens et al., 2005)
Cornflakes	Belgium	205	134 (66)	7.5-43	FB_2	LC/MS-MS	(Paepens et al., 2005)

Natural source	Country	n	Positive (%)	Range (μg kg^{-1})	Toxin	Method	Reference
Cornflakes	Belgium	205	134 (66)	12.5-90	FB_3	LC/MS-MS	(Paepens et al., 2005)
Rice	Korea	88	2 (2)	48-61	FB_1	HPLC	(Park et al., 2005
Wheat	South Africa	30	28 (93)	290-1700	Fs	HPLC	(Shephard et al., 2005a)
Home-brewed maize-based beer	South Africa	18	18 (100)	43-1329	Fs	HPLC	(Shephard et al., 2005b)
Cereals	Ethiopia	67	3 (4)	1370-2117	Fs	ELISA	(Ayalew et al., 2006)
Maize products	Brazil	74	70 (95)	20-8600	FB_1	HPLC	(Kawashima and Soares, 2006)
Wheat/wheat products	South Africa	210	4 (2)	1000-2000	FB_1	TLC	(Mashinini & 2006)
Dietary and medical wild plants	South Africa	49	8 (16)	34-524	FB_1	HPLC	(Sewram et al., 2006)
Maize	Morocco	20	10 (50)	>60-5960	FB_1	HPLC	(Zinedi et al., 2006)
Maize	Spain	60	7 (12)	>25-359	FB_1	HPLC	(Ariño et al., 2007)
Maize	Spain	60	5 (8)	>25-153	FB_2	HPLC	(Ariño et al., 2007)
Maize	Argentina	31	24 (77)	>10-34700	Fs	HPLC	(Broggi et al., 2007)
Maize-based products	Portugal	97	77 (79)	>50-1300	FB_1	HPLC	(Martin et al., 2008)
Maize-based products	Portugal	105	29 (28)	>100-450	FB_2	HPLC	(Martin et al., 2008)
Food samples	Tunisia	180	19 (11)	70-2130	FB_1+ FB_2	HPLC	(Ghall et al., 2009)
Feed samples	Tunisia	15	13 (87)	55-2800	FB_1+ FB_2	HPLC	(Ghall et al., 2009)
Foodstuffs	Jordan	55	1 (2)	250	Fs	ELISA	(Salem & Ahmad, 2010)

FB_1: Fumonisin B_1.
FB_2: Fumonisin B_2.
FB_3: Fumonisin B_3.
Fs: Fumonisins.
HPLC: High performance liquid chromatography.
ELISA: Enzyme-linked immonosorbent assay.
LC-MS: Liquid chromatography-mass spectrometry.
LC-MS/MS: Liquid chromatograhphy-tandem mass spectrometry.
TLC: Thin layer chromatography.

In humans, a link has been suggested between ingestion of fumonisin-contaminated maize and the occurrence of esophageal cancer in Transkei, South Africa (Rheeder et al., 1992; Sydenham et al., 1990) and in parts of China (Chu & Li, 1994; Yoshizawa et al., 1994). Fumonisins are also suggested to be a risk factor in the promotion of primary liver cancer in endemic areas of China, along with the trichothecene DON (Ueno et al., 1997). The IARC (IARC, 1993) concluded that there is limited evidence in experimental animals for the carcinogenicity of FB_1 and that toxins derived from *F. moniliforme* are possibly carcinogenic to humans (Group 2B). However, there is inadequate evidence in studies with experimental animals to classify FB_2 as a carcinogen.

The mean estimates of international intake of FB_1 have been reported to range from 0.2 μg kg^{-1} b.w. per day in the Europe to 2.4 μg kg^{-1} b.w. per day in Africa. A PMTDI has been fixed for fumonisins B_1, B_2 and B_3 alone or in combination, of 2 μg kg^{-1} b.w. per day on the basis of the NOAEL of 0.2 μg kg^{-1} b.w. day^{-1} and a safety factor of 100 (JECFA, 2001). The EU has set a limit for the sum of FB_1 and FB_2 at 2000 μg kg^{-1} in unprocessed maize; 1000 μg kg^{-1} in maize flour, maize meal, maize grits, maize germ and refined maize oil; 400 μg kg^{-1} in maize based foods for direct human consumption; and 200 μg kg^{-1} in processed maize-based foods and baby foods for infants and young children (European Commission, 2006).

3.3. Zearalenone

Zearalenone (ZEA), previously known as F-2 toxin, is a nonsteroidal estrogenic mycotoxin produced by several *Fusarium* species, primarily by *F. graminearum* (*Gibberella zeae* in sexual stage) and by *F. culmorum*. Other *Fusarium* species that produce ZEA include *F. cerealis (F. crookwellense)*, *F. equiseti* and *F. semitectum*. This mycotoxin is common in maize, but other important cereal crops such as barley, oats, wheat, rice, sorghum and soybeans and their derived products are also susceptible to contamination with ZEA, both in temperate and warmer climates zones (Table 6). ZEA occurs in pre-harvest grain and almost always co-occurs with other *Fusarium* toxins, particularly DON, NIV and fumonisins (EFSA, 2004b).

Chemically, ZEA (6-[10-hydroxy-6-oxo-trans-1-undecenyl]-β-resorcyclic acid lactone] is a phenolic resorcyclic acid lactone. It has a molecular formula of $C_{18}H_{22}O_5$ and a molecular weight of 318.36. It is a white crystalline compound, with a melting point of 164-165°C, which exhibits blue-green fluorescence when excited by long-wave UV light (360 nm), and appears greenish under short-wave UV light (260 nm). The maximum UV absorptions are at 236, 274 and 316 nm in methanol. Maximum fluorescence in ethanol occurs on irradiation at 314 nm with emission at 450 nm. The solubility of ZEA in water is only 0.002 g/100 ml. It is slightly soluble in hexane and progressively more soluble in benzene, acetonitrile, methylene chloride, methanol, ethanol and acetone. It is also soluble in aqueous alkali (Kuiper-Goodman et al., 1987).

Numerous *in vivo* and *in vitro* studies have indicated that ZEA binds to estrogen receptors, generating an estrogen-like response. Studies of pharmacokinetics and metabolism indicate that ZEA is fairly rapidly absorbed following oral administration and can be metabolized by intestinal tissues, particularly in the liver in pigs and possibly in humans during its absorption, with the formation of α- and β-zearalenol and α- and β-zearalanol (Figure 9), which are subsequently conjugated with glucuronic acid. The rate of conversion, and the ratio between α and β zearalenol varies, and may account for the recognized species differences in the sensitivity to ZEA, as α-zearalenol has a higher binding affinity to estrogen receptors (EFSA, 2004b; SCF, 2000a). The relative binding affinities to the rat uterine cytoplasmic receptor for ZEA and its derivatives can be ranked in the following order: α-zearalanol > α-zearalenol > β-zearalanol > ZEA > β-zearalenol (Kuiper-Goodman et al., 1987).

As previously stated ZEA has a potent estrogenic effect. This can cause reproductive problems in laboratory animals (mice, rats, guinea pigs) and in farm animals. ZEA consumption may cause decreased fertility, increased number of resorptions, reduced litter size, and changes in the weight of adrenal, thyroid and pituitary glands as well as changes in serum progesterone and estradiol levels. However, teratogenic effects have not been reported in experimental animals. The toxin has been implicated in numerous incidences of hyperestrogenism in farm animals, especially pigs. Pigs seem to be the most sensitive and the most frequently affected animals, followed by sheep. The NOAEL for ZEA in pigs is 40 mg kg^{-1} b.w. per day, while it is 100 mg kg^{-1} b.w. per day in rats (Kuiper-Goodman et al., 1987) .

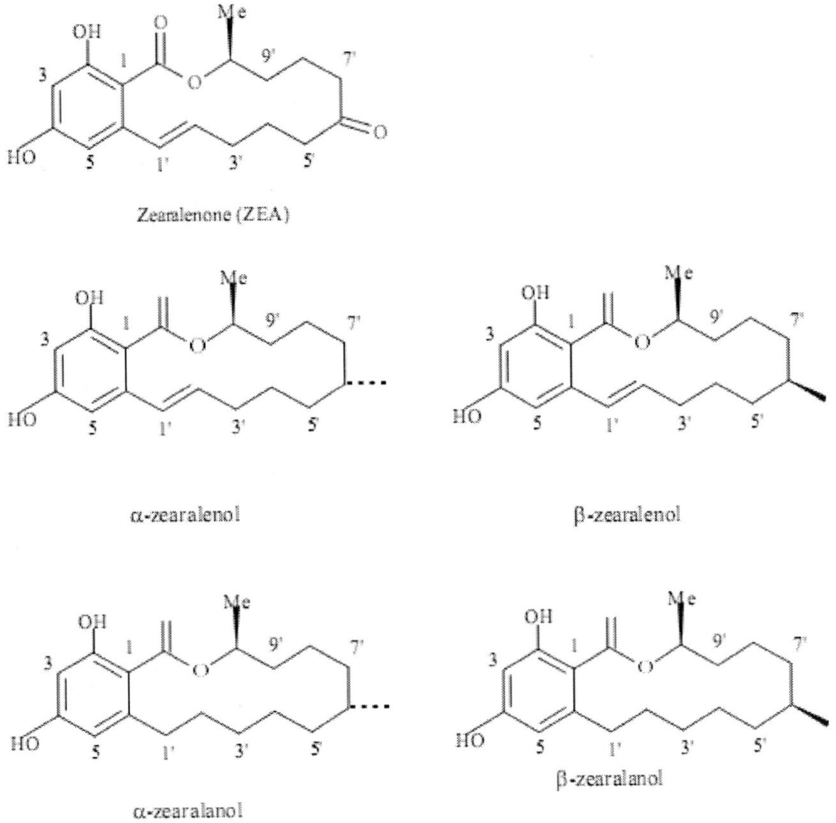

Figure 9. Structure of zearalenone and its derivatives.

ZEA has low acute toxicity after oral administration in mice (LD_{50} value of > 20000 mg kg^{-1} b.w.), rats (> 10000 mg kg^{-1} b.w.), chickens (> 10000 mg kg^{-1} b.w.) and guinea pigs (> 5000 mg kg^{-1} b.w). However, its intraperitoneal LD_{50} values for female mice and guinea pigs has been reported to be > 500 and 2500 mg kg^{-1} b.w., respectively (Kuiper-Goodman et al., 1987). The data available on the genotoxicity of ZEA is somewhat contradictory, but it has been suggested that ZEA is genotoxic in mice (Pfohl-Leszkowicz et al., 1995).

Long-term carcinogenicity studies have reported the presence of hepatocellular adenomas and pituitary adenomas in mice. However, these tumours were observed only at doses which greatly exceed concentrations that have hormonal effects, i.e at levels of 8-9 mg kg^{-1} b.w. day^{-1} or more and thus it can be concluded that these tumours are most likely as a consequence of the estrogenic effects of ZEA (EFSA, 2004b). The IARC has classified ZEA, together with other *Fusarium* toxins, as Group 3 (not classifiable as to their carcinogenicity to humans), based on inadequate evidence in humans and limited evidence in experimental animals ZEA (IARC (International Agency for Research on Cancer, 1993).

Table 6. Worldwide contamination of maize and other cereals with zearalenone

Natural source	Country	n	Positive (%)	Range (μg kg⁻¹)	Method	Reference
Cereals/cereal-based foods	Africa countries	40	5 (13%)	40-400	HPLC	(Doko et al., 1996)
Maize	Indonesia	16	2 (13)	11-12	HPLC	(Ali et al., 1998)
Maize meal/cornflakes	Argentina	38	-	-	TLC	(Solovey et al., 1999)
Cereals	Finland	23	-	-	HPLC	(Eskola et al., 2001)
Maize	Brazil	110	1 (1)	4640	TLC	(Machinski et al., 2001)
Maize	Brazil	214	65 (30)	37-719	HPLC	(Vargas et al., 2001)
Wheat	Germany	24	22 (92)	11-860	LC-MS	(Schneweis et al., 2002)
Wheat flour	Germany	60	22 (37)	1-24	HPLC	(Schollonberger et al.,2002)
Infant cereal foods	Canada	181	59 (33)	1-35	HPLC	(Lombaert et al., 2003)
Wheat and rye flours	Denmark	60	12 (20)	1-2	HPLC	(Rasmussen et al., 2003)
Cereals	Russia	839	58 (7)	10-1480	TLC/HPLC	(Tutelyan, 2004)
Beer	Kenya	75	75 (100)	4.3-10.2	ELISA	(Mbugua & Gathumbi, 2004)
Maize	Italy	46	13 (28)	8-969	LC-MS/MS	(Cavailere et al., 2005)
Maize	Croatia	49	41 (84)	0.4-39	HPLC	(Domijan et al., 2005)
Rice	Korea	88	3 (2)	22-47	HPLC	(Park et al., 2005)
Cereal-based foods	Germany	84	33 (38)	2-67	HPLC	(Schollenberger et al., 2005b)
Maize products	Brazil	74	-	-	TLC	(Kawashima and Soares, 2006)
Wheat/wheat products	South Africa	210	4 (2)	10-4000	TLC	(Mashinini & 2006)
Maize	Côte d'Ivoire	10	10 (100)	20-50	HPLC	(Sangare-Tigori et al., 2006)
Rice	Côte d'Ivoire	10	10 (100)	50-200	HPLC	(Sangare-Tigori et al., 2006)
Peanuts	Côte d'Ivoire	10	10 (100)	50-200	HPLC	(Sangare-Tigori et al., 2006)
Cereals	Etiopia	69	2 (3)	19-32	HPLC	(Ayalew et al., 2006)
Cereals	Lithuania	366	178 (49)	n.r.-193	ELISA	(Mankevičiene et al., 2006)
Maize	Morocco	20	3 (15)	>5-17	HPLC	(Zinedine et al., 2006)
Maize	Argentina	23	11 (48)	>50-2564	TLC	(Broggi et al., 2007)
Foods	Tunisia	209	31 (15)	1.8-41.6	ELISA	(Ghali et al., 2008)
Wheat	UK and Ireland	1624	309 (19)	>5-1292	HPLC	(Edwards, 2009)
Foodstuffs	Jordan	50	-	-	ELISA	(Salem & Ahmad, 2010)

n.r.: not reported.
HPLC: High performance liquid chromatography.
TLC: Thin layer chromatography.
LC-MS: Liquid chromatography-mass spectrometry.
ELISA: Enzyme-linked immonosorbent assay.
LC-MS/MS: Liquid chromatograhphy-tandem mass spectrometry.

ZEA has been suspected as a causative agent in sexual precocity in girls in Puerto Rico, early thelarche in South-eastern Hungary and episodes of breast enlargement in young boys in Italy (EFSA, 2004b; Pitt et al., 2000).

A risk assessment of ZEA has been conducted by SCF and JECFA. A t-TDI of 0.2 μg kg^{-1} b.w. was established by SCF, whereas the PMTDI established by JECFA was 0.5 μg kg^{-1} b.w., based on the NOAEL of 40 μg kg^{-1} b.w. per day obtained in a 15 day study with pigs and the LOAEL of 200 μg kg^{-1} b.w. per day in this study (SCF, 2000a). The EU has set a tolerance level of 20 μg kg^{-1} of ZEA for processed maize-based and other cereal-based foods for infants and young children; 50 μg kg^{-1} for bread (including small bakery wares), pastries, biscuits, cereal snacks and breakfast cereals, maize snacks and maize based breakfast cereals; 75 μg kg^{-1} for cereals intended for direct human consumption, cereal flour, bran as end product marketed for direct human consumption and germ; 100 μg kg^{-1} for unprocessed cereals other than maize; and 200 μg kg^{-1} for unprocessed maize, maize intended for direct human consumption, maize flour, maize meal, maize grits, maize germ and refined maize oil (European Commission, 2006).

3.4. Moniliformin

Moniliformin (MON) was first discovered by Cole et al. (1973) from *F. moniliforme (F. verticillioides)*, isolated from southern leaf blight-damaged maize seed in the United States. Subsequently, different *Fusarium* species have been tested for their ability to produce MON and the following *Fusarium* species have been found to be producers: *F. sporotrichoides*, *F. culmorum* (Scott et al., 1987), *F. fusarioides* (Rabie et al., 1978), *F. subglutinans* (Desjardins et al., 2006; Sewram et al., 1999; Thiel et al., 1982; Vesonder, 1986), *F. avaneceum* (Abramson et al., 2001), *F. proliferatum*, *F. anthophilum* (Martins et al., 2008), *F. acuminatum*, *F. concolor*, *F. equiseti*, *F. semitectum* (Rabie et al., 1982), *F. beomiforme*, *F. napiforme* (Marin et al., 1995) and *F. fujkuroi* (Desjardins et al., 1997). Among these however, *F. subglutinans*, *F. proliferatum* and *F. avenaceum* are the main producers of MON.

MON is found rarely in maize and other cereals, such as barley, oats, wheat and triticale. Although limited surveys are available, MON production appears to be distributed rather widely in the genus *Fusarium*, including species that also produce the trichothecene or fumonisin classes of mycotoxins (Desjardins et al., 2006). The natural occurrence of MON and its co-occurrence with DON and ZEA was first indicated in 1982, at levels of 16 and 25 mg kg^{-1} in two samples of mouldy maize (Thiel et al., 286). It has also been reported to naturally co-occur with fusarin C in maize samples in the U.S. (Thiel et al., 1986). In another report, a UK survey of 36 samples of maize products (principally meal and flour) showed detectable but low levels of MON ranging from 0.05 to 0.25 mg kg^{-1}, while sixty-four samples of maize from ten different countries showed generally higher levels of contamination, with samples from Gambia and South Africa containing 3.16 and 2.73 mg kg^{-1}, respectively. Samples of *Fusarium*-damaged oat, wheat and triticale were also found to be contaminated with MON, at levels from between 0.05 to 399.3 mg kg^{-1} (Sharman et al., 1991). In a South African study, MON has been reported at levels of 17 and 10 μg kg^{-1} in two *Fusarium*-infected maize samples (Sewram et al., 1999), while in a later study conducted in the United States, MON was found in 50 out of 100 maize samples tested at levels ranging from 26 to 774 μg kg^{-1}. The simultaneous occurrence of FB_1 and MON was observed in 34%

of maize samples and 53% of maize-based food products (Gutema et al., 2000). In another study, MON was present up to 1.72 mg kg^{-1} in Polish wheat samples, while average concentrations for different regions and seasons were between 0.08 and 0.34 mg kg^{-1} (Tomczak et al., 2002). In a Brazilian study however, MON was not found in any of 68 commercial maize products (Leoni et al., 2003), whereas it has been detected in 25, 32 and 76% of the barley, oats and wheat samples from Norway, up to concentrations of 380, 210 and 950 μg kg^{-1}, respectively (Uhlig et al., 2004).

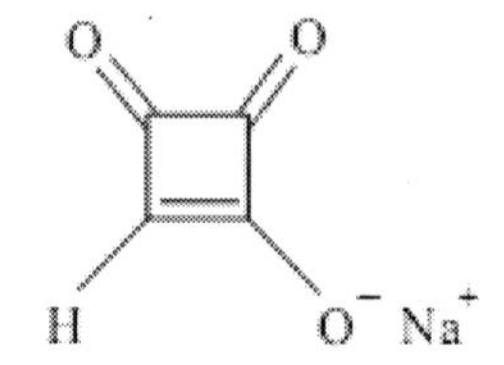

Figure 10. Structure of moniliformin.

MON has been structurally characterized as the sodium or potassium salt of 1-hydroxycyclobut-1-ene-3,4-dione (Figure 10). It has a molecular formula of C_4HO_3Na with a molecular weight of 120. It is soluble in both water and in polar solvents, with reported pKa values between 0.0 and 1.7. On heating, MON as the free acid decomposes at 150-153°C without melting. Its maximum UV absorption wavelengths are 229 and 269 nm in methanol (EMANc).

MON has been shown to be acutely toxic to animals at relatively high dosages. The oral LD_{50} of MON in 1-day old cockerels is 4 mg kg^{-1} b.w. (Cole et al., 1973). It is less toxic to rats, with an LD_{50} of 41.6 and 50 mg kg^{-1} b.w. for female and male rats, respectively (Ueno, 1985). The intraperitoneal LD_{50} values for male and female mice are 20.9 and 29.1 mg kg^{-1} b.w., respectively (Burmeister et al., 1979); whereas in 7-week old female broiler chickens it is 1.38 mg kg^{-1} b.w., following intravenous injection with the pure compound (Allen et al., 1981). In rats, MON causes progressive muscular weakness, respiratory distress, cyanosis, coma, and death (Kriek et al., 1977). Similarly, in studies in which rats were fed diets containing MON, four out of eight rats died within 10 days (Rabie et al., 1978). In sub-acute and chronic studies in experimental animals it has been shown that its principle target is the heart. It is a potent inhibitor of mitochondrial pyruvate and ketoglutarate oxidation. It is also cytotoxic to mammalian cells at higher concentration (EMANc). It has been shown that chicks fed diets containing 50 mg kg^{-1} MON consumed more feed but put on less weight (Bromhead et al., 2002). Moreover, MON has been reported to be potentially associated with the higher rates of Keshan heart disease among human populations in certain regions of China (Yu et al., 1995).

References

Abdelhamid, A. M. (1990). Occurrence of some mycotoxins (aflatoxin, ochratoxin A, citrinin, zearalenone and vomitoxin) in varraious Egyptian feeds. *Archiv für Tierernährung*, 40, 647-664.

Abramson, D., Clear, R. M., Gaba, D., Smith, D. M., Patrick, S. K., Saydak, D. (2001). Trichothecene and moniliformin production by *Fusarium* species from Western Canadian wheat. *Journal of Food Protection*, 64, 1220-1225.

Adejumo, T. O., Hettwer, U., Karlovsky, P. (2007). Occurrence of *Fusarium* species and trichothecenes in Nigerian maize. *International Journal of Food Microbiology*, 116, 350-357.

Afla-guard. (2005). Aflatoxin in Africa. Available from: http://www.circleoneglobal.com/aflatoxin_africa.htm.

Ali, N., Sardjono, Yamashita, A., Yoshizawa, T. (1998). Natural co-occurrence of aflatoxins and *Fusarium* mycotoxins (fumonisins, deoxynivalenol, nivalenol and zeralenone) in corn from Indonesia. *Food Additives and Contaminants*, 15, 377-384.

Allen, N. K., Burmeister, H. R., Weaver, G. A., Mirocha, C. J. (1981). Toxicity of dietary and intravenously administered moniliformin to broiler chickens. *Poultry Science*, 60, 1415-1417.

Almeida, A. P., Fonseca, H., Fancelli, A. L., Direito, G. M., Ortega, E. M., Corrêa, B. (2002). Mycoflora and fumonisin contamination in Brazilian corn from sowing to harvest. *Journal of Agricultural and Food Chemistry*, 50, 3877-38882.

Anderson, S. J. (1995). Compositional changes in surface mycoflora during ripening of naturally fermented sausages. *Journal of Food Protection*, 58, 426-429.

Arafat, M., Musa, M. N. (1995). Patulin-induced inhibition of protein synthesis in hepatoma tissue culture. *Research Communications in Molecular Pathology and Pharmacology*, 87, 177-186.

Arafat, W., Kern, D., Dirheimer, G. (1985). Inhibition of aminoacyl-tRNA syntheases by the mycotoxin patulin. *Chemico-Biological Interactions*, 56, 333-349.

Ariño, A., Estopañan, G., Juan, T., Herrera, A. (2007). Estimation of dietary intakes of fumonisins B_1 and B_2 from conventional and organic corn. *Food Control*, 18, 1058-1062.

Arranz, I., Baeyens, W. R. G., Van Der Weken, G., De Saeger, S., Van Peteghem, C. (2004). Review: HPLC determination of fumonisin mycotoxins. *Critical Reviews in Food Science and Nutrition*, 44, 195-203.

Ayalew, A., Fehrmann, H., Lepschy, J., Beck, R., Abate, D. (2006). Natural occurrence of mycotoxins in staple cereals from Ethiopia. *Mycopathologia*, 162, 57-63.

Aziz, N. H., Loutfy, A., Moussa, A. (2002). Influence of gamma-radiation on mycotoxin producing moulds and mycotoxins in fruits. *Food Control*, 13, 281-288.

Bailly, J. D., Querin, A., Le Bars-Bailly, S., Benard, G., Guerre, P. (2002). Citrinin production and stability in cheese. *Journal of Food Protection*, 65, 1317-1321.

Balachandran, C., Parthasarathy, K. R. (1996). Occurrence of cyclopiazonic acid in feeds and feedstuffs in Tamil Nadu, India. *Mycopathologia*, 133, 159-162.

Barkai-Golan, R. (2008). *Penicillium* mycotoxins. In: Barkai-Golan, R., Paster, N. (Eds.) *Mycotoxins in Fruits and Vegetables*, Academic Press, San Diego, USA, pp: 153-184.

Becroft, D. M. O., Webster, D. R. (1972). Aflatoxins and Reye's disease. *British Medical Journal*, 4, 117.

Bennet, J. W., Klich, M. (2003). Mycotoxins. *Clinically Microbiology Reviews*, 16, 497-516.

Bezuidenhout, G. C., Gelderblom, W. C. A., Gorst-Allam, C. P., Horak, R. M., Marasas, W. F. O., Spiteller, G., Vleggaar, R. (1988). Structure elucidation of the fumonisins, mycotoxins from *Fusarium moniliforme*. *Journal of the Chemical Society, Chemical Communications*, 743-745.

Bhat, R. V., Ramakrishna, Y., Beedu, S. R., Munshi, K. L. (1989). Outbreak of trcihothecene mycotoxicosis associated with consumption of mould-damaged wheat products in Kashmir Valley, India. *The Lancet*, 333, 35-37.

Blakley, B. R., Hancock, D. S., Rousseaux, C. G. (1987). Embryotoxic effects of prenatal T-2 toxin exposure in mice. *Canadian Journal of Veterinary Research*, 51, 399-403.

Blanc, P. J., Loret, M. O., Goma, G. (1995). Production of citrinin by various species of *Monascus*. *Biotechnology Letters*, 17, 291-294.

Boonzaaijer, G., Bobeldijk, I., Van Osenbruggen, W. A. (2005). Analysis of patulin in Dutch food, an evaluation of a SPE based method. *Food Control*, 16, 587-591.

Bottalico, A., Perrone, G. (2002). Toxigenic *Fusarium* species and mycotoxins associated with head blight in small-grain cereals in Europe. *European Journal of Plant Pathology*, 108, 611-624.

Boutrif, E. (1998). Prevention of aflatoxins in pistachios. *Food, Nutrition and Agriculture*, 21, 32-39.

Broggi, L. E., Pacin, A. M., Gasparovic, A., Sacchi, C., Rothermal, A., Gallay, A., Resnik, S. (2007). Natural occurrence of aflatoxins, deoxynivalenol, fumonisins and zearalenone in maize from Entre Ríos province, Argentina. *Mycotoxin Research*, 2, 59-64.

Bromhead, J. N., Ledoux, D. R., Bermudez, A. J., Rottinghaus, G. E. (2002). Chronic effects of moniliformin in broilers and turkeys fed dietary treatments to market age. *Avian Diseases*, 46, 901-908.

Bullerman, L. B. (1997). Fusaria and toxigenic moulds other than Aspergilli and Penicillia. In: Doyle, M. P., Beuchat, L. R., Montville, T. J. (Eds.), *Food Microbiology Fundamentals and Frontiers*, American Society for Microbiology, Washington, DC, USA, pp: 419-434.

Burda, K. (1992). Incidence of patulin in apple, pear and mixed fruit products marketed in New South Wales. *Journal of Food Protection*, 55, 796-798.

Burdock, G. A., Flamm, W. G. (2000). Review article: safety assessment of the mycotoxin cyclopiazonic acid. *International Journal of Toxicology*, 19, 195-218.

Burmeister, H. R., Ciegler, A., Vesonder, R. F. (1979). Moniliformin, a metabolite of *Fusarium moniliforme* NRRL 6322: Purification and toxicity. *Applied and Environmental Microbiology*, 37, 11-13.

Burmeister, H. R. (1971). T-2 toxin productionby *Fusarium tricinctum* on solid substrate. *Applied Microbiology*, 21, 739-742.

CAST (Council for Agricultural Science and Technology). (2003). *Mycotoxins: risks in plant, animal and human systems.* Report No. 139. Council for Agricultural Science and Technology, Ames, Iowa.

Castellá, G., Bragulat, M. R., Cabañes, F. J. (1999). Surveillance of fumonisins in maize-based feeds and cereals from Spain. *Journal of Agricultural and Food Chemistry*, 47, 4707-4710.

Castillo, M.-Á., Montes, R., Navarro, A., Segarra, R., Cuesta, G., Hernández, E. (2008). Occurrence of deoxynivalenol and nivalenol in Spanish corn-based food products. *Journal of Food Composition and Analysis*, 21, 423-427.

Cavailere, C., D'Ascenzo, G., Foglia, P., Pastorini, E., Samperi, R., Lagana, A. (2005). Determination of type B trichothecenes and macrocyclic lactone mycotoxins in field contaminated maize. *Food Chemistry*, 92, 559-568.

CDC (Center for Disease Control and Prevention). (2004). Outbreak of aflatoxin poisoning-Eastern and Central Provinces, Kenya, January-July, 2004. Available from: http://www.cdc.gov/mmwr/preview/mmwrhtml/mm533a4.htm.

Chang, P.-K., Ehrlich, K. C., Fujii, I. (2009). Cyclopiazonic acid biosynthesis of *Aspergillus flavus* and *Aspergillus oryzae*. *Toxins*, 1, 74-99.

Chen, J. P., Mirocha, C. J., Xie, W., Hogge, L., Olson, D. (1992). Production of the mycotoxin fumonisin B_1 by *Alternaria alternata* f. sp. *lycopersici*. *Applied and Environmental Microbiology*, 58, 3928-3931.

Cheraghali, A. M., Mohammadi, H. R., Amirahmadi, M., Yazdanpanah, H., Abouhossain, G., Zamanian, F., Khansari, M. G., Afshar, M. (2005). Incidence of patulin contamination in apple juice produced in Iran. *Food Control*, 16, 165-167.

Choudhary, P. L., Sharma, R. S., Borkhateria, V. N. (1998). Carry-over of aflatoxin B_1 from feed as aflatoxin M_1 in milk of Indian cows. *Milchwissenschaft*, 53, 513-515.

Chu, F. S., Li, G. Y. (1994). Simultaneous occurrence of fumonisin B_1 and other mycotoxins in mouldy corn collected from the People's Republic of China in regions with high incidence of esophageal cancer. *Applied and Environmental Microbiology*, 60, 847-852.

Ciegler, A., Detroy, R. W., Lillehoj, E. B. (1971). Patulin, penicillic acid, and other carcinogenic lactones. *Microbial Toxins*, 409-434.

Ciegler, A., Kurtzman, C. P. (1970). Penicillic acid production by blue-eye fungi on various agricultural commodities. *Applied Microbiology*, 20, 761-764.

Ciegler, A. (1978). Trichothecenes: occurrence and toxicoses. *Journal of Food Protection*, 41, 399-403.

Cirillo, T., Ritieni, A., Visone, M., Cocchieri, R. A. (2003). Evaluation of conventional and organic Italian foodstuffs for deoxynivalenol and fumonisins B_1 and B_2. *Journal of Agricultural and Food Chemistry*, 51, 8128-8131.

Codex Alimentarius Commission (2002). Proposed draft code of practice for the prevention (reduction) of mycotoxin contamination in cereals, including annexes on ochratoxin A, zearalenone, fumonisins and trichothecenes, CX/FAC 02/21, Joint FAO/WHO Food Standards Programme, Rotterdam,

Cole, R. J., Kirksey, J. W., Cutler, H. G., Doupnik, B. L., Peckham, J. C. (1973). Toxin from *Fusarium moniliforme*: effects on plants and animals. *Science*, 179, 1324-1326.

Cooray, R., Kiessling, K.-H., Lindahl-Kiessling, K. (1982). The effects of patulin and patulin-cysteine mixtures on DNA synthesis and the frequency of sister-chromatid exchanges in human lymphocytes. *Food and Chemical Toxicology*, 20, 893-898.

Cotty, P. J. (1994). Influence of filed application of an atoxigenic strain of *Aspergillus flavus* on the populations of *A. flavus* infecting cotton bolls and on the aflatoxin content of cottonseed. *Phytopathology*, 84, 1270-1277.

Cotty, P. J. (1989). Virulence and cultural characteristics of two *Aspergillus flavus* strains pathogenic on cotton. *Phytopathology*, 79, 808-814.

De Castro, M. F. P. M., Shephard, G. S., Sewram, V., Vicente, E., Mendoça, T. A., Jordan, A. C. (2004). Fumonisins in Brazilian corn-based foods for infant consumption. *Food Additives and Contaminants*, 21, 693-699.

De Nijs, M., Sizoo, E. A., Rombouts, F. M., Notermans, S. H. W., Van Egmond, H. P. (1998a). Fumonisin B_1 in maize for food production imported in the Netherlands. *Food Additives and Contaminants*, 15, 389-392.

De Nijs, M., Sizoo, E. A., Vermunt, A. E. M., Notermans, S. H. W., Van Egmond, H. P. (1998b). The occurrence of fumonisin B_1 in maize-containing foods in The Netherlands. *Food Additives and Contaminants*, 15, 385-388.

Deshpande, S. S. (2002). Fungal Toxins. In: *Handbook of Food Toxicology*. Marcel Dekker, New York, NY, USA, pp: 387-456.

Desjardins, A. E., Maragos, C. M., Proctor, R. H. (2006). Maize ear rot and moniliformin contamination by cryptic species of *Fusarium subglutinans*. *Journal of Agricultural and Food Chemistry*, 54, 7383-7390.

Desjardins, A. E., Plattner, R. D., Nelson, P. E. (1997). Production of fumonisin B_1 and moniliformin by *Gibberella fujikuroi* from rice from various geographic areas. *Applied and Environmental Microbiology*, 63, 1838-1842.

De Sylos, C. D., Rodriguez-Amaya, D. B. (1999). Incidence of patulin in fruits and fruit juices marketed in Campinas, Brazil. *Food Additives and Contaminants*, 16, 71-74.

Doko, M. B., Canet, C., Brown, N., Sydenham, E. W., Mpuchane, S., Siame, B. A. (1996). Naural co-occurrence of fumonisins and zearalenone in cereals and cereal-based foods from Eastern and Southern Africa. *Journal of Agricultural and Food Chemistry*, 44, 3240-3243.

Domijan, A.-M., Peraica, M., Jurjević, Z., Ivić, D., Cvjetkovic, B. (2005). Fumonisin B_1, fumonisin B_2, zearalenone and ochratoxin A contamination of maize in Croatia. *Food Additives and Contaminants*, 22, 677-680.

Dorner, J. W. (1983). Production of cyclopiazonic acid by *Aspergillus tamarii* Kita. *Applied and Environmental Microbiology*, 46, 1435-1437.

Dutton, M. F., Kinsey, A. (1995). Occurrence of mycotoxins in cereals and animal feedstuffs in Natal, South Africa 1994. *Mycopathologia*, 131, 31-36.

Edwards, S. G. (2009). *Fusarium* mycotoxin content of UK organic and conventional wheat. *Food Additives and Contaminants*, 26, 496-506.

EFSA (European Food Safety Authority). (2004a). Opinion on the scientific panel on contaminants in the food chain on a request from the commission related to aflatoxin B_1 as undesirable substance in animal feed. *The EFSA Journal*, 39, 1-27.

EFSA. (2004b). Opinion of the scientific panel on contaminants in the food chain on a request from the commission related to zearalenone as undesirable substance in animal feed. Question N^{o} EFSA-Q-2003-037. *The EFSA Journal*, 89, 1-35.

EFSA. (2006). Opinion of the scientific panel on contaminants in the food chain on a request from the commission related to ochratoxin A in food. Question N^{o} EFSA-Q-2005-154. *The EFSA Journal*, 365, 1-56.

Ehrlich, K. C., Chang, P. K., Yu, J., Cotty, P. J. (2004). Aflatoxin biosynthesis cluster gene cypA is required for G aflatoxin formation. *Applied and Environmental Microbiology*, 70, 6518-6524.

Ehrlich, K. C., Montalbano, B. G., Cotty, P. J. (2003). Sequence comparison of aflR from different *Aspergillus* species provides evidence for variability in regulation of aflatoxin production. *Fungal Genetics and Biology*, 38, 63-74.

El-Kady, I. A., El-Maraghy, S. S. M., Mostafa, M. E. (1995). Natural occurrence of mycotoxins in different species in Egypt. *Folia Microbiologica*, 40, 297-300.

El-Sayed, A. M. A., Metwally, M. M., Mehriz, A. M., Abu Sree, Y. H. (1996). Sterigmatocystin: incidence, fate and production by *Aspergillus versicolor* in Ras cheese. *Nahrung*, 40, 310-313.

EMANa (European Myxotoxin Awaraness Network). Basic factsheet 10. Cyclopiazonic acid. Available from http://services.leatherheadfood.com/mycotoxins.

EMANb. Basic factsheet 4. Deoxynivalenol. Available from http://services.leatherhead food.com/mycotoxins.

EMANc. Basic factsheet 11. Moniliformin. Available from http://services.leatherhead food.com/mycotoxins.

Englebrecht, J. C., Altenkirk, B. (1972). Comparison of some biological effects of sterigmatocystin and aflatoxin analogs on primary cell cultures. *J. Natl. Cancer Inst.*, 48, 1647-1653.

Eriksen, G. S., Pettersson, H. (2004). Toxicological evaluation of trichothecenes in animal feed. *Animal Feed Science and Technology*, 114, 205-239.

Eskola, M., Parikka, P., Rizzo, A. (2001). Trichothecenes, ochratoxin A and zearalenone contamination and *Fusarium* infection in Finnish cereal samples in 1998. *Food Additives and Contaminants*, 18, 707-718.

Essigmann, J. M., Barker, L. J., Fowler, K. W., Francisco, M. A., Reinhold, V. N., Wogan, G. N. (1979). Sterigmatocystin-DNA interactions: identification of a major adduct formed after metabolic activation *in vitro*. *Proc. Natl. Acad. Sci.*, 76, 179-183.

European Commission. (2002a). EC No 472/2002 of 12 March 2002 amending Regulation (EC) No 466/2001 setting maximum levels for certain contaminants in foodstuffs. *Official Journal of the European Union* L75, 18-20.

European Commission. (2002b). Report of experts participating in Task 3.2.7. Assessment of dietary intake of ochratoxin A by the population of EU Member States. Directorate-General Health and Consumer Protection.

European Commission. (2003). Reports on tasks for scientific co-operation in Task 3.2.10. Collection of occurrence data of *Fusarium* toxins in food and assessment of dietary intake by the population of EU Member States. Directorate-General Health and Consumer Protection.

European Commission. (2006). Commission Regulation (EC) No 1881/2006 of 19 December 2006 setting maximum levels for certain contaminants in foodstuffs. *Official Journal of the European Union,* L 364/5-L 364/24.

FAO. (2001). Manual on the application of the HACCP system in mycotoxin prevention and control. Food and Agricultural Organization of the United Nations, Food and Nutrition Paper, 73, Rome.

Flajs, D., Peraica, M. (2009). Toxicological properties of citrinin. *Arhiv Za Higijenu Rada I Toksikologiju*, 60, 457-64.

Forsell, J. H., Jensen, R., Tai, J.-H., Witt, M., Lin, W. S., Pestka, J. J. (1987). Comparison of acute toxicities of deoxynivalenol (vomitoxin) and 15-acetyldeoxynivalenol in the $B6C3F_1$ mouse. *Food and Chemical Toxicology*, 25, 155-162.

Frisvad, J. C., Samson, R. A. (1991). Mycotoxins produced by species of *Penicillium* and *Aspergillus* occurring in cereals. In: Chelkowski, J (Ed), *Cereal grain mycotoxins, fungi and quality in drying and storage*, Elsevier, Amsterdam.

Gelderblom, W. C. A., Jaskiewicz, K., Marasas, W. F. O., Thiel, P. G., Horak, R. M., Vleggaar, R., Kriek, N. P. J. (1988). Fumonisins-novel mycotoxins with cancer-promoting activity produced by *Fusarium moniliforme*. *Applied and Environmental Microbiology*, 54, 1806-1811.

Gelderblom, W. C. A., Jaskiewicz, K., Marasas, W. F. O., Thiel, P. G. (1991). Toxicity and carcinogenicity of the *Fusarium moniliforme* metabolite, fumonisin B_1 in rats. *Carcinogenesis*, 12, 1247-1251.

Gelderblom, W. C. A., Smuths, C. M., Abel, S., Snyman, S. D., Caewood, M. E., Van der Westhuizen, L., Swanevelder, S. (1996). Effect of fumonisin B_1 on protein and lipid synthesis in primary rat hepatocytes. *Food and Chemical Toxicology*, 34, 361-369.

Gelderblom, W. C. A., Snyman, S. D. (1991). Mutagenicity of potential carcinogenic mycotoxins produced by *Fusarium moniliforme. Mycotoxin Research*, 7, 46-52.

Ghali, R., Hmaissia-Khlifa, K., Ghorbel, H., Maaroufi, K., Hedili, A. (2008). Incidence of aflatoxins, ochratoxin A and zearalenone in Tunisian foods. *Food Control*, 19, 921-924.

Ghall, R., Ghorbel, H., Hedilli, A. (2009). Fumonisin determination in Tunisian foods and feeds. ELISA and HPLC methods comparison. *Journal of Agricultural and Food Chemistry*, 57, 3955-3960.

González-Osnaya, L., Soriano, J. M., Moltó, J. C., Mañes, J. (2007). Exposure to patulin from consumption of apple-based products. *Food Additives and Contaminants*, 24, 1268-1274.

Gökmen, V., Acar, J. (1998). Incidence of patulin in apple juice concentrates produced in Turkey. *Journal of Chraomatography A*, 815-99-102.

Gökmen, V., Acar, J. (1996). Rapid reversed-phase liquid chromatographic determination of patulin in apple juice. *Journal of Chromatography A*, 730, 53-58.

Gutema, T., Munimbazi, C., Bullerman, L. B. (2000). Occurrence of fumonisins and moniliformin in corn and corn-based food products of U.S. origin. *Journal of Food Protection*, 63, 1732-1737.

Harrison, L. R., Colvin, B. M., Greene, J. T., Newman, L. E., Cole, J. R. (1990). Pulmonary edema and hydrothorax in swine produced by fumonisin B_1 a toxic metabolite of *Fusarium moniliforme. Journal of Veterinary Diagnostic Investigation*, 2, 217-221.

Hayashi, Y., Yoshizawa, T. (2005). Analysis of cyclopiazonic acid in corn and rice by a newly developed method. *Food Chemistry*, 93, 215-221.

Hendrickse, R. G., Coulter, J. B. S., Lamplugh, S. M., Macfarlane, S. B. J., Williams, T. E., Omer, M. I. A., Suliman, G. I. (1982). Aflatoxins and kwashiorkor: a study in Sudanese children. *British Medical Journal*, 285, 843-846.

Hetherington, A. C., Raistrick, H. (1931). Studies in the biochemistty of microorganisms. Part XIV, on the production and chemical constitution of a yellow coloring matter, citrinin, produced from glucose by *Penicillium citrinum. Thom. Philos. Trans. R. Soc. Lond. Ser. B.*, 220: 269-271.

Hlywka, J. J., Bullerman, L. B. (1999). Occurrence of fumonisin B_1 and B_2 in beer. Food *Additives and Contaminants Part A*, 16, 319-324.

Holzapfel, C. W. (1968). The isolation and structure of cyclopiazonic acid, a toxic metabolite of *Penicillium cyclopium* Westling. *Tetrahedron*, 24, 2101-2119.

Hope, R., Aldred, D., Magan, N. (2005). Comparison of environmental profiles for growth and deoxynivalenol production by *Fusarium culmorum* and *F. graminearum* on wheat grain. *Letters in Applied Microbiology*, 40, 295-300.

Hsia, C. C., Wu, Z. Y., Li, Y. S., Zhang, F., Sun, Z. T. (2004). Nivalenol, a main *Fusarium* toxin in dietary foods from high-risk areas of cancer of esophagus and gastric cardia in China, induced benign and malignant tumours in mice. *Oncology Reports*, 12, 449-456.

IARC (International Agency for Research on Cancer). (1993). Monographs on the evaluation of carcinogenic risks to humans, some naturally occurring substances: Food items and constituents, heterocyclic aromatic amines and mycotoxins. Lyon: International Agency for Research on Cancer, 56, 489-521.

ICMSF (International Commission on Microbiological Specifications for Foods). (1996a). Toxigenic fungi: *Aspergillus*. In: *Microorganisms in Foods*. 5. Characteristics of Food Pathogens. Academic Press, London, pp. 347-381.

ICMSF. (1996b). Toxigenic fungi: *Penicillium*. In: *Microorganisms in foods*. 5. Characteristics of Food Pathogens. London: Blackie Academic and Professional, pp: 397-413.

Iha, M. H., Sabino, M. (2008). Indidence of patulin in Brazilian apple-based drinks. *Food Control*, 19, 417-422.

Ito, R., Yamazaki, H., Inoue, K., Yoshimura, Y., Kawaguchi, M., Nakazawa, H. (2004). Development of liquid chromatography-electrospray mass spectrometry for the determination of patulin in apple juice: Investigation of its contamination levels in Japan. *Journal of Agricultural and Food Chemistry*, 52, 7464-7468.

Jajić, I., Juric, V., Abromavić, B. (2008). First survey of deoxynivalenol occurrence in crops in Serbia. *Food Control*, 19, 545-550.

Jalali, A., Khorasgani, Z. N., Goudarzi, M., Khoshlesan, N. (2010). HPLC determination of patulin in apple juice: A single center study of southweast area of Iran. *Journal of Pharmacology and Toxicology*, 5, 208-214.

Jay, J. M. (1992). *Modern food microbiology*, Chapman and Hall, London, p.675.

JECFA (Joint FAO/WHO Expert Committee on Food Additives) (2001). Fifty-sixth meeting, 6-15 February, Geneva.

Kabak, B., Dobson, A. D. W., Var, I. (2006). Strategies to prevent mycotoxin contamination of food and animal feed: a review. *Critical Reviews in Food Science and Nutrition*, 46, 593-619.

Kabak, B. (2009). Ochratoxin A in cereal-derived products in Turkey: occurrence and exposure assessment. *Food and Chemical Toxicology*, 47, 348-352.

Kang, S. W., Park, C. H., Hong, S. I., Kim, S. W. (2007). Production of penicillic acid by *Aspergillus sclerotium* CGF. *Bioresource Technology*, 98, 191-197.

Karimi, G., Hassanzadeh, M., Yazdanpanah, H., Nazari, F., Iranshahi, M., Nili, A. (2008). Contamination of patulin in clear apple juice in Mashhad, Iran. *Journal of Food Safety*, 28, 413-421.

Kasali, O. B., Schiefer, H. B., Hancock, D. S., Blakley, B. R., Tomar, R. S., Greenhalgh, R. (1985). Subacute toxicity of dietary 3-acetyldeoxynivalenol in mice. *Canadian Journal of Comparative Medicine*, 49, 319-322.

Kawasaki, Y., Uchida, O., Sekita, K., Matsumoto, K., Ochiai, T., Usoi, A., Nakaji, Y., Furoya, L., Kurukawa, Y., Tobe, M. (1990). Single and repeated oral administration toxicity studies of nivalenol in F344rats. *Journal of the Food Hygienic Society of Japan*, 31, 144-154.

Kawashima, L. M., Soares, L. M. V. (2006). Occurrence of fumonisin B_1, aflatoxins B_1, B_2, G_1, and G_2, ochratoxin A and zearalenone in corn products. *Ciência e Technologia de Alimentos*, 26, 516-521.

Keromnes, J., Thouvenot, D. (1985). Role of penicillic acid in the phytotoxicity of *Penicillium cyclopium* and *Penicillium canescens* to the germination of corn seeds. *Applied and Environmental Microbiology*, 49, 660-663.

Khachatourians, G. G. (1990). Metabolic effects of trichothecene T-2 toxin. *Canadian Journal of Physiology and Pharmacology,* 68, 1004-1008.

Khera, K. S., Arnold, D. L., Whalen, C., Angers, G., Scott, P. M. (1984). Vomitoxin (4-deoxynivalenol): Effects on reproduction of mice and rats. *Toxicology and Applied Pharmacology*, 74, 345-356.

Kim, E.-K., Maragos, C. M., Kendra, D. F. (2004). Liquid chromatographic determination of fumonisins B_1, B_2 and B_3 in corn silage. *Journal of Agricultural and Food Chemistry*, 52, 196-200.

Kim, E.-K., Shon, D.-H., Chung, S.-H., Kim, Y.-B. (2002). Survey of fumonisin B_1 in Korean corn-based food products. *Food Additives and Contaminants*, 19, 459-464.

Koehler, P.E., Beuchat, L.R., Chinnan, M.S. (1985). Influence of temperature and water activity on aflatoxin production by *Aspergillus flavus* in cowpea seeds and meal. *Journal of Food Protection*, 48, 1040-1043.

Kononenko, G. P., Burkin, A. A. (2008). A survey on the occurrence of citrinin in feeds and their ingredients in Russia. *Mycotoxin Research*, 24, 3-6.

Kpodo, K., Sorensen, A. K., Jakobsen, M. (1996). The occurrence of mycotoxins in fermented maize products. *Food Chemistry*, 56, 147-153.

Kriek, N. P. J., Marasas, W. F. O., Steyn, P. S., Van Rensburg, S. J., Steyn, M. (1977). Toxicity of a moniliformin-producing strain of *Fusarium moniliforme* var. *subglutinans* isolated from maize. *Food and Cosmetics Toxicology*, 15, 579-587.

Krisnamachari, K.A.V.R., Bhat, R. V., N agarajon, V., Tilek, T. B. G. (1975). Hepatitis due to aflatoxicosis. *Lancet*, 305, 10631-1063.

Krysińska-Traczyk, E., Perkowski, E., Dutkiewicz, J. (2007). Levels of fungi and mycotoxins in the samples of grain and grain dust collected from five various cereal crops in eastern Poland. *Ann. Agric. Environ. Med.*, 14, 159-167.

Kuiper-Goodman, T., Scott, P. M., Watanabe, H. (1987). Risk assessment of the mycotoxin zearalenone. *Regulatory Toxicology and Pharmacology*, 7, 253-306.

Langesth, W., Rundberget, T. (1999). The occurrence of HT-2 toxin and other trichıothecenes in Norwegian cereals. *Mycopathologia*, 147, 157-165.

Lansden, J. A., Davidson, J. I. (1983). Occurrence of cyclopiazonic acid in penuts. *Applied and Environmental Microbiology*, 45, 766-769.

Lawley, R., Curtis, L., Davis, J. (2008). The food safety hazard guidebook. Royal Society of Chemistry, p.300.

Le Bars, P., Le Bars, J., Dupuy, J., Boudra, H. (1994). Biotic and abiotic factors in fumonisin B_1 production and stability. *Journal of Association of Official Analytical Chemists International*, 77, 517-521.

Ledoux, D. R., Brown, T. P., Weibking, T. S., Rottinghaus, G. S. (1992). Fumonisin toxicity in broiler chicks. *Journal Veterinary Diagnosis and Investigations*, 4, 330-334.

Lee, Y. J., Hagler, W. M. (1991). Aflatoxin and cyclopiazonic acid production by *Aspergillus flavus* isolated from contaminated maize. *Journal of Food Science*, 56, 871-872.

Leggott, N. L., Shephard, G. S. (2001). Patulin in South African commercial apple products. *Food Control*, 12, 73-76.

Leoni, L. A. B., Valente Soares, L. M. (2003). Survey of moniliformin in corn cultivated in the state of São Paulo and in corn products commercialized in the city of campinas, S.P. *Brazilian Journal of Microbiology*, 34, 13-15.

Li, F. Q., Xu, G. R., Li, Y. W., Chen, Y.,Ji, R. (2005). Natural occurrence of citrinin in *Monascus* products. *Wei Sheng Yan Jiu*, 34, 451-454.

Li, G., Shinozuka, J., Uetsuka, K., Nakayama, H., Doi, K. (1997). T-2 toxin-induced apoptosis in intestinal crypt epithelial cells os mice. *Experimental and Toxicologic Pathology,* 49, 447-450.

Lillehoj, E. B., Ciegler, A. (1968). Biological activity of sterigmatocystin. *Mycopathologia*, 35, 373-376.

Li, M. X. (1988). Mutagenicity and carcinogenicity of T-2 toxin, a trichothecene produced by *Fusarium* fungi. *Zhonghua Zhong Liu Za Zhi*, 10, 326-329.

Liu, B.-H., Wu, T.-S., Su, M.-C., Chung, C. P., Yu, F, F.-Y. (2005a). Evaluation of citrinin occurrence and cytotoxicity in *Monascus* fermentation products. *Journal of Agricultural and Food Chemistry*, 53, 170-175.

Liu, C., Liu, F., Xu, W., Kofoet, A., Humpf, H.-U., Jiang, S. (2005b). Occurrence of fumonisins B_1 and B_2 in asparagus from Shandong province, P.R. China. *Food Additives and Contaminants*, 22, 673-676.

Liu, F.-M-Chen, P.-C., Fu, Y.-M., Shih, D. Y.-C. (2005c). Determination of fumonisin B_1 and B_2 in corn products. *Journal of Food and Drug Analysis*, 13, 273-278.

Llorens, A., Mateo, R., Hinojo, M. J., Valle-Algarra, F. M., Jiménez, M. (2004). Influence of environmental factors on the biosynthesis of type B trichothecenes by isolates of *Fusarium* spp. from Spanish crops. *International Journal of Food Microbiology*, 94, 43-54.

Logrieco, A., Bottalico, A., Mulé, G., Moretti, A., Perrone, G. (2003). Epidemiology of toxigenic fungi and their associated mycotoxins for some Mediterranean crops. *European Journal of Plant Pathology*, 109, 645-667.

Lomax, L. G., Cole, R. J., Dorner, J. W. (1984). The toxicity of cyclopiazonic acid in weaned pigs. *Veterinary Pathology*, 21, 418-424.

Lombaert, G. A., Pellaers, P., Roscoe, V., Mankotia, M., Neil, R., Scott, P. M. (2003). Mycotoxins in infant cereal foods from the Canadian retail market. *Food Additives and Contaminants*, 20, 494-504.

Luchese, R. H., Harrigan, W. F. (1993). Biosynthesis of aflatoxin-the role of nutritional factors. *Journal of Applied Bacteriology*, 74, 5-14.

Luk, K. C., Kobbe, B., Townsend, J. M. (1977). Production of cyclopiazonic acid by *Aspergillus flavus* Link. *Applied and Environmental Microbiology*, 33, 211-212.

Lye, M. S., Ghazali, A. A., Mohan, J., Alwin, N., Nair, R. C. (1995). An outbreak of acute hepatic encephalopathy due to severe aflatoxicosis in Malaysia. *American Journal of Tropical Medicine and Hygiene*, 53, 68-72.

Machinski, M., Midio, A. F. (1996). Incidencia de patulina in jugo de manzana industrializado. *Alimentaria*, 33, 61-64.

Machinski, M., Valente Soares, L. M., Sawazaki, E., Bolonhezi, D., Castro, J. L., Bortolleto, N., 2001. Aflatoxin, ochratoxin A and zearalenone in Brazilian corn cultivars. *Journal of the Science of Food and Agriculture*, 81, 1001-1007.

Mahfoud, R., Maresca, M., Garmy, N., Fantini, J. (2002). The mycotoxin patulin alters the barrier function of the intestinal epithelium: mechanism of action of the toxin and protective effects of glutathione. *Toxicology and Applied Pharmacology*, 18, 1209-1218.

Mahrous, K. F., Khalil, W. K. B., Mahmoud, M. A. (2006). Assessment of toxicity and clastogenicity of sterigmatocystin in Egyptian Nile tilapia. *African Journal of Biotechnology*, 5, 1180-1189.

Mankevičiene, A., Gaurilčikienė, Dabkeivičiuc, Z., Semaskiene, R., Mačkinaitė, R., Supronienė, S. (2006). Mycotoxin contamination of Lithuanian-grown cereal grains and factors determining it. *Ekologija*, 3, 21-27.

Marasas, W. F. O., Kellerman, T. S., Gelderblom, W. C. A., Coetzer, J. A. W., Thiel, P. G., Van Der Lugt, J. J. (1988). Leukoencephalomalacia in horse induced by fumonisin B_1 isolated from *Fusarium moniliforme*. *Onderstepoort Journal of Veterinary Research*, 55, 197-203.

Marasas, W. F. O., Thiel, P. G., Rabie, C. J., Nelson, P. E., Toussoun, T. A. (1986). Moniliformin production in *Fusarium* section *Liseola*. *Mycologia*, 78, 242-247.

Marasas, W. F. O., Thiel, P. G., Sydenham, E. W., Rabie, C. J., Lübben, A., Nelson, P. E. (1991). Toxicity and moniliformin production by four recently described species of *Fusarium* and two uncertain taxa. *Mycopathologia*, 113, 191-197.

Marin, S., Sanchis, V., Vinas, I., Canela, R., Magan, N. (1995). Effect of water activity and temperature on growth and fumonisin B_1 and B_2 production by *Fusarium proliferatum* and *F. moniliforme* on maize grain. *Letters in Applied Microbiology*, 21, 298-301.

Martins, H. M., Almeida, I., Marques, M. F., Guerra, M. M. (2008). Fumonisins and deoxynivalenol in corn-based food products in Portugal. *Food and Chemical Toxicology*, 46, 2585-2587.

Martins, M. L., Gimeno, A., Martins, H. M., Bernardo, F. (2002). Co-occurrence of patulin and citrinin in Portuguese apples with rotten spots. *Food Additives and Contaminants*, 19, 568-574.

Martins, M. L., Martins, H. M., Bernardo, F. (2001a). Fumonisins B_1 and B_2 in black tea and medical plants. *Journal of Food Protection*, 64, 1268-1270.

Martins, M. L., Martins, H. M. (2001b). Determination of deoxynivalenol in wheat-based breakfast cereals marketed in Portugal. *Journal of Food Protection*, 11, 1848-1850.

Martins, M. L., Martins, H. M. (1999). Natural and *in vitro* co-production of cyclopiazonic acid and aflatoxins. *Journal of Food Protection*, 62, 292-294.

Mashinini, K., Dutton, M. F. (2006). The incidence of fungi and mycotoxins in South Africa wheat and wheat-based products. *Journal of Environmental Science and Health Part B*, 41, 285-296.

Mbugua, S. K., Gathumbi, J. K. (2004). The contamination of Kenyan lager beers with *Fusarium* mycotoxins. *Journal of Institute of Brewing*, 110, 227-229.

McKinley, E. R., Carlton, W. W. (1991). Patulin. In: Sharma R. P., Salunkhe, D. K. (Eds.), *Mycotoxins and Phytoalexins,* CRC Press, Boca Raton, FL, pp: 191-236.

McLean, M., Dutton, M. F. (1995). Cellular interactions and metabolism of aflatoxin: An update. *Pharmacology and Therapeutics*, 65, 163-192.

Medina-Martínez, M. S., Martínez, A. J. (2000). Mold occurrence and aflatoxin B_1 and fumonisin B_1 determination in corn samples in Venezuela. *Journal of Agricultural and Food Chemistry*, 48, 2833-2836.

Meister, U. (2008). Analysis of T-2 and HT-2 toxins in oats and other cereals by means of HPLC with fluorescence detection. *Mycotoxin Research*, 24, 31-39.

Meister, U. (2003). Detection of citrinin in ochratoxin A-containing products by a new HPLC method. *Mycotoxin Research*, 19, 27-30.

Milanez, T. V., Valente-Soares, L. M., Baptista, G. G. (2006). Occurrence of trichothecene mycotoxins in Brazilian corn-based food products. *Food Contol*, 17, 293-298.

Ministry of Agriculture, Fisheries and Foods. (1999). Survey of apple juice for patulin. Food information sheet, 173. London, http://archive.food.gov.uk/maff/archive/food/infsheet/ 1999 /no173/ 173pat.htm.

Mirocha, C. J., Chen, T., Xie, W., Xu, Y., Abbas, H. K., Hogge, L. R. (1996). Biosynthesis of fumonisin and AAL derivatives by *Alternaria* and *Fusarium* in laboratory culture. *Advances in Experimental Medicine and Biology*, 392, 213-224.

Moake, M. M., Padilla-Zakour, O. I., Worobo, R. W. (2005). Comprehensive review of patulin control methods in foods. *Comprehensive Reviews in Food Science and Food Safety*, 1, 8-21.

Molinié, A., Faucet, V., Castegnaro, M., Pfohl-Leszkowicz, A. (2005). Analysis of some breakfast cereals on the Fench market for their contents of ochratoxin A, citrinin and fumonisin B_1: development of a method for simultaneous extraction of ochratoxin A and citrinin. *Food Chemistry*, 92, 391-400.

Mortimer, D. N., Parker, I., Shepherd, M. J., Gilbert, J. (1985). A limited survey of apple and grape juices for the mycotoxin patulin. *Food Additives and Contaminants*, 2, 165-170.

Moss, M. O. (2002). Mycotoxin review-1. *Aspergillus* and *Penicillium*. *Mycologist*, 16, 116-119.

Moukas, A., Panagiotopoulou, V., Markaki, P. (2008). Determination of patulin in fruit juices using HPLC-DAD and GC-MSD techniques. *Food Chemistry*, 109, 860-867.

Mphande, F. A., Siame, B. A., Taylor, J. E. (2004). Fungi, aflatoxins, and cyclopiazonic acid associated with peanut retailing in Bostwana. *Journal of Food Protection*, 67, 96-102.

Munimbazi, G. T., Bullerman, L. B. (2000). Occurrence of fumonsins and moniliformin in corn and corn-based food products of U.S. origin. *Journal of Food Protection*, 63, 1732-1737.

Murillo-Arbizu, M., Amézqueta, S., González-Peñas, E., López de Cerain, A. (2009). Occurrence of patulin and its dietary intake through apple juice consumption by the Spanish population. *Food Chemistry*, 113, 420-423.

Murphy, P. A., Hendrich, S., Landgren, C., Bryant, C. M. (2006). Food mycotoxins: an update. *Journal of Food Science*, 71, 51-65.

Musser, S. M., Plattner, R. D. (1997). Fumonisin composition in cultures of *Fusarium moniliforme*, *Fusarium proliferatum*, and *Fusarium nygami*. *Journal of Agricultural and Food Chemistry*, 45, 1169-1173.

Nelson, P. E., Plattner, R. D., Shackelford, D. D., Desjardins, A. E. (1992). Fumonisin B_1 production by *Fusarium* species other than *F. moniliforme* in section *Liseola* and by some related species. *Applied and Environmental Microbiology*, 58, 984-989.

Ngindu, A., Kenya, P. R., Ocheng, D. M., Omondi, T. N., Ngare, W., Gatei, D., Johnson, B. K., Ngira, J. A., Nandwa, H., Jansen, A. J., Kaviti, J. N., Siongok, T. A. (1982). Outbreak of acute hepatitis caused by aflatoxin poisoning in Kenya. *The Lancet*, 319, 1346-1348.

Nguyen, M. T., Tozlovanu, M., Tran, T. L., Pfohl-Leszkowicz, A. (2007). Occurrence of aflatoxin B_1, citrinin and ochratoxin A in rice in five provinces of the central region of Vietnam. *Food Chemistry*, 105, 42-47.

Norred, W. P., Porter, J. K., Dorner, J. W., Cole, R. J. (1988). Occurrence of the mycotoxin cyclopiazonic acid in meat after oral administration to chickens. *Journal of Agriculture and Food Chemistry*, 36, 113-136.

Northolt, M. D., Bullerman, L. B. (1982). Prevention of mold growth and toxin production through control of environmental condition. *Journal of Food Protection*, 45, 519-525.

Northolt, M. D., Van Egmond, H. P., Paulsch, W. E. (1978). Patulin production by some fungal species in relation to water activity and temperature. *Journal of Food Protection*, 41, 885-890.

Northolt, M. D., Van Egmond, H. P., Soentoro, R., Deijll, E. (1980). Fungal growth and the presence of sterigmatocystin in hard cheese. *Journal Association of Official Analytical Chemists*, 63, 115-119.

Nuryono, C. T., Noviandi, C. T. Agus, A., Wedhastri, S., Maryudani, Y. B., Böhm, J., Razzazi, E. (2002). A survey of fumonisins (B_1, B_2, B_3) in Indonesian corn-based food and feed samples. *Mycotoxin Research*, 18, 117-120.

Ohmono, S., Sugita, M., Abe, M. (1973). Isolation of cyclopiazonic acid, cyclopiazonic acid imine and bissedehydrocyclopiazonic acid from the cultures of *Aspergillus versicolor* (Vuill.) Tiraboshi. *J. Agric. Chem. Soc.*, 47, 57-63.

Ohtsubo, K., Ryu, J. C., Nakamura, K., Izumayama, N., Tanaka, T., Yamamura, H., Kobayashi, T., Ueno, Y. (1989). Chronic toxicity of nivalenol in female mice: a 2 year feeding study with *Fusarium nivale* Fn 2b moulded rice. *Food and Chemical Toxicology*, 27, 591-598.

Oliveira, C. A. F., Sebastião, L. S., Fagundes, H., Rosim, R. E., Fernandes, A. M. (2008). Aflatoxins and cyclopiazonic acid in feed and milk from dairy farms in São Paulo, Brazil. *Food Additives and Contaminants Part B*, 1, 147-152.

Olsen, M., Jonsson, N., Magan, N., Banks, J., Fanelli, C., Rizzo, A., Haikara, A., Dobson, A., Frisvad, J., Holmes, S., Olkku, J., Persson, S. J., Börjesson, T. (2003). Prevention of ochratoxin A in cereals. Final report to project OTA PREV-QLK1-CT-1999-00433 from 1 February 2000 to 31 October 2003. Available from: http://www.slv.se/upload/dokument/fou/MIB/FINAL%20REPORT.pdf.

Omurtag, G. Z. (2001). Determination of fumonisin B_1 and B_2 in corn and corn-based products in Turkey by high performance liquid chromatography, *Journal of Food Protection*, 64, 1072-1075.

Omurtag, G. Z., Yazıcıoğlu, D. (2001). Occurrence of T-2 toxin in processed cereals and pulses in Turkey determined by HPLC and TLC. *Food Additives and Contaminants*, 18, 844-849.

Paepens, C., De Saeger, S., Sibanda, L., Barna-Vetró, I., Anselme, M., Larondelle, Y., Van Peteghem, C. (2005). Evaluation of fumonisin contamination in cornflakes on the Belgian market by "flow-through" assay screening and LC-MS/MS analyses. *Journal of Agricultural and Food Chemistry*, 53, 7337-7343.

Park, J. W., Choi, S.-Y., Hwang, H.-J., Kim, Y.-B. (2005). Fungal mycoflora and mycotoxins in Korean polished rice destined for humans. *International Journal of Food Microbiology*, 103, 305-314.

Park, J. W., Kim, E. K., Shon, D. H., Kim, Y. K. (2002). Natural co-occurrence of aflatoxin B_1, fumonisin B_1 and ochratoxin A in barley and corn foods from Korea. *Food Additives and Contaminants*, 19, 1073-1080.

Patel, S., Hazel, C. M., Winterton, A. G. M., Gleadle, A. E. (1997). Surveillance of fumonisins in UK maize-based foods and other cereals. *Food Additives and Contaminants*, 14, 187-191.

Petersen, A., Thorup, I. (2001). Preliminary evaluation of fumonisins by the Nordic countries and occurrence of fumonisins (FB_1 and FB_2) in corn-based foods on the Danish market. *Food Additives and Contaminants*, 18, 221-226.

Pfohl-Leszkowicz, A., Chekir-Ghedir, L., Bacha, H. (1995). Genotoxicty of zearalenone, an ostrogenic mycotoxin: DNA adduct formation in female mouse tissues. *Carcinogenesis*, 16, 2315-2320.

Piemontese, L., Solfrizzo, M., Visconti, A. (2005). Occurrence of patulin in conventional and organic fruit products in Italy and subsequent exposure assessment. *Food Additives and Contaminants*, 22, 437-442.

Pinto, V. F., Patriarca, A., Locani, O., Vaamonde, G. (2001). Natural co-occurrence of aflatoxin and cyclopiazonic acid in peanuts grown in Argentina. *Food Additives and Contaminants*, 18, 1017-1020.

Pittet, A., Parisod, V., Schellenberg, M. (1992). Occurrence of fumonisins B_1 and B_2 in corn-based products from the Swiss market. *Journal of Agricultural and Food Chemistry*, 40, 1352-1354.

Pitt, J. I., Basilico, J. C., Abarca, M. L., Lopez, C. (2000). Mycotoxins and toxigenic fungi. *Medical Mycology*, 38, 41-46.

Pitt, J. I., Cruickshank, R. H., Leistner, L. (1986). *Penicillium commune*, *Penicillium camaberti*, the origin of white cheese mould, and the production of cyclopiazonic acid. *Food Microbiology*, 3, 363-371.

Pitt, J. I., Hocking, A. D. (1997). Fungi and food spoilage, 2nd edition, London: Blackie Academic and Professional.

Pitt, J. I. (2000). Toxigenic fungi: which are important? *Medical Mycology*, 38, 17-22.

Pitt, J. I. (1997). Toxigenic *Penicillium* species. In: Doyle, M. P., Beuchat, L. R., Montville, T. J. (Eds.), *Food Microbiology Fundamentals and Frontiers*, American Society for Microbiology, Washington, DC, USA, pp: 406-418.

Placinta, C. M., D'Mello, J. P. F., Macdonald, A. M. C. (1999). A review of worldwide contamination of cereal grains and animal feed with *Fusarium* mycotoxins. *Animal Feed Science and Technology*, 78, 21-37.

Poapolathep, A., Ohtsuka, R., Kiatipattanasakul, W., Ishigami, N., Nakayama, H., Doi, K. (2002). Nivalenol-induced apoptosis in thymus, spleen and Peyer's patches of mice. *Experimental and Toxicologic Pathology*, 53, 441-446.

Prieta, J., Moreno, M. A., Díaz, S., Suárez, G., Domínguez, L. (1994). Survey of patulin in apple juice and children's apple food by the diphasic dialysis membrane procedure. *Journal of Agricultural and Food Chemistry*, 42, 1701-1703.

Purchase, I. F. H. (1971). The acute toxicity of the mycotoxin cyclopiazonic acid to rats. *Toxicology and Applied Pharmacology*, 18, 114-123.

Rabie, C. J., Lübben, A., Louw, A. I., Rathbone, E. B., Steyn, P. S., Vleggaar, R. (1978). Moniliformin, a mycotoxin from *Fusarium* fusarioides. *Journal of Agricultural and Food Chemistry*, 26, 375-379.

Rabie, C. J., Marasas, W. F. O., Thiel, P. G., Lübben, A., Vleggaar, R. (1982). Moniliformin production and toxicity of different *Fusarium* species from southern Africa. *Applied and Environmental Microbiology*, 43, 517-521.

Rabie, C. J., Sydenham, E. W., Thiel, P. G., Lübben, A., Marasas, W. F. O. (1986). T-2 toxin production by *Fusarium acuminatum* isolated from oats and barley. *Applied and Environmental Microbiology*, 52, 594-596.

Rafai, P., Pettersson, H., Bata, Á., Papp, Z., Glávits, R., Tuboly, S., Ványi, A., Soós, P. (2000). Effect of dietary T-2 fusariotoxin concnetrations on the health and production of white Pekin duck broilers. *Poultry Science*, 79, 1548-1556.

Rao, L. B., Husain, A. (1985). Presence of cyclopiazonic acid in kodo millet (*Paspalum scrobicalutum*) causing "kodua poisoning" in man and its production by associated fungi. *Mycopathologia*, 89, 177-180.

Rasmussen, P. H., Ghorbani, F., Berg, T. (2003). Deoxynivalenol and other *Fusarium* toxins in wheat and rye flours on the Danish market. *Food Additives and Contaminants*, 20, 396-404.

Rheeder, J. P., Marasas, W. F. O., Thiel, P. G., Sydenham, E. W., Shephard, G. S., Van Schalkyk, D. J. (1992). *Fusarium moniliforme* and fumonisisns in corn in relation to human esophageal cancer in Transkei. *Phytopathology*, 82, 353-357.

Rheeder, J. P., Marasas, W. F. O., Vismer, H. F. (2002). Production of fumonisin analogs by *Fusarium* species. *Applied and Environmental Microbiology*, 68, 2101-2105.

Riley, R. T., Goeger, D. E., Yoo, H., Showker, J. L. (1992). Comparison of three tetramic acids and their ability to alter membrane function in cultured skeletal muscle cells and sarcoplasmic reticulum vesicles. *Toxicology and Applied Pharmacology*, 114, 261-267.

Ritieni, A. (2003). Patulin in Italian commercial apple products. *Journal of Agricultural and Food Chemistry*, 51, 6086-6090.

Rogers, C. G., Héroux-Metcalf, C. (1983). Cytotoxicity and absence of mutagenic activity of vomitoxin (4-deoxynivalenol) in a hepatocyte-mediated mutation assay with V79 Chinese hamster lung cells. *Cancer Letters*, 20, 29-35.

Roland, J. O., Beuchat, L. R. (1984). Influence of temperature and water activity on growth and patulin production by *Byssochlamys nivea* in apple juice. *Applied and Environmental Microbiology*, 47, 205-207.

Ross, P. F., Nelson, P. E., Richard, J. L., Osweiler, G. D., Rice, L. G., Plattner, R. D., Wilson, T. M. (1990). Production of fumonisins by *Fusarium moniliforme* and *Fusarium proliferatum* isolates associated with equine leukoencephalomalacia and a pulmonary edema syndrome in swine. *Applied and Environmental Microbiology*, 56, 3225-3226.

Rotter, B. A., Perlusky, D. B., Pestka, J. J. (1996). Toxicology of deoxynivalenol (vomitoxin). *Journal of Toxicology and Environmental Health*, 48, 1-34.

Rotter, B. A., Thompson, B. K., Clarkin, S., Owen, T. C. (1993). Rapid colorimetric bioassay for screening of *Fusarium* mycotoxins. *Natural Toxins*, 1, 303-307.

Rovira, R., Ribera, F., Sanchis, V., Canela, R. (1993). Improvements in the quantitation of patulin in apple juice by high-performance liquid chromatography. *Journal of Agricultural and Food Chemistry*, 41, 214-216.

Ryu, J.-C., Ohtsubo, K., Izumiyama, N., Mori, M., Tanaka, T., Ueno, Y. (1987). Effects of nivalenol on the bone marrow in mice. *Journal of Toxicological Sciences*, 12, 11-21.

Ryu, J.-C., Ohtsubo, K., Izumiyama, N., Nakamura, K., Tanaka, T., Yamamura, H., Ueno, Y. (1988). The acute and chronic toxicities of nivalenol in mice. *Fundamental and Applied Toxicology*, 11, 38-47.

Saito, M., Enomoto, M., Tatsuno, T., Uraguchi, K. (1971). Yellowed rice toxins: Luteroskyrin and related compounds, chlorine-containing compounds, citrinin and citreoviridin. In: Ciegler, A., Kadis, S., Ajl, S. J. (Eds.), *Microbial Toxins*, vol. 6. *Fungal Toxins*, Academic Press, New York, pp: 299-380.

Salem, N. M., Ahmad, R. (2010). Mycotoxins in food from Jordan: Preliminary survey. *Food Control*, 21, 1099-1103.

Sanchis, V., Abadias, M., Oncins, L., Sala, N., Viñas, I., Canela, R. (1994). Occurrence of fumonisins B_1 and B_2 in corn-based products from the Spanish market. *Applied and Environmental Microbiology*, 60, 2147-2148.

Sangare-Tigori, B., Moukha, S., Kouadio, H. J., Betbeder, A.-M., Dano, D. S., Creppy, E. E. (2006). Co-occurrence of aflatoxin B_1, fumonisin B_1, ochratoxin A and zearalenone in cereals and peanuts from Côte d'Ivoire. *Food Additives and Contaminants*, 23, 1000-1007.

Saxena, N., Dwivedi, P. D., Ansari, K. M., Das, M. (2008). Patulin in apple juices: Incidence and likely intake in an Indian population. *Food Additives and Contaminants Part B*, 1, 140-146.

Scaff, R. M. C., Scussel, V. M. (2004). Fumonisins B_1 and B_2 in corn-based products commercialized in the state of Santa Catarina-Southern Brazil. *Brazilian Archives of Biology and Technology*, 47, 911-919.

SCF (Scientific Committee on Food). (1998). Opinion on ochratoxin A, expressed on 17 September 1998, European Commission.

SCF. (1999). Opinion on Fusarium toxins, part 1: Deoxynivalenol (DON). European Commission SCF/CS/CNTM/MYC/19 Final, Brussels, Belgium.

SCF. (2000a). Opinion of the scientific committee on food on *Fusarium* toxins, part 2: Zearalenone (ZEA), SCF/CS/CNTM/MYC22 Rev. 3 Final, 22 June 2000, pp: 1-12.

SCF. (2000b). Opininon of the Scientific Committee on Food on *Fusarium* toxins, Part 3: Fumonisin B_1 (FB_1). SCF/CS/CNTM/MYC/24 FINAL, Brussel, Belgium.

SCF. (2000c). Opinion of the Scientific Committee on Food on *Fusarium* toxins, part 4: Nivalenol, European Commission SCF/CS/CNTM/MYC/26 Final, Brussel, Belgium.

SCF. (2001). Opinion of the Scientific Committee on Food on *Fusarium* toxins, part 5: T-2 toxin and HT-2 toxin, European Commission SCF/CS/CNTM/MYC/25 Rev. 6 Final, Brussel, Belgium.

Schneweis, I., Meyer, K., Engelhardt, G., Bauer, J. (2002). Occurrence of zearalenone-4-β-D-glucopyranoside in wheat. *Journal of Agricultural and Food Chemistry*, 50, 1736-1738.

Schollonberger, M., Drochner, W., Rüfle, M., Suchy, S., Terry-Jara, H., Müller, H.-M. (2005). Trichothecene toxins in different groups of conventional and organic bread of the German market. *Journal of Food Composition and Analysis*, 18, 69-78.

Schollonberger, M., Jara, H. T., Suchy, S., Drochner, W., Müller, H.-M. (2002). *Fusarium* toxins in wheat flour collected in an area in southwest Germany. *International Journal of Food Microbiology*, 72, 85-89.

Schollenberger, M., Müller, H.-M., Rüfle, M., Suchy, S., Planck, S., Drochner, W. (2005). Survey of *Fusarium* toxins in foodstuffs of plant origin marketed in Germany. *International Journal of Food Microbiology*, 97, 317-326.

Scott, P. M., Abbas, H. K., Mirocha, C. J., Lawrance, G. A., Weber, D. (1987). Formation of moniliformin by *Fusarium sporotrichoides* and *Fusarium culmorum*. *Applied and Environmental Microbiology*, 53, 196-197.

Scott, P. M. (1993). Fumonisins. *International Journal of Food Microbiology*, 18, 257-270.

Scott, P. M., Van Walbeek, W., Kennedy, B., Anyeti, D. (1972). Mycotoxins (ochratoxin A, citrinin and sterigmatocystin) and toxigenic fungi in grains and other agricultural products. *Journal of Agricultural Food Chemistry*, 20, 1103-1109.

Scudamore, K. A., Hetmanski, M. T., Chan, H. K., Collins, S. (1997). Occurrence of mycotoxins in raw ingredients used for animal feeding stuffs in the United Kingdom in 1992. *Food Additives and Contaminants*, 14, 157-173.

Sewram, V., Nieuwoudt, T. W., Marasas, W. F. O., Shephard, G. S., Ritieni, A. (1999). Determination of the mycotoxin moniliformin in cultures of *Fusarium subglutinans* and in naturally contaminated maize by high-performance liquid chromatography-atmospheric pressure chemical ioinization mass spectrometry. *Journal of Chromatography A*, 848, 185-191.

Sewram, V., Shephard, G. S., Van der Merwe, L., Jacobs, T. V. (2006). Mycotoxin contamination of dietary and medical wild plants in the Eastern Cape province of South Africa. *Journal of Agricultural and Food Chemistry*, 54, 5688-5693.

Sharman, M., Gilbert, J., Chelkowski, J. (1991). A survey of the occurrence of the mycotoxin moniliformin in cereal samples from sources worldwide. *Food Additives and Contaminants*, 8, 459-466.

Shephard, G. S. (2008a). Impact of mycotoxins on human health in developing countries. *Food Additives and Contaminants,* 146-151.

Shephard, G. S., Marasas, W. F. O., Leggott, N. L., Yazdanpanah, H., Rahimian, H., Safavi, N. (2000). Natural occurrence of fumonisins in corn from Iran. *Journal of Agricultural and Food Chemistry*, 48, 1860-1864.

Shephard, G. S. (2008b). Risk assessment of aflatoxins in food in Africa. *Food Additives and Contaminants*, 25, 1246-1256.

Shephard, G. S., Van Der Westhuizen, L., Gatyeni, P. M., Katerere, D. R., Marasas, W. F. O. (2005a). Do fumonisin mycotoxins occur in wheat. *Journal of Agricultural and Food Chemistry*, 53, 9293-9296.

Shephard, G. S., Van Der Westhuizen, L., Gatyeni, P. M., Somdyala, N. I. M., Burger, H.-M., Marasas, W. F. O. (2005b). Fumonisin mycotoxins in traditional Xhosa maize beer in South Africa. *Journal of Agricultural and Food Chemistry*, 53, 9634-9637.

Shetty, P. H., Bhat, R. V. (1997). Natural occurrence of fumonisin B_1 and its co-occurrence with aflatoxin B_1 in Indian sorghum, maize and poultry feeds. *Journal of Agricultural and Food Chemistry*, 45, 2170-2173.

Shinozuka, J., Guanmin, L., Uetsuka, K., Nakayama, H., Doi, K. (1997). Process of the development of T-2 toxin-induced apoptosis in the lymphoid organs of mice. *Experimental Animals*, 46, 117-126.

Shinozuka, J., Suziki, H., Tsutsui, S., Nakayama, H., Doi, K. (2001). T-2 toxin-induced apoptosis and c-fos mRNA expression in con A-stimulated mouse thymocyte primary cultures. *Journal of Toxicologic Pathology*, 14, 247-251.

Smith, E. E., Kubena, L. F., Braithewaite, C. E., Harvey, R. B., Phillips, T. D., Reine, A. H. (1992). Toxicological evaluation of aflatoxin and cyclopiazonic acid in broiler chickens. *Poultry Science*, 71, 1136-1144.

Smith, J. E., Lewis, C. W., Anderson, J. G., Solomons, G. L. (1994). Mycotoxins in human health. Report EUR16048 EN. European Commission, Directorate-General XII, Brussels.

Solfrizzo, M., De Girolamo, A., Visconti, A. (2001). Determination of fumonisin B_1 and B_2 in cornflakes by high performance liquid chromatography and immunoaffinity clean-up. *Food Additives and Contaminants*, 18, 227-235.

Solovey, M. M. S., Somoza, C., Cano, G., Pacin, A., Resnik, S. (1999). A survey of fumonisins, deoxynivalenol, zearalenone and aflatoxins contamination in corn-based food products in Argentina. *Food Additives and Contaminants*, 16, 325-329.

Sorenson, W. G., Simpson, J. (1986). Toxicity of penicillic acid for rat alveolar macrophages *in vitro*. *Environmental Research*, 41, 505-513.

Spadaro, D., Garibaldi, A., Gullino, M. L. (2008). Occurrence of patulin and its dietary intake through pear, peach, and apricot juices in Italy. *Food Additives and Contaminants Part B*, 1, 134-139.

Stockmann-Juvala, H. (2007). Neuro- and immunotoxic effects of fumonisin B_1 in cells. Academic Dissertation, Faculty of Pharmacy of the University of Helsinki, 75p, Helsinki.

Stoloff, L. (1983). Aflatoxin as a cause of primary liver-cell cancer in the United States a probability study. *Nutrition and Cancer*, 5, 165-186.

Sudakin, D. L. (2003). Trichothecenes in the environment: relevance to human health. *Toxicology Letters*, 143, 97-107.

Sweeney, M. J., Dobson, A. D. W. (1998). Mycotoxin production by *Aspergillus*, *Fusarium* and *Penicillium* species. *International Journal of Food Microbiology*, 43, 141-158.

Sydenham, E. W., Shephard, G. S., Thiel, P. G., Marasas, W. F. O., Rheeder, J. P., Sanhueza, C. E. P., González, H. H. L., Resnik, S. L. (1993). Fumonisins in Argentinian field-trial corn. *Journal of Agricultural and Food Chemistry*, 41, 891-895.

Sydenham, E. W., Thiel, P. G., Marasas, W. F. O., Shephard, G. S., Van Schalkwyk, D. J., Koch, K. R. (1990). Natural occurrence of some mycotoxins in corn from low and high esophageal cancer prevalence areas of the Transkei, Sothern Africa. *Journal of Agricultural and Food Chemistry*, 38, 1900-1903.

Takahashi, M., Shibutani, M., Sugita-Konishi, Y., Aihara, M., Inoue, K., Woo, G.-H., Fujimoto, H., Hirose, M. (2008). A 90-day subchronic toxicity study of nivalenol, a trichothecene mycotoxin, in F344 rats. *Food and Chemical Toxicology*, 46, 125-135.

Tangni, E. K., Theys, R., Mignolet, E., Maudoux, M., Michelet, J. Y., Larondelle, Y. (2003). Patulin in domestic and imported apple-based drinks in Belgium: occurrence and exposure assessment. *Food Additives and Contaminants*, 20, 482-489.

Terao, K. (1983). Stergimatocystin-a masked potent carcinogenic mycotoxin. *Journal of Toxicology-Toxin Reviews*, 2, 77-110.

Thiel, P. G., Gelderblom, W. C. A., Marasas, W. F. O., Nelson, P. E., Wilson, T. M. (1986). Natural occurrence of moniliformin and fusarin C in corn screenings known to be hepatocarcinogenic in rats. *Journal of Agricultural and Food Chemistry*, 34, 773-775.

Thiel, P. G., Meyer, C. J., Marasas, W. F. O. (1982). Natural occurrence of moniliformin together with deoxynivalenol and zearalenone in Transkeian corn. *Journal of Agricultural and Food Chemistry*, 30, 308-312.

Thompson, W. L., Wannamacher, R. W. (1990). *In vivo* effects of T-2 mycotoxin on synthesis of proteins and DNA in rat tissues. *Toxicology and Applied Pharmacology*, 105, 483-491.

Thuvander, A., Möller, T., Enghardt Barbieri, H., Jansson, A., Salomonsson, A.-C., Olsen, M. (2001). Dietary intake of some important mycotoxins by the Swedish population. *Food Additives and Contaminants*, 18, 696-706.

Tomczak, M., Wisniewska, H., Stepien, L., Kostecki, M., Chelkowski, J., Golinski, P. (2002). Deoxynivalenol, nivalenol and moniliformin in wheat samples with head blight (scab) symptoms in Poland (1998-2000). *European Journal of Plant Pathology*, 108, 625-630.

Torres, A. M., Reynoso, M. M., Rojo, F. G., Ramirez, M. L., Chulze, S. N. (2001). *Fusarium* species (section *Liseola*) and its mycotoxins in maize harvested in northern Argentina. *Food Additives and Contaminants*, 18, 836-843.

Torres, M. R., Sanchis, V., Ramos, A. J. (1998). Occurrence of fumonisins in Spanish beers analyzed by an enzyme-linked immunosorbent assay of method. *International Journal of Food Microbiology*, 39, 139-143.

Trucksess, M. W., Tang, Y. (1999). Solid-phase extraction method for patulin in apple juice and unfiltered apple juice. *Journal of AOAC International*, 82, 1109-1113.

Trucksess, M. W., Thomas, F., Young, K., Stack, M. E., Fulgueras, W. J., Page, S. W. (1995). Survey of deoxynivalenol in U.S. 1993 wheat and barley crops by enzyme-linked immunosorbent assay. *Journal of AOAC International*, 78, 631-636.

Tryphonas, H., Bondy, G., Miller, J. D., Lacroix, F., Mcguire, P., Fernie, S., Miller, D., Hayward, S. (1997). Effects of fumonisin B_1 on the immune system of Sprague-Dawley rats following a 14-day oral (gavage) exposure. *Fundamental and Applied Toxicology*, 39, 53-59.

Tseng, T.-C., Liu, C.-Y. (1999). Natural occurrence of fumonisins B_1 and B_2 in domestic maize of Taiwan. *Journal of Agricultural and Food Chemistry*, 47, 4799-4801.

Tseng, T.-C., Liu, C.-Y. (1997). Occurrence of fumonisin B_1 and B_2 in corn-based foodstuffs in Taiwan market. *Mycopathologia*, 137, 57-61.

Tutelyan, V. A. (2004). Deoxynivalenol in cereals in Russia. *Toxicology Letters*, 153, 173-179.

Ueno, Y., Hjima, K., Wang, S.-D., Sugiura, Y., Sekijima, M., Tanaka, T., Chen, C., Yu, S.-Z. (1997). Fumonisins as a possible contributory risk factor for primary liver cancer: A 3-year study of corn harvested in Haimen, China, by HPLC and ELISA. *Food and Chemical Toxicology*, 35, 1143-1150.

Ueno, Y., Sato, N., Ishii, K., Sakai, K., Tsunoda, H., Enomoto, M. (1973). Biological and chemical detection of trichothecene mycotoxins of *Fusarium* species. *Applied Microbiology*, 25, 699-704.

Ueno, Y. (1985). The toxicology of mycotoxins. *Critical Reviews in Toxicology*, 14, 99-132.

Ueno, Y. (1984). Toxicological features of T-2 toxin and related trcihothecenes. *Fundamental Applied Toxicology*, 4, 124-132.

Ueno, Y., Umemori, K., Nilimi, E., Tanuma, S., Nagata, S., Sugamata, M., Ihara, T., Sekijima, M., Kawai, K., Ueno, I., Tashiro, F. (1995). Induction of apoptosis by T-2 toxin and other natural toxins in HL-60 human promyelotic leukemia cells. *Natural Toxins*, 3, 129-137.

Uhlig, S., Torp, M., Jarp, J., Parich, A., Gutleb, A. C., Krska, R. (2004). Moniliformin in Norwegian grain. *Food Additives and Contaminants*, 21, 598-606.

Urano, T., Trucksess, M. W., Baever, R. W., Wilson, D. M., Dorner, J. W., Dowell, F. E. (1992). Co-occurrence of cyclopiazonic acid and aflatoxins in corn and peanuts. *Journal of AOAC International*, 75, 838-841.

Usleber, E., Straka, M., Terplan, G. (1994). Enzyme immunoassay for fumonisin B_1 applied to corn-based foods. *Journal of Agricultural and Food Chemistry*, 42, 1392-1396.

Vargas, E. A., Preis, R. A., Castro, L., Silva, C. M. G. (2001). Co-occurrence of aflatoxins B_1, B_2, G_1, G_2, zearalenone and fumonisin B_1 in Brazilian corn. *Food Additives and Contaminants*, 18, 981-986.

Var, I., Kabak, B. (2007). Occurrence of ochratoxin A in Turkish wines. *Microchemical Journal*, 86, 241-247.

Velluti, A., Marín, S., Sanchis, V., Ramos, A. J. (2001). Occurrence of fumonisin B_1 in Spanish corn-based foods for animal and human consumption. *Food Science and Technology International*, 7, 433-437.

Veršilovskis, A., Bartkevičs, V., Mikelsone, V. (2008a). Sterigmatocystin presence in typical Latvian grains. *Food Chemistry*, 109, 243-248.

Veršilovskis, A., De Saeger, S., Mikelsone, V. (2008b). Determination of sterigmatocystin in beer by high performance liquid chromatography with ultraviolet detection. *World Mycotoxin Journal*, 1, 161-166.

Veršilovskis, A., De Saeger, S. (2010). Sterigmatocystin: Occurrence in foodstuffs and analytical methods-an overview. *Molecular Nutrition and Food Research*, 54, 136-147.

Veršilovskis, A., Mikelsone, V. (2008). Stergimatocystin presence in different Latvian bread samples. *Foodbalt*, 156-160.

Veršilovskis, A., Van Peteghem, C., De Saeger, S. (2009). Determination of sterigmatocystin in cheese by high-performance liquid chromatography-tandem mass spectrometry. *Food Additives and Contaminants*, 26, 127-133.

Vesonder, R. F., Ellis, J. J., Kwolek, W. F., DeMarini, D. J. (1982). Production of vomitoxin on corn by *Fusarium graminearum* NRRL 5883 and *Fusarium roseum* NRRL 6101. *Applied and Environmental Microbiology*, 43, 967-970.

Vesonder, R. F., Horn, B. (1985). Sterigmatocystin in dairy cattle feed contaminated with *Aspergillus versicolor*. *Applied and Environmental Microbiology*, 49, 234-235.

Vesonder, R. (1986). Moniliformin produced by cultures of *Fusarium moniliforme* var. *subglutinans* isolated from swine feed. *Mycopathologia*, 95, 149-153.

Vrabcheva, T., Usleber, E., Dietrich, R., Märtlbauer, E. (2000). Co-occurrence of ochratoxin A and citrinin in cereals from Bulgarian villages with a history of Balkan Endemic Nephropathy. *Journal of Agricultural and Food Chemistry*, 48, 2483-2488.

Wagacha, J. M., Muthomi, J. W. (2007). *Fusarium culmorum*: Infection process, mechanisms of mycotoxin production and their role in pathogenesis in wheat. *Crop Protection*, 26, 877-885.

Walker, R. (1999). Mycotoxins of growing interest, ochratoxins. Third Joint FAO/WHO/UNEP international conference on mycotoxins, MYC-CONF/99/5b, 3-6 March, Tunisia.

Wang, J.-S., Groopman, J. D. (1999). DNA damage by mycotoxins. *Mutation Research*, 424, 167-181.

Wang, Z. G., Feng, J. N., Tong, Z. (1993). Human toxicosis caused by mouldy rice contaminated with *Fusarium* and T-2 toxin. *Biomedical and Environmental Sciences*, 6, 65-70.

Wheeler, J. L., Harrison, M. A., Koehler, P. E. (1987). Presence and stability of patulin in pasteurized apple cider. *Journal of Food Science*, 52, 479-480.

Wheeler, K. A., Hurdman, B. F., Pitt, J. I. (1991). Influence of pH on the growth of some toxigenic species of *Aspergillus*, *Penicillium* and *Fusarium*. *International Journal of Food Microbiology*, 12, 141-150.

WHO (World Health Organization). (1995). Evaluation of certain food additives and contaminants. *Forty-fourth Report of the Joint FAO/WHO Expert Committee on Food Additives*. Technical report series 859, Geneva, Switzerland, pp: 36-38.

Widiastuti, R., Maryam, R., Blaney, B. J., Stoltz, S., Stoltz, D. R. (1988). Cyclopiazonic acid in combination with aflatoxins, zearalenone and ochratoxin A in Indonesian corn. *Mycopathologia*, 104, 153-156.

Wilson, D. M., Mubatanhema, W., Jurjevic, Z. (2002). Biology and ecology of mycotoxigenic *Aspergillus* species as related to economic and health concerns. In: Devries J. W., Trucksess, M. W., Jackson, L. S. (Eds), *Mycotoxins and Food Safety*, Kluwer Academic/Plenum Publishers, New York, USA, pp: 3-18.

Yoshizawa, T., Mirocha, C. J., Behrens, J. C., Swanson, S. P. (1981). Metabolic fate of T-2 toxin in a lactating animals. *Food and Cosmetics Toxicology*, 19, 31-39.

Yoshizawa, T., Yamashita, A., Luo, Y. (1994). Fumonisin occurrence in corn from high- and low-risk areas of human esophageal cancer in China. *Applied and Environmental Microbiology*, 60, 1626-1629.

Yurdun, T., Omurtag, G. Z., Ersoy, Ö. (2001). Incidence of patulin in apple juices marketed in Turkey. *Journal of Food Protection*, 64, 1851-1853.

Yu, S.-R., Liu, X.-J., Wang, Y.-H., Liu, J. A. (1995). A survey of moniliformin contamination of rice and corn from Keshan disease endemic and non-KSD areas in China. *Biomedical and Environmental Sciences*, 8, 330-334.

Zinedine, A., Brera, C., Elakhdari, S., Catano, C., Debegnach, F., Angelini, S., De Santis, B., Faid, M., Benlemlih, M., Minardi, V., Miraglia, M. (2006). Natural occurrence of mycotoxins in cereals and spices commercialized in Morocco. *Food Control*, 17, 868-874.

In: Nutritional Insights and Food Safety
Editor: Jaroslava Švarc-Gajiæ
ISBN: 978-1-61122-130-5

Chapter XII

Milk Production and Safety Food

Valente Velàzquez-Ordoñez[1a], Benjamin Valladares Carranza[b], Adriana Del Carmèn Gutìerrez Castillo[c], Martìn Talavera Rojas[c], Nazario Pescador Salas[c] and Roxana Valdès Ramos[d]

[a]Área de Inocuidad Alimentaria y Salud Pública, Centro de Investigación y Estudios Avanzados en Salud animal, Facultad de Medicina Veterinaria y Zootecnia, Universidad Autónoma del Estado de México, (CIESA-FMVZ-UAEM), Autopista de cuota Toluca-Atlacomulco Km 15.5, San Cayetano de Morelos, Toluca Estado de México CP 50200 México

[b]Área de Toxicología, Centro de Investigación y Estudios Avanzados en Salud animal, Facultad de Medicina Veterinaria y Zootecnia, Universidad Autónoma del Estado de México, CIESA-FMVZ-UAEM.

[c]Facultad de Medicina Veterinaria y Zootecnia, Universidad Autónoma del Estado de México, FMVZ-UAEM.

[d]Centro de investigación y estudios avanzados en Ciencias de la Salud, Facultad de Medicina, Universidad Autónoma del Estado de México (CIEACS-FM-UAEM)

Abstract

The safety of milk and dairy products is an important aspect in public health and milk industry puts a lot of efforts in the prevention and control of milk borne diseases, as well as in avoiding the toxic residues in milk products. In order to explain the complex relationship between the risk factors involved in milk production and the safety of dairy products, this paper consideres and elaborates several important topics: microbial aspects of the quality of dairy products, raw and pasteurized milk contamination, the relationship between the cow feeding conditions and milk composition, as well as the impact of environmental pollutants and agricultural pesticides residues on the quality of dairy products. Other aspects such as analytical methods are considered as well in order to present the means of controlling the milk quality in dairy industry management.

[1]vvo @uaemex.mx.

Introduction

The World milk production is a complex activity involving the sustainable production system of the dairy cattle husbandry with main priorities of maintaining a productive and healthy herd as well as providing the safety of dairy products (Smith et al., 2001). The main role of the modern dairy herd is to maintain the productivity and competitiveness in the milk market industry.

Milk is a basic food in human diet, in its original form or in the form of different dairy products. Considering the availability and the variety of milk products, the consumers have an opportunity to give the prevalence to safe and healthy products. Consumer behavior patterns may significantly vary depending on demographic, cultural and socioeconomic variations among human population (Gomes et al., 2008; Patilk et al., 2005).

Milk has a great value as a nutritious food; it is an important nutritional factor in the first stages of human life. However milk can also be an important source of bacterial infections and may threaten the human's health, especially when milk is consumed without pasteurization (Frank et al., 2001; Jayarao et al., 1999; Oliver et al., 2009). The sources of milk contamination by pathogens may arise from poor herd management and poor milk hygiene practice and mastitis (Callaway & Oliver, 2009; Gillespie et al., 2009; Oliver et al., 2009). In addition, mammary glands participate in the excretion of numerous xenobiotic substances, such as veterinary drug residues and environmental pollutants that can be found in grass lands, animal feedstuffs, and field crops. This factors affect the raw milk production and the quality of milk products and can further influence the consumer's health and nutrition (Murinda et al., 2002a). The milk market requires the safe and high quality products, free from pathogens and drug residues.

Contaminated farm environment can be a source of pathogens which can strongly affect the animal population, milk quality and emerge public health risk (Murinda et al., 2004). Presence of pathogens and chemical residues in milk is a principal indicator of the quality of milk and dairy products. The status of milk bulk tank offers quick information's about udder health status, environmental pathogens and chemical residues. When milk borne disease outbreaks occur in humans, there are many reasons to trace back and analyze the pasteurized and unpasteurized milk, as well as fresh cheeses produced from non-pasteurized milk. The pathogens from raw milk can persist in production systems a long time in the form of biofilms and can subsequently contaminate the processed milk products. Inadequate milk pasteurization allows survival of food borne pathogens in milk and dairy products (Barker et al., 1998; Oliver et al., 2009).

Important aspect that assures the sustainability of the milk quality involves the health educational programs which offer knowledge to consumers on how to handle the milk and dairy products and prevent the risk of food borne diseases from non-pasteurized raw milk and unsafe hygiene practices (Cremonesi et al., 2007; Tsegmed et al., 2007; Vernozy-Rozand et al., 2005).

In order to explain the relationship between dairy production and safety, this paper consideres different topics including the microbial aspects of the quality of dairy products, the routes of raw and pasteurized milk contamination, as well as the relationship between the cow feeding conditions and milk composition. Occurrence of environmental pollutants and agricultural residues in dairy products is also elaborated, as well as the analytical methods for controlling the milk quality. In this chapter the main principles of the dairy industry management are described.

1. Microbial Aspects of the Quality of Dairy Products

Milk products are characterized by high susceptibility to contamination by microorganisms. In recent years the incidence of viral food borne infections in human population increased. Therefore new strategies have to be developed to reduce the presence of infectious as well as environmental pathogens in bulk milk (Jørgensen et al., 2005). Among bacterial infections the *Salmonella* infections are the most frequent food diseases in food borne outbreaks. Considering that the frequent source of food borne diseases arises from the raw milk, food markets should pay a specific attention to control the risk of microbial milk contamination (Baumann & Sadkowska-Todys, 2008).

Semi hard cheese can keep microbial contaminants for a few months. Normally *Staphylococcus sciuri, Staphylococcus epidermidis, Staphylococcus saprophyticus, Staphylococcus aureus* are not detected in old cheese.

Herd health status is an important issue in milk production. The maintance of herd hygiene, disease control programmes, and preventive herd management are oriented to reduce the prevalence of contagious diseases in dairy cattle (Koskinen et al., 2009; Riyaz-Ul-Hassan et al., 2008; Velázquez-Ordoñez et al., 2008). Special attention is given to controlling the udder pathogens and mastitis in herds due to their significant sanitary and economical impact.

The intrammary infections in dairy cows can be caused by numerous microorganisms, which can be classified as infectious pathogens (*Staphylococcus aureus, Streptococcus agalactiae*), environmental pathogens (*Escherichia coli* and *Streptococcus* none agalactiae), and minor pathogens (coagulase negative *Staphylococcus*). The udder infections (subclinical and clinical mastitis) (Figure 1) may significantly increase the costs of herd management. Even for mild subclinical mastitis in dairy herd, indicated by the milk somatic cell count about 200,000 cells/mL, the milk losses are estimated to be 3 to 5 % of the milk yield production (Barker et al., 1998; Oliver et al., 1984). Mammary gland inflammation results in the reduction of milk yield by impaired glandular secretion.

The changes in milk yields and milk composition caused by mastitis depend on the severity and duration of the infection. Uninfected mammary gland contains <100,000 somatic cells per milk milliliter. Somatic cells counts >200,000/mL suggests an incipient mammary gland inflammatory response (Smith et al., 2001).

Bovine mastitis in dairy herds' affects milk composition by increasing the counts of milk somatic cells in milk, as well as serum proteins and enzymes; while sodium, chloride ion, calcium and casein are decreased in such milk (Bunning et al., 1988). The chemical changes observed in milk depend on the disease severity. Other undesirable mastitis effects include numerous bacterial toxins and abnormal proteins deriving from inflammatory tissue response. These compounds can influence the milk flavor and taste as well as the stability of milk product (Oliver & Calvinho, 1995). Affecting the milk quality and safety, bovine mastitis is considered as a disease with high economic impact to dairy production.

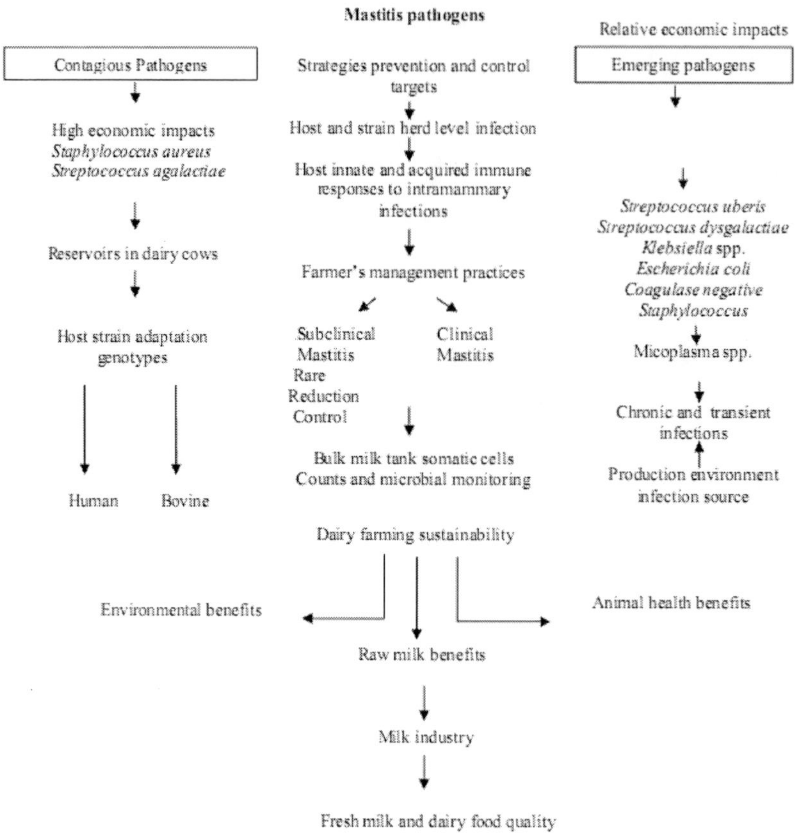

Figure 1. Economic impact of mastitis in dairy herds.

The most prevalent contagious pathogens isolated from dairy herds that produce long-term intramammary infections in dairy cows, include *Staphylococcus aureus* (Figure 2) and *Streptococcus agalactiae*. *Streptococcus uberis* and other bacterial coliforms are considered environmental pathogens affecting the milk safety mostly in dry periods and during lactation (Velázquez-Ordoñez et al., 2005a).

The prevention and control strategies combating mastitis in dairy herds include situational diagnostic and regular control of somatic cell counts as well as microbial agents in different stages of milk production. Such approach provides the strategic information's on the herd hygiene status and milking hygiene practices. Regular maintance of milk machines is mandatory. Monitoring the somatic cell counts in the bulk milk tanks and dairy cows during fresh and dry lactation periods provide the informations about the mammary health status in herds (Jayarao, 1999; Oliver et al., 1999; Rea et al., 1992; Ruegg & Tabone, 2000).

The mean values of somatic cells/mL >500,000 in milk indicates a serious mastitis problem in cow population. In such serious inflammations the occurrence of antibiotic residues in the bulk tank milk can be expected (Table 1). For preventing the milk contamination by veterinary drug resides the maintenance of udder health and milk hygiene practices are of high important as well as cow genetic selection programs (Ruegg & Tabone, 2000; Velázquez-Ordoñez et al., 2005b).

Pre and post milking disinfectant routines help reduce dramatically the sources of microbial infections, while udder hygiene in the milking practice directly reduces pathogen transmission by cows (Oliver et al., 1999). Reliable and prudent antibiotic use in herd medication schemes supports the effectiveness in the treatment of clinical mastitis, however such practice contributes to antibiotic residues in milk and to the development of bacterial resistance to antibiotics (Ruegg & Tabone, 2000; Tan et al., 2009). Antibiotic therapy used with neglecting the directions and prescriptions might be a significant public health concern. Antibiotic residues in milk may provoke allergic reactions and hypersensitivity in humans, and may induce resistance of bacteria leading to low response to antibiotherapy in humans.

Pasteurization has variable effects on antibiotic drug residues, influencing the quality of raw milk, fermented dairy products and cheeses. The possibility of some people to develop allergic type responses to milk and dairy products may be linked to antibiotics in milk. In order to minimize the content of antibiotics and other veterinary drug residues in milk, the milk discard period after veterinary treatment must be respected.

Table 1. Xenobiotics in Milk and Dairy Products

Xenobiotic	Residues and Contaminants	Contamination Source	Prevention Measures
Antibiotics	Aminoglycocide antibiotics; Neomycin, Dihidro streptomycin and Gentamycin. Tetracyclines; chlortetracycline, oxytetracicline, doxycicline. B-lactactam; penicillin and cephalosporin. Macrolyde antibiotics; erythromycin	Dairy cattle diseases treatment	Approved antibiotic use for milking dairy cattle. Observe milk withdrawal period. Preventive and reproductive management in fresh cow period and mastitis program.
Antihelmintics	Benzimidazole compounds and others	Nematode,cestode and trematode parasite protecting and treating control programs	Restricted antihelmintic drugs for milking dairy cattle. Observe use according to label directions and milk withdrawal period. Preventive herd management.
Pesticides	Compounds Pyrethroids	Insects control; adult, larvae protection develops in slowrry. Vectors control. Hygienic treatments directly on animal and the house farm. Field protection crops and stored grain conserving.	Observe use according to label directions. Legal limits. Agricola use licensed products. Food animal licensed products. Vector prevention and control.
Other veterinary drug products	Corticosteroids, Non-steroidal anti-inflammatory drugs (NSAID´s). Diuretics, Prostaglandins, hormones like and others products.	Special restricted drug treatment	Restricted and prohibited products for milking dairy cows.
Chemicals	Disinfectants; Iodine compounds	Thyroid gland effects	Iodine disinfectant for long periods use. Teat disinfectant over application, and over dosage in milking hygiene. Legal limits. Special formulated Iodinated products, observe use according to label directions.

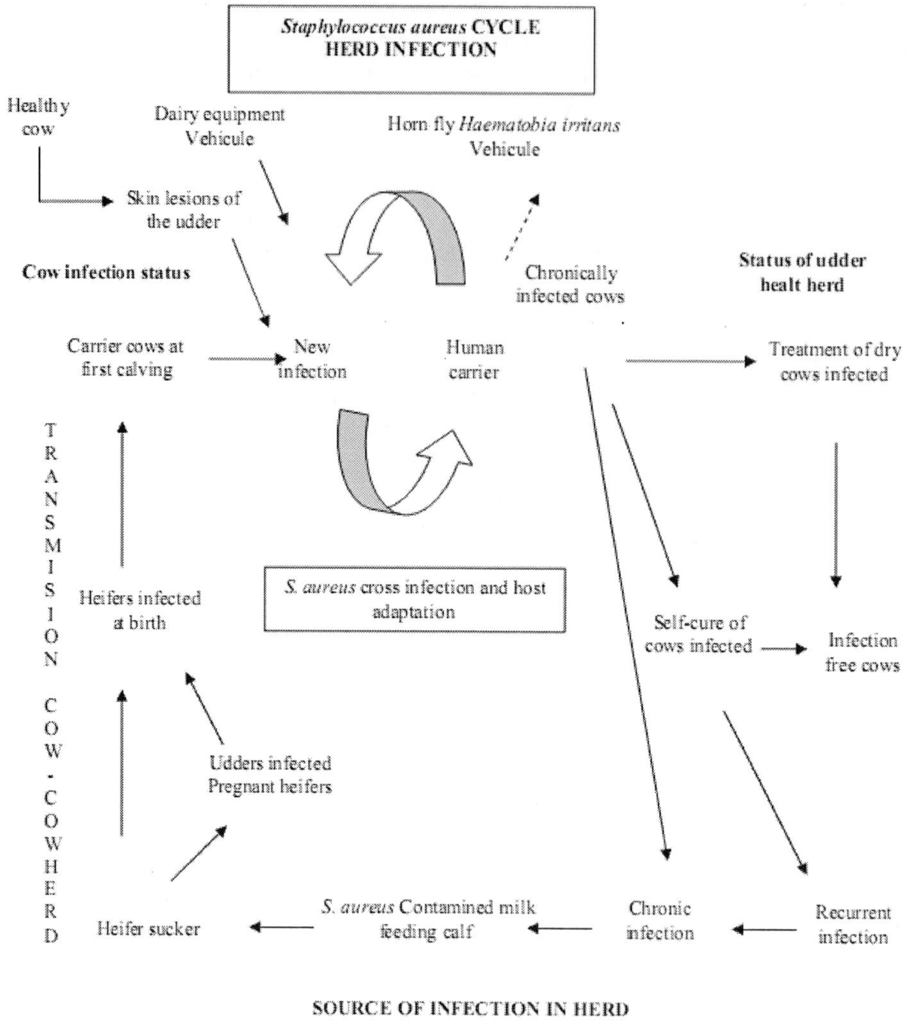

Figure 2. *Staphylococcus aureus* cycle of infection in small holder dairy herds.

The milk withdrawal period which reduces the residues of antibiotics and other drugs in raw milk is regulated by low in most of the countries. Some of the antibiotics which have shown to be very effective in veterinary treatment of herds are not yet officially approved and are suggested not to be used during lactating period (Gallo et al., 2008; Karlström et al., 2007).

The emerging public health concerns linked to veterinary treatment of the dairy herds is the development of antibiotic resistance of different bacterial pathogens. *Staphylococcus aureus* methicilline resistant strains (MRSA) and *Staphylococcus aureus* fluoroquinolone resistant strains (Velázquez-Ordoñez et al., 2005) have been identified in small dairy herds. The possibility of transmission of such strains (exotic *Staphylococcus aureus*) to human population is main public concern (Zamora et al., 1994). Other effects of antibiotic residues in milk to be considered include the decrease in the effectiveness of antibiotics in humans. The overall effects of the treatment of the dairy cows by antibiotics on human health, especially in prolonged antibiotic use, include the development of the antibiotic resistance and potential transfer of this resistance to other pathogens capable of producing human diseases, thereby decreasing therapeutic effectiveness of antibiotics in animal and human populations. Exposure of bacteria to antibiotics can result in selection of bacteria with broad antibiotic resistance patterns (Chao et al., 2007). Examples of antibiotic resistant animal bacterial pathogens include vancomicyn-resistant *Enterococcus* strains, DT 104 *Salmonella Typhimurium* and oxacillin/methicillin-resistant *Staphylococcus aureus* (ORSA/MRSA), which became the important subject of surveillance programmes in human health control (Moon et al., 2007; Trakulsonboon et al., 2001). The main mechanism of transmission of multi-resistant strains like MRSA is person-to-person contact, although domestic pets and farm animals are also implicated. The use of fluoroquinolones antibiotics in herd treatment should be avoided due to the rapid development of *S.aureus* resistance. Instead, linezolid, daptomycin or intrahospital can be used. Still, adequate hygiene practices are the most efficient measures to prevent the spread of nosocomial infections (Cercenado & Ruiz de Gopegui, 2008).

The potential development of antimicrobial resistance of bacteria in dairy cattle increased the awareness and concerns about the use of antimicrobials. In developing countries the antibiotic and veterinary drug administration is the subject of surveillance by agricultural department authorities (Committee on drug use in food animals, 1999). Many different routes of pathogens transmission in herds and microbial milk contamination have been documented. The ingestion of fresh dairy products contaminated with soil-borne or water-borne *Escherichia coli* and other pathogens provokes mainly enteric diseases. Currently numerous biotic and abiotic factors that may affect the survival and enhance the dissemination of pathogens in dairy farms are being investigated (Doyle et al., 2001; Srinivasan et al., 2007).

Food borne pathogens that can be found in milk and dairy products represent an important public health risk particularly in rural communities. Food borne infections and intoxications most often occur in family's living in small villages. The zoonotic bacterial pathogens identified in raw milk are *Brucella ssp.*, mainly *Brucella mellitensis*, *Listeria monocytogenes*, *Yersinia enterocolitica*, *Salmonella ssp.*, *Mycobacterium bovis, M Mycobacterium paratuberculosis, Streptococcus pyogenes, Streptococcus agalactiae* and more recently *Escherichia coli* O157:H7 and *Enterobacter sakasakii* (Entis, 2007; Lal et al., 2005; Riffon et al., 2001). New identified emerging pathogens in milk which deserve public health concerns are *Cryptosporidium parvum, Citrobacter freundii, Corynebacterium ulcerans*, hepatitis A virus, *Mycobacterium paratuberculosis, Streptococcus zooepidemicus* (B-hemolytic *Streptococcus* Lancefield C group) and *Campylobacter jejuni* (Riffon et al., 2001; Skovgaard, 2007;Van Kessel et al., 2008).

Staphylococcus aureus is considered one of the major food borne pathogens in the dairy industry due to its capability to produce a wide range of virulence factors (Reij & Waitering, 2008). The enterotoxigenic *Staphylococcus aureus* from raw milk produces dangerous heat-stable enter toxins (Zouharova & Rysanek, 2008). *S.aureus* enterotoxins are expressed by the genes (sea, seb, sec, sed, see, seg, seh, sei), and sej and 1 gene (tst). In larger farms the prevalence of enterotoxin genes in *Staphylococcus aureus* is estimated to be about of $6.0x10^3$ CFU/ml counts in bulk milk (Peles et al., 2007). The multiple antibiotic resistant *Staphylococcus aureus* strains produce enterotoxins (Chao et al., 2007); Cremonesi et al., 2007; Tsegmed et al., 2007).

In human nutrition bovine colostrum can be considered an excellent source of bioactive proteins and the product beneficial for improving general health. The content of *Salmonella ssp.,* Streptococcus *agalactiae, Staphylococcus aureus*, coagulase negative staphylococci, and streptococci non-agalactiae, as well as coliforms and non-coliforms in colostrum depends mainly on herd health status. The counts of these bacteria in fresh colostrums are considerably higher than in the raw milk. Herd size and location normally do not influence the bacteriological quality of colostrum (Kagkli et al., 2007).

Several new spore-forming bacteria that can survive food-processing were recently detected in dairy products. The shelf life of heat-treated milk products mostly depend on *Bacillus* and *Clostridium* species providing that post-process contamination is avoided. The shelf life of final dairy products is largely determined by the production processes management which controls all steps of the production process including raw materials, ingredients and environmental sources.

1.1. Microbial Contamination of Raw and Pasteurized Milk

Bacterial contamination of raw milk from production environment may include different sources: air, milking equipment, feed, soil, feces and grass. The dairy farm environment and animal population may represent serious reservoirs of pathogens, which can contaminate raw milk during milking, as well as bulk milk tanks. The pathogens may be transmitted to milking machines and bring to risk future activities.

Raw milk and dairy products produced from unpasteurized milk are often involved in food borne diseases in humans. Microbially contaminated raw milk produces serious gastroenteric diseases in humans. Occasionally pasteurized milk may be also contaminated (Frank et al., 2001).

The microbiological quality of row milk reflects good hygienic practices. Raw milk contamination may occur from infected and diseased cows, or may be caused by environmental bacteria (Kongo et al., 2008).

Non-contaminated raw milk normally contains high bacteria counts. Milk preservation procedures normally allow the survival of normal milk microflora. Pasteurization reduces dramatically the number of bacteria and the risk of milk borne disease in consumers, in particular the diseases like salmonelosis, tuberculosis, brucelosis, campylobacteriosis and listeriosis (Center of diseases control, 1996; Frank et al., 2001). The outbreaks of diseases caused by the consumption of fresh cheeses that were produced with non-pasteurized milk have been reported and the recognized causes were linked to contamination post-pasteurization, faulty pasteurization equipment or improper conservation of dairy products (Johnson et al., 1990). Prompt detection of the *Salmonella typhimurium* phage type 561 (STM DT7 international typing scheme) may reduce the risk of poisoning by homemade cheese (Van Duynhoven et al., 2009).

Milk production parameters favor certain microbial species. Eventually a particular yeast community develops, which either stimulates or inhibits the growth of normal milk bacteria. The interaction between yeasts and bacteria influences the quality of the final dairy products (Viljoen, 2001).

Monitoring and identifying the bacteria in raw milk is of high importance. The Enterobacteriacea; *Klebsiella* species and *Enterobacter* ssp., might be normally present in raw milk, while the presence of *Salmonella ssp.,* depends on hygienic practices in the herd (Kongo et al., 2008).

Raw milk samples should be tested for *L. monocytogenes* and *Salmonella spp.*, and the indicator microorganisms (mesophilic aerobes and total coliforms), as well as for *Echerichia coli* (Nero et al., 2008). The majority of antagonistic bacteria to the pathogens were identified as lactic acid bacteria species, mainly *Lactococcus lactis subsp. lactis* and *Enterococcus faecium* (Kagkli et al., 2007).

Somatic cell counts (SCC) and total bacterial counts (TBC) in raw milk vary during different seasonal periods (Gillespie et al., 2009). The presence of coliforms in milk bulk samples, such as *Salmonella ssp.,Yersinia enterocolitica, Listeria monocytogenes* and others, can give the useful informations about the production environment and the quality of raw milk (Ackers et al., 2000; Rea & Tobin, 1992).

The dairy cattle can be a serious source of salmonellae. The animal carriers of this infection agent are often asymptomatic and difficult to identify. Infections with *Salmonella* show the fluctuation over seasonal periods. Frequent route of infection includes the transfer the bacteria from water contaminated with feces to bulk milk and milk filters.

The contamination of the row milk by *Yersinia enterocolitica* O is usually linked to post-pasteurization contamination. The cases where the contamination occurred due to rinsing the milk bottles with untreated water prior to filling has been reported (Ackers et al., 2000).

Escherichia coli (STEC) is one of the most important food pathogens. Shiga toxin-producing STEC are common as colonizers in the intestine of healthy cattle and are spread into the environment by fecal shedding and the use of manure. The bacteria can be transmitted to humans by consuming the food, such as in the case of inadequately cooked ground beef or unpasteurized milk. The persistency of bacteria in cattle production environments contributes to the contamination and recontamination of cattle, as well as to human infections. In order to limit the entry of STEC strains into the environment, effective control strategies must be applied in farms (Fremaux et al., 2008). The prevalence of shiga like toxin produced by *Escherichia coli* (STEC) in cheeses produced from raw milk including soft, hard, unripened and blue mould cheeses, is mostly related to serotypes, O6, O174, O175, O176, O109, O76, O162 and in minor frequency to O22 serogroup (Vernozy-Rozand et al.,2005).

Escherichia coli infection is frequent in small communities which are close to the source of infection. Specific epidemiologic studies suggested that namely O157:H7 was the causative agent since it was isolated from both raw milk samples and environmental samples (Denny et al., 2008).

Enterohemorrhagic *Escherichia coli* (EHEC), EHEC O26: H- is an emerging cause of hemolytic-uremic syndrome (HUS). The sources of milk contamination with EHEC O26 often remain identified. In order to confirm that *E. coli* O26 is responsible for infection it is recommended to analyze fecal samples from cows producing the incriminating milk (Allerberger et al., 2003).

The presence of *Brucella* species in raw milk, cheese, and ewes' cheese has been frequently reported. In general, the ewes' milk cheese is an important source of *Brucella spp* and should be regarded with the precaution (Kasimoğlu, 2002).

Different feeding and housing strategies may influence the microbial quality of milk, especially the presence of *Bacillus licheniformis, Bacillus pumilus, Bacillus circulans, Bacillus subtilis* and strain types of the species belonging to the *Bacillus cereus* group.

Bacillus licheniformis and *Bacillus pallidus* can act as entry points for highly heat-resistant spores into raw milk. The spore content of psychotropic *Bacillus cereus* affects the milk quality even after pasteurization. The milk contamination with spores usually occurs during grazing seasons and is linked to contamination by soil or dirty farm accessories (Christiansson et al., 1999). Good hygienic measures reduce the contamination level of raw milk, minimizing the number of aerobic spore-forming bacteria that can lead to spoilage of milk and dairy products (Scheldeman et al., 2005). When comparing the milk quality originating from conventional dairy farms and organic farms, higher number of thermo tolerant sporulated organisms are usually found in milk samples produced in conventional farms (Coorevits et al., 2008).

Bacillus cereus and *Bacillus licheniformis* contamination is frequent in raw and pasteurized milk and yoghurt, and usually occurs during milk processing (Banykó & Vyletelová, 2009). The enterotoxins of both enterotoxigenic *Bacillus cereus* (hemolytic) and *B. cereus* (non-hemolytic) were identified in row milk and milk products (Ombui & Nduhiu, 2005). The contamination of raw milk with *Bacillus cereus* spores, suggested an environmental contamination. Large number of spores was found in free stalls, bedding material, especially sawdust beds. A positive relationship was observed between the number of spores in the feed, feces, and raw milk (Magnusson et al., 2007).

The silage can be a significant source of contamination of raw milk with spores. Preventive management of outgrowth of aerobic spores in silage includes the application of lactic acid bacteria or the use of chemical additives. This can improve the silage fermentation and reduce the total spore loads in the raw milk (Te Giffel et al., 2002).

The contamination of dairy products by *Pseudomonas spp.* has a direct affects on the shelf life of dairy products. *Pseudomonas fluorescens,* and *Pseudomonas putida* provoke the degradation of milk components in raw and pasteurized milk via different enzyme systems, mostly proteases, lecithinase, and lipase. The contamination sources are mostly linked to herd environment (Dogan & Boor, 2003).

Milk contamination by *Clostridium disporicum,* can derive from soil, forage, grass silage, maize silage and dry hay. The consistent occurrence of the *Clostridium tyrobutyricum* in milk indicated that the presence of clostridia was related to bad farm management rather than to feed contamination (Julien et al., 2008).

The enterococci and lactobacilli are part of the normal microflora of the gastrointestinal tract of dairy cows and other food animals. The contamination of the milking equipment by these bacteria is usually caused by fecal contamination. The Lactobacilli that were identified in bovine feces were predominantly *Lactobacillus mucosae* and *Lactobacillus brevis* and were also detected in raw milk and the milking machines. Small number of other lactobacilli and enterococci were found in the milk. The majority of the bovine fecal enterococcal isolation was identified as *Aerococcus viridans* (Kagkli et al., 2007).

The important indicator of hygienic quality of raw milk includes the presence of bifidobacteria species because fecal contamination of raw milk is indicated by the bifidobacteria presence (*Bifidobacterium pseudolongum* subsp. *globosum* (Beerens et al., 2000).

2. The Cow Feeding Conditions and Milk Composition

Environmental pollution and contaminant deposition on grassland increase the animal feeding risks and cause the transfer of pollutants to raw milk. Agricultural practices like the use of fertilizers and pesticides may contaminate the grass corn and silage. The agricultural chemical residues may appear in milk after the animal has consumed the contaminated feed. The composition of the bulk milk is therefore a good indicator of milk production conditions and farm feeding practices. In some cases the variability in the composition of the bulk milk among herds may be significant due to different feeding conditions and environmental pollutants, such as heavy metals or dioxins (Table 2). The residues of agricultural pesticides carry a serious public health risk, especially to nursing infants (atrazine residues and 2, D-a acidic herbicides) who are receiving contaminated infant formulas (Gupta, 2007; Hyde et al., 1977).

In some geographical areas with predominant toxic plant species in the grasslands the safety of the milk may be significantly compromised due to toxicants presence in milk (Table 3). Depending on the ingested amount and toxin blood concentration, primary compound and its metabolites are able to diffuse into mammary gland tissue and to be excreted in milk. The content of plant toxins in milk is associated with seasonal periods. Besides grazing the toxin producing species the contamination might arise via silage or dried pasture contaminated with toxic plants or feeding grains contaminated with toxic plant seeds.

In small dairy farms and home-produced milk the transfer of plant toxins to milk occurs via green pasture and hay pasture administered in the barn. In these cases raw milk and homemade dairy products could potentially be contaminated with the plant toxins. Babies and young children will be most affected though drinking contaminated milk (Panter & James, 1990).

Table 2. Milk and Dairy Products Contamination by Mycotoxins and Environmental Pollutants

Xenobiotic	Residues and contaminants	Human health risk	Source
Mycotoxins	Aflatoxins; B1 (AFB1), and AFB1 metabolites to M1(AFM1) Citricina,ciclopiazonic acid, penitrem A, roquefortine C	AFM1 carcinogenic hepatic metabolites, antimetabolic effects. Inmmunodepletion and bone marrow depletion. Estrogenic effects none widely probed	Toxic metabolites from fungi growing originated in pasture, animal foodstuffs, AFM1 milk excretion, and mycotoxins synthesis and fungi contamination in dairy products, and poor hygiene dairy process
Heavy metals and others	Lead, arsenic, mercury, chromiun,cadmiun, nickel,cobalt, manganese, copper and zinc	Chronically effects by chromium and lead ingestion in the children, bone marrow myelodisplasia and other morbid syndromes	Road way traffic, industrial activities and environmental contamination and agriculture activities
Dioxins	Organochlorine compounds; 1, 3, 5- polychlorinated dibenzo furans (PCDF), and 75 polychlorinated dibenzo-*p*-dioxins (PCDD)	Adverse health affects cancer-causing agents	Live stock environmental exposure. Contaminated milk and dairy products from over exposed grazing dairy cows and contaminated feed grains

In the intensive production systems the excretion of plant toxins in milk by lactating cows represents a minor risk to human heath because of the low exposure of grazing cows in the grassland due to good agricultural management. The public health and food safety measures consider the regular control of xenobiotics in bulk milk in regions indigenious to toxic plants. Besides the amount of the ingested toxin, the amount of the plant toxins excreted in milk is influenced by milk composition and pH, as well as the polarity of the toxin. The examples of recognized plant threats include the white snakeroot (*Europoium rogosum*) and ray less goldenrod (*Haplopappus heterophyllus*) which has shown to be main causes of toxicosis in livestock and humans in the southwestern U.S and northern Mexico. This can be prevented by changing feeding and management practices in milk production. There are other poisonous plants rich in alkaloids and glucosinolates that have been identified in grasslands. The toxins like piperidine from hemlock (*Coninum maculatum*), *Lobelia. Cassia* and Pinnus, are considered to be teratogenic in cattle. The loco weed plant (*Astragalus lenttiginosus*) produces toxic indolizidine compound. The castan (*Castan osperm* and *C.australe*) produces toxins such as castanospermine which is highly toxic to ruminants of different ages. Quinolizidine compounds are present in toxic plants such as "golden chain" (*Laburnusum spp.*) and "mountain thermopsis" (*Laburnusum cystus*).

Table 3. Natural Plant Toxicants Excreted in Milk

Toxicant Compound	Plant Common Name	Taxonomy	Affected Population	Clinical Signs In Humans
Tremetol and tremetona	White snakeroot, Raykess golden rod	*Eupatorium rugosum, Haplopapaus[1] heterophyllus*	Dairy cattle, human beans, mainly others	Milk sickness, trembles. Ataxia, cetonunemia, delirium and coma
Pyrrolizidine and other alkaloids	Tasty ragwort (*Senecio spp*), and others. Tussilago and Borage	*Senecio* different species, *Cynoglossum* spp., *Crotalaria* spp., *Symphytum* spp, *Heliottropium* spp., From in to the other species; *Borrago officinallis* and , *Tussilago farfara*	Dairy cattle, other species and human beans occasionally	Minimal public health risk by acute toxicosis. Chronic milk excretion may ocurr in carcinogenic effects
Glucosinolates, goinitrin, thiocyanates and nitrates	Meadow foam. Mustard, radish and others	*Limanthes spp., Brassica spp.,* Horse radish	Different animal species, less effects to human population.	Different effects, affects microsomal activity and iodine transport
Glucosinolates, goinitrin, thiocyanates and nitrates	Meadow foam. Mustard, radish and others	*Limanthes spp., Brassica spp.,* Horse radish	Different animal species, less effects to human population	Different effects, affects microsomal activity and iodine transport

These are closely related to a nervous sinology and the poisoning with them is characterized by seizures in exposed sucking calves. Pregnant ewes and lambs fed on the plants produce the offspring with skeletal abnormalities.

Other considerations concerning the poisonous plants that must be taken into account is that some plants preserve their toxins even after drying. Such are colchicines present in autumn crocus (*Colchicum autumnal*), or selenocompounds derived from astragalus (*Astragalus stanleya*). These compounds' are gastro-intestinally well absorbed and transferred to milk. The green grass rich in amino acid L-tryptophan is metabolized in grazing cows to indole and 3-methylindole derivatives provoking pulmonary edema in grazing cattle. There are no confirmed cases of human population poisoning with L-tryptophan (Panter et al., 2007).

The proper conserving methods of silages, forages and grains used for animal feed are an important production steps oriented to reduce the contamination with environmental microbial pathogens. The evidence of the presence of aflatoxin M1 in milk appears to be a serious public health problem, since aflatoxin M1 has shown to be a possible hepatotoxic carcinogen. Frequent contamination of the corn and concentrated feeds by aflatoxin B1 poses a need to limit the exposure to aflatoxins in dairy cattle by imposing regulatory limits (Tajik et al., 2007).

The grazing conditions might have also beneficial influence on the composition of the milk by enriching the milk with beta-carotene, lutein, vitamin E and sesquiterpenes (Agabriel et al., 2007).

3. Enviromental Contamination Pollutants and Agricultural Pesticides Residues in Dairy Production

The presence of pesticide residues in milk results from common agricultural practices and persistency of the used compounds (triazine herbicides) (Pecníková et al., 2002) as well as from corn and forage conserving methods (Beerens et al., 2000; Donaghy et al., 2008; Te Giffel et al., 2002). In addition to pesticide presence in milk, the monitoring of lead and cadmium content is very important especially in regions located near a highway. The use of fertilizers and manure further influence the metal accumulation in the soil and plants in different seasonal periods and might contribute to high total daily metal intake by cows. To reduce the milk contamination with heavy metals the farm management must consider the reduction of the levels of lead and cadmium in soil and plants (Parkpian et al., 2003). As an example supporting the fact that environment is the main source of milk contamination by heavy metals serves evidence that in a providence of Turkey, raw milk samples were collected from an industrial region with intensive traffic. High amounts of heavy metal contents like lead, arsenic, copper, zinc, and iron were found in raw milk, while no mercury was detected (Simsek et al., 2000).

The international agencies and the European Union (European commission for dioxin-like PCBs), regulated the dioxin levels and PCBs in food. The dietary intake of non-dioxin-like polychlorinated biphenyls (NDL-PCBs) has been estimated in foodstuffs. The level of exposure to these compounds is highly affected by the dietary habits of consumers. Fishery products as well as milk and dairy products are marked as the major contributors to the total dietary intake of NDL-PCBs (Fattore et al., 2008). In Japan the surveillance and environmental monitoring of PCDDs, PCDFs, and dioxin like PCBs follows a very consistent sampling programs of air and soil, sea water, fresh water, ground water, water purification plants and raw water. It was shown that the soil sediments, aquatic organisms, raw milk, animal foods, human breast milk, and human blood contain measurable levels of PCBs, PCDDs and PCDFs (Mato et al., 2007).

In addition, nuclear pollution of herbages and grass of agroecosystems is also possible. This might occur after the nuclear accidents (Pickerell, 2007). The lands remain contaminated by radiation for a long time. In a restricted zone of the Chernobyl accident, the composition of grass and herbages and the biodiversity shows significant variations in comparison to botanical patterns in the zone before the accident. The soil and air-dry herbage from a region showed a mass contamination by ^{137}Cs and 90Sr radioneuclotides of herbages and grass. Consequently the use of meadow agroecosystem herbages in the zone is restricted due to their high level of soil contamination with ^{90}Sr (Sapegin et al., 2008).

4. Analytical Methods for Controlling the Milk Quality

The main task of milk industry is to produce a high quality milk as well as safe and healthy dairy products. Good manufacture practices and hazard critical control points (HACCP), contribute to the traceability and insurance of the quality of dairy products preventing at the same time the food borne diseases in humans and exposure to chemical contaminants (Nauta, 2008; Ray & Bhunia, 2008). The occurrence of pathogens in food is prevented by controlling the herd health status and the milk pasteurization, as well as applying a good manufacturing practices.

As a part of the quality control in dairy industry the presence of eubiotics deriving from grazing cows, conserved feed or feeding grains, like aflatoxins AFB1 and AFM1 is routinely monitored in milk (Roussi et al., 2002). Heavy metals are monitored in the graze lands close to highway roads and industrial activities. The concerns about dioxins are an actual and controversial subject in the food industry. Due to their high toxicity and bioconcentration these compounds demand a continuous environment monitoring and the residues tracking in both feed and raw milk (Fattore et al., 2008).

The food-borne diseases are etiologically and epidemiologically usually difficult to investigate. The predominant infectious pathogens originating from dairy products that are causing human diseases are the microorganisms of subclinical mastitis and include *Salmonella* species, Campylobacter species, *Yersinia enterocolitica*, *Listeria* species, *Aeromona hydrophila, E.coli* O157:H7, *Leptospira interrogans* and *Mycobaterium* species. In contrast, *Coxiella brunetti, Cryptosporidium parvum* and *Toxoplasma gondii* may be infrequent (Doyle et al., 2001; Entis, 2007). *Campylobacter* infections are reported seasonally by public health services (Murinda et al., 2002b). It is not uncommon to detect *Salmonella* species in icecream and fresh cheeses, as well as *Brucella mellitensis* in non-pasteurized milk and homemade dairy products like goat cheese (Hoob & Roberts, 1990).

In recent years food borne outbreaks are very often associated with the consumption of raw milk and dairy products prepared without milk pasteurization. The infections often arise as a result of improper manipulation of the dairy products. The actual causes of infections are identified by conventional microbial laboratory tests, which include the tests for *Salmonella* species, *Listeria* species and *Staphylococcus aureus* enterotoxins as well as multiple resistant strains (Srinivasan et al., 2006). For identifying the infectious agents, microbial and other toxins, highly specific enzyme linked assays may be used (Center of diseases control, 1996; Srinivasan et al., 2007). The microbial contamination of raw milk is evaluated by determining the total microbial charge and somatic cell counts.

The adverse effects of antibiotics from milk on human health require a continuous monitoring program and residue detection in raw milk and dairy products. This is performed by different conventional methods such as the agar diffusion test with *Bacillus stearothermophilus* variety *calidolactis*, very sensitive to b-lactamic antibiotics. The test is less effective for the detection of spiramycin, sulphonamides or chlorampenicol residues (Bruhn et al., 1985; Committee on drug use in food animals, 1999). The test with *Streptococcus termophilus, Bacillus subtilis, Bacillus megaterius, Bacillus cereus* and *Micrococcus luteus* slightly increases the sensitivity of the test for macrolydes and sulphonamides (Bruhn et al., 1985). Methods such as electrophoresis and ELISA tests detect drug residues in milk at low concentrations (ppm). Nuclear magnetic resonance and high-resolution liquid chromatography (HPLC) are very useful to detect antibiotic residues in milk at very low concentrations (ppb) (Cerkvenik et al., 2002; Gallo et al., 2008; Karlström et al., 2007). Use of fluorometry for determination of adulterations in fresh milk (Guan et al., 2005). Melamine detection in untreated milk by mass spectrometry (Zhu et al., 2009).Gas chromatography can be used to detect antiparasitic drugs (Cerkvenik et al., 2002; Mato et al., 2007; Sugiyama et al., 2008). The traces of heavy metals in milk might be detected by atomic absorption spectrophotometry. Thin layer liquid chromatography is useful to detect other xenobiotics like plant toxins and mycotoxins.

In many countries agricultural and public health regulations require high performance liquid chromatography (HPLC) protocols to evaluate how antibiotic residues and other xenobiotics are distributed in milk and tissues of food animals. The drugs are traced after the drug has been radio labeled and administered to animals. The distribution of the drug is monitored by radioactivity tests in feces, urine and milk. On the basis of these investigations the maximum tolerant level of residue (MRL) and maximum daily ingested drug without adverse effects for food animal (ADI_{tox}) are defined.

5. Dairy Industry Management

The bacteriological status of the milk consideres the occurrence of the microbial resistant strains (Skovgaard, 2007). Herd, pasteurization and distribution management assures a good milk production hygiene (Spreer & Mixa, 1998). Neglecting a sanitary management, homemade dairy products made of raw non-pasteurized milk are often reported as a source of infections (Rohrbach et al., 1992). Some outbreaks of milk borne diseases have been associated to infection after pasteurization (Straley et al., 2006).

The safety of dairy products is controlled and regulated by joined activities of the governmental agencies, dairy farmers and veterinarians. The milk industry can contribute to the safety of dairy products by preventing drug residues in milk and by monitoring the milk quality (Cerkvenik et al., 2002). The principal strategies of quality assurance in dairy industry include:

1. Disease prevention and milking management by sustaining the healthy herd

2. Proper drug use by veterinarian's guidance
3. The use of licensed drugs for milking cows
4. Following the drug administration protocols and milk retention periods
5. Drug-residue screening tests
6. Educational programs among small dairy farmers about milk contaminants and residues

The microbial milk quality and drug residue programs are the responsibilities of the agricultural departments, public health agencies and milk industry (Gallo et al., 2008; Seiber, 2001). Collaborative action of these provides the establishment of the safety tolerance levels and sanitary protocols.

The first step in assuring the milk free of antibiotic residues is to control the dairy processing plants, bulk milk tanks and tanker truck milk loads. The screen testing of *Bacillus stearothermophilus* cultures is routinely performed. Milk sampling for physicochemical tests and somatic cell counts are the responsibility of milk hullers. The collection of representative samples from each milk bulk tank in the dairy farm must be ensured (Bruhn et al., 1985; Chao et al., 2007).

The rough estimation of milk quality is performed by measuring the electrical conductivity, somatic cells counts, as well as lactoferrin and lyzosome activity in suspicious milk. The improper administration and over dosage or chronic administration of certain veterinary drugs increases the risk of antibiotic residues in milk (Committee on drug use in food animals, 1999). Among the most important agricultural chemicals in milk to be considered are 2,4-D acidic herbicides, atrazine and paraquat. These could be detected by gas chromatography. The same analytical technique is used to evaluate the contamination level by organochlorine, organophosphous and carbamates pesticides (Hyde et al., 1977).

Conclusion

The main priorities of dairy industry are to produce high quality milk and safe dairy products. Microbial milk contamination sources are mostly related to production environment, herd hygiene, and the udder health status. In addition, numerous xenobiotic substances can be detected in milk including veterinary drugs, agricultural chemicals, and environmental pollutants. At present, dairy farms put many efforts in reducing the milk contamination from production environment and poor udder health status. The environmental pollutants are considered the challenge for food producers particularly with the respect to dioxins levels. By careful monitoring of the production systems it is possible to define which factors are compromising the raw milk production and the quality of the dairy products. The control of milk bulk tanks in farms offers fast informations about possible mastitis in cows, environmental pathogens and chemical residues in milk. When milk borne disease outbreaks occur in human population, it is necessary to identify the actual cause by investigating the principal sources of contamination and by tracking back the process to pasteurized and non-pasteurized milk.

Good milk production management assures the milk quality and prevents the food borne diseases and exposure to chemical residues. Due to new emerging pathogens and eubiotics found in milk, public health programs of many countries gives a priority to milk borne diseases. Now the strategies for preventing and controlling the milk borne diseases have strict regulations in North America, United Kingdom, European Union and Japan. Dairy industry management oriented towards preventing the risks in critical points in the production process is considerably reducing the food borne outbreaks.

Educational programs have an important role in reducing the exposure to unsafe food products, and provide a knowledge important for adequate handling of milk and dairy products, food distribution and consumption. The actual goal of milk industry and dairy farms is to act responsibly, to withstand the new challenges arising in the production of the safe food and to provide a sustainability in milk production.

References

Ackers, M.L; Schoenfeld, S; Markman, J; Smith, M.G; Nicholson, M.A; De Witt, W; Cameron, D.N; Griffin, P.M and Slutsker, L. An outbreak of *Yersinia enterocolitica* O:8 infections associated with pasteurized milk. *J. Infect. Dis.*, (2000). 181(5), 1834-1837.

Agabriel, C; Cornu, A; Journal, C; Sibra, C; Grolier, P and Martin, B. Tanker milk variability according to farm feeding practices: vitamins A and E, carotenoids, color, and terpenoids. *J. Dairy. Sci.,* (2007). 90(10), 4884-4896.

Allerberger, F; Friedrich, A.W; Grif, K; Dierich, M.P; Dornbusch, H.J; Mache, C.J; Nachbaur, E; Freilinger, M; Rieck, P; Wagner, M; Caprioli, A; Karch, H and Zimmerhackl, L.B. Hemolytic-uremic syndrome associated with enterohemorrhagic *Escherichia coli* O26:H infection and consumption of unpasteurized cow's milk. *Int. J. Infect. Dis.*, (2003). 7(1), 42-45.

Banykó, J and Vyletelová, M. Determining the source of Bacillus cereus and Bacillus licheniformis isolated from raw milk, pasteurized milk and yoghurt. *Lett. Appl. Microbiol.,* (2009). 48(3), 318-323.

Barker, AR; Schrick, FN; Lewis, MJ; Dowlen, HH and Oliver, SP. Influence of clinical mastitis during early lactation on reproductive performance of Jersey cows. *J. Dairy Sci.*, (1998). 81(5), 1285-1290.

Baumann, A and Sadkowska-Todys, M. Foodborne infections and intoxications in Poland in 2006. *Przegl. Epidemiol.*, (2008). 62(2), 275-286.

Beerens, H; Hass Brac de la Perriere, B and Gavini, F. Evaluation of the hygienic quality of raw milk based on the presence of bifidobacteria: the cow as a source of faecal contamination. *Int. J. Food Microbiol.*, (2000). 54(3), 163-169.

Bruhn, J.C; Ginn, R.E; Messer, J.W and Mikolajcik, E.M. Detection of antibiotic residues in milk and dairy products: In: Richarson,G.M. Editor. *Standard methods for the examination of dairy products:* Washington, D.C; American Public Health Association. (1985); 265-287.

Bunning, V. K; Donnelly, C. W; Peter, J. T; Briggs, E. H; Bradshaw, J. G; Crawford,R.G; Beliveau, C. M and Tierney, L. T. Thermal inactivation of *Listeria monocytogenes* within bovine macrophages. *Appl. Environ. Microbiol.*, (1988). 54, 364-370.

Callaway TR and Oliver, SP. On-farm strategies to reduce foodborne pathogen contamination. *Foodborne Pathog Dis.*, (2009). 6(7), 753.

Center of diseases control. Surveillance for foodborne-disease outbreaks in the United States, 1988-1992. *Morbib. Mortal. Weekly.*, (1996). 45 (SS-5), 1-66.

Cercenado, E and Ruiz de Gopegui, E. Community-acquired methicillin-resistant *Staphylococcus aureus* Enferm. *Infecc. Microbiol. Clin.*, (2008). Suppl 13, 19-13.

Cerkvenik, V. Analysis and monitoring of cholanphenicol residues in food of animal origin in Slovenia from 1991 to 2000. *Food Addit. Contam.*, (2002). 19(4), 357-367.

Chao,G; Zhou,X; Jiao,X; Quian,X and Xu,L. Prevalence and antimicrobial resistance of food borne pathogens isolated from food products in China. *Food Borne Pathog. Dis.* (2007). 5(3), 277-284.

Christiansson, A; Bertilsson, J and Svensson, B. *Bacillus cereus* spores in raw milk: factors affecting the contamination of milk during the grazing period. *J. Dairy. Sci.*, (1999). 82(2), 305-314.

Committee on drug use in food animals, Panel of animal health, Food safety, and Public Health, Board on Agriculture, National Research Council. *The use of drugs in food animals: benefits and risks*, National Academy of Sciences(Ed), Washington, D.C : National Academic Press; (1999). 63.

Coorevits, A; De Jonghe, V; Vandroemme, J; Reekmans, R; Heyrman, J; Messens, W; De Vos, P and Heyndrickx, M. Comparative analysis of the diversity of aerobic spore-forming bacteria in raw milk from organic and conventional dairy farms. *Syst. Appl. Microbiol.*, (2008). 31(2), 126-140.

Cremonesi, P ; Perez, G ; Pisoni, G; Moroni, P; Morandi, S; Luzzana, M; Brasca, M and Castiglioni, B. Detection of enterotoxigenic *Staphylococcus aureus* isolates in raw milk cheese. *Lett. Appl. Microbiol.*, (2007). 45 (6), 586-591.

Denny, J; Bhat, M and Eckmann, K. Outbreak of *Escherichia coli* O157:H7 associated with raw milk consumption in the Pacific Northwest. *Foodborne. Pathog. Dis.*, (2008). 5(3), 321-328.

Dogan, B and Boor, K.J. Genetic diversity and spoilage potentials among *Pseudomonas* spp. isolated from fluid milk products and dairy processing plants. *Appl. Environ. Microbiol.*, (2003). 69(1), 130-138.

Donaghy, J.A; Rowe, M.T; Rademaker, J.L; Hammer, P; Herman, L; De Jonghe, V; Blanchard, B; Duhem, K and Vindel, E. An inter-laboratory ring trial for the detection and isolation of *Mycobacterium avium* subsp. paratuberculosis from raw milk artificially contaminated with naturally infected faeces. *Food. Microbiol.*, (2008). 25(1), 128-135.

Doyle, M.P; Beuchant, L and Monteville, T.J. *Food microbiology: Fundamentals and frontiers*. 2nd Edition.Washington, D.C : ASM Press, (2001).

Entis,P. *Food safety: old habits new perspectives*. Washington, D.C: ASM press. (2007).

Fattore, E; Fanelli, R; Dellatte, E; Turrini, A and di Domenico, A. Assessment of the dietary exposure to non-dioxin-like PCBs of the Italian general population. *Chemosphere.*, (2008). 73(1 Suppl), S278-283.

Frank,JF. Milk and dairy products. In: Doyle, PM; Beuchant, LR and Monteville, T.J, editors. *Food microbiology: fundamentals and frontiers* Washington, D.C. ASM press, 2nd edition; 2001; 111.

Fremaux, B; Prigent-Combaret, C and Vernozy-Rozand, C. Long-term survival of Shiga toxin-producing *Escherichia coli* in cattle effluents and environment: an updated review. *Vet. Microbiol.*, (2008). 132(1-2), 1-18.

Gallo, P; Fabbrocino, S; Vinci,F; Fiori ,M; Danese,V and Serpe, L. Confirmatory identification of sixteen non-steroidal anti-inflammatory drug residues in raw milk by liquid choomatography couplrd with ion trap mass spectrometry. *Rapid. Commun. Mass. Spectrom.*, (2008). 22(6), 841-854.

Gillespie, BE; Headrick, SI; Boonyayatra, S and Oliver, SP. Prevalence and persistence of coagulase-negative *Staphylococcus* species in three dairy research herds. *Vet Microbiol.*, (2009). 134(1-2), 65-72.

Gomes, B.C; Esteves, C.T; Palazzo, I.C; Darini, A.L; Felis, G.E; Sechi, L.A; Franco, B.D and De Martinis, E.C. Prevalence and characterization of *Enterococcus* spp. Isolated from Brazilian foods. *Food. Microbiol.*, (2008). 25(5), 668-675.

Guan, R.F; Liu, D.H; Ye X.Q and Yang, K. Use of fluorometry for determination of skim milk powder adulteration in fresh milk. *J. Zhejiang. Univ. Sci. B.*, (2005). 6(11), 1101-1106.

Gupta, P.K. Toxicity of herbicides. In: Gupta, R.C, editor. *Veterinary Toxicology*. Oxford, UK: Elsevier; 2007; 567-574.

Hyde, W; Kiesey, J; Ross P.F and Stahr, H.M. In: Stahr, H.M, editor. *Analytical toxicology methods manual*. Ames, Iowa, USA: Iowa State University Press; 1977; 90-123.

Hoob, BC and Roberts, D. *Food poisoning and food hygiene* (6th edition). London, UK: Edward Arnolds Publishers Limited. (1990).

Houser, B.A; Donaldson, S.C; Kehoe, S.I; Heinrichs, A.J and Jayarao, B.M. A survey of bacteriological quality and the occurrence of Salmonella in raw bovine colostrum. *Foodborne Pathog. Dis.*, (2008). 5(6), 853-888.

Jayarao, B. M. A study on the prevalence of pathogens in bulk tank milk. In: *Proc. Natl. Mastitis. Counc*; 1999; 148-149.

Johnson, E. A. Microbiological safety of cheese made from heat-treated milk. I. Executive summary, introduction and history. *J. Food. Prot.*, (1990). 53, 441.

Jørgensen, H.J; Mørk, T and Rørvik, L.M. The occurrence of *Staphylococcus aureus* on a farm with small-scale production of raw milk cheese. *J. Dairy. Sci.*, (2005). 88(11), 3810-3817.

Julien, M.C; Dion, P; Lafrenière, C; Antoun, H and Drouin, P. Sources of clostridia in raw milk on farms. *Appl. Environ. Microbiol.*, (2008). 74(20), 6348-6357.

Kagkli, D.M; Vancanneyt, M; Hill, C; Vandamme, P and Cogan, T.M. Enterococcus and Lactobacillus contamination of raw milk in a farm dairy environment. *Int J. Food. Microbiol* . (2007). 114(2), 243-251.

Karlström,U; Nuotio,L; Lindfords, E and Maijala, R. Simulation of human exposure to benzylpenicillin residues via pork originating from pigs fed a dairy by-product. *Food Addit. Contam.*, (2007). 24(3), 266-273.

Kasimoğlu, A. Determination of *Brucella* ssp in raw milk and turkish white cheese in Kirikkale. *Dtsch Tierarztl Wochenschr.*, (2002). 109(7), 324-326.

Kongo, J.M; Gomes, A.P and Malcata, F.X. Monitoring and identification of bacteria associated with safety concerns in the manufacture of São Jorge, a Portuguese traditional cheese from raw cow's milk. *J. Food. Prot.*, (2008). 71(5), 986-992.

Koskinen, M.T; Holopainen, J; Pyörälä, S; Bredbacka, P; Pitkälä, A; Barkema, H.W; Bexiga, R; Roberson, J; Sølverød, L; Piccinini, R; Kelton, D; Lehmusto, H; Niskala, S; and Salmikivi, L. Analytical specificity and sensitivity of a real-time polymerase chain reaction assay for identification of bovine mastitis pathogens. *J. Dairy. Sci.*, (2009). 92(3), 952-959.

Lal, M; Kaur, H; Gupta, L.K and Sood, N.K. Isolation of *Yersinia enterocolitica* from raw milk and pork in Ludhiana. I*ndian. J. Pathol. Microbiol.*, (2005).48(2),286-287.

Magnusson, M; Christiansson, A and Svensson, B. *Bacillus cereus* spores during housing of dairy cows: factors affecting contamination of raw milk. *J. Dairy. Sci.*, (2007), 90(6), 2745-2754.

Mato, Y; Suzuki, N; Katatani, N; Kadokami, K; Nakano, T; Nakayama, S; Sekii, H; Komoto, S; Miyake, S and Morita, M. Human intake of PCDDs, PCDFs, and dioxin like PCBs in Japan. *Chemosphere.*, (2007). 67(9), S247-S255.

Moon, J.S; Lee, A.R; Jaw, S.H; Kang, H.M; Joo, Y.S; Park, Y.H; Kim, M.N and Koo, H.C. Comparison of antibiogram, staphylococcal enterotoxin productivity, and coagulase genotypes among *Staphylococcus aureus* isolated from animal and vegetable sources in Korea. *J. Food. Prot.*, (2007). 70(11), 2541-2548.

Murinda, S. E; Nguyen, L. T; Ivey, S. J; Gillespie, B. E; Almeida, R. A and Oliver S. P. Prevalence and molecular characterization of *Escherichia coli* O157:H7 in bulk tank milk and fecal samples from cull dairy cows: a 12-month survey of dairy farms in East Tennessee. *J. Food Prot.*, (2002a). 65, 752-759.

Murinda, S. E; Nguyen, L. T; Ivey, S. J; Gillespie, B. E; Almeida, R. A; Draughon F. A and Oliver S. P. Molecular characterization of *Salmonella* spp. isolated from bulk tank milk and cull dairy cow fecal samples. *J. Food Prot.*, (2002b). 65, 1100-1105.

Murinda, S.E; Nguyen, L.T; Nam, H.M; Almeida, R.A; Headrick, S.J and Oliver SP. Detection of sorbitol-negative and sorbitol-positive Shiga toxin-producing *Escherichia coli*, *Listeria monocytogenes*, *Campylobacter jejuni*, and *Salmonella* spp. in dairy farm environmental samples. *Foodborne Pathog Dis.*, (2004). 1(2), 97-104.

Nauta, M.J. Modular process risk model (MPRM). In: Schaffner, WD, editor. *A structurated approach to food chain exposure assessment: microbial risk analysis of foods.* Washington,DC: ASM press; 2008; 99.

Nero L.A; de Mattos, M.R; Barros, M de A; Ortolani,M.B; Beloti, V and Franco, B.D. *Listeria monocytogenes* and *Salmonella* spp. in raw milk produced in Brazil: occurrence and interference of indigenous microbiota in their isolation and development. *Zoonoses Public Health.*, (2008). 55(6), 299-305.

Oliver, SP; Boor KJ; Murphy SC and Murinda, SE. Food safety hazards associated with consumption of raw milk. *Foodborne Pathog Dis.*, (2009). 6(7), 793-806.

Oliver, S. P and L. F. Calvinho. Influence of inflammation on mammary gland metabolism and milk composition. In: 2nd International Workshop on the Biology of Lactation in Farm Animals, *J. Animal Sci.*, (1995). 73,18-33.

Oliver, S.P; Lewis, M.J; Gillespie, B.E; Ivey, S.J; Coleman, L.H; Almeida, R.A; Fang, W and Lamar, K. Evaluation of a postmilking teat disinfectant containing a phenolic combination for the prevention of mastitis in lactating dairy cows. *J Food Prot.*, (1999). 62(11), 1354-1357.

Oliver, S. P and Mitchell, B. A. Prevalence of mastitis pathogens in herds participating in a mastitis control program. *J. Dairy Sci.*, (1984). 67, 2436-2440.

Ombui, J.N and Nduhiu, J.G. Prevalence of enterotoxigenic *Bacillus cereus* and its enterotoxins in milk and milk products in and around Nairobi. *East. Afr. Med. J.*, (2005). 82(6), 280-284.

Panter, KE; Garder,D.R; Lee, S.T; Pfister, J.A; Ralphs, M.H; Stegelmeier, B.L and James L.F. Important poisonous plants of the United Satates. In: Gupta, R.C,editor. *Veterinary Toxicology*. Oxford, UK: Elsevier; 2007; 825-854.

Panter, K.E and James, LF. Natural plant toxicants in milk: A review. *J. Anim. Sci.*, (1990). 68, 892-904.

Parkpian, P; Leong, S.T; Laortanakul, P and Thunthaisong, N. Regional monitoring of lead and cadmium contamination in a tropical grazing land site, Thailand. *Environ. Monit. Assess*. (2003). 85(2), 157-173.

Patilk, S.R; Cates, S.A and Morales, R. Consumer food safety knowledge, practices, and demographic differences: findings from a meta-analysis., *J. Food. Prot.*, (2005).68(9), 1884-1994.

Pecníková, K; Tekel, J and Fulmeková, M. Infant formulas based on dried milk and risks of its contamination with residual pesticides. *Ceska.Slov. Farm.*, (2002). 51(2), 68-72.

Peles, F; Wagner, M; Varga, L; Hein, I; Rieck, P; Gutser, K; Keresztúri, P; Kardos, G; Turcsányi, I; Béri, B and Szabó, A. Characterization of Staphylococcus aureus strains isolated from bovine milk in HungaryInt. *J. Food. Microbiol.*, (2007). 118(2), 186-193.

Pickerell, J.A. Readiation and radioactive materials. In: Gupta, R.C, editor. *Veterinary Toxicology*. Oxford, UK: Elsevier; 2007; 339-340.

Ray, B and Bhunia, A. Fundamental food Microbiology. Boca Ratòn, Fla.USA: CRC Press; (2008), 471-474.

Rea, M.C; Cogan, T.M and Tobin, S. Incidence of pathogenic bacteria in raw milk in Ireland, *J. Appl. Bacteriol.*, (1992). 73(4), 331-336.

Riffon,R; Sayasith,K; Khalil; Dubreil,P; Drolet, M and Lagace,J. Development of rapid and sensitive test for identification of major pathogens in bovine mastitis by PCR. *J. Clin. Microbiol.*, (2001). 37(7), 2584-2589.

Riyaz-Ul-Hassan, S; Verma, V and Qazi, G.N. Evaluation of three different molecular markers for the detection of *Staphylococcus aureus* by polymerase chain reaction. *Food Microbiol.*, (2008). 25(3), 452-459.

Reij, M.W and Waitering. M.H.R. Integrating concepts: a case study using Enterobacter sakasakii in infant formula. In: Schaffner,W.D, editor. *A structurated approach to food chain exposure assessment: microbial risk analysis of foods*. Washington,DC: ASM press;2008;117.

Rohrbach, B. W; Draughon, F. A; Davidson, P. M and Oliver, S. P. Prevalence of *Listeria monocytogenes*, *Campylobacter jejuni*, *Yersinia enterocolitica*, and *Salmonella* in bulk tank milk: risk factors and risk of human exposure. *J. Food Prot.*, (1992). 55: 93-97.

Roussi V; Govaris, A; Varagouli, A and Botsoglou, N.A. Occurrence of aflatoxin M(1) in raw and market milk commercialized in Greece. *Food Addit Contam.*, (2002). 19(9), 863-868.

Ruegg, P. L and Tabone, T. J. The relationship between antibiotic residue violations and somatic cell counts in Wisconsin dairy herds. *J. Dairy Sci.*, (2000). 83: 2805-2809.

Sapegin, L.M; Daĭneko, N.M and Timofeev, S.F. The agroecosystems flora status in restricted zone 20 years after the Chernobyl NPP accident. *Radiats. Biol. Radioecol.*, (2008). 48(1), 67-75.

Scheldeman, P; Pil, A; Herman, L; De Vos, P and Heyndrickx, M. Incidence and diversity of potentially highly heat-resistant spores isolated at dairy farms. *Appl. Environ. Microbiol.*, (2005). 71(3), 1480-1494.

Seiber, J.N. Analysis of chemical toxicant and contaminants in food:In Heiferich,W and Winter, C.K, editors. *Food toxicology*. Boca Ratòn, Fla.USA: CRC Press; 2001; 203-218.

Simsek, O; Gültekin, R; Oksüz, O and Kurultay, S. The effect of environmental pollution on the heavy metal content of raw milk. *Nahrung*., (2000). 44(5), 360-363.

Skovgaard, N. New trends in emerging pathogens. *Int. J. Food Microbiol*., (2007). 120(3), 217-224.

Smith, K. L., J. E. Hillerton, and Harmon, R. J. National Mastitis Council guidelines on normal and abnormal raw milk based on somatic cell counts and signs of clinical mastitis. 2001. (2009, july 24th consulted).Available from: http://www.nmconline.org/ docs/a bmilk.pdf.

Spreer, E and Mixa, A. *Milk and dairy products technology*. New York.USA. Marcel Dekker, Inc; 1998; 39-48.

Srinivasan, V; Gillespie, B.E; Lewis, M.J; Nguyen, L.T; Headrick, S.I; Schukken, Y.H and Oliver S.P. (2007). Phenotypic and genotypic antimicrobial resistance patterns of *Escherichia coli* isolated from dairy cows with mastitis. *Vet. Microbiol*., 124(3-4), 319-328.

Srinivasan, V; Sawant, A.A; Gillespie, B.E; Headrick ,S.J; Ceasaris, L and Oliver, S.P. Prevalence of enterotoxin and toxic shock syndrome toxin genes in Staphylococcus aureus isolated from milk of cows with mastitis. *Foodborne Pathog Dis*., (2006). 3(3), 274-83.

Straley, B.A; Donaldson, S.C; Hedge, N.V; Sawant, A.A; Srinivasan, V; Oliver, S.P and Jayarao, B.M. Public health significance of antimicrobial-resistant gram-negative bacteria in raw bulk tank milk. *Foodborne. Pathog. Dis*., (2006). 3(3), 222-223.

Sugiyama,K; Hiraoka, H.,V; and Sugita-Konishi, Y. Aflatoxin M1 contamination in raw bulk tank milk and the presence of aflatoxin B1 in corn supplied to dairy cattle in *Japan. Shokuhin Eiseigaku Zasshi*., (2008). 49(5), 352-355.

Tajik, H; Rohani, S.M and Moradi, M. Detection of aflatoxin M1 in raw and commercial pasteurized milk in Urmia, *Iran. Pak. J. Biol. Sci*., (2007), 10(22), 4103-4107.

Tan, X; Jiang, Y.W; Huang, Y.J and Hu, S.H. Persistence of gentamicin residues in milk after the intramammary treatment of lactating cows for mastitis. *J. Zhejiang Univ. Sci. B*., (2009). 10(4), 280-284.

Te Giffel, M.C; Wagendorp, A; Herrewegh, A and Driehuis, F. Bacterial spores in silage and raw milk. *Antonie Van Leeuwenhoek*., (2002). 81(1-4), 625-630.

Trakulsonboon, S; Danchaivijitr, S; Rongrun-Granugruang,Y; Dhiraputra,C; Susaegrant, W; Ito, T and Iramatsu, K. Firsth report of methicillin-resistant *Staphylococcus aureus* with reduced susceptibility to vancomicyn in Thailand. *J. Clin. Microbiol*., (2001). 32(2); 591-595.

Tsegmed, U; Normanno, G; Pringle, M and Krovacek, K. Occurrence of enterotoxic Staphylococcus aureus in raw milk from yaks and cattle in Mongolia., *J. Food Prot*., (2007). 70(7), 1726-1729.

Van Duynhoven, Y.T; Isken, L.D; Borgen, K; Besselse, M; Soethoudt, K; Haitsma, O; Mulder, B; Notermans, D.W; De Jonge, R; Kock, P; Van Pelt, W; Stenvers, O and Van Steenbergen, J. A prolonged outbreak of *Salmonella Typhimurium* infection related to an uncommon vehicle: hard cheese made from raw milk. *Epidemiol. Infect*. (2009). 19, 1-10.

Van Kessel, J.S; Karns, J.S; Wolfgang, D.R; Hovingh, E; Jayarao, B.M; Van Tassell, C.P and Schukken, Y.H. Environmental sampling to predict fecal prevalence of *Salmonella* in an intensively monitored dairy herd. *J. Food. Prot.*, (2008). 71(10), 1967-1973.

Velázquez-Ordoñez, V; Lagunas, B.S; Gutiérrez, G.B; Talavera, R.M; Alonso, F.U and Saltijeral , O.J. *Staphylococcus aureus* methicillin resistant strain (MRSA) mínimum inhibitory enrofloxacin concentration in *Staphylococcus aureus* isolations obtained from cows with subclinical mastitis in family dairy farms. In: Krynsky, A., and Wrzesien, R, editors. Proceedings XIIth International congress ISAH 2005. Warsaw, Poland: International Society for Animal Hygiene, Faculty of Animal Science, Agricultural University; 2005a; 338-341.

Velázquez-Ordoñez, V; Pescador, S.N; Gorodezky, C and Saltijeral, O.J. *In vitro* differential neutrophil phagocytosis activity on *Staphylococcus aureus* when obtained from blood and milk dairy cows in early lactation period. *Rev. Latin. Microbiol.*, (2008), 50(3-4), 66-71.

Velázquez-Ordoñez, V; Pescador, S.N; Saltijeral , O.J; and Gorodezky, L.C. Epidemiología y control de la mastitis bovina por *Staphylococcus aureus* en vacas lecheras. In: Rodríguez-Vivas R.I, editor: *Enfermedades de importancia en la producción animal*, México, D.F: Editorial Mc Graw Hill; 2005; 355-377.

Velázquez-Ordoñez, V; Vázquez, CH. J.C; Pescador, S.N; and Saltijeral, O.J. Niveles de células somáticas en leche y resistencia a la mastitis. *Producción animal.*, (2005b), 207,15-23.

Vernozy-Rozand, C; Montet, M.P; Berardin, M; Bavai, C and Beutin, L. Isolation and characterization of Shiga toxin-producing *Escherichia coli* strains from raw milk cheeses in France. *Lett. Appl. Microbiol.*, (2005). 41(3), 235-241.

Viljoen, B.C. The interaction between yeasts and bacteria in dairy environments. *Int. J. Food. Microbiol.*, (2001). 69(1-2), 37-44.

Zamora, E.J.L; Velazquez, O.V; Montes de Oca, J.R; Phillipe, G.F; Produccion de B-lactamasa y hemolisina en biotipos humano y bovino en cepas de *Staphylococus aureus* aisladas de vacas lecheras con mastitis subclinica. Acapulco, México: Resúmenes XIV Congreso Panamericano de Ciencias Veterinarias. PANVET. (1994), 44.

Zhu, L; Gamez, G; Chen, H; Chingin, K and Zenobi, R. Rapid detection of melamine in untreated milk and wheat gluten by ultrasound-assisted extractive electrospray ionization mass spectrometry (EESI-MS). *Chem. Commun (Camb).*, (2009). 7(5), 559-561.

Zouharova, M and Rysanek, D. Multiplex PCR and RPLA Identification of *Staphylococcus aureus* enterotoxigenic strains from bulk tank milk. *Zoonoses Public Health.*, (2008). 55(6), 313-313.

In: Nutritional Insights and Food Safety
Editor: Jaroslava Švarc-Gajiæ
ISBN: 978-1-61122-130-5

Chapter XIII

Food Allergens

Anamarija Mandić and Nebojša Ilić
Institute for Food Technology in Novi Sad, Bulevar cara Lazara 1, University of Novi Sad, Serbia

Abstract

Food allergy is characterized by abnormal immunological reactions to a food or food ingredient in sensitive individuals. The immune system of such individuals recognizes allergenic proteins by allergen specific immunoglobulin E (IgE) antibodies and triggers immunological reactions that result in a variety of symptoms that range from mild to life-threatening. For that reason food allergy is recognized as an important food safety issue. Major serious food allergens that account for more than 90% of all allergic reactions are so called the „big eight“. The only efficient way to prevent food allergies is to avoid specific food, since no effective treatment has been found. The most common reason for allergic reaction is the incidence of hidden food allergens, which have not been specified on food labels.

A list of foods and ingredients that should always be declared on labels has been adopted by Codex Alimentarius Commission. The recommended approach to control the possibility of allergen contamination is through a HACCP program. This control system relies heavily on the availability and development of modern food allergen detection methods. Selection of the specific method depends on the type of food matrix and on the nature of food allergen. Most commonly used method is enzyme-linked immunosorbent assay (ELISA) and most recently there is a big increase in the application of mass spectrometry-based proteomics as the most modern method in food allergen detection and analysis.

Introduction

Adverse reactions to food may occur in the form of food allergies, non-allergenic responses, microbial and chemical food poisoning. Food allergy is recognized as an important food safety issue, since it is estimated that 2-4% of adults and 5-8% of children suffer from food allergies worldwide.

Food sensitivies can be divided into food allergies and food intolerances, and the distinction between these two types of adverse reactions has practical implication from clinical and regulatory perspective. Food allergies include abnormal response of the immune system to certain food component, while food intolerances do not involve immunologic reaction. Reactions caused by food allergens range from mild to severe or even life-threatening. More than 150 food products have been identified to cause allergies in sensitive individuals. Major serious food allergens proposed by the Food and Agriculture Organization (FAO) of the United Nations and the World Health Organization (WHO), that account for more than 90% of all allergic reactions, are so called the „big eight":

- soy
- egg
- milk
- wheat
- fish (such as bass, cod, flounder)
- shellfish (such as crab, lobster, shrimp)
- peanuts
- tree nuts: walnuts, cashews, almonds, macadamia nuts, brazil nuts, pecans, pistachios, chestnuts, beechnuts, hazelnuts, pine nuts, gingko nuts and hickory nuts.

Other than above mentioned, there is the „second eight" which includes: sesame seeds, sunflower seeds, cottonseed meal, poppy seeds, molluscs, beans (other than green beans), peas and lentils. Tartrazine, sulphites and latex are considered also as major serious allergens. The „second eight" list may vary among countries, depending on usually consumed foodstuffs.

Codex Alimentarius Commission (CAC) adopted a list of foods and ingredients that should always be declared on labels. These include the „big eight" and products of these, and sulphites in concentration of 10 mg/kg or more. The only efficient way to prevent food allergies is to avoid specific food, since no effective treatment has been found.

1. Hidden Sources of Allergens

The most common reason for allergic reaction is the incidence of hidden food allergens, which have not been declared on food labels. Contamination of safe food with allergens could occur in many ways, but more often includes:

- cross contamination, when the same equipment or production line is used in a plant to make different products (chocolate with and without nuts), or when in the same plant the allergen free and other food products are processed (gluten free and bakery products containing wheat)

- misleading labels of ingredients, added for the specific purposes such as binders, emulsifiers, flavoring agents, etc. (not listed in a user friendly way to inform the consumer, but declared as E number or its chemical structure).

Food processing affects food allergens. Protein denaturation and/or hydrolysis during food processing can be used to produce hypoallergenic products. Sathe and Sharma (2009) give an overview of the effects of food processing on food allergen stability.

2. The Labeling of Food Allergens

The most common labeling problems occur when a food allergen is present in another ingredient compound in a small amount and is not listed, or even when is listed, it is given in the fashion not easily recognized by the consumer. Failure to list an ingredient as an allergen may cause a product recall. Additional problem could arise from the fact that food allergen may be unnoticed by the consumer, because the majority of packed food products possess the small declarations\` font size. Precautionary statements such as „may contain", indicate the manufacturers\` concern that the product could possibly contain ingredients not listed on the label of the final product. On the other hand, for the consumers, precautionary labeling may mean even more restricted food choice. Regulations and Directives on food allergens labeling are permanently improving, but still there is a lack of uniformity of labeling among countries.

3. Threshold Doses of Allergenic Foods

The lowest observed adverse effect level (LOAEL) is a value which defines a threshold dose for allergenic foods which causes mild and objective symptoms in highly sensitive individuals. Also, there is a need to define the non observed adverse effect level (NOAEL), the quantity of allergen in food which does not affect the individuals highly sensitive to the particular food. Double-blind, placebo-controlled food challenges should be used for the determination of the threshold doses for allergenic foods (Taylor et al., 2004).

The determination of LOAEL and NOAEL for the specific foods containing allergen may enable the establishment of maximum levels of allergen in foods that figures in the Regulation concerning allergens. Additionally, these values could provide the food industry the aim to be achieved through good manufacturing practices and sanitation programs for the food production. LOAEL and NOAEL differ among allergens and individuals. For peanut-allergic individuals, individual threshold doses ranged from 2 to more than 50 mg. The level of 100 μg of peanut proteins can trigger a mild reaction such as itching.

For the allergic individuals even low doses of allergenic foods could present a risk. Therefore, the zero tolerance would be the ideal solution. On the other hand, that goal is unachievable for the food industry, especially because of the use of the same processing facility or equipment for different food products.

4. Allergen Management in Food Industry

Allergen control strategies involve aspects of the manufacturing process, from raw material acquisition to labeling. Key areas for the allergen risk control include: raw material sourcing and storage, employee training and supervision, production scheduling, equipment and premises design, manufacturing, labeling and post-manufacturing controls. The recommended approach to control the possible allergen contamination is through HACCP program, which establishes the system to monitor the defined critical control points.

5. Methods for Detection of Food Allergens

Food allergen detection, characterization and quantification is of huge importance in order to ensure consumer`s safety and to comply with food labeling regulations. This is not an easy task considering the complex nature of allergens and food matrixes. Most of allergens are proteins or glycoproteins (Poms et al., 2005) and they are numerous and heterogeneous, often with several variants of the same protein which makes detection and characterization difficult. Also, the nature of food matrix in which allergen is present strongly influences allergen detection and isolation and greatly affects method sensitivity (Monaci & Visconti, 2009). Another issue is that food allergen detection can be hampered by thermal and biochemical procedures as a part of technological food processing and preservation (van Hengel, 2007). Under these conditions the suspected allergenic protein structure can be altered making the detection and characterization more difficult and demanding. Additionally, there is possibility of food contamination from another sources via machinery used in food processing chain.

In general, food allergies are allergic reactions that are characterized by production of allergen specific immunoglobulin E (IgE) and onset of allergenic symptoms (Taylor & Hefle, 2006). Using IgE from sera of allergenic individuals that binds to specific allergen, allergenicity of food or food product can be determined. After offending allergen is identified, purified and characterized, it constitutes an antigen on which antibodies can be raised in appropriate animal (rat, rabbit, sheap, or goat are most often used) and then these antibodies can be applied for allergen detection in various food items and products. This is just one of the technical approaches in detection of offending allergenic substance where it is a protein that constitutes an allergenic marker that is characteristic for particular food or food product. Theoretically, any compound that is present in allergenic food could be used as a marker but in reality most often employed and analyzed are proteins that are allergens themselves and they constitute ideal markers. However, in some cases where, for example, an abundance of allergenic proteins exists and allergen isolation is not feasible, other type of markers could be selected. That is most often DNA present in food and selected as a marker. Depending on which of these two types of markers is employed for food allergen detection, the methods for food allergen detection are divided into protein and DNA based methods.

Protein-based methods can be divided into two groups: immunological (antibody-based methods) and protein separation (for example mass spectrometry) methods. As mentioned above, immunological methods use antibodies raised in animals against purified allergens (antigens) isolated from offending food. These methods are most often used because of high specificity and sensitivity of the produced antibodies. Protein separation methods relay on protein separation due to their difference in size and they are mostly used for identification of allergenic proteins and its structure confirmation.

DNA-based methods are indirect methods because they do not deal with specific allergen (mainly protein) but rather employ the amplification of specific DNA fragments present in offending food by application of the polymerase chain reaction (PCR) technique. The specificity of method is based on the use of primers that are characteristic for offending food enabling the amplification of DNA fragment (van Hengel, 2007; Rossi et al., 2006).

Selection of the detection method depends on food or food product in question and knowledge on its allergen(s), on the availability of the antibodies/DNA primers, on allergen concentrations, on the type of food processing (if any) and on the type of food matrix. A food matrix composition can greatly influence the efficiency of protein or DNA extraction and consequently affecting allergen quantification (Poms et al., 2004; Keck-Gassenmeier et al., 1999). Currently, the ELISA immunoanalytical technique is the only one used in food industry laboratories and food-control bodies for routine food analysis. Its high specificity and precision, rather simple handling and good potential for standardization are the main reasons for this.

The following section describes in more detail some of the most commonly used methods for food allergens detection.

5.1. Enzyme-Linked Immunosorbent Assay (ELISA)

At present, ELISA is the most commonly used method for analysis of allergens in food and food commodities. The assay is carried out in multiple-well strips or more commonly 96-well microtiter plates. These plates contain immobilized antibody (for specific allergen) labeled by specific enzyme and visualized by an enzymatic reaction producing a colored product. The color of product is read on spectrophotometer and measured absorption is directly proportional to the concentration of allergenic compound which can be determined from the calibration curve. This assay allows analysis of multiple samples for a single allergen in rather short time (from 0.5 to 3 hours, depending on type of ELISA assay). Many ELISA kits became available in recent years for the analysis of main allergens. For example, ELISA assay for detection of eggs in food products employs polyclonal antibodies raised against total egg protein, egg white protein or a specific egg allergen (ovalbumin and/or ovomucoid) respectively. The detection range is between < 1 and 5 mg/kg. ELISA is also used for the analysis of gluten, main allergen from cereals. A method to trace gluten in various food products was first introduced by Skerritt and Hill (1991). The method was highly specific thus limited to specific cultivars and for that reason was later modified. Currently, there are several ELISA assay kits that target gliadin fraction of gluten with detection range between 1 and 2 mg/kg. In a similar way there are kits for the majority of main food allergens. ELISA kits have a rather good reliability even though difference exists from the supplier to supplier and there is a need for the method validation and common experimental protocol (Poms et al., 2005; Park et al., 2005).

5.2. SDS – PAGE and Immunoblotting

This method employs one dimensional sodium dodecyl sulphate (SDS) polyacryl gel electrophoresis (PAGE) to separate suspected proteins-allergens according to their molecular mass. It is then followed by transfer of separated proteins onto a membrane and detection by antibodies (immunoblotting). Specific antibody reacts with a particular protein band and in that way detects specific allergen. The drawback of the method is a long and complex procedure even though it can detect food allergens down to 5 mg/kg (Scheibe et al., 2001). For example, detection of bovine milk proteins in soy protein was performed by this methodology (Molina et al., 1998). Similar to this method is *Dot immunoblotting* where protein extracts are spotted onto nitrocellulose or polyvynylidene fluoride membrane and incubated with enzyme- or radio-labeled specific antibodies that bind to the proteins-antigens. The ensuing enzymatic reaction produces colored product whose intensity is proportional to the concentration of antigen. In the case of radio-labeled antibodies, the radioactivity is measured.

5.3. Polymerase Chain Reaction (PCR)

PCR is DNA based method and represents an indirect method for food allergen analysis. It does not detect or measure the allergen itself but rather a specific fragment of DNA characteristic for an allergen or allergenic food. This fragment coupled with primers (oligonucleotides on each end of the fragment) is amplified by series of reactions by enzyme polymerase at appropriate temperatures and number of cycles producing amplified quantity of original DNA fragment. Amplification is followed by agarose gel electrophoresis to separate the obtained DNA fragment and visualization by staining with a fluorescent dye or by southern blotting. The method is qualitative, not quantitative. Quantification is achieved by using Real-time PCR method. It allows detection of product during a whole process of amplification in real-time. This is accomplished by using fragment specific olegonucleotide probe labelled with a fluorescent reporter dye which permits detection only after hybridization of the probe with its complementary DNA target. In that way by measuring the intensity of the fluorescence the quantity of the amplification product is measured. Several commercially available PCR kits are present on the market for allergens like almond, celery, gluten, hazelnut, milk, peanut and soya (Poms et al., 2004.).

5.4. Biosensors

Biosensors are rather new technology used for food allergens analysis. These are instruments that are capable of measuring specific molecular interactions in real-time. In the case of food allergens, the target molecule, allergenic protein antibody or single stranded DNA fragment, are usually immobilized on the surface of biosensor chip and binding of complementary molecules (e.g. allergens) is observed in real-time by monitoring the changes in refractive index. Quantification is usually performed form the calibration curves. Major advantage of this methodology is short assay time, automation and convenient detection without using the labels. On other hand the instruments are rather expensive and only a single sample can be tested at the time. In practice, biosensors have been applied for the analysis of various allergens as for example hazelnut protein in olive oil (Bremer et al., 2009).

5.5. Mass Spectrometry-Based Proteomics

This is a new emerging methodology that couples proteomics (study of proteins) with mass spectrometry, a powerful analytical tool. In general, proteomics part of this methodology involves protein extraction from the sample matrix, protein cleavage to obtain constitutive peptides and then mass spectrometry part where these peptides or whole proteins are analyzed to obtain their structure and to identify the allergenic protein (Monaci & Visconti, 2009). Protein isolation and separation techniques like two-dimensional polyacrilamide gel electrophoresis (2D-PAGE) and liquid chromatography (LC) are mostly used to isolate, separate and prepare the proteins for the analysis by mass spectrometry (MS). Proteins can be analyzed as a whole, intact, or they can be subjected to proteolytic digestion to obtain peptides, separated by LC and then analyzed by one of the mass spectrometry methods. Obtained MS spectra can be scanned against bases of protein sequence data to identify obtained peptides and final protein structure (Lane, 2005). There is a variety of mass spectrometry techniques used for protein identification and they differ mostly in the types of ionization and detection used. This is described in more details by Monaci and Visconti (2009). The advantage of this modern method is unambiguous identification of protein-allergen structure and low level of detection, on the other hand, the instrumentation is expensive and sample preparation is rather long. Despite this, MS-based methods are receiving more and more application in food allergen detection. Several proteins and peptides from peanuts, milk and milk whey have been isolated and detected using this methodology (Shefcheck & Musser, 2004; Weber et al., 2006; Monaci & van Hengel, 2008).

Conclusion

Emerging issues of food allergens relate to genetically modified (GM) food due to introduction of novel proteins comparing to the original food from which genetically modified food was derived. There is some possibility that some of those novel proteins could be or become food allergens (Taylor, 2000). Currently, it is highly unlikely that many of the health risks from GM food can be identified and eliminated, since data on allergies caused by GM food are still limited. Definitions in this area are necessary from the food safety point of view (van Tassel, 2009; FAO/WHO, 2001).

Rise in the number of people with food allergy and further development of novel foods and food ingredients will require a development of even more sensitive and easy to use food allergen detection methods.

References

Bremer, M.G.E.G., Smits, N.G.E. and Haasnoot, W. (2009). Biosensor immunoassay for traces of hazelnut protein in olive oil. *Analytical and Bioanalytical Chemistry, 395,* 119-126.

FAO/WHO (2001). Evaluation of allergenicity of genetically modified foods. In: Report of a Joint FAO/WHO Expert Consultation of Allergenicity of Foods.

Keck-Gassenmeier, B., Benet, S., Rosa, C. and Hischenhuber, C. (1999). Determination of peanut traces in food by a commercially available ELISA test. *Food and Agricultural Immunology, 11,* 243-250.

Lane, C.S. (2005). Mass spectrometry-based proteomics in the life sciences. *Cellular and Molecular Life Sciences, 62,* 848-869.

Molina, E., Amigo, L. and Ramos, M. (1998). Detection of bovine milk proteins in soymilk by Western blotting. *Journal of Food Protection, 61,* 1691-1694.

Monaci, L. and van Hengel, A.J. (2008). Development of a method for the quantification of whey allergen traces in mixed-fruit juices based on liquid chromatography with mass spectrometric detection. *Journal of Chromatography A, 1192,* 113-120.

Monaci, L. and Visconti, A. (2009). Mass spectrometry-based proteomics methods for analysis of food allergens. *Trends in Analytical Chemistry, 28,* 581-591.

Park, D.L., Coates, S., Brewer, V.A., Garber, E.A., Abouzied, M., Johnson, K., Ritter, B. and Mckenzie, D. (2005). Performance tested method SM multiple laboratory validation study of ELISA-based assays for the detection of peanuts in food. *Journal of AOAC International, 88,* 156-160.

Poms, R.E., Capelletti, C. and Anklam, E. (2004). Effect of roasting history and buffer composition on peanut protein extraction efficiency. *Molecular Nutrition and Food Research, 48,* 459-464.

Poms, R.E., Klein, C.L. and Anklam, E. (2004). Methods for allergen analysis in food: a review. *Food Additives and Contaminants, 21,* 1-31.

Poms, R.E., Agazzi, M.E., Bau, A., Brohee, M., Capelletti, C., Norgaard, J.V and Anklam, E. (2005). Inter-laboratory validation of five commercial ELISA test kits for the determination of peanut proteins in biscuits and dark chocolate. *Food Additives and Contaminants, 22,* 104-112.

Rossi, S., Scaravelli, E., Germini, A., Corradini, R., Fogher, C. and Marchelli, R. (2006). A PNA-array platform for the detection of hidden allergens in foodstuffs. *European Food Research and Technology, 223,* 1-6.

Sathe, S.K. and Sharma, G.M. (2009). Effects of food processing on food allergens. *Molecular Nutrition and Food Research, 53,* 970-978.

Schefcheck, K.J. and Musser, S.M. (2004). Confirmation of the Allergenic Peanut Protein, Ara h 1, in a Model Food Matrix Using Liquid Chromatography/Tandem Mass Spectrometry (LC/MS/MS). *Journal of Agricultural and Food Chemistry, 52,* 2785-2790.

Scheibe, B., Weiss, W., Rueff, F., Przybilla, B. and Gorg, A. (2001). Detection of trace amounts of hidden allergens: hazelnut and almond proteins in chocolate. *Journal of Chromatography B Biomedical Science and Applications, 756,* 229-237.

Skerritt, J.H. and Hill, A.S. (1991). Enzyme immunoassay for determination of gluten in foods: collaborative study. *Journal of Association of Official Analytical Chemists, 74,* 257-264.

Taylor, S. L. (2000). Emerging problems with food allergens. Food Nutrition and Agriculture, FAO, 26, 14–21.

Taylor, S. L., Hefle, S. L., Bindslev-Jensen, C., Atkins, F. M., Andre, C., Bruijnzeel-Koomen, C., Burks, A. W., Bush, R. K., Ebisawa, M., Eigenmann, P. A., Host, A., Hourihane, J. O'B., Isolauri, E., Hill, D. J., Knulst, A., Lack, G., Sampson, H. A., Moneret-Vautrin, D. A., Rance, F. and Vadas, P. A. (2004). A consensus protocol for the determination of the threshold doses for allergenic foods: how much is too much? *Clinical and Experimental Allergy, 34,* 689-695.

Taylor, S.L. and Hefle, S.L. (2006). Food allergen labeling in the USA and Europe. *Current Opinion in Allergy and Clinical Immunology, 6,* 186-190.

van Hengel, A.J. (2007). Food allergen detection methods and the challenge to protect food-allergic consumers. *Analytical and Bioanalytical Chemistry, 389,* 111-118.

Van Tassel, K. A. (2009). Genetically Modified Plants Used for Food, Risk Assessment and Uncertainty Principles: Does the Transition from Ignorance to Indeterminacy Trigger the Need for Post-Market Surveillance. *Boston University Journal of Science and Technology Law, 15,* 220-251.

Weber, D., Raymond, P., Ben-Rejeb, S. and Lau, B. (2006). Development of a Liquid Chromatography–Tandem Mass Spectrometry Method Using Capillary Liquid Chromatography and Nanoelectrospray Ionization–Quadrupole Time-of-Flight Hybrid Mass Spectrometer for the Detection of Milk Allergens. *Journal of Agricultural and Food Chemistry, 54,* 1604-1610.

In: Nutritional Insights and Food Safety
Editor: Jaroslava Švarc-Gajiæ

ISBN: 978-1-61122-130-5

Appendix I

Comparative list of EU and Codex Alimentarius MRLs (Council Directive 2377/90/EC, Anex I, III, consolidated version, updated 2009, Codex Alimentarius Commission, Updated as at the 32nd session of the Codex Alimentarius Commission, July 2009).

Annex I. LIST OF PHARMACOLOGICALLY ACTIVE SUBSTANCES USED IN VETERINARY MEDICINAL PRODUCTS FOR WHICH MAXIMUM RESIDUE LIMITS HAVE BEEN FIXED

Pharmacologically active substances	Animal species	Target tissues	EU MRLs	Codex Alimentarius MRLs
Sulfonamides	All food-producing species	Muscle	100 μg/kg	100 μg/kg – sulfadimidine only
		Fat	100 μg/kg	100 μg/kg – sulfadimidine only
		Liver	100 μg/kg	100 μg/kg – sulfadimidine only
		Kidney	100 μg/kg	100 μg/kg – sulfadimidine only
	Bovine, ovine	Milk	100 μg/kg	Bovine 25 μg/kg – sulfadimidine only
Baquiloprim	Bovine	Fat	10 μg/kg	
		Liver	300 μg/kg	
		Kidney	150 μg/kg	
		Milk	30 μg/kg	
	Porcine	Skin and fat	40 μg/kg	
		Liver	50 μg/kg	
		Kidney	50 μg/kg	
Trimethoprim	All food-producing species	Fat	50 μg/kg	
		Muscle	50 μg/kg	
		Liver	50 μg/kg	
		Kidney	50 μg/kg	
		Milk	50 μg/kg	
	Equidae	Muscle	100 μg/kg	
		Fat	100 μg/kg	
		Liver	100 μg/kg	
		Kidney	100 μg/kg	
Amoxicyllin	All food-producing species	Muscle	50 μg/kg	
		Fat	50 μg/kg	

Annex I. (Continued)

Pharmacologically active substances	Animal species	Target tissues	EU MRLs	Codex Alimentarius MRLs
		Liver	50 µg/kg	
		Kidney	50 µg/kg	
		Milk	4 µg/kg	
Ampicillin	All food-producing species	Muscle	50 µg/kg	
		Fat	50 µg/kg	
		Liver	50 µg/kg	
		Kidney	50 µg/kg	
		Milk	4 µg/kg	
Benzylpenicillin	All food-producing species	Muscle	50 µg/kg	
		Fat	50 µg/kg	
		Liver	50 µg/kg	
		Kidney	50 µg/kg	
		Milk	4 µg/kg	
	Chicken/Pig	Muscle		50 µg/kg
		Liver		50 µg/kg
		Kidney		50 µg/kg
	Cattle	Muscle		50 µg/kg
		Liver		50 µg/kg
		Kidney		50 µg/kg
		Milk (µg/l)		4 µg/kg
Cloxacillin	All food-producing species	Muscle	300 µg/kg	
		Fat	300 µg/kg	
		Liver	300 µg/kg	
		Kidney	300 µg/kg	
		Milk	30 µg/kg	
Dicloxacillin	All food-producing species	Muscle	300 µg/kg	
		Fat	300 µg/kg	
		Liver	300 µg/kg	
		Kidney	300 µg/kg	
		Milk	30 µg/kg	
Nafcillin	All ruminants	Muscle	300 µg/kg	
		Fat	300 µg/kg	
		Liver	300 µg/kg	
		Kidney	300 µg/kg	
		Milk	30 µg/kg	
Oxacillin	All food-producing species	Muscle	300 µg/kg	
		Fat	300 µg/kg	
		Liver	300 µg/kg	
		Kidney	300 µg/kg	
		Milk	30 µg/kg	
Penethemate	Bovine	Muscle	50 µg/kg	
		Fat	50 µg/kg	
		Liver	50 µg/kg	
		Kidney	50 µg/kg	
		Milk	4 µg/kg	
	Porcine	Muscle	50 µg/kg	
		Fat	50 µg/kg	
		Liver	50 µg/kg	
		Kidney	50 µg/kg	
	All mammalian-food	Muscle	50 µg/kg	

Pharmacologically active substances	Animal species	Target tissues	EU MRLs	Codex Alimentarius MRLs
	producing species			
		Fat	50 µg/kg	
		Liver	50 µg/kg	
		Kidney	50 µg/kg	
		Milk	4 µg/kg	
Phenoxymethylpenicillin	Porcine	Muscle	25 µg/kg	
		Liver	25 µg/kg	
		Kidney	25 µg/kg	
	Poultry	Muscle	25 µg/kg	
		Skin and fat	25 µg/kg	
		Liver	25 µg/kg	
		Kidney	25 µg/kg	
Cefacetrile	Bovine	Milk	125 µg/kg	
Cefalexin	Bovine	Muscle	200 µg/kg	
		Fat	200 µg/kg	
		Liver	200 µg/kg	
		Kidney	1000 µg/kg	
		Milk	100 µg/kg	
Cefalonium	Bovine	Milk	20 µg/kg	
Cefapirin	Bovine	Muscle	50 µg/kg	
		Fat	50 µg/kg	
		Kidney	100 µg/kg	
		Milk	60 µg/kg	
Cefazolin	Bovine, ovine, caprine	Milk	50 µg/kg	
Cefoperazone	Bovine	Milk	50 µg/kg	
Cefquinome	Bovine	Muscle	50 µg/kg	
		Fat	50 µg/kg	
		Liver	100 µg/kg	
		Kidney	200 µg/kg	
		Milk	20 µg/kg	
	Porcine	Muscle	50 µg/kg	
		Skin and fat	50 µg/kg	
		Liver	100 µg/kg	
		Kidney	200 µg/kg	
	Equidae	Muscle	50 µg/kg	
		Fat	50 µg/kg	
		Liver	100 µg/kg	
		Kidney	200 µg/kg	
Ceftiofur	All mammalian food-producing species	Muscle	1000 µg/kg	1000 µg/kg
		Fat	2000 µg/kg	2000 µg/kg
		Liver	2000 µg/kg	2000 µg/kg
		Kidney	6000 µg/kg	6000 µg/kg
		Milk	100 µg/kg	100 µg/l
Danofloxacin	All food-producing species except bovine, ovine, caprine, porcine and poultry	Muscle	100 µg/kg	
		Fat	50 µg/kg	
		Liver	200 µg/kg	
		Kidney	200 µg/kg	
	Bovine, ovine, caprine	Muscle	200 µg/kg	
		Fat	100 µg/kg	
		Liver	400 µg/kg	
		Kidney	400 µg/kg	

Annex I. (Continued)

Pharmacologically active substances	Animal species	Target tissues	EU MRLs	Codex Alimentarius MRLs
		Milk	30 µg/kg	
	Poultry	Muscle	200 µg/kg	
		Skin and fat	100 µg/kg	
		Liver	400 µg/kg	
		Kidney	400 µg/kg	
Difloxacin	All food-producing species except bovine, ovine, caprine, porcine and poultry	Muscle	300 µg/kg	
		Fat	100 µg/kg	
		Liver	800 µg/kg	
		Kidney	600 µg/kg	
	Bovine, ovine, caprine	Muscle	400 µg/kg	
		Fat	100 µg/kg	
		Liver	1400 µg/kg	
		Kidney	800 µg/kg	
	Porcine	Muscle	400 µg/kg	
		Skin and fat	100 µg/kg	
		Liver	800 µg/kg	
		Kidney	800 µg/kg	
	Poultry	Muscle	300 µg/kg	
		Skin and fat	400 µg/kg	
		Liver	1900 µg/kg	
		Kidney	600 µg/kg	
Enrofloxacin	All food-producing species except bovine, ovine, caprine, porcine, rabbits and poultry	Muscle	100 µg/kg	
		Fat	100 µg/kg	
		Liver	200 µg/kg	
		Kidney	200 µg/kg	
	Bovine, ovine, caprine	Muscle	100 µg/kg	
		Fat	100 µg/kg	
		Liver	300 µg/kg	
		Kidney	200 µg/kg	
		Milk	100 µg/kg	
	Porcine, rabbits	Muscle	100 µg/kg	
		Fat	100 µg/kg	
		Liver	200 µg/kg	
		Kidney	300 µg/kg	
	Poultry	Muscle	100 µg/kg	
		Skin and fat	100 µg/kg	
		Liver	200 µg/kg	
		Kidney	300 µg/kg	
Flumequine	All food-producing species except bovine, ovine, caprine, porcine, poultry and fin fish	Muscle	200 µg/kg	
		Fat	250 µg/kg	
		Liver	500 µg/kg	

Pharmacologically active substances	Animal species	Target tissues	EU MRLs	Codex Alimentarius MRLs
		Kidney	1000 µg/kg	
	Bovine, porcine, ovine, caprine	Muscle	200 µg/kg	
		Fat	300 µg/kg	
		Liver	500 µg/kg	
		Kidney	1500 µg/kg	
		Milk	50 µg/kg	
	Poultry	Muscle	400 µg/kg	
		Skin and fat	250 µg/kg	
		Liver	800 µg/kg	
		Kidney	1000 µg/kg	
	Fin fish	Muscle and skin in natural proportion	600 µg/kg	
Marbofloxacin	Bovine	Muscle	150 µg/kg	
		Fat	50 µg/kg	
		Liver	150 µg/kg	
		Kidney	150 µg/kg	
		Milk	75 µg/kg	
	Porcine	Muscle	150 µg/kg	
		Skin and fat	50 µg/kg	
		Liver	150 µg/kg	
		Kidney	150 µg/kg	
Oxolinic acid	Porcine	Muscle	100 µg/kg	
		Skin and fat	50 µg/kg	
		Liver	150 µg/kg	
		Kidney	150 µg/kg	
	Chicken	Muscle	100 µg/kg	
		Skin and fat	50 µg/kg	
		Liver	150 µg/kg	
		Kidney	150 µg/kg	
	Fin fish	Muscle and skin in natural proportion	100 µg/kg	
	All food-producing species	Muscle	100 µg/kg	
		Fat	50 µg/kg	
		Liver	150 µg/kg	
		Kidney	150 µg/kg	
Sarafloxacin	Chicken	Skin and fat	10 µg/kg	20 µg/kg
		Liver	100 µg/kg	80 µg/kg
		Kidney		80 µg/kg
		Muscle		10 µg/kg
	Turkey	Muscle		10 µg/kg
		Liver		80 µg/kg
		Kidney		80 µg/kg
		Fat		20 µg/kg
	Salmonidae	Muscle and skin in natural proportion	30 µg/kg	
Erythromycin	All food-producing species	Muscle	200 µg/kg	
		Fat	200 µg/kg	
		Liver	200 µg/kg	
		Kidney	200 µg/kg	
		Milk	40 µg/kg	
		Eggs	150 µg/kg	
Gamithromycin	Bovine	Fat	20 µg/kg	

Annex I. (Continued)

Pharmacologically active substances	Animal species	Target tissues	EU MRLs	Codex Alimentarius MRLs
		Liver	200 μg/kg	
		Kidney	100 μg/kg	
Spiramycin	Bovine	Muscle	200 μg/kg	200 μg/kg
		Fat	300 μg/kg	300 μg/kg
		Liver	300 μg/kg	600 μg/kg
		Kidney	300 μg/kg	300 μg/kg
		Milk	200 μg/kg	200 μg/kg
	Chicken	Muscle	200 μg/kg	200 μg/kg
		Skin and fat	300 μg/kg	300 μg/kg
		Liver	400 μg/kg	600 μg/kg
		Kidney		800 μg/kg
	Porcine	Muscle	250 μg/kg	200 μg/kg
		Liver	2000 μg/kg	600 μg/kg
		Kidney	1000 μg/kg	300 μg/kg
		Fat		300 μg/kg
Tilmicosin	All food-producing species except poultry	Muscle	50 μg/kg	
		Fat	50 μg/kg	
		Liver	1000 μg/kg	
		Kidney	1000 μg/kg	
		Milk	50 μg/kg	
	Poultry	Muscle	75 μg/kg	
		Skin and fat	75 μg/kg	
		Liver	1000 μg/kg	
		Kidney	250 μg/kg	
Tulathromycin	Bovine	Fat	100 μg/kg	
		Liver	3000 μg/kg	
		Kidney	3000 μg/kg	
	Porcine	Skin and fat	100 μg/kg	
		Liver	3000 μg/kg	
		Kidney	3000 μg/kg	
Tylosin	All food-producing species	Fat	100 μg/kg	100 μg/kg
		Muscle	100 μg/kg	100 μg/kg
		Liver	100 μg/kg	100 μg/kg
		Kidney	100 μg/kg	100 μg/kg
		Milk	50 μg/kg	100 μg/kg
		Eggs	200 μg/kg	300 μg/kg
Tylvalosin	Porcine	Muscle	50 μg/kg	
		Fat	50 μg/kg	
		Liver	50 μg/kg	
		Kidney	50 μg/kg	
	Poultry	Fat	50 μg/kg	
		Liver	50 μg/kg	
Thiamphenicol	All food-producing species	Muscle	50 μg/kg	
		Fat	50 μg/kg	
		Liver	50 μg/kg	
		Kidney	50 μg/kg	
		Milk	50 μg/kg	
Chlortetracycline	All food-producing species	Muscle	100 μg/kg	200 μg/kg
		Liver	300 μg/kg	600 μg/kg
		Kidney	600 μg/kg	1200 μg/kg

Pharmacologically active substances	Animal species	Target tissues	EU MRLs	Codex Alimentarius MRLs
		Milk	100 μg/kg	100 μg/kg
		Eggs	200 μg/kg	400 μg/kg
Doxycycline	Bovine Not for use in animals from which milk is produced for human consumption	Muscle	100 μg/kg	
		Liver	300 μg/kg	
		Kidney	600 μg/kg	
	Porcine	Muscle	100 μg/kg	
		Skin and fat	300 μg/kg	
		Liver	300 μg/kg	
		Kidney	600 μg/kg	
	Poultry Not for use in animals from which eggs are produced for human consumption	Muscle	100 μg/kg	
		Skin and fat	300 μg/kg	
		Liver	300 μg/kg	
		Kidney	600 μg/kg	
Oxytetracycline	All food-producing species	Muscle	100 μg/kg	200 μg/kg
		Liver	300 μg/kg	600 μg/kg
		Kidney	600 μg/kg	1200 μg/kg
		Milk	100 μg/kg	100 μg/kg
		Eggs	200 μg/kg	400 μg/kg
	Fish	Muscle		200 μg/kg
Tetracycline	All food-producing species	Muscle	100 μg/kg	200 μg/kg
		Liver	300 μg/kg	600 μg/kg
		Kidney	600 μg/kg	1200 μg/kg
		Milk	100 μg/kg	100 μg/kg
	Fish	Muscle		200 μg/kg
		Eggs	200 μg/kg	400 μg/kg
Rifaximin	Bovine	Milk	60 μg/kg	
Tiamulin	Porcine	Muscle	100 μg/kg	
		Liver	500 μg/kg	
	Chicken	Muscle	100 μg/kg	
		Skin and fat	100 μg/kg	
		Liver	1000 μg/kg	
	Rabbits	Muscle	100 μg/kg	
		Liver	500 μg/kg	
	Turkey	Muscle	100 μg/kg	
		Skin and fat	100 μg/kg	
		Liver	300 μg/kg	
		Eggs	1000 μg/kg	
Valnemulin	Porcine	Muscle	50 μg/kg	
		Liver	500 μg/kg	
		Kidney	100 μg/kg	
Linomycin	All food-producing species	Fat	50 μg/kg	
		Muscle	100 μg/kg	
		Liver	500 μg/kg	
		Kidney	1500 μg/kg	
		Milk	150 μg/kg	
		Eggs	50 μg/kg	
	Cattle	Milk		150 μg/l
	Chicken	Muscle		200 μg/kg
		Liver		500 μg/kg

Annex I. (Continued)

Pharmacologically active substances	Animal species	Target tissues	EU MRLs	Codex Alimentarius MRLs
		Kidney		500 μg/kg
		Fat		100 μg/kg
	Pig	Muscle		200 μg/kg
		Liver		500 μg/kg
		Kidney		1500 μg/kg
		Fat		100 μg/kg
Pirlimycin	Bovine	Muscle	100 μg/kg	
		Fat	100 μg/kg	
		Liver	1000 μg/kg	
		Kidney	400 μg/kg	
		Milk	100 μg/kg	
	Porcine	Muscle	100 μg/kg	
		Skin and fat	50 μg/kg	
		Liver	500 μg/kg	
		Kidney	1500 μg/kg	
	Chicken	Muscle	100 μg/kg	
		Skin and fat	50 μg/kg	
		Liver	500 μg/kg	
		Kidney	1500 μg/kg	
		Eggs	50 μg/kg	
Apramycin	Bovine	Muscle	1000 μg/kg	
		Fat	1000 μg/kg	
		Liver	10000 μg/kg	
		Kidney	20000 μg/kg	
Dihydrostreptomycin	All ruminants	Muscle	500 μg/kg	
		Fat	500 μg/kg	
		Liver	500 μg/kg	
		Kidney	1000 μg/kg	
		Milk	200 μg/kg	
	Porcine	Muscle	500 μg/kg	
		Skin and fat	500 μg/kg	
		Liver	500 μg/kg	
		Kidney	1000 μg/kg	
	Rabbits	Muscle	500 μg/kg	
		Fat	500 μg/kg	
		Liver	500 μg/kg	
		Kidney	1000 μg/kg	
Gentamicin	Bovine	Muscle	50 μg/kg	100 μg/kg
		Fat	50 μg/kg	100 μg/kg
		Liver	200 μg/kg	2000μg/kg
		Kidney	750 μg/kg	5000 μg/kg
		Milk	100 μg/kg	200 μg/l
	Porcine	Muscle	50 μg/kg	100 μg/kg
		Skin and fat	50 μg/kg	100 μg/kg
		Liver	200 μg/kg	2000 μg/kg
		Kidney	750 μg/kg	5000 μg/kg
Kanamycin	All food-producing species except fish	Muscle	100 μg/kg	
		Fat	100 μg/kg	
		Liver	600 μg/kg	
		Kidney	2500 μg/kg	
		Milk	150 μg/kg	
Neomycin (including framycetin)	All food-producing species	Fat	500 μg/kg	500 μg/kg
		Muscle	500 μg/kg	500 μg/kg

Pharmacologically active substances	Animal species	Target tissues	EU MRLs	Codex Alimentarius MRLs
		Liver	500 µg/kg	500 µg/kg
		Kidney	5000 µg/kg	10000 µg/kg
		Milk	1500 µg/kg	1500 µg/kg
		Eggs	500 µg/kg	500 µg/kg
Paromomycin	All food-producing species	Muscle	500 µg/kg	
		Liver	1500 µg/kg	
		Kidney	1500 µg/kg	
Spectinomycin	All food-producing species except ovine	Fat	500 µg/kg	
		Muscle	300 µg/kg	
		Liver	1000 µg/kg	
		Kidney	5000 µg/kg	
		Milk	200 µg/kg	
	Ovine	Muscle	300 µg/kg	
		Fat	500 µg/kg	
		Liver	2000 µg/kg	
		Kidney	5000 µg/kg	
		Milk	200 µg/kg	
	Cattle, Chicken, Pig, Sheep	Muscle		500 µg/kg
		Liver		2000 µg/kg
		Kidney		5000 µg/kg
		Fat		2000 µg/kg
	Cattle	Milk (µg/l)		200 µg/l
Streptomycin	All ruminants	Muscle	500 µg/kg	
		Fat	500 µg/kg	
		Liver	500 µg/kg	
		Kidney	1000 µg/kg	
		Milk	200 µg/kg	
	Porcine	Muscle	500 µg/kg	
		Skin and fat	500 µg/kg	
		Liver	500 µg/kg	
		Kidney	1000 µg/kg	
	Rabbits	Muscle	500 µg/kg	
		Fat	500 µg/kg	
		Liver	500 µg/kg	
		Kidney	1000 µg/kg	
Novobiocin	Bovine	Milk	50 µg/kg	
Bacitracin	Bovine	Milk	100 µg/kg	
	Rabbits	Muscle	150 µg/kg	
		Fat	150 µg/kg	
		Liver	150 µg/kg	
		Kidney	150 µg/kg	
Clavulanic acid	Bovine	Muscle	100 µg/kg	
		Fat	100 µg/kg	
		Liver	200 µg/kg	
		Kidney	400 µg/kg	
		Milk	200 µg/kg	
	Porcine	Muscle	100 µg/kg	
		Skin and fat	100 µg/kg	
		Liver	200 µg/kg	
		Kidney	400 µg/kg	
Colistin	All food-producing species	Fat	150 µg/kg	
		Muscle	150 µg/kg	
		Liver	150 µg/kg	
		Kidney	200 µg/kg	

Annex I. (Continued)

Pharmacologically active substances	Animal species	Target tissues	EU MRLs	Codex Alimentarius MRLs
		Milk	50 μg/kg	
		Eggs	300 μg/kg	
Avilamycin	Porcine	Muscle	50 μg/kg	200 μg/kg
		Fat	100 μg/kg	200 μg/kg
		Liver	300 μg/kg	300 μg/kg
		Kidney	200 μg/kg	200 μg/kg
	Rabbit	Muscle	50 μg/kg	200 μg/kg
		Fat	100 μg/kg	200 μg/kg
		Liver	300 μg/kg	300 μg/kg
		Kidney	200 μg/kg	200 μg/kg
	Poultry	Muscle	50 μg/kg	200 μg/kg
		Fat	100 μg/kg	200 μg/kg
		Liver	300 μg/kg	300 μg/kg
		Kidney	200 μg/kg	200 μg/kg
	Turkey	Muscle		200 μg/kg
		Liver		300 μg/kg
		Kidney		200 μg/kg
		Fat/Skin		200 μg/kg
Monensin	Bovine	Muscle	2 μg/kg	10 μg/kg
		Fat	10 μg/kg	100 μg/kg
		Liver	30 μg/kg	20 μg/kg
		Kidney	2 μg/kg	10 μg/kg
		Milk	2 μg/kg	2 μg/kg
	Sheep, goats	Muscle		10 μg/kg
		Liver		20 μg/kg
		Kidney		10 μg/kg
		Fat		100 μg/kg
	Chicken, turkey, quail	Muscle		10 μg/kg
		Liver		10 μg/kg
		Kidney		10 μg/kg
		Fat		100 μg/kg
Lasalocid	Poultry	Muscle	20 μg/kg	
		Fat	100 μg/kg	
		Liver	100 μg/kg	
		Kidney	50 μg/kg	
		Eggs	150 μg/kg	
Closantel	Bovine	Muscle	1000 μg/kg	1000 μg/kg
		Fat	3000 μg/kg	3000 μg/kg
		Liver	1000 μg/kg	1000 μg/kg
		Kidney	3000 μg/kg	3000 μg/kg
	Ovine	Muscle	1500 μg/kg	1500 μg/kg
		Fat	2000 μg/kg	2000 μg/kg
		Liver	1500 μg/kg	1500 μg/kg
		Kidney	5000 μg/kg	5000 μg/kg
Rafoxanide	Bovine	Muscle	30 μg/kg	
		Fat	30 μg/kg	
		Liver	10 μg/kg	
		Kidney	40 μg/kg	
	Ovine	Muscle	100 μg/kg	
		Fat	250 μg/kg	
		Liver	150 μg/kg	
		Kidney	150 μg/kg	
Levamisole	Bovine, ovine, porcine, poultry	Muscle	10 μg/kg	10 μg/kg

Pharmacologically active substances	Animal species	Target tissues	EU MRLs	Codex Alimentarius MRLs
		Fat	10 μg/kg	10 μg/kg
		Liver	100 μg/kg	100 μg/kg
		Kidney	10 μg/kg	10 μg/kg
Albendazole	All ruminants	Muscle	100 μg/kg	100 μg/kg
		Fat	100 μg/kg	100 μg/kg
		Liver	1000 μg/kg	5000 μg/kg
		Kidney	500 μg/kg	5000 μg/kg
		Milk	100 μg/kg	100 μg/kg
Albendazole oxide	Bovine, ovine	Muscle	100 μg/kg	
		Fat	100 μg/kg	
		Liver	1000 μg/kg	
		Kidney	500 μg/kg	
		Milk	100 μg/kg	
Febantel	All ruminants	Muscle	50 μg/kg	100 μg/kg
		Fat	50 μg/kg	100 μg/kg
		Liver	500 μg/kg	500 μg/kg
		Kidney	50 μg/kg	100 μg/kg
		Milk	10 μg/kg	100 μg/kg
Fenbendazole	All ruminants	Muscle	50 μg/kg	100 μg/kg
		Fat	50 μg/kg	100 μg/kg
		Liver	500 μg/kg	500 μg/kg
		Kidney	50 μg/kg	100 μg/kg
		Milk	10 μg/kg	100 μg/l
Flubendazole	Poultry, porcine	Muscle	50 μg/kg	
		Skin and fat	50 μg/kg	
		Liver	400 μg/kg	
		Kidney	300 μg/kg	
	Pig	Muscle		10 μg/kg
		Liver		10 μg/kg
	Poultry	Muscle		200 μg/kg
		Liver		500 μg/kg
Flubendazole	Poultry	Eggs	7000 μg/kg	7000 μg/kg
Mebendazole	Ovine, caprine, equidae	Muscle	60 μg/kg	
		Fat	60 μg/kg	
		Liver	400 μg/kg	
		Kidney	60 μg/kg	
Netobimin	Bovine, ovine	Muscle	100 μg/kg	
		Fat	100 μg/kg	
		Liver	1000 μg/kg	
		Kidney	500 μg/kg	
		Milk	100 μg/kg	
Oxfendazole	All ruminants	Muscle	50 μg/kg	100 μg/kg
		Fat	50 μg/kg	100 μg/kg
		Liver	500 μg/kg	500 μg/kg
		Kidney	50 μg/kg	100 μg/kg
		Milk	10 μg/kg	100 μg/l
Oxibendazole	Porcine	Muscle	100 μg/kg	
		Skin and fat	500 μg/kg	
		Liver	200 μg/kg	
		Kidney	100 μg/kg	
Thiabendazole	Caprine	Muscle	100 μg/kg	
		Fat	100 μg/kg	
		Liver	100 μg/kg	
		Kidney	100 μg/kg	
		Milk	100 μg/kg	
	Cattle, goat, pig, sheep	Muscle		100 μg/kg

Annex I. (Continued)

Pharmacologically active substances	Animal species	Target tissues	EU MRLs	Codex Alimentarius MRLs
		Liver		100 μg/kg
		Kidney		100 μg/kg
		Fat		100 μg/kg
		Milk		100 μg/l
Triclabendazole	All ruminants	Muscle	225 μg/kg	
		Fat	100 μg/kg	
		Liver	250 μg/kg	
		Kidney	150 μg/kg	
	Cattle	Muscle		250 μg/kg
		Liver		850 μg/kg
		Kidney		400 μg/kg
		Fat		100 μg/kg
	Sheep	Nuscle		200 μg/kg
		Liver		300 μg/kg
		Kidney		200 μg/kg
		Fat		100 μg/kg
Nitroxinil	Bovine, ovine	Muscle	400 μg/kg	
		Fat	200 μg/kg	
		Liver	20 μg/kg	
		Kidney	400 μg/kg	
Oxyclozanide	All ruminants	Muscle	20 μg/kg	
		Fat	20 μg/kg	
		Liver	500 μg/kg	
		Kidney	100 μg/kg	
		Milk	10 μg/kg	
Clorsulon	Bovine	Muscle	35 μg/kg	
		Liver	100 μg/kg	
		Kidney	200 μg/kg	
Piperazine	Porcine	Muscle	400 μg/kg	
		Skin and fat	800 μg/kg	
		Liver	2000 μg/kg	
		Kidney	1000 μg/kg	
	Chicken	Eggs	2000 μg/kg	
Morantel	Bovine, ovine	Muscle	100 μg/kg	
		Fat	100 μg/kg	
		Liver	800 μg/kg	
		Kidney	200 μg/kg	
		Milk	50 μg/kg	
	All ruminants	Muscle	100 μg/kg	
		Fat	100 μg/kg	
		Liver	800 μg/kg	
		Kidney	200 μg/kg	
		Milk	50 μg/kg	
Monepantel	Ovine	Muscle	700 μg/kg	
		Fat	7000 μg/kg	
		Liver	5000 μg/kg	
		Kidney	2000 μg/kg	
Coumafos	Bees	Honey	100 μg/kg	
Diazinon	Bovine, ovine, caprine	Milk	20 μg/kg	
	Bovine, porcine, ovine, caprine	Muscle	20 μg/kg	
		Fat	700 μg/kg	
		Liver	20 μg/kg	
		Kidney	20 μg/kg	

Pharmacologically active substances	Animal species	Target tissues	EU MRLs	Codex Alimentarius MRLs
Phoxim	Ovine, Caprine	Muscle	50 µg/kg	50 µg/kg
		Fat	400 µg/kg	400 µg/kg
		Kidney	50 µg/kg	50 µg/kg
		Liver		50 µg/kg
	Porcine	Muscle	20 µg/kg	50 µg/kg
		Skin and fat	700 µg/kg	400 µg/kg
		Liver	20 µg/kg	50 µg/kg
		Kidney	20 µg/kg	50 µg/kg
	Chicken	Muscle	25 µg/kg	
		Skin and fat	550 µg/kg	
		Liver	50 µg/kg	
		Kidney	30 µg/kg	
		Eggs	60 µg/kg	
Amitraz	Bovine	Fat	200 µg/kg	
		Liver	200 µg/kg	
		Kidney	200 µg/kg	
		Milk	10 µg/kg	
	Ovine	Fat	400 µg/kg	
		Liver	100 µg/kg	
		Kidney	200 µg/kg	
		Milk	10 µg/kg	
	Porcine	Skin and fat	400 µg/kg	
		Liver	200 µg/kg	
		Kidney	200 µg/kg	
	Bees	Honey	200 µg/kg	
	Caprine	Fat	200 µg/kg	
		Liver	100 µg/kg	
		Kidney	200 µg/kg	
		Milk	10 µg/kg	
Cyhalothrin	Bovine, pig, sheep	Fat	500 µg/kg	400 µg/kg
		Kidney	50 µg/kg	20 µg/kg
		Liver		20 µg/kg
		Muscle		20 µg/kg
	Bovine	Milk	50 µg/kg	30 µg/kg
Cyfluthrin	Bovine, caprine	Fat	50 µg/kg	
		Liver	10 µg/kg	
		Kidney	10 µg/kg	
		Milk	20 µg/kg	
Deltamethrin	All ruminants	Muscle	10 µg/kg	
		Fat	50 µg/kg	
		Liver	10 µg/kg	
		Kidney	10 µg/kg	
		Milk	20 µg/kg	
	Fin fish	Muscle and skin in natural proportion	10 µg/kg	
Fenvalerate	Bovine	Muscle	25 µg/kg	
		Fat	250 µg/kg	
		Liver	25 µg/kg	
		Kidney	25 µg/kg	
		Milk	40 µg/kg	
Flumethrin	Bovine	Muscle	10 µg/kg	
		Fat	150 µg/kg	
		Liver	20 µg/kg	
		Kidney	10 µg/kg	
		Milk	30 µg/kg	
	Ovine	Muscle	10 µg/kg	
		Fat	150 µg/kg	

Annex I. (Continued)

Pharmacologically active substances	Animal species	Target tissues	EU MRLs	Codex Alimentarius MRLs
		Liver	20 μg/kg	
		Kidney	10 μg/kg	
Permethrin	Bovine	Muscle	50 μg/kg	
		Fat	500 μg/kg	
		Liver	50 μg/kg	
		Kidney	50 μg/kg	
		Milk	50 μg/kg	
Cypermethrin	Salmonidae	Muscle and skin in natural proportion	50 μg/kg	
	All ruminants	Muscle	20 μg/kg	50 μg/kg
		Fat	200 μg/kg	1000 μg/kg
		Liver	20 μg/kg	50 μg/kg
		Kidney	20 μg/kg	50 μg/kg
		Milk	20 μg/kg	100 μg/kg
Alphacypermethrin	Bovine, ovine	Muscle	20 μg/kg	50 μg/kg
		Fat	200 μg/kg	1000 μg/kg
		Liver	20 μg/kg	50 μg/kg
		Kidney	20 μg/kg	50 μg/kg
		Milk	20 μg/kg	100 μg/kg
Diflubenzuron	Salmonidae	Muscle and skin in natural proportion	1000 μg/kg	
Fluazuron	Bovine	Muscle	200 μg/kg	200 μg/kg
		Fat	7000 μg/kg	7000 μg/kg
		Liver	500 μg/kg	500 μg/kg
		Kidney	500 μg/kg	500 μg/kg
Teflubenzuron	Salmonidae	Muscle and skin in natural proportion	500 μg/kg	
Dicyclanil	Ovine	Muscle	200 μg/kg	150 μg/kg
		Fat	150 μg/kg	200 μg/kg
		Liver	400 μg/kg	125 μg/kg
		Kidney	400 μg/kg	125 μg/kg
Cyromazine	Ovine	Muscle	300 μg/kg	
		Fat	300 μg/kg	
		Liver	300 μg/kg	
		Kidney	300 μg/kg	
Abamectin	Bovine	Fat	10 μg/kg	100 μg/kg
		Liver	20 μg/kg	100 μg/kg
		Kidney		50 μg/kg
	Ovine	Muscle	20 μg/kg	
		Fat	50 μg/kg	
		Liver	25 μg/kg	
		Kidney	20 μg/kg	
Doramectin	All mammalian food-producing species	Muscle	40 μg/kg	
		Fat	150 μg/kg	
		Liver	100 μg/kg	
		Kidney	60 μg/kg	
	Cattle	Muscle		10 μg/kg
		Liver		100 μg/kg
		Kidney		30 μg/kg
		Fat		150 μg/kg
		Milk		15 μg/kg

Pharmacologically active substances	Animal species	Target tissues	EU MRLs	Codex Alimentarius MRLs
	Pig	Muscle		5 μg/kg
		Liver		100 μg/kg
		Kidney		30 μg/kg
		Fat		150 μg/kg
Emamectin	Fin fish	Muscle and skin in natural proportion	100 μg/kg	
Eprinomectin	Bovine	Muscle	50 μg/kg	100 μg/kg
		Fat	250 μg/kg	250 μg/kg
		Liver	1500 μg/kg	2000 μg/kg
		Kidney	300 μg/kg	300 μg/kg
		Milk	20 μg/kg	20 μg/l
Ivermectin	Bovine	Fat	40 μg/kg	40 μg/kg
		Liver	100 μg/kg	100 μg/kg
		Milk		10 μg/kg
	Porcine, ovine, equidae	Fat	20 μg/kg	20 μg/kg
		Liver	15 μg/kg	15 μg/kg
	Deer, including reindeer	Muscle	20 μg/kg	
		Fat	100 μg/kg	
		Liver	50 μg/kg	
		Kidney	20 μg/kg	
	All mammalian food-producing species	Fat	100 μg/kg	
		Liver	100 μg/kg	
		Kidney	30 μg/kg	
Moxidectin	Bovine, ovine	Muscle	50 μg/kg	
		Fat	500 μg/kg	
		Liver	100 μg/kg	
		Kidney	50 μg/kg	
	Bovine	Milk	40 μg/kg	
	Equidae	Muscle	50 μg/kg	
		Fat	500 μg/kg	
		Liver	100 μg/kg	
		Kidney	50 μg/kg	
	Ovine	Milk	40 μg/kg	
	Cattle, deer	Muscle		20 μg/kg
		Liver		100 μg/kg
		Kidney		50 μg/kg
		Fat		500 μg/kg
	Sheep	Muscle		50 μg/kg
		Liver		100 μg/kg
		Kidney		50 μg/kg
		Fat		500 μg/kg
Toltrazuril	Chicken	Muscle	100 μg/kg	
		Skin and fat	200 μg/kg	
		Liver	600 μg/kg	
		Kidney	400 μg/kg	
	Turkey	Muscle	100 μg/kg	
		Skin and fat	200 μg/kg	
		Liver	600 μg/kg	
		Kidney	400 μg/kg	
	Porcine	Muscle	100 μg/kg	
		Skin and fat	150 μg/kg	
		Liver	500 μg/kg	
		Kidney	250 μg/kg	

Annex I. (Continued)

Pharmacologically active substances	Animal species	Target tissues	EU MRLs	Codex Alimentarius MRLs
	All mammalian food-producing species	Muscle	100 μg/kg	
		Fat	150 μg/kg	
		Liver	500 μg/kg	
		Kidney	250 μg/kg	
	Poultry	Muscle	100 μg/kg	
		Skin and fat	200 μg/kg	
		Liver	600 μg/kg	
		Kidney	400 μg/kg	
Halofuginone	Bovine	Muscle	10 μg/kg	
		Fat	25 μg/kg	
		Liver	30 μg/kg	
		Kidney	30 μg/kg	
Imidocarb	Bovine	Muscle	300 μg/kg	300 μg/kg
		Fat	50 μg/kg	50 μg/kg
		Liver	2000 μg/kg	1500 μg/kg
		Kidney	1500 μg/kg	2000 μg/kg
		Milk	50 μg/kg	50 μg/kg
	Ovine	Muscle	300 μg/kg	
		Fat	50 μg/kg	
		Liver	2000 μg/kg	
		Kidney	1500 μg/kg	
Azaperone	Porcine	Muscle	100 μg/kg	60 μg/kg
		Skin and fat	100 μg/kg	60 μg/kg
		Liver	100 μg/kg	100 μg/kg
		Kidney	100 μg/kg	100 μg/kg
Carazolol	Porcine	Muscle	5 μg/kg	5 μg/kg
		Skin and fat	5 μg/kg	5 μg/kg
		Liver	25 μg/kg	25 μg/kg
		Kidney	25 μg/kg	25 μg/kg
	Bovine	Muscle	5 μg/kg	
		Fat	5 μg/kg	
		Liver	15 μg/kg	
		Kidney	15 μg/kg	
		Milk	1 μg/kg	
Clenbuterol hydrochloride	Bovine	Muscle	0,1 μg/kg	0.2 μg/kg
		Liver	0,5 μg/kg	0.6 μg/kg
		Kidney	0,5 μg/kg	0.6 μg/kg
		Milk	0,05 μg/kg	0.05 μg/l
		Fat		0.2 μg/kg
	Equidae	Muscle	0,1 μg/kg	0.2 μg/kg
		Liver	0,5 μg/kg	0.6 μg/kg
		Kidney	0,5 μg/kg	0.6 μg/kg
		Fat		0.2 μg/kg
Carprofen	Bovine	Muscle	500 μg/kg	
	Not for use in animals from which milk is produced for human consumption	Fat	1000 μg/kg	
		Liver	1000 μg/kg	
		Kidney	1000 μg/kg	
	Equidae	Muscle	500 μg/kg	
		Fat	1000 μg/kg	
		Liver	1000 μg/kg	

Pharmacologically active substances	Animal species	Target tissues	EU MRLs	Codex Alimentarius MRLs
		Kidney	1000 μg/kg	
Vedaprofen	Equidae	Muscle	50 μg/kg	
		Fat	20 μg/kg	
		Liver	100 μg/kg	
		Kidney	1000 μg/kg	
Carprofen	Bovine, equidae	Muscle	500 μg/kg	
		Fat	1000 μg/kg	
		Liver	1000 μg/kg	
		Kidney	1000 μg/kg	
Flunixin	Bovine	Muscle	20 μg/kg	
		Fat	30 μg/kg	
		Liver	300 μg/kg	
		Kidney	100 μg/kg	
		Milk	40 μg/kg	
	Porcine	Muscle	50 μg/kg	
		Skin and fat	10 μg/kg	
		Liver	200 μg/kg	
		Kidney	30 μg/kg	
	Equidae	Muscle	10 μg/kg	
		Fat	20 μg/kg	
		Liver	100 μg/kg	
		Kidney	200 μg/kg	
Tolfenamic acid	Bovine	Muscle	50 μg/kg	
		Liver	400 μg/kg	
		Kidney	100 μg/kg	
		Milk	50 μg/kg	
	Porcine	Muscle	50 μg/kg	
		Liver	400 μg/kg	
		Kidney	100 μg/kg	
Meloxicam	Equidae	Muscle	20 μg/kg	
		Liver	65 μg/kg	
		Kidney	65 μg/kg	
Meloxicam	Porcine, equidae, rabbit	Muscle	20 μg/kg	
		Liver	65 μg/kg	
		Kidney	65 μg/kg	
	Bovine, caprine	Muscle	20 μg/kg	
		Liver	65 μg/kg	
		Kidney	65 μg/kg	
		Milk	15 μg/kg	
Metamizole	Bovine	Muscle	100 μg/kg	
		Fat	100 μg/kg	
		Liver	100 μg/kg	
		Kidney	100 μg/kg	
		Milk	50 μg/kg	
	Porcine	Muscle	100 μg/kg	
		Skin and fat	100 μg/kg	
		Liver	100 μg/kg	
		Kidney	100 μg/kg	
	Equidae	Muscle	100 μg/kg	
		Fat	100 μg/kg	
		Liver	100 μg/kg	
		Kidney	100 μg/kg	
Diclofenac	Bovine	Muscle	5 μg/kg	
		Fat	1 μg/kg	
		Liver	5 μg/kg	
		Kidney	10 μg/kg	
		Milk	0,1 μg/kg	

Annex I. (Continued)

Pharmacologically active substances	Animal species	Target tissues	EU MRLs	Codex Alimentarius MRLs
	Porcine	Muscle	5 μg/kg	
		Skin and fat	1 μg/kg	
		Liver	5 μg/kg	
		Kidney	10 μg/kg	
Firocoxib	Equidae	Muscle	10 μg/kg	
		Fat	15 μg/kg	
		Liver	60 μg/kg	
		Kidney	10 μg/kg	
Betamethasone	Bovine	Muscle	0,75 μg/kg	
		Liver	2 μg/kg	
		Kidney	0.75 μg/kg	
		Milk	0.3 μg/kg	
	Porcine	Muscle	0.75 μg/kg	
		Liver	2 μg/kg	
		Kidney	0.75 μg/kg	
Dexamethasone	Bovine	Milk	0.3 μg/kg	0.3 μg/l
	Bovine, porcine, equidae	Muscle	0.75 μg/kg	1μg/kg
		Liver	2 μg/kg	2 μg/kg
		Kidney	0.75 μg/kg	1 μg/kg
	Caprine	Muscle	0.75 μg/kg	
		Liver	2 μg/kg	
		Kidney	0.75 μg/kg	
		Milk	0.3 μg/kg	
Methylprednisolone	Bovine	Muscle	10 μg/kg	
		Fat	10 μg/kg	
		Liver	10 μg/kg	
		Kidney	10 μg/kg	
Prednisolone	Bovine	Muscle	4 μg/kg	
		Fat	4 μg/kg	
		Liver	10 μg/kg	
		Kidney	10 μg/kg	
		Milk	6 μg/kg	
Chlormadinone	Bovine	Fat	4 μg/kg	
		Liver	2 μg/kg	
		Milk	2.5 μg/kg	
Flugestone acetate	Ovine	Milk	1 μg/kg	
	Caprine	Milk	1 μg/kg	
	Ovine, caprine	Muscle	0.5 μg/kg	
		Fat	0.5 μg/kg	
		Liver	0.5 μg/kg	
		Kidney	0.5 μg/kg	
Altrenogest	Porcine	Skin and fat	1 μg/kg	
		Liver	0.4 μg/kg	
	Equidae	Fat	1 μg/kg	
		Liver	0.9 μg/kg	
Norgestomet	Bovine	Muscle	0.2 μg/kg	
		Fat	0.2 μg/kg	
		Liver	0.2 μg/kg	
		Kidney	0.2 μg/kg	
		Milk	0.12 μg/kg	

In: Nutritional Insights and Food Safety
Editor: Jaroslava Švarc-Gajiæ

ISBN: 978-1-61122-130-5

Appendix II

ANNEX III. LIST OF PHARMACOLOGICALLY ACTIVE SUBSTANCES USED IN VETERINARY MEDICINAL PRODUCTS FOR WHICH PROVISIONAL MAXIMUM RESIDUE LIMITS HAVE BEEN FIXED

Pharmacologically active substances	Animal species	Target tissues	EU MRLs	Codex MRLs
Clorsulon	Bovine	Muscle	50 µg/kg	
		Liver	150 µg/kg	
		Kidney	400 µg/kg	
Clavulanic acid	Bovine, ovine	Milk	200 µg/kg	
	Bovine, ovine, porcine	Muscle	200 µg/kg	
		Fat	200 µg/kg	
		Liver	200 µg/kg	
		Kidney	200 µg/kg	
Acetylisovaleryltylosin	Porcine	Muscle	100 µg/kg	
		Skin and fat	100 µg/kg	
		Liver	100 µg/kg	
		Kidney	100 µg/kg	
Acetylisovaleryltylosin	Poultry	Skin and fat	50 µg/kg	
		Liver	50 µg/kg	
Erythromycin	Bovine, ovine	Milk	40 µg/kg	
	Bovine, ovine, porcine, poultry	Muscle	400 µg/kg	
		Fat	400 µg/kg	
		Liver	400 µg/kg	
		Kidney	400 µg/kg	
	Poultry	Eggs	200 µg/kg	50 µg/kg
	Chicken	Muscle		100 µg/kg
		Liver		100 µg/kg
		Kidney		100 µg/kg
		Fat		100 µg/kg
	Turkey	Muscle		100 µg/kg
		Liver		100 µg/kg
		Kidney		100 µg/kg
		Fat		100 µg/kg
Josamycin	Chicken	Muscle	200 µg/kg	
		Fat	200 µg/kg	
		Liver	200 µg/kg	
		Kidney	400 µg/kg	
		Eggs	200 µg/kg	

Annex III. (Continued)

Pharmacologically active substances	Animal species	Target tissues	EU MRLs	Codex MRLs
	Porcine	Muscle	200 μg/kg	
		Skin and fat	200 μg/kg	
		Liver	200 μg/kg	
		Kidney	400 μg/kg	
Tilmicosin	Bovine	Milk	40 μg/kg	
	Cattle, sheep	Muscle		100 μg/kg
		Liver		1000 μg/kg
		Kidney		300 μg/kg
		Fat		100 μg/kg
	Pig	Muscle		100 μg/kg
		Liver		1500 μg/kg
		Kidney		1000 μg/kg
		Fat		100 μg/kg
Tulathromycin	Bovine	Fat	100 μg/kg	
		Liver	3000 μg/kg	
		Kidney	3000 μg/kg	
	Porcine	Skin and fat	100 μg/kg	
		Liver	3000 μg/kg	
		Kidney	3000 μg/kg	
Gamithromycin	Bovine	Fat	20 μg/kg	
		Liver	200 μg/kg	
		Kidney	100 μg/kg	
Cefacetrile	Bovine	Milk	125 μg/kg	
Cefalonium	Bovine	Milk	10 μg/kg	
Cefoperazone	Bovine	Milk	50 μg/kg	
Cefquinome	Porcine	Muscle	50 μg/kg	
		Skin and fat	50 μg/kg	
		Liver	100 μg/kg	
		Kidney	200 μg/kg	
Cephapirin	Bovine	Muscle	50 μg/kg	
		Fat	50 μg/kg	
		Liver	50 μg/kg	
		Kidney	100 μg/kg	
		Milk	10 μg/kg	
Aminosidine	Bovine, porcine, rabbits, chicken	Muscle	500 μg/kg	
		Liver	1500 μg/kg	
		Kidney	1500 μg/kg	
Apramycin	Bovine	Muscle	1000 μg/kg	
	For use in non-lactating cattle only	Fat	1000 μg/kg	
		Liver	10000 μg/kg	
		Kidney	20000 μg/kg	
	Porcine	Muscle	1000 μg/kg	
		Skin and fat	1000 μg/kg	
		Liver	1000 μg/kg	
		Kidney	5000 μg/kg	
Dihydrostreptomycin	Bovine, ovine	Muscle	500 μg/kg	600 μg/kg
		Fat	500 μg/kg	600 μg/kg
		Liver	500 μg/kg	600 μg/kg
		Kidney	1000 μg/kg	1000 μg/kg
		Milk	200 μg/kg	200 μg/kg

Pharmacologically active substances	Animal species	Target tissues	EU MRLs	Codex MRLs
	Porcine	Muscle	500 μg/kg	600 μg/kg
		Skin and fat	500 μg/kg	600 μg/kg
		Liver	500 μg/kg	600 μg/kg
		Kidney	1000 μg/kg	1000 μg/kg
	Chicken	Muscle		600 μg/kg
		Liver		600 μg/kg
		Kidney		1000 μg/kg
		Fat		600 μg/kg
Gentamicin	Bovine	Milk	100 μg/kg	
	Bovine, porcine	Muscle	50 μg/kg	
		Fat	50 μg/kg	
		Liver	200 μg/kg	
		Kidney	750 μg/kg	
Kanamycin	Rabbits	Muscle	100 μg/kg	
		Fat	100 μg/kg	
		Liver	600 μg/kg	
		Kidney	2500 μg/kg	
	Bovine, ovine	Muscle	100 μg/kg	
		Fat	100 μg/kg	
		Liver	600 μg/kg	
		Kidney	2500 μg/kg	
		Milk	150 μg/kg	
	Porcine, chicken	Muscle	100 μg/kg	
		Skin and fat	100 μg/kg	
		Liver	600 μg/kg	
		Kidney	2500 μg/kg	
Neomycin (including framycetin)	Bovine, porcine, chicken	Muscle	500 μg/kg	
		Fat	500 μg/kg	
		Liver	500 μg/kg	
		Kidney	5000 μg/kg	
	Bovine	Milk	500 μg/kg	
	Chicken	Eggs	500 μg/kg	
Spectinomycin	Bovine	Milk	200 μg/kg	
	Bovine, porcine, poultry	Muscle	300 μg/kg	
		Fat	500 μg/kg	
		Liver	2000 μg/kg	
		Kidney	5000 μg/kg	
	Ovine	Muscle	300 μg/kg	
	Not for use in animals from which milk is produced for human consumption	Fat	500 μg/kg	
		Liver	2000 μg/kg	
		Kidney	5000 μg/kg	
	Chicken	Eggs	200 μg/kg	
Streptomycin	Bovine, ovine	Muscle	500 μg/kg	600 μg/kg
		Fat	500 μg/kg	600 μg/kg
		Liver	500 μg/kg	600 μg/kg
		Kidney	1000 μg/kg	1000 μg/kg
		Milk	200 μg/kg	200 μg/l
	Porcine	Muscle	500 μg/kg	600 μg/kg
		Skin and fat	500 μg/kg	600 μg/kg
		Liver	500 μg/kg	600 μg/kg
		Kidney	1000 μg/kg	1000 μg/kg

Annex III. (Continued)

Pharmacologically active substances	Animal species	Target tissues	EU MRLs	Codex MRLs
	Chicken	Muscle		600 μg/kg
		Liver		600 μg/kg
		Kidney		1000 μg/kg
		Fat		600 μg/kg
Danofloxacin	Porcine	Muscle	100 μg/kg	100 μg/kg
		Skin and fat	50 μg/kg	100 μg/kg
		Liver	200 μg/kg	50 μg/kg
		Kidney	200 μg/kg	200 μg/kg
	Cattle, chicken	Muscle		200 μg/kg
		Liver		400 μg/kg
		Kidney		400 μg/kg
		Fat		100 μg/kg
Decoquinate	Bovine, ovine	Muscle	500 μg/kg	
		Fat	500 μg/kg	
		Liver	500 μg/kg	
		Kidney	500 μg/kg	
Difloxacin	Bovine	Muscle	400 μg/kg	
	Not for use in animals from which milk is produced for human consumption	Fat	100 μg/kg	
		Liver	1400 μg/kg	
		Kidney	800 μg/kg	
	Porcine	Muscle	400 μg/kg	
		Skin and fat	100 μg/kg	
		Liver	800 μg/kg	
		Kidney	800 μg/kg	
Enrofloxacin	Ovine	Muscle	100 μg/kg	
		Fat	100 μg/kg	
		Liver	300 μg/kg	
		Kidney	200 μg/kg	
Flumequine	Bovine, ovine, porcine, chicken	Muscle	50 μg/kg	500 μg/kg
		Fat or skin and fat	50 μg/kg	1000 μg/kg
		Liver	100 μg/kg	500 μg/kg
		Kidney	300 μg/kg	3000 μg/kg
	Salmonidae	Muscle and skin	150 μg/kg	
	Trout	Muscle		500 μg/kg
Marbofloxacin	Bovine	Muscle	150 μg/kg	
		Fat	50 μg/kg	
		Liver	150 μg/kg	
		Kidney	150 μg/kg	
		Milk	75 μg/kg	
	Porcine	Muscle	150 μg/kg	
		Skin and fat	50 μg/kg	
		Liver	150 μg/kg	
		Kidney	150 μg/kg	
Oxolinic acid	Bovine	Muscle	100 μg/kg	
		Fat	50 μg/kg	
		Liver	150 μg/kg	
		Kidney	150 μg/kg	
	Porcine	Muscle	100 μg/kg	
		Skin and fat	50 μg/kg	

Pharmacologically active substances	Animal species	Target tissues	EU MRLs	Codex MRLs
		Liver	150 μg/kg	
		Kidney	150 μg/kg	
	Chicken	Muscle	100 μg/kg	
		Skin and fat	50 μg/kg	
		Liver	150 μg/kg	
		Kidney	150 μg/kg	
		Eggs	50 μg/kg	
	Fin fish	Muscle and skin in natural proportions	300 μg/kg	
Colistin	Bovine, ovine	Milk	50 μg/kg	50 μg/kg
	Bovine, ovine, porcine, chicken, rabbits, turkey	Muscle	150 μg/kg	150 μg/kg
		Fat	150 μg/kg	150 μg/kg
		Liver	150 μg/kg	150 μg/kg
		Kidney	200 μg/kg	200 μg/kg
	Chicken	Eggs	300 μg/kg	300 μg/kg
Nafcillin	Bovine	Muscle	300 μg/kg	
		Fat	300 μg/kg	
		Liver	300 μg/kg	
		Kidney	300 μg/kg	
		Milk	30 μg/kg	
Penethamate	Ovine	Muscle	50 μg/kg	
		Fat	50 μg/kg	
		Liver	50 μg/kg	
		Kidney	50 μg/kg	
		Milk	4 μg/kg	
	Porcine	Muscle	50 μg/kg	
		Fat	50 μg/kg	
		Liver	50 μg/kg	
		Kidney	50 μg/kg	
Florfenicol	Fish	Muscle and skin in natural proportions	1000 μg/kg	
Thiamphenicol	Ovine	Muscle	50 μg/kg	
		Fat	50 μg/kg	
		Liver	50 μg/kg	
		Kidney	50 μg/kg	
	Porcine	Muscle	50 μg/kg	
		Skin and fat	50 μg/kg	
		Liver	50 μg/kg	
		Kidney	50 μg/kg	
	Fin fish	Muscle and skin in natural proportions	50 μg/kg	
Thiamphenicol	Porcine	Muscle	50 μg/kg	
		Skin and fat	50 μg/kg	
		Liver	50 μg/kg	
		Kidney	50 μg/kg	
Bacitracin	Bovine	Milk	150 μg/kg	
Lincomycin	Ovine	Muscle	100 μg/kg	
		Fat	50 μg/kg	
		Liver	500 μg/kg	
		Kidney	1500 μg/kg	
		Milk	150 μg/kg	
	Porcine	Muscle	100 μg/kg	
		Skin and fat	50 μg/kg	
		Liver	500 μg/kg	
		Kidney	1500 μg/kg	
	Chicken	Muscle	100 μg/kg	

Annex III. (Continued)

Pharmacologically active substances	Animal species	Target tissues	EU MRLs	Codex MRLs
		Fat	50 μg/kg	
		Liver	500 μg/kg	
		Kidney	1500 μg/kg	
		Eggs	50 μg/kg	
Pirlimycin	Bovine	Muscle	100 μg/kg	100 μg/kg
		Fat	100 μg/kg	100 μg/kg
		Liver	1000 μg/kg	1000 μg/kg
		Kidney	400 μg/kg	400 μg/kg
		Milk	100 μg/kg	100 μg/kg
Tiamulin	Turkey	Muscle	100 μg/kg	
		Skin and fat	100 μg/kg	
		Liver	300 μg/kg	
Oxyclozanide	Bovine	Muscle	20 μg/kg	
		Fat	20 μg/kg	
		Liver	500 μg/kg	
		Kidney	100 μg/kg	
		Milk	10 μg/kg	
	Ovine	Muscle	20 μg/kg	
		Fat	20 μg/kg	
		Liver	500 μg/kg	
		Kidney	100 μg/kg	
Albendazole sulphoxide	Bovine, ovine	Milk	100 μg/kg	
	Bovine, ovine, pheasant	Muscle	100 μg/kg	
		Fat	100 μg/kg	
		Liver	1000 μg/kg	
		Kidney	500 μg/kg	
Mebendazole	Ovine, caprine, equidae	Muscle	60 μg/kg	
	Not for use in animals from which milk is produced for human consumption	Fat	60 μg/kg	
		Liver	400 μg/kg	
		Kidney	60 μg/kg	
Netobimin	Bovine, ovine, caprine	Muscle	100 μg/kg	
		Fat	100 μg/kg	
		Liver	1000 μg/kg	
		Kidney	500 μg/kg	
		Milk	100 μg/kg	
Morantel	Bovine, ovine	Muscle	100 μg/kg	
		Fat	100 μg/kg	
		Liver	800 μg/kg	
		Kidney	200 μg/kg	
		Milk	100 μg/kg	
	Porcine	Muscle	100 μg/kg	
		Skin and fat	100 μg/kg	
		Liver	800 μg/kg	
		Kidney	200 μg/kg	
Piperazine	Porcine	Muscle	400 μg/kg	
		Skin and fat	800 μg/kg	

Pharmacologically active substances	Animal species	Target tissues	EU MRLs	Codex MRLs
		Liver	2000 μg/kg	
		Kidney	1000 μg/kg	
	Chicken	Eggs	2000 μg/kg	
Rafoxanide	Bovine	Muscle	30 μg/kg	
	Not for use in animals from which milk is produced for human consumption	Fat	30 μg/kg	
		Liver	10 μg/kg	
		Kidney	40 μg/kg	
	Ovine	Muscle	100 μg/kg	
	Not for use in animals from which milk is produced for human consumption	Fat	250 μg/kg	
		Liver	150 μg/kg	
		Kidney	150 μg/kg	
Monepantel	Caprine	Muscle	700 μg/kg	
		Fat	7000 μg/kg	
		Liver	5000 μg/kg	
		Kidney	2000 μg/kg	
Amitraz	Bees	Honey	200 μg/kg	
Cymiazole	Bees	Honey	1000 μg/kg	
Cyfluthrin	Bovine	Muscle	10 μg/kg	20 μg/kg
		Fat	50 μg/kg	200 μg/kg
		Liver	10 μg/kg	20 μg/kg
		Kidney	10 μg/kg	20 μg/kg
		Milk	20 μg/kg	40 μg/l
Alphacypermethrin	Bovine, ovine	Muscle	20 μg/kg	50 μg/kg
		Fat	200 μg/kg	1000 μg/kg
		Liver	20 μg/kg	50 μg/kg
		Kidney	20 μg/kg	50 μg/kg
		Milk	20 μg/kg	100 μg/l
	Chicken	Muscle	50 μg/kg	
		Skin and fat	50 μg/kg	
		Liver	50 μg/kg	
		Kidney	50 μg/kg	
		Eggs	50 μg/kg	
Cypermethrin	Bovine	Muscle	20 μg/kg	
		Fat	200 μg/kg	
		Liver	20 μg/kg	
		Kidney	20 μg/kg	
		Milk	20 μg/kg	
	Ovine	Muscle	20 μg/kg	
		Fat	200 μg/kg	
		Liver	20 μg/kg	
		Kidney	20 μg/kg	
	Porcine	Muscle	20 μg/kg	
		Skin and fat	200 μg/kg	
		Liver	20 μg/kg	
		Kidney	20 μg/kg	
	Chicken	Muscle	50 μg/kg	
		Skin and fat	50 μg/kg	
		Liver	50 μg/kg	

Annex III. (Continued)

Pharmacologically active substances	Animal species	Target tissues	EU MRLs	Codex MRLs
		Kidney	50 μg/kg	
		Eggs	50 μg/kg	
	Salmonidae	Muscle and skin in natural proportions	50 μg/kg	
Deltamethrin	Bovine	Muscle	10 μg/kg	30 μg/kg
		Fat	50 μg/kg	500 μg/kg
		Liver	10 μg/kg	50 μg/kg
		Kidney	10 μg/kg	50 μg/kg
		Milk	20 μg/kg	30 μg/kg
	Ovine	Muscle	10 μg/kg	30 μg/kg
	Not for use in animals from which milk is produced for human consumption	Fat	50 μg/kg	500 μg/kg
		Liver	10 μg/kg	50 μg/kg
		Kidney	10 μg/kg	50 μg/kg
	Chicken	Muscle	10 μg/kg	30 μg/kg
		Skin and fat	50 μg/kg	500 μg/kg
		Liver	10 μg/kg	50 μg/kg
		Kidney	10 μg/kg	50 μg/kg
		Eggs	50 μg/kg	30 μg/kg
	Fin fish	Muscle and skin in natural proportions	10 μg/kg	
	Salmon	Muscle		30 μg/kg
Fenvalerate	Bovine	Muscle	25 μg/kg	
		Fat	250 μg/kg	
		Liver	25 μg/kg	
		Kidney	25 μg/kg	
		Milk	40 μg/kg	
Permethrin	Chicken, porcine	Muscle	50 μg/kg	
		Skin and fat	500 μg/kg	
		Liver	50 μg/kg	
		Kidney	50 μg/kg	
	Bovine, caprine	Muscle	50 μg/kg	
		Fat	500 μg/kg	
		Liver	50 μg/kg	
		Kidney	50 μg/kg	
		Milk	50 μg/kg	
	Chicken	Eggs	50 μg/kg	
Azamethiphos	Salmonidae	Muscle and skin in natural proportions	100 μg/kg	
Coumafos	Bees	Honey	100 μg/kg	
Phoxim	Porcine	Muscle	20 μg/kg	
		Skin and fat	700 μg/kg	
		Liver	20 μg/kg	
		Kidney	20 μg/kg	
	Ovine	Muscle	50 μg/kg	
		Fat	400 μg/kg	
		Kidney	50 μg/kg	
	Chicken	Muscle	50 μg/kg	
		Skin and fat	550 μg/kg	
		Liver	25 μg/kg	
		Kidney	50 μg/kg	

Pharmacologically active substances	Animal species	Target tissues	EU MRLs	Codex MRLs
		Eggs	60 µg/kg	
Propetamphos	Ovine Not for use in animals from which milk is produced for human consumption	Fat	90 µg/kg	
		Kidney	90 µg/kg	
Teflubenzuron	Salmonidae	Muscle and skin in natural proportions	500 µg/kg	
Diflubenzuron	Salmonidae	Muscle and skin in natural proportions	1000 µg/kg	
Fluazuron	Bovine	Muscle	200 µg/kg	
		Fat	7000 µg/kg	
		Liver	500 µg/kg	
		Kidney	500 µg/kg	
Dicyclanil	Ovine	Muscle	200 µg/kg	
		Fat	50 µg/kg	
		Liver	400 µg/kg	
		Kidney	400 µg/kg	
Cyromazine	Ovine	Muscle	300 µg/kg	
		Fat	300 µg/kg	
		Liver	300 µg/kg	
		Kidney	300 µg/kg	
Abamectin	Ovine	Muscle	20 µg/kg	
		Fat	50 µg/kg	
		Liver	25 µg/kg	
		Kidney	20 µg/kg	
Doramectin	Deer, including reindeer	Muscle	20 µg/kg	
		Fat	100 µg/kg	
		Liver	50 µg/kg	
		Kidney	30 µg/kg	
Moxidectin	Equidae	Muscle	50 µg/kg	
		Fat	500 µg/kg	
		Liver	100 µg/kg	
		Kidney	50 µg/kg	
Imidocarb	Bovine, ovine	Muscle	300 µg/kg	
		Fat	50 µg/kg	
		Liver	2000 µg/kg	
		Kidney	1500 µg/kg	
		Milk	50 µg/kg	
Halofuginone	Bovine	Muscle	10 µg/kg	
		Fat	25 µg/kg	
		Liver	30 µg/kg	
		Kidney	30 µg/kg	
Toltrazuril	Porcine	Muscle	100 µg/kg	
		Skin and fat	150 µg/kg	
		Liver	500 µg/kg	
		Kidney	250 µg/kg	
Toltrazuril	Bovine	Muscle	100 µg/kg	
		Fat	150 µg/kg	
		Liver	500 µg/kg	
		Kidney	250 µg/kg	
Amprolium	Chicken, turkey	Muscle	200 µg/kg	
		Skin and fat	200 µg/kg	
		Liver	200 µg/kg	
		Kidney	400 µg/kg	

Annex III. (Continued)

Pharmacologically active substances	Animal species	Target tissues	EU MRLs	Codex MRLs
		Eggs	1000 μg/kg	
Lasalocid	Poultry	Eggs	150 μg/kg	
Clenbuterol hydrochloride	Bovine	Muscle	0.1 μg/kg	
	Indication: solely for tocolysis in parturient cows	Liver	0.5 μg/kg	
		Kidney	0.5 μg/kg	
		Milk	0.05 μg/kg	
	Equidae	Muscle	0.1 μg/kg	
	Indication: tocolysis and the treatment of respiratory ailments	Liver	0.5 μg/kg	
		Kidney	0.5 μg/kg	
Carazolol	Bovine	Muscle	5 μg/kg	
		Fat	5 μg/kg	
		Liver	15 μg/kg	
		Kidney	15 μg/kg	
		Milk	1 μg/kg	
Carprofen	Bovine	Muscle	500 μg/kg	
		Fat	500 μg/kg	
		Liver	1000 μg/kg	
		Kidney	1000 μg/kg	
	Equidae	Muscle	50 μg/kg	
		Fat	100 μg/kg	
		Liver	1000 μg/kg	
		Kidney	1000 μg/kg	
Meloxicam	Bovine	Muscle	25 μg/kg	
		Liver	60 μg/kg	
		Kidney	35 μg/kg	
Metamizole	Bovine, porcine, equidae	Muscle	200 μg/kg	
		Fat	200 μg/kg	
		Liver	200 μg/kg	
		Kidney	200 μg/kg	
Firocoxib	Equidae	Muscle	10 μg/kg	
		Fat	15 μg/kg	
		Liver	60 μg/kg	
		Kidney	10 μg/kg	
Altrenogest	Porcine	Skin and fat	3 μg/kg	
		Liver	3 μg/kg	
		Kidney	3 μg/kg	
	Equidae	Fat	3 μg/kg	
		Liver	3 μg/kg	
		Kidney	3 μg/kg	
Flugestone acetate	Ovine, caprine	Muscle	0.5 μg/kg	
		Fat	0.5 μg/kg	
		Liver	0.5 μg/kg	
		Kidney	0.5 μg/kg	
Norgestomet	Bovine	Muscle	0.5 μg/kg	
		Fat	0.5 μg/kg	
		Liver	0.5 μg/kg	
		Kidney	0.5 μg/kg	

Pharmacologically active substances	Animal species	Target tissues	EU MRLs	Codex MRLs
		Milk	0.15 µg/kg	
Methylprednisolone	Bovine	Muscle	10 µg/kg	
		Fat	10 µg/kg	
		Liver	10 µg/kg	
		Kidney	10 µg/kg	
Diclazuril	Poultry, rabbit, sheep	Muscle		500 µg/kg
		Liver		3000 µg/kg
		Kidney		2000 µg/kg
		Fat		1000 µg/kg
Diminazene	Cattle	Muscle		500 µg/kg
		Liver		12000 µg/kg
		Kidney		6000 µg/kg
		Milk (µg/l)		150 µg/l
Estradiol-17beta	Cattle	Muscle		Not appllicable - Residues resulting from the use of this substances as a growth promoter in accordance with good animal husbandry practice are unlikely to pose a hazard to human health
		Liver		
		Kidney		
		Fat		
Procaine benzylpenicillin	Cattle, chicken, pig	Muscle		50 µg/kg
		Liver		50 µg/kg
		Kidney		50 µg/kg
	Chicken	Milk		4 µg/l
Isometamidium	Cattle	Muscle		100 µg/kg
		Liver		500 µg/kg
		Kidney		1000µg/kg
		Fat		100 µg/kg
		Milk (µg/l)		100 (µg/l)
Melengestrol acetate	Chicken	Muscle		1 µg/kg
		Liver		10 µg/kg
		Kidney		2 µg/kg
		Fat		18 µg/kg
Narasin	Chicken	Muscle		15 µg/kg
		Liver		50 µg/kg
		Kidney		15 µg/kg
		Fat		50 µg/kg
Nicarbazin	Chicken	Muscle		200 µg/kg
		Liver		200 µg/kg
		Kidney		200 µg/kg
		Fat/skin		200 µg/kg
Progesterone	Cattle	Muscle		Not applicabe - Residues resulting from the use of this substances as a growth promoter in accordance with good animal husbandry practice are unlikely to pose a hazard to human health
		Liver		
		Kidney		
		Fat		

Annex III. (Continued)

Pharmacologically active substances	Animal species	Target tissues	EU MRLs	Codex MRLs
Testosterone	Cattle	Muscle Liver Kidney Fat		Not applicable - Residues resulting from the use of this substances as a growth promoter in accordance with good animal husbandry practice are unlikely to pose a hazard to human health
Trenbolone acetate	Cattle	Muscle Liver		2 μg/kg 10 μg/kg
Trichlorfon	Cattle	Milk		50 μg/kg
Zeranol	Cattle	Muscle Liver		2 μg/kg 10 μg/kg

Index

C

D

E

F

G

H

I

N

O

P

Q

R

S

U

V